CONTRIBUTORS

Herbert H. Butler, MD

Emergency Department Physician, Underwood-Memorial Hospital, Woodbury, New Jersey; Immediate Past President, New Jersey Chapter American College of Emergency Physicians.

James F. Elam PhD

Clinical Biochemist, Pathology Department, Alexandria Hospital, Alexandria, Virginia

Joseph B. Mizgerd, MD

Director, Department of Pulmonary Medicine, Washington Adventist Hospital, Takoma Park, Maryland

Kathleen C. Morton, MD FAAP

President, New York Medical College, Valhalla, New York; formerly Dean for Primary Care Education, John Hopkins School of Medicine

Alfred Munzer, MD

Associate Director, Department of Pulmonary Medicine, Washington Adventist Hospital, Takoma Park, Maryland

Becky A. Winslow, RN MSN

Assistant Director, Nursing Education Programs, School Health Services, Johns Hopkins University, Baltimore, Maryland

THE LIPPINCOTT MANUAL OF PAEDIATRIC NURSING
SECOND EDITION

Adapted for the UK by

Barbara F. Weller, RSCN, SRN, RNT

*Nursing Officer,
Department of Health and Social Security;
formerly Nurse Tutor,
Hospital for Sick Children, Great Ormond Street, and
St Mary's Hospital, London*

Harper & Row, Publishers
London

Cambridge
Philadelphia
New York
San Francisco

Mexico City
São Paulo
Singapore
Sydney

Copyright © 1986 Harper & Row Ltd, London
First published 1981
Reprinted 1983, 1984
Second edition 1986

Adapted from The Lippincott Manual of Nursing Practice,
Second Edition

Copyright © 1978 J B Lippincott Company

Published by arrangement with Harper and Row Inc, New York, 1986

Harper & Row Ltd
28 Tavistock Street
London WC2E 7PN

British Library Cataloguing in Publication Data

Weller, Barbara F.
  The Lippincott manual of paediatric nursing.—
  2nd ed.
  1. Pediatric nursing
  I. Title   II. Brunner, Lillian Sholtis.
  Lippincott manual of nursing practice. 2nd ed.
  610.73'62   RJ245

  ISBN 0-06-318329-3

Typeset by Gedset, Cheltenham
Printed and bound by Butler & Tanner Ltd, Frome and London

NOTE:
The Publishers wish to state that, whilst every effort has been made to
ensure the accuracy and correctness of the information contained herein,
the authors of the original work from which this adaption is taken cannot
be held responsible for any changes made to the original text in the course
of the adaptation.

CONTENTS

Preface   1

Preface to second edition   3

Acknowledgements   5

1 PAEDIATRIC CONCEPTS

Growth and development   7

Preventative paediatrics   44

Safety   48

The hospitalized child   56

Transcultural knowledge of ethnic minority
   groups' health-illness behaviours   87

The dying child   89

Further reading   96

2 PAEDIATRIC TECHNIQUES

Measuring vital signs in children   99

Nursing management of the child with fever   105

Administering medications to children   109

Enema   113

Protective measures to limit movement (restraints)   115

Infant feeding and nutrition   120

Specimen collection 139
Fluid and electrolyte balance in children 149
Chest physiotherapy 174
Cardiac and respiratory monitoring 196
Cardiopulmonary resuscitation 198
The child undergoing dialysis 206
Traction 219
Casts 228
Further reading 237

3 PROBLEMS OF INFANTS
Management of the preterm infant 240
Small for gestational age (light for dates) infant 262
Postmature infant 268
Infant of a diabetic mother 271
Jaundice in the newborn (hyperbilirubinaemia) 275
Failure to thrive 282
Septicaemia neonatorum 286
Infant of a drug-addicted mother 293
Neonatal or prolonged sleep apnoea of infancy 299
Further reading 305

4 CONDITIONS OF THE RESPIRATORY TRACT
Overview of childhood respiratory disorders 307
Asthma 318
Respiratory distress syndrome (hyaline membrane
    disease) 327
Cystic fibrosis 334
Further reading 341

5 BLOOD DISORDERS

Anaemia   343
Sickle cell disease (sickle cell anaemia)   351
Haemophilia   358
Further reading   365

6 CARDIOVASCULAR DISORDERS

Congenital heart disease   367
Congestive heart failure   390
Nursing care of the child undergoing cardiac
   catheterization   394
Cardiac surgery   396
Myocarditis   400
Infective endocarditis   403
Further reading   404

7 ALIMENTARY TRACT DISORDERS

Dental caries   407
Cleft lip and palate   410
Oesophageal atresia and tracheo-oesophageal fistula   418
Hypertrophic pyloric stenosis   425
Coeliac disease   429
Diarrhoea   436
Hirschsprung's disease   445
Intussusception   454
Imperforate anus   457
Abdominal hernia   461
Appendicitis   463
Meckel's diverticulum   465
Intestinal obstruction   466

Hepatitis 469
Jaundice 472
Threadworm (enterobiasis, oxyuriasis) 474
Further reading 475

8 KIDNEYS, URINARY TRACT, AND REPRODUCTIVE SYSTEM CONDITIONS
Acute glomerulonephritis 477
Nephrotic syndrome 485
Urinary tract infection 494
Abnormalities of the genitourinary tract which require
  surgery 499
Further reading 512

9 SKIN PROBLEMS
Burns 515
Atopic eczema (infantile and childhood eczema) 523
Impetigo 528
Ringworm of the scalp (Tinea capitis) 530
Pediculosis 532
Scabies 534
Oral candidiasis (thrush) and candidal nappy dermatitis 535
Further reading 538

10 METABOLIC DISORDERS
Juvenile diabetes mellitus 539
Diabetes insipidus 548
Hypothyroidism 552
Hyperthyroidism (thyrotoxicosis) 556
Further reading 559

11 EYE, EAR, NOSE & THROAT CONDITIONS

The blind child	561
Eye defects requiring surgery	568
Tonsillectomy and adenoidectomy	574
Otitis media	578
The child with impaired hearing	582
Further reading	591

12 CONNECTIVE TISSUE DISEASE

Juvenile rheumatoid arthritis	594
Henoch-Schönlein purpura (anaphylactoid purpura)	600
Acute rheumatic fever	603
Further reading	610

13 NEUROLOGICAL SYSTEM CONDITIONS

Diagnostic evaluation of neurological disease	611
Cerebral palsy	616
Hydrocephalus	625
Spina bifida	634
Bacterial meningitis	645
Convulsive disorders (seizure disorders, epilepsy)	651
Febrile convulsions	665
Subdural haematoma	667
Reye's syndrome	674
Further reading	678

14 THE MENTALLY HANDICAPPED CHILD

Mental handicap	680
Down's syndrome	689

Further reading 697

15 ORTHOPAEDIC CONDITIONS
Fractures 700
Osteomyelitis 705
Congenital dislocation of the hip 709
Congenital clubfoot (Talipes equinovarus) 712
Perthes disease 715
Structural scoliosis 718
Rickets 724
Genuvalgum (knock-knee) 725
Further reading 726

16 PAEDIATRIC ONCOLOGY
General considerations 727
Acute lymphoblastic leukaemia 729
Brain tumours 743
Wilms' tumour 750
Further reading 754

17 SPECIAL PAEDIATRIC PROBLEMS — POISONING, NONACCIDENTAL INJURY, GENETIC COUNSELLING
Poisoning 756
Lead poisoning 763
Nonaccidental injury (the battered child — abuse and neglect) 771
Genetic counselling 780
Further reading 789

INDEX 791

PREFACE

'Nursing terminology written by Americans is not always familiar to us when it crosses the Atlantic.'

Charlotte Kratz

It has been said that England and America are separated by a common language. For us as nurses, this is a pity. Because our professional concerns, wherever we happen to live and work, are focused on the quality of care that we give to our patients, we have much in common to share in achieving our mutual goals.

Never was this more so than in the field of paediatrics, where we need to plan and provide care for the child in relation to his family and his community. The authors of this book have been most scholarly and caring in their approach to providing a framework for the provision of this care. Their dynamic and positive awareness of all the needs of the child and his family sets a level of excellence to us all.

It is particularly appropriate that this book should be made more readily available to nurses in the United Kingdom at this time. There is now active discussion, consideration, and implementation of the nursing process for the care of sick children, Nursing cannot be static, but must react to new knowledge, and the evolving society allows for nursing care to be provided within a logical and problem-solving framewok using nursing care plans, with the aim of enhancing the quality of care given to our patients and their families, which for us as nurses remains a permanent challenge.

I am delighted to have had the opportunity of 'anglicizing' this book. My role has been to provide the local dialect and change Webster spelling to Concise Oxford. The essential theme of the book remains unchanged. The bibliography has been extended to include appropriate English texts for further reading and reference.

I am most grateful to many colleagues who gave me every encouragement to proceed with this work. Special acknowledgement must go to Miss D. Saunders, Principal Nursing Officer (Education) and Miss Debbie Collinson, Librarian, Charles West School of Nursing, The Hospital for Sick Children, Great Ormond Street, London, for their support and help. I should also like to acknowledge the help and advice received from Miss A. Blake, Nursing Officer, University College Hospital, London, and P. Hales, Nursing Officer, The City Hospital, Nottingham.

Barbara F. Weller
1980

PREFACE
TO THE SECOND EDITION

One of the nicest things about writing or adapting a nursing textbook is to have comments and suggestions from student or nurse readers. Without exception these have been constructive and helpful. It is with these comments in mind that changes made to the text have concentrated on new clinical material and the implications for individualized nursing care. The publishing format has been changed to make for easier reading and a more comprehensive index has been introduced to provide the reader with a quick reference guide. I hope it will prove as popular as the previous edition with new readers.

Barbara F. Weller
1986

ACKNOWLEDGEMENTS

With very special thanks for their support and wisdom, without which this book would never have been adapted, to Daphne Learmont, David Russell-Fisher and Cathy Peck.

1

PAEDIATRIC CONCEPTS

GROWTH AND DEVELOPMENT

Reflexes of the Newborn

1   *Pupillary reflexes*   Ipsilateral (pertaining to the same side) constriction to light.
2   *Rooting*   When corner of mouth is touched and object is moved towards cheek, infant will turn head towards object and open mouth.
3   *Palmar grasp*   Pressure on palm of hand will elicit grasp.
4   *Plantar grasp*   Pressure on sole of foot behind toes will cause flexion of toes.
5   *Tonic neck reflex*   Sudden jolt will cause head to turn to one side with leg and arm on that side extended, while the extremities on the other side flex.
6   *Neck righting*   When head is turned to one side, the shoulder and trunk, followed by the pelvis, will turn to that side.
7   *Moro reflex*   Response to sudden loud noise, causing body to stiffen and arms to go up and out, then forward and towards each other. Thumb and index finger will assume C-shape.
8   *Positive-supporting reflex*   When held in an erect position, baby will stiffen lower extremities and support his weight.
9   *Babinski's sign*   Scratching sole of foot causes big toe to flex and toes to fan.
10   *Crossed extensor reflex*   When one leg is extended and the knee is held straight, while the sole of the foot is stimulated, the opposite leg will flex.
11   *Landau's sign*   When baby is suspended horizontally with head depressed against trunk and neck flexed, legs will flex and be drawn up to trunk.
12   *Optical blink reflex*   When light is suddenly shone into open eyes, the eyes will close quickly with a quick dorsal flexion of head.

13   *Auditory blink reflex*   Eyes quickly close if examiner loudly claps her hands about 30 cm from infant's head.

14   *Recoil of arm*   When both arms are extended simultaneously by pulling outward grasping wrists, both arms will flex at the elbows when released.

15   *Withdrawal reflex*   Pricking sole of foot will result in the baby's leg being flexed at hip, knee, and ankle.

16   *Stepping reflex*   When infant is held upright with dorsum of foot gently touching edge of table, he will bend his hips and knees and put foot on table. This will elicit stepping response in the opposite foot. Series of alternating stepping actions will result when infant is moved forward so that one foot at a time touches the firm surface.

17   *Parachute reflex*   While the infant is held prone and lowered quickly towards a surface, he will extend arms and legs.

18   *Side-turning*   Placing baby prone with head in midline will elicit the baby's turning his head to the side.

19   Other characteristics of the newborn:

    a Cries

    b Sucks

    c Has extremely sensitive skin

    d Makes discriminating sounds

    e Sleeps for long intervals

    f Has little head control (head lag).

Infant to Adolescent Growth and Development

See Table 1.1, pp. 9-27

Childhood Diseases

See Table 1.2, pp. 28-35

Nutrition in Paediatrics

See Table 1.3, pp. 36-43

Table 1.1 Growth and development

Age and physical characteristics	Behaviour patterns	Nursing implications/ parental guidance
Birth–4 weeks (1 month)	*Motor development* Momentary visual fixation on objects and adult face Eyes follow bright moving objects Lies awake on back with head averted Immediately drops objects placed in hands Responds to sounds of bell and other similar noises Keeps hands fisted *Socialization and vocalization* Mews and makes throaty noises Shows interest in human face *Cognitive and emotional development* Reflexive External stimuli are meaningless Responses are generally limited to tension states or discomfort Gains satisfaction from feeding and being held, rocked, fondled, and cuddled Has an intense need for sucking pleasure Quietens when picked up	*Play stimulation* Use human face-smile and talk Dangle bright and moving object in field of vision (mobile) Hold, touch, caress, fondle, kiss Rock, pat, change position Play soft music or have infant listen to ticking clock, sing Talk to infant, call him by name. *Parental guidance* Begin to expose infant to different household sounds Change cot location in room Use bright-coloured clothing and linen Keep infant nearby Allow him to sleep Play with him when he is awake Hold him during feeding
8 weeks (2 months) Crossed extensor reflex disappears	*Motor development* Reflexive behaviour is slowly being replaced by voluntary movements Turns from side to back Begins to lift head momentarily from prone position Shows eye coordination to light and objects	*Play stimulation* Arrange mobile over cot so infant's movement will set it in motion Hang wind chimes near infant Hang bright-coloured pictures on wall (yellow and red coloured stripes for example) Hang dangley cot toys and use infant seat

(continued)

Table 1.1 Growth and development (*continued*)

Age and physical characteristics	Behaviour patterns	Nursing implications/ parental guidance
	If bell is sounded near him, he will stop activity and listen Eyes follow better, both vertically and horizontally	Use rattles Hold infant and walk around room Allow freedom of kicking with clothes off
	Socialization and vocalization Begins vocalization-coos, especially to a voice Crying becomes differentiated Visually looks for sounds May squeal with delight when stimulated by touching, talking, or singing Begins social smile Eyes follow person or object more intently	*Parental guidance* Talk to him and smile, get excited when he coos Place infant seat near mother's activities but where he cannot fall off or tip over Put in prone position in bed or on floor Expose infant to different textures Exercise infant's arms and legs Sing to infant Provide tactile experience during bathing, nappy changing, feeding
	Cognitive and emotional development Recognizes familiar face Becomes more aware and interested in environment Anticipates being fed when in feeding position Enjoys sucking-puts hand in mouth	
12 weeks (3 months)	*Motor development* When prone, he will rest on forearms and keep head in midline-makes crawling movements	*Play stimulation* Encourage socialization, smiling, laughing Place on mat on floor Continue to introduce new sounds
Landau reflex appears at 3-4 months; stepping reflex disappears Positive support reflex disappears Posterior fontanelle closes	with legs, arches back, and holds head high, he may get chest off surface Indicates preference for prone or supine position Discovers hands-strikes at objects while watching hands Holds objects in hands and brings to mouth Has fairly good head control	*Parental guidance* Take on daily outing as weather permits Bounce on bed Play with infant during feeding Rattles can be used effectively for visual following and for hand play

First dose of diptheria, tetanus, pertussis and poliomyelitis vaccines should be given

Socialization and vocalization
Smiles more readily
Babbles and coos
Stops crying when mother enters room or when he is caressed
Enjoys playing during feeding
Stays awake longer without crying
Turns head to follow familiar person

Cognitive and emotional development
Shows active interest in environment
Recognizes familiar faces and objects
Focuses and follows objects
Shows repetitiveness in play activity
Is aware of strange situations
Derives pleasure from sucking-purposefully gets hand to mouth
Begins to establish routine preceding sleep

16 weeks (4 months)

Stepping reflex disappears
Rooting reflex disappears
By 4-5 months infant's weight approximately doubles birth weight

Motor development
Eyes focus on small objects; he may pick a dangling ring
Holds head up (when being pulled to sitting position)
Becomes more interested in environment
Hand comes to meet rattle
Listens-turns head to familiar sound
Sits with minimal support
Intentional rolling over, back to side
Reaches for offered objects
Grasps objects with both hands and everything goes into mouth

Socialization and vocalization
Laughs and chuckles socially
Demands social attention by fussing
Recognizes mother

Play stimulation
Encourage mirror play
Provide soft squeeze toys in vivid colours of varying texture
Allow infant to splash in bath
Infant still enjoys holding and playing with rattles
Enjoys old-fashioned clothes-pegs and playing pat-a-cake, peek-a-boo

Parental guidance
Be certain button eyes on toys and other small objects cannot be pulled off
Hold rattle for him and let him reach and grasp it
When baby is in highchair, strap in
Let him play with food; give finger foods
Move mobile out of reach-he may grab it and cause injury
Repeat child's sounds to him

(continued)

Table 1.1   Growth and development (*continued*)

Age and physical characteristics	Behaviour patterns	Nursing implications/ parental guidance
	Begins to respond to 'No, no' Enjoys being propped in sitting position	Talk in varying degrees of loudness Begin looking at and naming pictures in book Begin roughhousing play by both parents Second dose of diptheria, tetanus, pertussis and polio vaccines should be given
	Cognitive and emotional development Actively interested in environment Enjoys attention; becomes bored when alone for long periods of time Recognizes bottle More interested in mother Indicates increasing trust and security Sleeps through night; has defined nap time	
26 weeks (7 months) By 5-6 months, tonic neck reflex disappears By 6-7 months, palmar grasp disappears By 7-9 months, develops eye-to-eye contact while talking; engages in social games Two central lower incisors erupt	*Motor development* Shows momentary sitting, with hand support Bounces and bears some weight when held in standing position Transfers and mouths objects in one hand Discovers feet Bangs objects together Rolls over well May begin some form of mobility *Socialization and vocalization* Discriminates between strangers and familiar figures Crows and squeals Starts to say 'Ma', 'Da' Self-play is self-contained Laughs out loud	*Play stimulation* Enjoys social games, 'hide-and-seek' with adult, toys, large blocks Likes to bang objects Plays in bounce chair, walker Enjoys large nesting toys (round rather than square) Likes to drop and retrieve things Likes metal cups, wooden spoons, and things to bang with Loves crumpled paper Enjoys squeeze toys in bath Likes peek-a-boo, bye-bye, and pat-a-cake *Parental guidance* Will play as long as you can Tie toys to chair with short string

Makes 'talking' sounds in response to others' talking

Cognitive and emotional development
Secures objects by pulling on string
Searches for lost objects that are out of sight
Inspects objects; localizes sounds
Likes to sit in highchair
Drops and picks up objects
Displays exploratory behaviour with food
Exhibits beginning fear of strangers
Becomes fretful when mother leaves
Shows much mouthing and biting

Let play with extra spoon at feeding
Give soft finger foods
Since infant puts everything in mouth, *use safety precautions*; keep small items away from him, he could choke on them
Show excitement at his achievements
Supply kitchen items for toys

40 weeks (10 months)

Four upper incisors erupt around 9 months
By 9-12 months, plantar reflex disappears
By 9-12 months, neck-righting reflex disappears

Motor development
Sits without support
Recovers balance
Manipulates objects with hands
Unwraps objects
Creeps
Pulls self upright at cot sides
Uses index finger and thumb to hold objects
Rings a bell
Can feed himself a rusk and can hold bottle
Can control lips around cup
Does not like supine position
Can hold index finger and thumb in opposition

Socialization and verbalization
Claps hands on request
Responds to own name
Is very aware of social environment
Imitates gestures, facial expressions, and sounds
Smiles at image in mirror
Offers toy to adult, but does not release it
Begins to test parental reaction during feeding and at bedtime

Play stimulation
Encourage use of motion toys-rocking horse
Water play
Imitate animal sounds
Allow exploration outdoors
Provide for learning by imitation
Offer new objects (blocks)
Child likes freedom of creeping and walking, but closeness of family is important
Good toys; milk carton; bean bag for tossing; fabric books; things to move around, fill up, empty out; pile-up and knock-down toys

Parental guidance
Do things with him
Protect him from dangerous objects-cover electrical outlets, block stairs, remove breakable objects from tables
Use plastic bottle or feeding cup
Have child with family at mealtime
Offer cup

(continued)

Table 1.1 Growth and development (*continued*)

Age and physical characteristics	Behaviour patterns	Nursing implications/ parental guidance
	Will entertain self for long periods of time	
	Cognitive and emotional development Begins to imitate Shows more interest in picture books Enjoys achievements Has strong urge towards independence- locomotion, feeding, dressing	
12 months (1 year)	*Motor development* Cruises around furniture Beginning to stand alone and toddle Turns pages in book Tries tossing object Shows hand dominance Navigates stairs; climbs on chairs Builds a tower of two blocks Puts ball in box May use spoon Can release objects at will Has regular bowel movements	*Play stimulation* Ball play Cloth doll Motion objects and toys Transporting objects Name and point to body parts 'Put-in' and 'take-out' toys Sand box with spoons and other similar objects Blocks Music
By 12-18 months, Babinski sign disappears By 12-24 months, Landau reflex disappears By 10-14 months, anterior fontanelle closes Weight should approximately triple birth weight Two lower lateral incisors appear Four first molars appear by 14 months	*Socialization and verbalization* Uses jargon Points to indicate wants Loves give-and-take game Responds to music Enjoys being centre of attention and will repeat laughed-at activities	*Parental guidance* Allow self-directed play rather than adult-directed play Continue to expose to foods of different textures, taste, smell, substance Offer cup Show affection and encourage child to return affection

(continued)

Cognitive and emotional development
Shows fear, anger, affection, jealousy, anxiety, and sympathy
Experiments to reach new goals
Displays intense determination to remove barriers to action
Begins to develop concepts of space, time, and causality
Has increased attention span

18 months
Note: Between 1 and 3 years the child is called a 'toddler'
Anterior fontanelle closed
Abdomen protrudes
Big muscles become well developed
Four cuspids appear by 18 months
Fine muscle coordination begins to develop

Motor development
Walks up stairs with help, creeps downstairs
Walks without support and with balance
Falls less frequently
Throws ball
Stoops to pick up toys, look at insects
Turns pages of book
Holds and lifts cup
Builds three block tower
Picks up and places small beads in container
Begins to use spoon

Cognitive and emotional development
Has vocabulary of 10 words which have meanings
Uses phrases, imitates words
Points to objects named by adult
Follows directions and requests
Imitates adult behaviour
Retrieves toy from several hiding places
Is beginning to develop symbolic thought

Psychosocial development
Develops new awareness of strangers
Wants to explore everything in reach
Plays alone, but near others
Is dependent upon parents, but begins to reach out for autonomy
Finds security in a blanket, toy, or thumbsucking

Play stimulation
Allow unrestricted motor activity (within safety limits)
Offer push-pull toys
Child selects favourite toy
Child likes blocks, pyramid toys, teddy bears, dolls, pots and pans, cloth picture books with colourful large pictures, telephone, musical top, nested blocks

Parental guidance
Begin to teach tooth brushing to establish good dental habits
Safety teaching: child gets into everything within his reach; place medications in safe, locked place; create a safe environment for child
Limits need to be set that give toddler sense of security, yet encourage exploration

Table 1.1 Growth and development (*continued*)

Age and physical characteristics	Behaviour patterns	Nursing implications/ parental guidance
2 years Protruding abdomen less noticeable Landau reflex disappears During first 2 years 35 cm are added to height	*Motor development* Walks up and down stairs Opens doors; turns knobs Has steady gait Holds drinking cup well with one hand Uses spoon without spilling food (may prefer fingers) Kicks a ball in front of him without support Builds a tower of four to six blocks Scribbles Rides tricycle or kiddie car (without pedals) *Cognitive development* Has 200–300 words in vocabulary Begins to use short sentences Refers to self by pronoun Obeys simple commands Does not know right from wrong Begins to learn about time sequences *Psychosocial development* Uses word 'mine' constantly Is possessive with toys Displays negativism–uses 'no' as assertion of self Routine and rituals are important Begins cooperation in toilet training Resists restrictions on freedom Has fear of parents' leaving Shows parallel play Dawdles	*Play stimulation* Shows parallel play, although he enjoys having other children around him Has very short attention span Enjoys same toys as child of 18 months Likes doll play, ball Imitates parents in domestic activities Likes swing, hammering, paper, large crayons *Parental guidance* Has need for peer companionship, although he displays his immaturity by his inability to share and take turns A decrease in appetite normally occurs at this stage Toilet training should be started (each child follows his own pattern) Begin to have child eat his meals with family if he has not already done so Begin to read to child; child likes storybooks with large pictures

(continued)

Resists bedtime-uses transitional objects (blanket, toy)
Vacillates between dependence and independence

2-3 years

Height approximates half his adult height
Legs are about 34% of body length
Begins 2+ kg weight gain per year until 5 years old
At 2½ years has full set (20) of baby teeth
Four second molars appear by 2½ years

Motor development
Throws objects overhead
Pedals tricycle
Walks backward
Washes and dries hands
Begins to use scissors
Can string large beads
Can undress himself
Feeds himself well
Tries to dance
Jumps in place
Builds tower of eight blocks
Balances on one foot
Swings and climbs
Can eat an ice-cream cone
Drinks from a straw

Cognitive development
Shows increased attention span
Gives first and last name
Begins to ask 'why'
Is egocentric in thought and behaviour
Beginning ability to reflect on own behaviour
Talks in short sentences
Uses plurals
May attempt to sing simple songs
Has vocabulary of 900 words
Begins to understand what it means to take turns
Can repeat three numbers
Shows interest in colours

Psychosocial development
Negativism grows out of child's sense of developing independence- says 'no' to every command

Play stimulation
Plays simple games with other children
Enjoys story-telling and dress-up play
Plays 'house'
Colours
Uses scissors and paper
Rides tricycle
Read simple books to him
Will assist in developing memory skills, visual discrimination skills, and language

Parental guidance
From 2-3 years the child develops a seeming maturity; do not expect more of him than he is able to do
Arrange first visit to the dentist to have teeth checked
Be aware that negativistic and ritualistic behaviour is normal
Be consistent in discipline
Control temper tantrums
Begin to teach road safety
Supervise outdoor play

Table 1.1 Growth and development (*continued*)

Age and physical characteristics	Behaviour patterns	Nursing implications/ parental guidance
	Ritualism is important to toddler for his security (follows certain pattern, especially at bedtime)	
	Temper tantrums may result from toddler's frustration in wanting to do everything himself	
	Shows parallel play as well as beginning interaction with others	
	Engages in associative play	
	Fears become pronounced	
	Continues to react to separation from parents but shows increasing ability to handle short periods of separation	
	Has daytime bladder control and is beginning to develop night-time bladder control	
	Becomes more independent	
	Begins to identify sex (gender) roles	
	Explores environment outside the home	
	Can create different ways of getting desired outcome	
3–4 years	*Motor development*	*Play stimulation*
	Drawings have form and meaning, not detail	Plays and interacts with other children
	Buttons front and side of clothes	Shows creativity
	Laces shoes	'Helps' adults
	Bathes self, but needs direction	Likes costumes and enjoys dramatic play
	Brushes teeth	Toys and games: record player, nursery rhymes, housekeeping toys, transportation toys (tricycle, trucks, cars, wagon), blocks, hammer and peg bench, floor trains, blackboard and chalk, easel
	Show continuous movement going up and down stairs	
	Climbs, and jumps well	

Attempts to print letters

Cognitive development
Awareness of body is more stable; child becomes more aware of own vulnerability
Is less negativistic
Learns some number concepts
Begins naming colours
Can identify longer of two lines
Has vocabulary of 1500 words
Uses mild profanities and name-calling
Uses language aggressively
Asks many questions
Can be given simple explanations as to cause and effect

Psychosocial development
Is more active with peers and engages in cooperative play
Performs simple tasks
Frequently has imaginary companion
Dramatizes experiences
Is proud of accomplishments
Exaggerates, boasts, and 'tells tales' on others
Can tolerate separation from mother longer without feeling anxiety
Is keen observer
Has good sense of 'mine' and 'yours'

4-5 years

By 2-5 years adds 25 cm to height
At age 4, legs comprise about 44% of body length

Motor development
Hops two or more times
Dresses without supervision
Has good motor control-climbs and jumps well
Walks up stairs without grasping handrail
Walks backwards
Washes self without wetting clothes
Prints first name and other words
Adds three or more details in drawings

and brushes, clay, crayon and finger paints, outside toys (sandbox, swing, small slide), books (short stories, action stories), drum, scrapbook

Parental guidance
Base your expectations within child's limitations
Provide limited frustrations from environment to assist him in coping
Give small errands to do around the house (putting cutlery on table, drying a dish)
Expand child's world with trips to the zoo, to the supermarket, to restaurant, etc.
Prevent accidents
Provide for brief, nonthreatening separation from parents and home

Play stimulation
Demonstrates gross motor activity-likes to jump rope, skip, climb on jungle gyms, etc.
Prefers group play and cooperates in projects
Plays simple letter, number, form, and picture games
Plays with cars and trucks
Still likes being read to

(continued)

Table 1.1 Growth and development (*continued*)

Age and physical characteristics	Behaviour patterns	Nursing implications/ parental guidance
	Cognitive development	*Parental guidance*
	Has 2100-word vocabulary	Child no longer takes an afternoon nap
	Talks constantly	Prepare child for kindergarten
	Uses adult speech forms	Tell him stories
	Participates in conversations	Provide opportunities and reassurance for group
	Asks for definitions	play; have his friends visit for lunch and an
	Knows age and residence	afternoon of playing
	Identifies heavier of two objects	Prevent accidents
	Knows weeks as time units	At about the age of 5 years, when commencing
	Names days of week	school, booster immunizations of diptheria,
	Begins to understand kinship	tetanus and polio vaccines
	Knows primary colours	
	Can count to 10	
	Can copy a triangle	
	Has high degree of imagination	
	Questioning is at a peak	
	Psychosocial development	
	May have an imaginary companion	
	Has a sense of order (likes to finish what he has started)	
	Is obedient and reliable	
	Is protective towards younger children	
	Begins to develop an elementary conscience with some influence in governing his behaviour	
	Has increased self-confidence	
	Accepts responsibility for acts	
	Is less rebellious	
	Has dreams and nightmares	
	Is cooperative and sympathetic	
	Shows generosity with toys	

Middle childhood 5-9 years

Growth rate is slow and steady
Child gains an average of 3.18 kg per year; height increases approximately 6.25 cm per year
Among children there is considerable variation in height and weight
Child appears taller and slimmer
Early lordosis disappears
Child begins to lose baby teeth; permanent teeth appear at a rate of about four teeth per year from 7-14 years
Neuromuscular and skeletal development allows improved coordination
Eyes become fully developed; vision approaches 20/20

Motor development

6 years
Is active and impulsive
Balance improves
Uses hands as manipulative tools in cutting pasting, hammering
Can draw large letters or figures

7 years
Has lower activity level
Capable of fine hand movements; can print sentences
Nervous habits such as nail-biting are common
Muscular skills such as ball throwing have improved

8 years
Moves with less restlessness
Has developed grace and balance, even in active sports
Has developed coordination of fine muscles, allowing him to write in script rather than to print

9 years
Uses both hands independently
Has become skilful in manual activities because of improved eye-hand coordination

Cognitive development

6 years
Begins to learn to read; defines objects in terms of use; time sense is as much in past as present
Is interested in relationship between home and neighbourhood; knows some streets

Family atmosphere continues to have impact on child's emotional development and his future response within the family

The child needs ongoing guidance in an open, inviting atmosphere; limits should be set with conviction; deal with only one incident at a time; when punishment is necessary, the child should not be humiliated; he should know that it was the *act* that the adult found undesirable, not the child

Needs assistance in adjusting to new experiences and demands of school; should be able to share experiences with family; parents need to have communication with the teacher in order to work together for the health of the child

Convey love and caring in communication; the child understands language directed at feelings better than at intellect; get down to eye level with the child

Parental guidance
Child is sex-conscious; he should be able to discuss his questions at home rather than with his friends; requires simple, honest answers to questions

(continued)

Table 1.1   Growth and development (continued)

Age and physical characteristics	Behaviour patterns	Nursing implications/ parental guidance
	Uses sentences, well; uses language to share other's experiences; may swear or use slang Distinguishes morning from afternoon	Common problems include teasing, quarrelling, nail-biting, enuresis, whining, poor manners, swearing: these are usually fleeting phases and should not be handled negatively; the causes for such behaviour should be investigated and dealt with constructively
	7 years More reflective and has deeper understanding of meanings Interested in conclusions and logical endings; begins to have scientific interests in cause and effect More responsible in relation to time; is more punctual; sense of space is more realistic; child wants some space of own Knows value of coins	
	8 years Thinking is less animistic; is aware of impersonal forces of nature; begins to understand logical reasoning, conclusions, implications Less self-centred in thinking; personal space is expanding, goes places on own; aware of time; plans events of day; understands right from left	
	9 years Intellectually energetic and curious; realistic; reasonable in thinking; able to plan in advance; breaks complex activities into steps	

Focuses on detail
Sense of space includes the entire Earth
Participates in family discussions
Likes to have secrets

Psychosocial development
(The following characteristics apply to the child in
the 5-9 year group)
Still requires parental support, but pulls away from
overt signs of affection
Peer groups provide companionship in widening
circle of persons outside the home; child learns
more about self as he learns about others
'Chum' stage occurs at about 9-10 years of age:
child chooses a special friend of same sex and age
in whom to confide; this is usually child's first
love relationship outside of home, when someone
becomes as important to him as himself
Play teaches the child new ideas and independence;
he progressively utilizes tools of competition,
compromise, cooperation, and beginning
collaboration

Patterns of play
6-7 years
Child acts out ideas of family and occupational
groups with which he has contact
Painting, pasting, reading, simple games,
watching TV, digging, running games, riding
bicycle, and swimming, are all enjoyed
activities

8 years
Child enjoys collections; loosely formed, short-lived
clubs; table games; card games; books; TV; records
Body image and self-concept are quite fluid

The child needs order and consistency in his life to
help him cope with doubts, fears, unacceptable
impulses, and unfamiliar experiences
Encourage peer activities as well as home
responsibilities and give recognition to child's
accomplishments and unique talents
Television may stimulate learning in several
spheres, but should be monitored
Accidents are a major cause of disability and
death; safety practices should be continued
(refer to section on safety, pp. 42-49)
Exercise is essential to promote motor and
psychosocial development; the child should
have a safe place to play and simple pieces of
equipment
A school health programme should be available
and concerned with the child's physical,
emotional, mental, and social health; this
should be augmented by information and
example at home
Medical supervision should continue to detect
developmental delay, disease; appropriate
immunizations should be administered.
Child frequently has 'quiet days'-periods of
shyness, which should be tolerated as part of
growing up and deciding who he is
Child may be subject to nightmares, a situation
which requires reassurance and understanding

(continued)

Table 1.1 Growth and development (*continued*)

Age and physical characteristics	Behaviour patterns	Nursing implications/parental guidance
	because of rapid physical, emotional, social changes Latency stage-sexual drive is controlled and repressed; emphasis is on the development of skills and talent	Parents, teachers, and health professionals should be available and able to provide information and answer questions about the physical changes which occur
Late childhood (9-12 years) Vital signs approach adult values Loses childish appearance of face and takes on features that will characterize him as an adult Growth spurt occurs, and some secondary sex characteristics appear: in females at age 10-12 years; in males at age 12-14 years Physical changes of puberty: increased height and weight, increased perspiration, activity of sebaceous glands, vasomotor instability, increased fat deposition Physical changes in female: pelvis increases in transverse diameter; hips broaden;	*Motor development* Energetic, restless, active movements such as finger-drumming or foot-tapping appear Has skilful manipulative movements nearly equal to those of adults Works hard to perfect physical skills *Cognitive development* 10 years Likes to reason, enjoys learning; thinking is concrete, matter of fact; wants to measure up to challenge; likes to memorize; identify facts. attention span may be short; space is rather specific (i.e where things are) Can write for relatively long time with speed 11 years Thinking is concrete and specific, not reflective Likes action in learning Concentrates well when working competitively Can understand relational terms such as weight and size Perceives space as nothingness that goes on forever	*Parental guidance* Continue sex education and preparation for adolescent body changes Lying and stealing are more serious problems; again, the causes must be determined (Usually these are attempts to gain recognition or remedy inadequacies) Harsh and severe punishment should be avoided Understanding is important Encourage participation in organized clubs, youth groups Democratic guidance is essential as child works through a conflict between dependence (on his parents) and independence; child needs realistic limits set Needs help channelling energy in proper direction — work and sports Requires adequate explanation of body changes

tenderness in developing
breast tissue, enlargement
of areola diameter;
appearance of pubic hair
Physical changes in male:
size of testes increases;
scrotum colour changes;
breasts enlarge,
temporarily; height and
shoulder breadth increase;
appearance of lightly
pigmented hair at base of
penis; increase in length and
width of penis

Able to discuss problems

12 years
Enjoys learning
Considers all aspects of a situation
Motivated more by inner drive than by
 competition
Able to classify, arrange, generalize
Likes to discuss and debate
Begins conceptual thinking
Verbal, formal reasoning now possible
Can recognize moral of a story
Defines time as duration; likes to plan ahead
Understands that space is abstract
Can be critical of own work

Psychosocial development
The group becomes important, and gang or club
code takes precedence over nearly everything;
often gang codes are characterized by
collective action against the mores of the adult world;
here children begin to work out own social patterns
without adult interference; early gangs may include
both sexes; later gangs are separated by sex

Patterns of play
Continues to enjoy reading, TV, table games
More interested in active sports as a means to
 improve skills
Creative talents may appear; may enjoy drawing,
modelling clay; by age 10, sex differences in play
become profound
Occasional privacy is important
May reach puberty; resurgence of sexual drives
causes recapitulation of Oedipal struggle

Special understanding required for the child who
lags in physical development

(continued)

Table 1.1 Growth and development (*continued*)

Age and physical characteristics	Behaviour patterns	Nursing implications/ parental guidance
Adolescence	*Motor development*	Stresses frequently result from conflicting value systems between generations; parents may need help to see that the adolescent is a product of the times and that his actions reflect what is happening around him
Phase of development begins when reproductive organs become functionally operative; phase ends when physical growth is completed	Often uncoordinated; has poor posture Tires easily	
	Cognitive development	Parent's limits and rules should be realistic and consistent; they should convey the love and concern of parents and should be a source of comfort and reassurance, protecting the child from activities for which he is not ready
Skeletal system grows faster than supporting muscles Hands and feet grow proportionally faster than rest of body	Mind has great ability to acquire and utilize knowledge Categorizes thoughts into usable forms May project thinking into the future Is capable of highly imaginative thinking	The home should be an accepting, emotionally stable environment
Large muscles develop more quickly than small muscles	*Psychosocial development*	Continue sex education, including discussion of ovulation, fertilization, menstruation, pregnancy, masturbation, nocturnal emissions, hygiene, make-up, and health
Females:physical changes include appearance of menarche; growth of axillary and perineal hair; deepened voice, ovulation, further development of breasts	Interest in opposite sex increases Often revolts from adult authority to conform to peer-group standards Continues to rework feelings for parent of opposite sex and unravel the ambivalence toward parent of same sex	Adolescents have an increased need for rest and sleep, because they are expending large amounts of energy and are functioning with an inadequate oxygen supply
Males: physical changes include growth of axillary, perineal, facial, chest hair; deepening of voice; production of spermatozoa, nocturnal emissions	Affection may turn temporarily to an adult outside of the family (for example, crush on family friend, neighbour, or teacher) Utilizes peer-group dialect-highly informal language or specially coined terminology Peer groups are especially important and help adolescent to define own identity, to adapt to changing body image, to establish more mature relationships with others, and to deal with heightened sexual feelings; cliques may develop Dating generally progresses from groups of couples to double dates and finally single couples	Recreational interests should be fostered; favourite activities include sports, dating, dancing, reading, hobbies, and TV; talking on the telephone, listening to records are favourite pastimes Adolescent health problems which require preventive education are accidents, obesity, acne, pregnancy, venereal disease, drug abuse Allow adolescent to handle his own affairs as

Teenage 'hangouts' become important centres of activity

much as possible, but be aware of physical and psychosocial problems with which he will need help; encourage independence but allow child to lean on parents for support when frightened or unable to attain his goals

Adolescents with special problems should have access to specialists such as adolescent clinics, and psychologists

Requires reassurance and help in accepting his changing body image; parents should make the most of his positive qualities

Give gentle encouragement and guidance regarding dating; avoid strong pressures in either direction

Understand his conflicts as he attempts to deal with social, moral, and intellectual issues

Provide opportunities for adolescents to earn their own money; allow some financial independence

Provide safety education-especially regarding driving

Provide assistance to develop good attitudes towards health-smoking, drinking, drugs, nutrition, etc.

Table 1.2 Childhood diseases

Disease (**a**, agent; **b**, mode of transmission; **c**, age when most common)	Incubation (*I*) and communicability (*C*) periods	Symptoms
Rubella (German/3-day measles) **a** Rubella virus **b** Droplets or direct contact with infected persons or articles freshly contaminated with nasopharyngeal secretions, faeces, urine **c** School age, young adult *Diagnostic tests:* Tissue culture of throat, blood or urine *Passive immunity:* Birth to about 1 year of age (if mother is immune prior to pregnancy)	*I:* 14-21 days after exposure *C:* Virus can be passed areas from 7 days before to 5 days after rash appears	**a** Rash-enlarged lymph nodes in postauricular, suboccipital and cervical **b** In adolescents — headache anorexia, low-grade fever, sore throat, coyza, conjunctivitis, before rash appears generalized malaise 1-5 days before rash appears *Duration:* 3-5 days *Rash characteristics:* Pinpoint (or larger) red spots on soft palate (Forchheimer's spots) spread to face and downward towards the feet, covering entire body at end of first day; rash begins to subside on second day in same order
Roseola infantum (exanthema subitum) **a** Presumably caused by virus **b** Transmission not known **c** 6 months-2 years	Not known — believed not to be highly contagious	**a** Fever of 40-40.5°C, either intermittent or sustained 3-4 days; decrease in appetite; slightly irritable **b** Fever suddenly drops and rash of red measles or maculopapules 2-3 mm appears *Duration* 1-2 days Rash fades on pressure; it appears first on trunk and spreads upward and downward
Rubeola (hard, red, 7-day measles) **a** Measles virus, RNA-containing paramyxovirus **b** Direct contact with droplets from infected persons	*I:* 10-12 days *C:* 5th day of incubation to first 5-7 days of rash	**a** Fever, lethargy **b** 48h-Koplik's spots on buccal mucosa (spots are reddened areas with greyish-blue centre)

Table 1.2 Childhood diseases *(continued)*

Nursing care and treatment	Complications	Special considerations
Symptomatic	In adolescent and adult: arthritis, encephalitis, purpura	Exposure of nonimmune pregnant women in first trimester results in high percentage of affected fetuses and infants born with various birth defects: cataracts, heart murmur, deafness, 'the rubella syndrome'
Symptomatic-antipyretic	Convulsions due to high fever	
Bed rest; isolation from onset of catarrh through 3rd day of rash Darkened room if child is photophobic; plenty of fluids	Otitis media, pneumonia, laryngitis, mastoiditis, encephalitis	Immunoglobulin is indicated for children at particular risk, for those with leukaemia, receiving corticosteroids or on immunosuppressive therapy

(continued)

Table 1.2 Childhood diseases *(continued)*

Disease (**a**, agent; **b**, mode of transmission; **c**, age when most common)	Incubation (*I*) and communicability (*C*) periods	Symptoms
Diagnostic tests: Serological procedures *Passive immunity:* Birth to about 1 year of age if mother is immune prior to pregnancy		**c** 2 days later, rash appears at hairline and spreads to feet in 1 day **d** Lymphadenopathy **e** Anorexia **f** Pruritis
Mumps **a** Mumps virus, paramyxovirus **b** Urine, blood, and saliva by direct contact or droplets *Diagnostic tests:* Complement fixation *Passive immunity:*Birth to 3-4 months of age if mother had antibodies against mumps prior to pregnancy	*I*: 14-28 (average 18 days) *C*: Until all swelling has disappeared, not usually less than 14 days from start of illness; virus in saliva greatest just before and after parotitis onset	**a** Headache, anorexia, generalized malaise; fever 1 day before glandular swelling; fever lasts 1-6 days **b** Glandular swelling, usually of parotid **c** Enlargement and reddening of Wharton's duct and Stensen's duct
Chickenpox **a** Varicella virus **b** Highly communicable; acquired via direct contact, indirect contact, droplet spread, airborne transmission **c** 2-8 years *Diagnostic tests:* Scrapings from vesicle; staining reveals multinucleated giant cells *Passive immunity:* Possibly some, but uncertain	*I*: 14-21 days after exposure *C*: Onset of fever 1 day prior to first lesion) until last vesicle is dried (5-7 days)	**a** General malaise and fever for 24 h **b** Rash-macules to papules and vesicles to crusts within several hours **c** Itching of lesions may be severe and scratching may cause scarring *Rash characteristics:* Rash appears first on head and mucous membranes, then becomes concentrated on body and sparse on extremities
Diptheria **a** *Corynebacterium diptheriae* **b** Acquired through secretions of carrier or infected	*I*: 2-6 days *C*: 2-4 weeks untreated; shorter period with antibiotic treatment	**a** Pharyngeal and tonsillar diptheria: (1) General malaise, low-grade fever, anorexia

Nursing care and treatment	Complications	Special considerations
and diet as desired. Frequent mouth care *Treatment of itching:* Application of calamine lotion to lesions, keeping fingernails trimmed, suitable play activities Keep child coolly dressed in loose cotton clothing		
Isolation until swelling has subsided Frequent mouth care Nourishing liquid diet at commencement of illness Analgesics to ease any discomfort	Meningoencephalitis Auditory nerve involvement, resulting in deafness Orchitis (if disease occurs after puberty)	
Symptomatic: Short fingernails to prevent scratching Oral antihistamines to decrease pruritis Isolation until all lesions have crusted-about 5-6 days Keep child cool, wear loose soft clothing Apply dusting powder or calamine lotion to skin	Complications are rare in normal children Haemorrhagic varicella, encephalitis, pneumonia, and bacteria skin infection are not common, but they can occur	Severe in neonate and pregnant women Specific immunoglobulin is available for high risk susceptible children, e.g. those with leukaemia or receiving corticosteroids
Diphtheria antitoxin Antibiotic therapy (penicillin) Supportive treatment, bedrest Respiratory support	Myocarditis Neuritis Bronchopneumonia Otitis media	

(continued)

Table 1.2   Childhood diseases *(continued)*

Disease (**a**, agent; **b**, mode of transmission; **c**, age when most common)	Incubation (*I*) and communicability (*C*) periods	Symptoms
individual by direct contact with contaminated articles and environment **c** Incidence increased in autumn and spring *Diagnostic tests:* Cultures of nose and throat	patient not clear until 2 consecutive throat cultures	(2) 1-2 days later, whitish-grey membranous patch on tonsils, soft palate and uvulva (3) Lymph node swelling, fever, rapid pulse **b** Nasal diptheria: (1) Choryza with increasing viscosity, possibly epistaxis, low-grade fever (2) Whitish-grey membrane may appear over nasal septum **c** Laryngeal diptheria: (1) Usually spread from pharynx to larynx (2) Fever, harsh voice, barking cough; respiratory difficulty with inspiratory retraction **d** Nonrespiratory diptheria: affects eye, ear, genitals or rarely, skin
Pertussis (whooping cough) **a** *Bordetella pertussis* **b** Direct contact, droplet spread; indirect contact with contaminated articles **c** Infants and young children; incidence higher in spring and summer	*I:* 5-14 days *C:* 7 days after exposure (greatest just before catarrhal stage) to 3 weeks after onset of paroxysms	**a** Stage I (catarrhal stage) (1) Lasts 1-2 weeks (2) Choryza, sneezing, tearing, tickling/dry cough, fever, loss of appetite **b** Stage II (paroxysmal stage) (1) Last 4-6 weeks (2) Severe, violent coughing attacks occurring in clusters leading to vomiting, cyanosis, and exhaustion **c** Stage III (convalescent stage) (1) Lasts 4 months-2 years (2) Coughing attacks decrease, but they return with each respiratory infection *Duration:* 9 months-2 years

Nursing care and treatment	Complications	Special considerations
Isolation until 2-3 cultures are negative after antibiotic therapy is completed Light nourishing diet; tube feeding may become necessary Intravenous fluids to maintain electrolyte equilibrium		
Symptomatic Bed rest Suctioning of nasopharyngeal secretions Antipyretics Antibiotics Increase fluids; nutrition and electrolyte balance; tube feeds may be necessary for small infants; older children require smaller, highly nourishing meals more frequently-best given immediately after a bout of whooping Place in an environment with reduced stimuli to reduce coughing. Sedation Isolation 4 weeks after coughing begins	Respiratory: pneumonia, atelectasis, emphysema Neurological: brain damage Convulsions Conjunctival haemorrhages Rectal prolapse, rare	

(continued)

Table 1.2   Childhood diseases *(continued)*

Disease (**a**, agent; **b**, mode of transmission; **c**, age when most common)	Incubation (*I*) and communicability (*C*) periods	Symptoms
Tetanus (lockjaw) **a** *Clostridium tetani*-prevalence in soil and animal faeces; can be introduced into body through any break in skin or intestinal tract **b** Direct or indirect contact with wound **c** All ages *Diagnostic tests:* Wound culture anaerobically for *Clostridium tetani*	*I:* 3 days to 3 weeks *C:* None	**a** Stiffening of striated muscles, usually the jaw **b** 1-2 days later, stiffening leads to spastic rigidity and spreads down body to the extremities
Poliomyelitis (polio) **a** Virus serotypes 1 − 3 + 2; incidence is higher in summer and autumn **b** Virus is haboured in gastrointestinal tract and is transmitted through saliva, vomitus and faeces. **c** Predisposing factors that increase risk of disease: recent tonsillectomy, tooth extraction or DTP injections, pregnancy, physical exhaustion *Diagnostic tests:* Isolation of polio virus from faeces and throat	*I:* 7-14 days, paralytic or nonparalytic; 3-5 days for prodromal or minor illness *C:* Increases around onset when virus is in throat and is excreted in faeces; virus is present in throat 1 week after onset, in stool 4-6 weeks after	**a** Nonparalytic polio: (1) Headache, lethargy, anorexia, vomiting, fever (2) Muscle pain and stiffness **b** Paralytic polio (1) Same and non-paralytic type, lasting about a week (2) Then 1-2 days of CNS symptoms: loss of deep tendon reflexes, positive. Kernig's and Brudinski's signs, lethargy (3) 1-2 days later, weakening of muscles and paralysis
Streptococcal pharyngitis ('strep throat') **a** Beta-haemolytic streptococcus-group A strain **b** Direct or indirect contact with nasopharyngeal secretion of infected person or recently established carrier **c** Not under 3 years of age, 5-16 years, incidence higher in winter and spring *Diagnostic tests:* Nasopharyngeal (throat) culture	*I:* 2-5 days *C:* Greatest during acute phase of illness	**a** Onset is generally acute: high fever, headache vomiting, scarlatina rash **b** After 12-24 hours, sore throat of varying degrees of severity, dryness of throat, cervical lymphadenopathy, white tongue coating that gives way to strawberry-red tongue

Nursing care and treatment	Complications	Special considerations
Reduce muscular spasm with medication, quiet, dark room Antibiotics: penicillin or tetracycline Tetanus immune globulin or antitoxin Debridement of wound Fluid and nutrition	Convulsion with laryngospasms leading to death Asphyxia from dysphagia and secretions	
Symptomatic, i.e. relief of pain Analgesics, heat Complete bed rest in early stages Planned nursing care to avoid unnecessary disturbance Isolation until 3 weeks after child has become apyrexial Excreta should be disposed of antiseptically	Respiratory paralysis Hypertension	*Note:* A careful watch must be kept for dyspnoea, restlessness and anxiety that can herald the onset of respiratory paralysis. A ventilator should be readily available
Isolation for 1 day while starting prescription Antibiotic therapy: penicillin G Symptomatic	Acute glomerulonephritis, 1-2 weeks after acute stage Rheumatic fever, 2-3 weeks after acute stage Peritonsillar abcscess, cervical adenitis Pneomonia, otitis media, meningitis	Throat cultures of entire household (i.e. parents, siblings) 2-3 days after patient started therapy and treated if culture was positive Repeat throat culture done 2-3 days after completion of 10-day course

Table 1.3 Nutrition in paediatrics

Age and developmental influence on nutritional requirements and feeding patterns	Feeding pattern/diet	Nursing implications/ parental guidance
Neonate (birth–4 weeks) Newborn's rapid growth makes him especially vulnerable to dietary inadequacies, dehydration, and iron deficiency anaemia Feeding process is basis for infant's first human relationship, his formation of trust; feeding reinforces mother's sense of 'motherliness' Because of limited nutritional stores, neonates require vitamin and mineral supplements Neonates require more fluid relative to their size than do adults Sucking ability is influenced by individual neuromuscular maturity	Breast milk or modified milk formula is generally given in 6–8 feedings per day, spaced 3–4 h apart Feeding schedules should be individualized according to infant's needs	Provide information to help parents make decision concerning breast or bottle feeding Support parents in their decision *Breast-fed infant* (see page 120): 1 Help mother assume comfortable and satisfying position for self and baby 2 Help mother to determine schedule, timing and when infant is satisfied 3 Provide specific information about the following: **a** Feeding technique: position, frequency of burping **b** Care of breasts **c** Manual expression of milk from breast **d** Importance of good maternal diet *Bottle-fed infant:* 1 Provide specific information concerning **a** Type of infant formula **b** Preparation of infant formula; measuring and sterilization **c** Equipment — types of bottles, teats, etc. **d** Sterilization of equipment **e** Technique of feeding: position, 'burping' 2 Help mother to determine when infant is satisfied, develop schedule for feeding Provide information concerning normal

Infant
(3 months-1 year)

Increased neuromuscular development allows infant to make transition from a totally liquid diet to a diet of milk and solid foods as well as to more active participation in the feeding process

3-6 months
Sucking reflex becomes voluntary and chewing action begins; infant can approximate lips to rim of cup and may begin drinking from cup at 6 months

Number of feedings per day decreases through the first year
By 1 year of age, most infants are satisfied with three meals and additional fluids throughout the day
By 4 months of age, the infant is generally ready to begin eating strained foods; the usual sequence of foods is cereal followed by fruits, vegetables, and meats; this sequence may vary according to individual preferences of paediatrician and family
Mashed table foods or junior foods generally are started at 6-8 months, when infant begins chewing action
Infant begins to enjoy finger foods at 10-12 months

characteristics of stools, signs of dehydration, constipation, colic, milk allergy
Discuss need for vitamin supplements and how to administer
Discuss need for additional fluids during periods of hot weather, and with fever, diarrhoea, and vomiting
Observe for evidence of common problems and intervene accordingly:
1 Overfeeding
2 Underfeeding
3 Difficulty digesting infant formula because of its particular composition
4 Improper feeding technique; holes in teats too large or too small; infant formula too hot or too cold; uncomfortable feeding position; failure to 'burp'; improper sterilization
5 Emotional problems in family may cause irritability, colic and other similar disturbances

New foods should be offered one at a time and early in the feeding while the infant is still hungry
The person feeding should be calm, gentle, relaxed, and patient in approach
When the child is first offered puréed foods with a spoon, he expects and wants to suck; the protrusion of his tongue, which is needed in sucking, makes it appear that he is pushing the food out of his mouth; this response should not be interpreted as dislike for the food, it is a result of immature muscle coordination and surprise at the taste and feel of the new food
The baby foods selected should be those which are high in nutrients without providing excessive calories; personal and cultural preferences should be considered

(continued)

Table 1.3 Nutrition in paediatrics (*continued*)

Age and developmental influence on nutritional requirements and feeding patterns	Feeding pattern/diet	Nursing implications/parental guidance
6-12 months Eyes and hands can work together; infant is able to sit without support and has developed grasp; able to feed itself a rusk; bangs objects on table; able to hold own bottle at 9-12 months; has 'pincher' approach to food; able to be weaned as child becomes developmentally able to take sufficient fluids from the cup Food provides the infant with a variety of learning experiences: motor control and coordination in self-feeding; recognition of shape, texture, colour; stimulation of speech movement through use of mouth muscles Mealtime allows the infant to continue his development of trust in a consistent, loving atmosphere; the infant is forming his lifetime eating habits; it is therefore important to make mealtime a positive experience		Infants should be observed for allergic reactions when new foods are added; common allergies are to citrus fruits and egg white Finger foods should be selected for their nutritional value: good choices include teething rusks, cooked vegetables, meat, cheese sticks, and enriched cereals; avoid nuts, raisins, and raw vegetables, which can cause choking Weaning is a gradual process 1 Assist parents to recognize indications of readiness 2 Do not expect the infant to completely drop his old pattern of behaviour while learning a new one; allow overlap of old and new techniques 3 Evening feedings are usually the most difficult to eliminate, because the infant is tired and in need of sucking comfort 4 During illness or household disorganization, the infant may regress and return to sucking to relieve his discomfort and frustration **Special considerations:** Hospitalized infant Obtain a thorough nursing history that includes the following: feeding pattern and schedule; types of foods that have been introduced; likes and dislikes; breast- or bottle-fed; type of bottle; temperature at which infant prefers food and fluids

Toddler
(1-3 years)

Growth slows at the end of the first year, and weight gain is small; the slower growth rate is reflected in a decreased appetite

The toddler has a total of 14-16 teeth, making him more able to chew foods

Increased self-awareness causes the toddler to want to do more for himself; refusals of food or of assistance in feeding are common ways in which the toddler asserts himself

Since body tissues, especially muscles, continue to grow quite rapidly, protein needs are high

Appetite is sporadic; specific foods may be favoured exclusively or refused from time to time

Child may be ritualistic concerning food preferences, schedule, manner of eating, etc.

Diet should include a full range of foods: milk, meat, fruits, vegetables, breads, and cereals

Older toddler can be expected to consume about one-half the amount of food that an adult consumes

Provide foods with a variety of colour, texture, and flavour; toddlers need to experience the feel of foods

Offer small portions; it is fun for the child to ask for more; it is more effective to give small helpings than to insist that he eat a specific amount

Maintain a regular mealtime schedule

Provide appropriate equipment:

1 Small-sized cutlery or spoon and fork only
2 Dishes — colourful, unbreakable; shallow round bowls are preferable to flat plates
3 Plastic bibs, placemats, and floor coverings, permit a relaxed attitude toward child's self-feeding attempts
4 Comfortable seating at good height and distance from table

Adults who help toddlers at mealtimes should be calm and relaxed; avoid bribes or force feeding, because this reinforces negative behaviour and may lead to a dislike for mealtime; encourage independence, but provide assistance when necessary; do not be concerned about table manners.

Avoid the use of fizzy drinks or 'sweets;' as rewards or between-meal snacks; instead, substitute fruit or juice

Toddlers who show little interest in eggs, meat, or vegetables should not be permitted to appease their appetite with carbohydrates or milk, because this may lead to iron-deficiency anaemia (see page 348).

Special considerations: Hospitalized toddler Nursing history should include the following: feeding pattern and schedule; food likes and dislikes; food allergies, special eating equipment and utensils; whether or not child is

(continued)

Table 1.3 Nutrition in paediatrics (*continued*)

Age and developmental influence on nutritional requirements and feeding patterns	Feeding pattern/diet	Nursing implications/parental guidance
		weaned and whether he takes bottle to bed; what child is fed when ill
3-5 years of age	Appetite tends to be sporadic	Emphasis should be placed on the quality rather than the amount of food ingested
Increased manual dexterity enables child to have complete independence at mealtime	Child requires the same basic four foods groups as the adult, but in smaller quantities	Foods should be attractively served, mildly flavoured, plain, as well as being separated and distinctly identifiable in flavour and appearance.
Psychosocially, this is a period of increased imitation and sex identification; the child identifies with parents at the table and will enjoy what parents enjoy	Generally likes to eat one food from plate at a time	Nutritional foods (e.g. biscuits and cheese, yoghurt, fruit) should be offered as snacks
Additional nutritional habits are developed which become part of the child's lifetime practices	Likes vegetables that are crisp, raw, and cut into finger-sized pieces; often dislikes strong-tasting foods	Desserts should be nutritious and a natural part of the meal, not used as a reward for finishing the meal or omitted as punishment
Slower growth rate and increased interest in exploring his environment may decrease the child's interest in eating		Unless they persist, periods of overeating or not wanting to eat certain foods should not cause concern; the overall eating pattern from month to month is more pertinent to assess
Eating assumes increasing social significance; mealtime promotes socialization and provides the child with opportunities to learn		Frequent causes of insufficient eating:
		1 Unhappy atmosphere at mealtime
		2 Overeating between meals
		3 Parental example
		4 Attention-seeking
		5 Excessive parental expectations
		6 Inadequate variety or quantity of foods
		7 Tooth decay
		8 Physical illness
		9 Fatigue
		10 Emotional disturbance

appropriate mealtime behaviour, language skills, and understanding of family rituals

Measures to increase food intake:
1 Allow child to help with preparations, planning menu, setting table, and other simple chores
2 Maintain calm environment with no distractions
3 Avoid between-meal snacks
4 Provide rest period before meal
5 Avoid coaxing, bribing, threatening
Special considerations: Hospitalized under-fives
Consider cultural differences
Allow parents to bring in favourite foods or eating utensils from home
Encourage family members to be present at mealtime
Place children in small groups, preferably at tables during mealtime
Provide simple foods in small portions; peanut butter and jam sandwiches are often favourites
Allow and encourage children to feed themselves
Utilize nursing histories as described for toddlers (see page 60)
Do not punish children who refuse to eat; offer alternative foods

School-age child
Slowed rate of growth during middle childhood results in gradual decline in food requirements per unit of body weight
The preadolescent growth spurt occurs about age 10 in girls and about age 12 in boys; at this time energy needs increase and approach those of the adult; intake is increased and approaches that of the adult; intake is

By this time, food practices are generally well established, a product of the eating experiences of the toddler and preschool period
Many children are too busy with other affairs to take time out to eat; play readily takes priority unless a firm understanding is reached and mealtime is relaxed and enjoyable

Nutrition education should help the child to select foods wisely and to begin to plan and prepare meals
Parental attitudes continue to be important as the child copies parental behaviour (e.g. skipping breakfast, not eating certain foods)
Most children require a nutritious breakfast to avoid lassitude in late morning
Mealtime should continue to be relaxed and enjoyable; diversions such as the TV being on should be avoided

(continued)

Table 1.3 Nutrition in paediatrics (*continued*)

Age and developmental influence on nutritional requirements and feeding patterns	Feeding pattern/diet	Nursing implications/parental guidance
particularly important, since reserves are laid down for the demands of adolescence The child becomes dependent on peers for approval and makes food choices accordingly The child experiences increased socialization and independence through opportunities to eat away from home—for example, at school and homes of peers		Calcium and vitamin D intake warrant special consideration; they must be adequate to support the rapid enlargement of bones Parents and health professionals should be alert to signs of developing obesity; intake should be altered accordingly Table manners should not be overemphasized; the young child often stuffs his mouth, spills foods, and chatters incessantly while eating; time and experience will improve his habits Provide some companionship and coversation at the child's level during meals; peers should be invited occasionally for meals **Special considerations:** Hospitalized child Nursing history should include the following: food preferences; mealtime patterns and snacks, food allergies; food preferences when ill Provide opportunities for children to eat in small groups at tables Consider cultural differences Allow parents to bring in favourite foods from home Allow child to order his own meal
Adolescent (roughly 11-17 years of age) Dietary requirements vary according to stage of sexual	Previously learned dietary patterns are difficult to change Food choices and eating habits may be quite unusual and are related to the adolescent's	Continue nutrition education, with special emphasis on the following: 1 Selecting nutritious foods 2 Nutritional needs related to growth

maturation, rate of physical growth, and extent of athletic and social activity

When rapid growth of puberty appears, there is a corresponding increase in energy requirements and appetite

psychological and social milieu

Generally, a significant percentage of the daily energy intake of the adolescent comes from snacks

3 Preparing favourite 'adolescent foods'

4 Avoiding the kinds of foods that aggravate acne

5 The importance of foods and physical fitness

Informal sessions are generally more effective than lectures on nutrition

Special problems requiring intervention: obesity; excessive dieting; extreme fads-eccentric and grossly restricted diets; anorexia; adolescent pregnancy

Provide nutritious foods relevant to the adolescent's lifestyle

Discourage cigarette smoking, which may contribute to poor nutritional status by decreasing appetite and increasing the body's metabolic rate

Special considerations: Hospitalized adolescent

Allow patient to choose own foods, especially if on a special diet

If possible, allow patient to prepare beverages and snacks in ward kitchen

Serve foods that appeal to adolescents

Utilize a nursing history similar to that for the school-aged child

PREVENTATIVE PAEDIATRICS

Immunization

Table 1.4   Immunization schedule for infants and children

Age	Immunization	
3 months	1st dose	diptheria, tetanus, pertussis, and vaccine
4½-5 months	2nd dose	poliomyelitis
9-11 months	3rd dose	
15-18 months	Measles	
5 years	Booster of diptheria, tetanus and poliomyelitis vaccine	
10-13 years	BCG vaccine if tuberculin skin test negative	
Girls 11-13 years	Rubella vaccine if seronegative	

Source: Prevention in the Child Health Services, DHSS, 1980.

General Considerations

1   A good nursing history will include determining whether or not the child has been exposed to any communicable disease or has experienced such. Surveillance in this area will prevent unnecessary disease and allow for proper immunization for the child and his family.

2   Immunizations may be started at any age. If an immunization programme is not begun in infancy, a slightly different schedule may be followed, depending upon the child's age and the prevalence of specific infections at the time.

3   An interrupted primary series of immunizations need not be restarted; it need only be continued, regardless of the length of time that has elapsed.

4   The immunoresponse is limited in a significant proportion of young infants, and the recommended booster doses are designed to ensure and maintain immunity.

5   **a** The combination of depot antigens is preferred, because it is more immunogenic.
   b Because of the increased risk of possible reactions to either diphtheria or pertussis, Td (adult-type tetanus and diphtheria toxins) is recommended for children over 6 years of age.
   c For contaminated wounds, a booster dose of tetanus should be given if more than 5 years have elapsed since the last dose.
   d Parents who refuse pertussis vaccine should be encouraged to accept diphtheria and tetanus vaccine.

6   Immunizations should be deferred if child has an acute febrile infection or illness. The common cold, without fever, is not a contraindication to immunization.

7   Contraindications to receiving measles and rubella vaccines include the following: pregnancy, generalized malignancy, cell-mediated immunodeficiency disorders, current immunosuppressive therapy, sensitivity to animal

species used in vaccine preparation, transfusion of immune serum globulin, plasma or blood. If any of these contraindications exist, immunizations may be temporarily deferred or an alternative vaccine preparation may be used.

8   Strict adherence to the manufacturer's storage recommendations is vital. Failure to observe these precautions and recommendations may reduce the potency and effectiveness of the specific vaccine.

9   *Pertussis:*
   a Protection of infant against pertussis should begin early.
   b In newborn infant the best protection against pertussis is avoidance of household contacts by adequate immunization of older siblings.

10 Tuberculin test
   a Tuberculin testing depends upon the following:
   (1) Risk of exposure of the child
   (2) Prevalence of tuberculosis in the population group
   (3) High-risk situations; intervals between routine testing should not exceed 6 months
   b *BCG vaccine* (Bacillus of Calmette-Guérin): BCG vaccine is given as a routine to children aged 11-13 years who are tuberculin negative, irrespective of whether there is a history of BCG vaccination at an earlier age BCG vaccine should be given at birth to children who come from environments where there is a high risk of contracting tuberculosis, e.g. certain immigrant families. Tuberculin-negative contacts of known cases of tuberculosis should be given BCG vaccine. Certain virus infections, such as measles, rubella and chickenpox, can suppress the tuberculin test for about 4-6 weeks. For this reason, the tuberculin test should not be carried out in the 6 weeks after rubella or measles vaccinations nor should BCG vaccine be given within 3 weeks after these vaccinations.
   It is recommended that BCG vaccine should have been given on entry into the UK to immigrant children, who are negative reactors, from the Indian subcontinent and Africa and to those born into these communities.

11. *Measles vaccine:* Measles vaccine should be offered to all susceptible children from the second year of life to puberty. It is important to recognize that the following groups are at special risk.
   a Children from the age of one year upwards in residential care
   b Children entering nursery school or other establishment accepting children for day care
   c Children with serious physical incapacity who are likely to develop severe illness as the result of natural measles infection. The use of immunoglobulin with the vaccination should be considered in these cases. Contraindications to vaccination should be observed, especially in immune deficient states.

12 *Poliomyelitis vaccine:* Live trivalent oral polio virus vaccine is preferred to the inactivated form, because administration is easier and the immunologic effects are broader and longer.

13 *Rubella vaccine:* The Joint Committee on Vaccination and Immunization (Health Services Development, Rubella vaccination, DHSS, HC(79)14,

1979) recommends that routine rubella vaccination should be offered to girls between 11 and 13 years.

14 *Smallpox vaccination:* No longer internationally required. The world-wide eradication of smallpox was declared by the World Health Organization 1980.

Dental Care

Primary Teeth

1 *Eruption*
   a Two lower central incisors — by 6-7 months
   b Four upper incisors — by 9 months
   c Two lower lateral incisors — by 1 year
   d Four first molars — by 14 months
   e Four cuspids — by 18 months
   f Four second molars — by 2-2½ years:

2 *Importance of primary teeth and dental care for primary teeth*
   a At about 2 years of age, toothbrushing should be started At this age, most of the primary teeth have erupted, and the child's muscle coordination has developed enough to allow some form of brushing.
   b By age 3, the child should be examined by a dentist when all primary teeth have erupted.
   c When decayed primary teeth are neglected, they endanger the child's health and may cause abscesses, fever, and excessive pain. The infected teeth may damage the permanent tooth that is forming within the jaw. A child with advanced tooth decay finds it difficult to chew some foods that are essential to a well-balanced diet.
   d Primary teeth act as a guide for the proper positioning of permanent teeth. Each primary tooth is holding the space for a permanent tooth that will replace it. If a primary tooth is lost permanently, there will be a loss of space. This usually results in crowding of permanent teeth, ultimately requiring orthodontic work when a child is older.
   e Primary teeth serve as a stimulus for growth of the jaws, aid in the development of speech, and serve a cosmetic function.
      (1) A young person can become very self-conscious when he loses a tooth in the front of his mouth and realizes that he looks different.
      (2) Indirectly, a child's speech may be affected if self-consciousness about his loss of teeth prevents him from opening his mouth for proper talking.
      (3) Ability to use the teeth for pronunciation is acquired entirely with the aid of the primary teeth. Early loss of front teeth may lead to difficulty in pronouncing 's', 'f', 'l', 'z' and 'th'.
      (4) Even after the permanent teeth erupt, difficulty in pronouncing 's', 'z' and 'th' may persist to the point that the child requires speech therapy.

Permanent Teeth

1 *Eruption*
  a Four '6-year molars' appear between the age of 6 and 7 years.
  b From this point onward, until 12-13 years of age, the primary teeth loosen, one by one, and each is replaced by a permanent tooth.
  c Four additional molars appear at 12-13 years of age.
  d Four molars ('wisdom teeth') appear at 17-21 years.
2 *Importance of early dental care:* Care of teeth during infancy and childhood is necessary in order to
  a Promote proper development of teeth.
  b Prevent dental caries.

Nursing Management

1 Take advantage of incidental opportunities to teach children and their parents information that will promote dental health.
  a Emphasize that inflammatory periodontal disease and dental caries are the results of dental plaque. Dental plaque is a mass composed primarily of microorganisms that adhere to the tooth surface. As these microorganisms grow, they form products that are destructive to the underlying tissue. Removal of this plaque and prevention of its collection is a major part of dental care.
  b Provide a well-balanced diet that is necessary for tooth development. Stress the importance of diet control in dental care. The microorganisms that form dental plaque need a sucrose substrate which comes from refined sugars for rapid growth. Therefore, decreasing the intake of such refined sugars is important.
  c Start child on the correct procedure by having a good attitude towards brushing. Parents serve as role models as well as assist the young child to care for his teeth.
2 Provide supplemental fluoride if the local drinking water supply does not contain fluoride. Fluoride makes the tooth surface more resistant to disease.
  a Topical application of fluoride should be done twice a year.
  b Daily fluoride rinse after brushing is effective in decreasing dental caries in children.
  c Daily use of a dentifrice containing fluoride is another source of protection.
3 Maintain the child's general health.
4 Encourage parents to arrange a dental visit when child is $2\frac{1}{2}$-3 years old
5 Teach child and parents good brushing technique and dental habits.
  a Use soft-bristle nylon brush with polished ends.
  b Place bristles at the gingival margin at a 45° angle to the tooth. Brush by using a scrubbing or horizontal motion.
  c Stress that the length of time and thoroughness of brushing are important.
  d Disclosing tablets can be used during teaching programme to show the location of dental plaque before and after brushing.

6   The adolescent needs special encouragement and attention to maintain good dental habits.

   a Stress importance of diet control of refined sugars.

   b Encourage proper brushing technique (see above).

   c Encourage daily flossing in which floss is used correctly. (Improper use can cause traumatic injury to the gingiva.) Flossing is accomplished by passing the floss between the teeth with a back and forth motion. Place floss against tooth and move it up and down six or seven times against the tooth as far as the gingiva permits. Repeat process on side of adjacent tooth. Repeat until all sides of all teeth are cleaned.

7   Practice measures that will aid in avoiding cavities.

   a Bottle mouth syndrome — high incidence of dental caries in child 18 months-3 years is the result of taking bottle of milk or juice to bed. This syndrome can be prevented. Do not let child take a bottle to bed with him; if child does take a bottle, put plain water in it.

   b Have the child brush teeth after every meal and at bedtime.

   c Reduce the amounts of sugar and sweets eaten by the child.

   d Beware of foods that contain large amounts of sugar:

Bubble and chewing gum

Cola drinks

Peanut butter and jam on white
   bread

Sweets, biscuits, cakes

Jelly, jam, honey

Malted and sweet chocolate drinks

Synthetic orange juice (artificially sweetened)

White bread and currant bread

Sugar-coated cereals.

SAFETY

Incidence of Childhood Accidents

Some 56,000 children were discharged from hospital following treatment for accidental injury in England and Wales in 1981. (*Useful address:* The Royal Society for the Prevention of Accidents, Cannon House, The Priory, Queensway, Birmingham B4 6BS.

Role of the Nurse

1   Identify environmental hazards and take action to reduce or eliminate them.

2   Identify behavioural characteristics in individual children which may be related to accident liability and caution parents accordingly. Pay particular attention to children who show the following:

a Characteristics which increase exposure to hazards, such as excessive curiosity, inability to delay gratification, hyperactivity, and daring.
b Characteristics which reduce the child's ability to cope with hazards, i.e. aggressiveness, stubborness, poor concentration, low frustration threshold, lack of self-control.
3 Provide anticipatory guidance about child development as it relates to accidents. Direct preventive teaching towards individuals or groups, towards children or adults.
4 Participate in accident prevention in hospitals. Participate in education of staff, visitors, and parents to promote a greater awareness of possible hazards as well as preventing and avoiding accidents.

Principles of Safety
1 The child's developmental stage influences the types of accidents that are likely to occur. Potential accident situations may be foreseen by parents who have knowledge of their own child's typical pattern of growth and development.
2 Children are naturally curious, impulsive, and impatient. The young child needs to touch, feel, and investigate.
   a Patient adult supervision will enable the child to learn what he wants to know within the limits of safety for his stage of growth and development.
   b Young children should never be left alone at home.
3 Children copy the behaviour of their parents and absorb parental attitudes. Parents and other adults should be certain that their ways of doing things are safe.
4 Children become less careful and less willing to listen to warnings and to observe routine safety precautions when they are tired or hungry.
5 An estimated 90% of all accidents are preventable.

General Areas of Adult Safety Responsibility

Motor Vehicles
1 All motor cars should be maintained in good mechanical condition.
2 Seat belts should be worn at all times. Special safety seats for young children should be provided. All children should sit in the back seat of the car.
3 Drivers should look carefully in the front and in the back of the car before accelerating.
4 All car doors should be locked when a child travels in the vehicle.
5 Young children should never be left alone in a car.
6 Heavy or sharp objects should not be placed on the same seat with a child.

Sports and Recreation
1 Keep equipment in good condition and proper working order.
2 Wear appropriate clothing for the activity.

3   Do not attempt activities beyond one's physical endurance.
4   Keep firearms and ammunition locked up.

Electrical and Mechanical Equipment

1   All electrical items should be inspected periodically by a qualified electrician.
2   Dry hands before touching appliances. Keep radios, fans, portable heaters, and hair dryers out of the bathroom.
3   Disconnect appliances after use or before attempting minor repairs.
4   Keep garden equipment and machinery in a restricted area. Teach proper use of the equipment as soon as the child is old enough.
5   Avoid overloading electrical circuits.
6   Discourage children from playing with or being in area where appliances or power tools (e.g. washing machine, clothes dryer, saw, lawn mower) are in operation.

Prevention of Falls

1   Keep stairs well lighted and free from clutter.
2   Provide sturdy railings.
3   Anchor small rugs securely.
4   Use rubber mats in the bath and shower.
5   Use only sturdy ladders for climbing.

Poisonings and Ingestions

1   Do not mix bleaches with ammonia, vinegar, and other household cleaners.
2   See section on ingested poisons (page 756).

Fire

1   Maintain an adequate fire escape plan and routinely conduct home fire drills. Teach the child escape routes as soon as he is old enough.
2   Keep a pressure-type hand fire extinguisher on each floor. Instruct all family members who are old enough in its use.
3   Fit fireplaces with snug fireplace guards.
4   Flame-retardant nightwear should be worn.
5   Mark children's rooms so that they are obvious to firemen.
6   Teach children about the danger of smoke inhalation.

Emergency Precautions

1   Record emergency phone numbers in an obvious and easily accessible place.
2   Keep a well-stocked first-aid kit immediately available for emergencies.
3   Give instruction in principles of first aid to all family members who are old enough.
    a Responsible adults should enroll in first-aid courses offered by the Red Cross, adult education programmes, etc.
    b Be aware of first-aid procedures for:

Burns
Electric shock
Poisoning
Bites and stings
Cuts, scrapes, and punctures
Drowning
Fractures.
4 Know the location of gas, water, and electrical switches and how to turn them off in an emergency.

Miscellaneous

1 Take advantage of preventive health care.
 a Obtain recommended immunizations.
 b Have regular physical examinations.
2 Seek immediate treatment of all diseases and health problems.
3 Balance periods of work, rest, and excercise in daily living.

Specific Safety Concerns Related to Child's Stage of Growth and Development

Infants

Newborn babies are helpless and need absolute protection. When they begin to move about they need close supervision.
1 Infants may wiggle, roll and shift position.
 a The sides of the cot should be kept up at all times.
 b The bars of the cot should be spaced so that the infant cannot catch his head between them.
 c The cot should not be placed near a radiator or heating unit.
 d The cot should be away from windows with venetian blinds, because the infant may become fatally entangled in a dangling cord.
 e Babies should not be left unattended on anything from which they might fall. Infant seats should not be left on tables, beds, or other furniture.
 f Infants should be strapped carefully in feeding chairs, infant seats, etc. A means should be provided to prevent the child from slipping down and being strangled by his waist strap.
 g Well-constructed infant carriers should be used for travelling.
  (1) Infant car seats and car beds should meet the vehicle safety standards of the British Standards Authority. All children's safety belts and harnesses are 'kitemarked'.
   (a) There should be a means of anchoring the device to the seat of the vehicle with the standard lap belt.
   (b) A harness should keep the child contained within the device.
   (c) The device should include a head support to minimize the danger of whiplash injury.
   Note: Harnesses designed for prams and high chairs must *not* be used in cars.

(2) For older infants and toddlers, special devices are available which dispense with the harness and instead surround the child with a protective shield that distributes collision forces evenly.

h Nappy pins should always be kept closed, even when not in use.

2   Infants may start to suck on toys, cot sides, and other objects.

a Paints containing lead should not be used on toys, furniture, or any other objects that the child is likely to put into his mouth.

b Stuffed toys should be checked carefully to be certain that button eyes and other small, attached parts cannot be pulled off and eaten by the child.

c Small objects should not be left within the reach of the infant.

d All plastic bags should be tied in knots and discarded to avoid danger of suffocation. Under no circumstances should mattresses be covered with thin plastic.

3   Children are helpless in water for the next several years.

a The temperature of the bath water should be checked carefully to avoid scalding.

b The child should never be left unattended in the bath for any reason.

4   They should be carried from one place to another. The adult who carries the infant should avoid walking on slippery floors or where toys or other small objects have been scattered.

Toddlers

Toddlers are adventurous and are eager to explore everything around them. Although they sometimes seem very mature and independent, they still require close adult supervision.

1   They want to roam all over the house.

a Gates should be used at the head and foot of stairways to prevent falls.

b Fireplaces should be screened.

c Radiators should be enclosed or covered.

d Cords on blinds or curtains should be tied or cut so that children cannot get their heads through the loops.

2   They poke and probe with their index fingers.

a Sharp objects such as scissors and nail files should be kept out of reach.

b Bureau drawers and cabinets with anything potentially dangerous in them should be locked.

c Unused light sockets should be taped or capped.

d Electric fans or heaters should be out of reach.

e Electrical cords should be kept in good repair.

3   They are curious about many things, especially those things higher than their eye level.

a They should be lifted occasionally to satisfy their curiosity.

b Furniture should be balanced to prevent the child from pulling it over on himself.

c Hot, scalding foods should be kept out of the reach of children.

d All handles of pots and pans should be turned to the back of the stove.

e Tablecloths should not hang over the edge of the table.

f A small child should never be left alone in the kitchen. Appliances such as hot ovens, toasters, coffee pots, and irons pose a special threat to small children.

4 They put almost anything into their mouth.

a Medicines, disinfectants, and household cleaning products should be locked up out of the reach of children.

b Pins, buttons, and needles should be put away.

c Unbreakable toys that have no small removable parts should be used.

d The child should be closely supervised if he plays with a balloon. Aspiration of rubber from broken balloons can be fatal.

e Foods such as popcorn, peanuts, and carrot sticks should not be offered to toddlers because of the danger of aspiration.

5 They climb on to things.

a Toddlers should be protected from falls.

(1)Windows should have guards on them.

(2)Screens should be firm and securely fastened.

b Car doors should be locked.

c Special equipment for climbing (e.g. small wooden crates or boxes) should be provided, and climbing should be done under adult supervision.

6 They like to play outside and in water.

a The toddler must have close supervision while playing outside.

b His play area should be fenced.

c Ponds, pools, wells, and other similar outdoor structures should be fenced or covered. Paddling pools should be emptied immediately after use.

d The child should never be left alone in a paddling pool.

e Caution should be used in allowing the toddler to play with older children. He may easily be injured by bats, hard balls, bicycles, and rough play.

Preschool Children

Preschool children are very active and inquisitive. They begin to develop increased self-control, but still have an immature understanding of danger. They are at an ideal age to learn simple safety routines:

1 They can reach doorknobs and are eager to explore the world beyond.

a Doors that open to potential danger should be locked.

b Bathroom doors should have locks which can be opened from the outside to prevent the child from locking himself in the room.

c Unused refrigerators, freezers, and trunks should have doors, handles, and/or hinges removed to prevent small children from climbing into them and becoming trapped inside.

2 They enjoy taking things apart and putting them together again and experimenting with their use.

a Dangerous items such as knives and electrical equipment should be put away.

b Matches and lighters should be kept well out of the child's reach.

3   They are nimble on their feet and usually in a hurry.

a The child should not be allowed to walk or run while eating a lollipop or ice cream.

b Stairs should have strong railings. They should be clear of objects or defective coverings on which a child can trip.

c Stairs and floors should not be highly polished.

d Rugs should be fixed.

4   They often enjoy cooperative play with others.

a Toy trucks or wagons should be strong enough to bear their weight as well as that of their playmates.

b They should be taught to ride tricycles on the pavement and to watch for cars in driveways.

c They should be cautioned not to run after the ball if it rolls into the street or driveway.

d Clothes should allow the child freedom of action and shoes should be suitable for running and climbing.

e The play area should be checked for such hazards as old refrigerators, deep holes, construction, broken glass, and rubbish heaps.

f Swings and other equipment should be properly installed and maintained.

5   They are proud to run simple errands. They should not be asked to do anything hazardous such as crossing the street or carrying a knife or glass container.

6   They can take verbal directions and their attention span is lengthening. They can be instructed in the following areas:

a Personal safety

(1) To supply information such as their name, address, and telephone number

(2) To identify firemen, policemen, and other safety officials

(3) Not to accept gifts or rides from strangers

b Home safety

(1) The reasons for various safety measures such as keeping the floor clear of their toys

(2) The safe way to use tools

(3) Kitchen safety

(4) The danger of matches, open flames, hot objects, and gas and electric equipment

c Recreational safety, e.g. swimming instructions

d Motor vehicle and pedestrian safety

(1) Safety rules and the dangers of traffic

(2) Obedience to the rules.

School-age Children

School-age children are usually fairly independent. They still need discipline and rules but they also need to know *why* precautions are necessary and what the consequences are for failing to follow the rules.

1 They are eager to make things and participate in household activities.

   a They should be taught the proper use and storage of equipment such as those listed below:

     (1) Saws

     (2) Nails and hammers

     (3) Kitchen implements

     (4) Sewing machines

     (5) Gas and electric appliances

   b They should be taught to wear protective devices over their eyes when doing anything potentially dangerous to their vision.

2 They enjoy holding and attending parties, carnivals, and other similar gatherings. Party costumes and equipment should be checked to be certain that they are flameproof.

3 They enjoy sports and outdoor play.

   a Their whereabouts should be known at all times.

   b The play areas should be inspected for broken glass, rusty nails, etc.

   c They should be instructed regarding the dangers of playing in sandpits, old refrigerators, excavations, rickety shacks, and deserted buildings.

   d They must learn the rules of the sports that they play. They should have the proper equipment and keep it in good working condition.

   e Ice skating and water sports should always be closely supervised.

   f They should be taught how to climb a tree safely. Tree houses that are sturdily constructed under adult supervision may help prevent falls from trees.

4 Areas for teaching:

   a The rules of cycling safety should be emphasized. A child with a bicycle must learn the rules of the road as well as respect for the traffic officers and their directions.

   b Pedestrian safety rules should also be stressed, because motor accidents are the most common cause of accidental injury in this age group.

   c Swimming instruction should be continued.

   d The older child should be taught respect for fire, its uses, and its dangers.

Adolescents

Adolescents are increasingly independent. They should be able to build on their past experiences and accept responsibility for their own safety. Limits must still be set and direction given by adults, because adolescents may lack emotional maturity.

1 In motor cars they must know that:

   a Seat belts should be worn at all times.

   b They must be aware of traffic regulations and the penalty for not obeying them.

   c They should be encouraged to participate in driver education and safety programmes at school.

d Proper clothes should be worn while riding on motorcycles, motor scooters, or motorbikes. A safety helmet is compulsory and must be worn at all times.

2   They enjoy competing in competitive sports. Safeguards should be taken to prevent physical trauma when they want to do something beyond their physical endurance.

3   Their values and habits are greatly influenced by their peer groups and cliques:

a Parents should be aware of their child's activities.

b Constructive group activities should be encouraged.

c Formal instructions should be continued in the areas of sex education, drug and alcohol abuse, and smoking. Open discussions with responsible adults should be encouraged.

4   Older adolescents are capable of assuming some responsibility for family safety measures.

a They should be included in safety planning.

b Their opinions and suggestions should be considered.

c Specific areas of responsibility may be delegated to them.

THE HOSPITALIZED CHILD

General Principles of Care

Emotional and Social Needs

1   The child has the same basic emotional and social needs during hospitalization as he does at home.

a He needs a chance to develop the following:

(1) Motor skills

(2) Social skills

(3) Language skills

(4) Psychological strengths

(a) A sense of autonomy

(b) Ego strength

(c) A sense of identity

(5) Patterns of behaviour.

b To help him accomplish these skills and strengths, he needs:

(1) The continuing and reliable presence of someone who is important to him

(2) An appropriately stimulating environment

(3) Opportunities to explore and play

(4) Information and explanations concerning the hospital, treatments, procedures, routines, people, and expectations of him both before and during hospitalization.

2 The hospitalized child has special needs — to deal with the many new problems that confront him.
 a Separation from home — implying loss of:
  (1) Consistent person who nurtures
  (2) Family associations
  (3) Familiar environment
  (4) Daily activities and routines
  (5) Peer associations
  (6) Independence
 b Problems concerning the illness itself
 c Hospital rules and regulations
 d Surgery
 e Death.

Essential Elements

1 Parents must be closely involved with the child's hospitalization and the plan for his care. Parent participation is to be encouraged.
2 Nursing care should allow the child dependence, thereby helping him to develop confidence and trust in the situation and at the same time assisting him to develop independence.
3 Nursing histories should be taken when child is admitted to the hospital. Questions should be asked to obtain information related to the following:
 a Family home situation
 b Toilet habits and means of communicating
 c Dietary habits
 d Home routines and rituals
 e Schooling
 f Friends, peers
 g Experience with illness
 h Preparation for hospitalization
 i Favourite toy, object, etc.
 j How child handles frustration or stressful situations
 k Disciplinary practices at home
 l Comforting practices at home.
4 Explanation and repeat explanation of the treatment plan and preparation for special tests, procedures, and surgery are essential. These should be appropriate to:
 a The child's age
 b His level of comprehension.
5 Play is a natural part of nursing care. It is a means to help the child cope with an unpleasurable experience; it allows him to project his fears to the outside world, and it helps him to attain a feeling of independence and control of the situation. It is important for the child's physical, emotional, and social development.
6 Nursing care should relate illness to the child's personality, individual

reaction, and previous experiences. Recognition must be given to:
a What the child comes from
b What he is returning to
c What he is experiencing during his hospitalization.
7   The ultimate goal in paediatric nursing is directed towards:
a Reduction of stress
b Increase in the child's feeling of well-being.
8   Nursing care is successful when its outcome is therapeutic and encompasses growth.

Impact of Hospitalization on the Child's Stage of Development

Neonate: Birth-1 Month

Primary Concern

1   Bonding: Hospitalization interrupts the early stages of the development of a healthy mother-child relationship.
2   Sensory-motor deprivation: Tactile, visual, auditory, kinesthetic.
3   Sensory bombardment.

Reactions

1   Impairment of attachment between mother and child.
2   Impairment of mother's ability to love and care for her baby.
3   Risking of infant's emotional and physical well-being.

Nursing Intervention

1   Provide for continual contact between baby and his parents (eye-to-eye contact and touch).
2   Minimize isolation and strangeness by explaining and re-explaining equipment, procedures, etc., to parents.
3   Actively involve parents in caring for their baby.
4   Foster good neonate-sibling relationships if apppropriate.
5   Identify areas of infant deprivation and/or overstimulation.
6   Provide sensory-motor stimulation as appropriate.
7   Allow individuality to begin to emerge.

Infant 1-4 Months

Primary Concern

1   Separation: Mother is learning to identify and meet the needs of her infant. Infant is learning to make his needs known and to trust his mother to meet them.
2   Sensory-motor deprivation.

Reactions

1 Separation anxiety is different from that of older child, because for infant his mother is part of him. Sense of developing trust is disturbed when infant is separated from mother.

Nursing Intervention

1 Encourage mother to stay and care for her baby, thus minimizing separation. When mother is absent, give infant attention and frequent handling from a limited number of personnel.
2 Provide opportunity for sensory stimulation and motor development.
3 Help parents to work through their anxieties. Remember, a mother's touch communicates her comfort or discomfort to her infant.

4-8 Months

Primary Concern

1 Separation from mother: Mother is now recognized as a person separate from himself, but important to him. He rejects strangers.

Reactions

1 Separation anxiety: Crying, terror.

Nursing Intervention

1 Encourage mother to stay and care for her baby.
2 Attempt to adjust the ward schedule to home routines.
3 Become friends with the infant through the mother.
4 The infant is beginning to develop purposeful activities and to strive towards independence. Provide opportunities and encouragement for this development to continue and provide ways for him to use newly acquired skills.

8-12 Months

Primary Concern

1 Separation: Infant becomes more possessive of mother and clings to her at the time of separation.

Reactions

1 Separation anxiety: Tolerance is very limited.
2 Relieve some of his tensions and loneliness with 'transference' object (i.e. blanket, toy).

Nursing Intervention

1 Have mother stay and care for her child.
2 Prepare child for procedures; allow him to become familiar with simple equipment. Have mother comfort child during procedures.
3 Provide for sensory stimulation and motor development appropriate for age. Provide for opportunities for child to continue using skills he has acquired, such as feeding himself and drinking from cup.

Toddler (1-3 years)

Primary Concerns

1 Separation anxiety: Relationship with mother is intense. Separation represents the loss of family and familiar surroundings, resulting in feelings of insecurity and grief.
2 Changes in rituals and routines, all of which are important to his sense of security, become a source of concern.
3 Inability to communicate: Beginning use and understanding of language affords him unlimited communication between himself and the world.
4 Loss of autonomy and independence: His egocentric view of life helps him develop a sense of autonomy.
5 Body integrity: Incomplete and inaccurate understanding of the body results in fear, anxiety, frustration, and anger.
6 Decrease in mobility: Restricting his mobility causes frustration. He wants to keep moving for the pleasure it gives him as well as for the feeling of independence, the opportunity to learn about his world, and the route it provides for coping with frustrations that cannot be verbally expressed.

Reactions

1 Protest:
   a Has urgent desire to find mother
   b Expects that she will answer his cries, 'I want mummy'
   c Frequently cries and shakes cot
   d Rejects attention of nurses
   e When with mother, child shows signs of distrust and anger, tears
2 Despair:
   a Feels increasingly hopeless about finding his mother
   b Becomes apathetic and looks sad
   c May cry continuously or intermittently
   d Uses comfort measures — thumbsucking, fingering lip, tightly clutching a toy
3 Denial:
   a Represses all feelings for his mother
   b Does not cry when she leaves
   c May seem more attached to nurses — will go to anyone

   d Finds little satisfaction in relationships with people
   e Accepts care without protest
   f Regresses to an earlier state of development
4   Regression: Temporarily ceases use of newly acquired skills in an attempt to retain or regain control of a stressful situation.

Nursing Intervention

1   Provide accommodation for mother or father to live in. Unrestricted visiting including siblings. Parental visits provide:
   a Opportunity for child to express some of his feelings about his situation
   b Assurance that his parents are not abandoning him or punishing him
   c Periods of comfort and reassurance that allow for the re-establishment of family bonds.
2   Attempt to continue routines used at home, especially with regard to sleeping, eating, and bathing.
3   Obtain from parents key words in communicating with child. Find out about his nonverbal behaviour as well.
4   Allow child to make choices when possible. Arrange physical setting to encourage independence. Allow child to explore the environment.
5   A Band-Aid or Elastoplast dressing may give the child security of wholeness after an injection.
6   Replace lost mobility with another form of motion: moving about in a wheel chair, cart, or bed. Exercise restrained extremity. Provide opportunity for the child to release energy suppressed by decreased mobility, i.e. by pounding, throwing. Provide opportunity to continue learning about world through sensory modalities such as water play and diversional play.
7   Discharge: If living-in has not occurred during hospitalization parents must be prepared for the possible post hospital behaviour of their toddler. They will need support in understanding and handling these behaviours. The child may do any of the following:
   a Show lack of affection or resist close physical contact. Parents may interpret this as rejection.
   b Regress to an earlier stage of development.
   c Cling to mother, unable to tolerate any separation from her. Show excessive need for love and affection.
8   Parents' response to child's behaviour is vital if relationships are to be re-established.
   a Extra love and understanding will help restore child's trust.
   b Hostility and withdrawal of love will cause child further loss of trust, self-esteem, and independence.

Preschool child (3-5 years)

Primary Concerns

1   Separation: Although cognitive and coping capabilities have increased and

the child responds less violently to separation from parents, separation and hospitalization represent stress beyond the coping mechanisms and adaptive capabilities of the preschool child. Loneliness and insecurities are experienced.

2 Unfamiliar environment: This requires coping with a change in daily routine and represents a loss of control and security.

3 Abandonment and punishment: Fantasies and thought may contain vengeful wishes for other persons, for which the child expects retribution. Illness may be interpreted as punishment for thoughts. Enforced parental separation may be interpreted as loss of parental love and represents abandonment by them.

4 Body image and integrity: Hospitalization and intrusive procedures provide a multitude of threats of both bodily mutilation and loss of identity.

5 Immobility: Mobility is the child's dominant form of self-expression and adaptation to the environment. He has a great urge for locomotion and exercise of large muscles. It represents his main expression of emotion and release of tension.

Reactions

1 Regression: Child temporarily stops using newly acquired skills in an attempt to retain or regain control of a stressful situation. Child may return to behaviour of the infant or toddler.

2 Repression: Child may attempt to exclude the undesirable and unpleasant stresses from consciousness.

3 Projection: The child may transfer his own emotional state, motives, and desires to others in his environment.

4 Displacement/sublimation: Emotions are permitted to be redirected and expressed in other situations such as art or play.

5 Identification: The child assumes characteristics of the aggressor in an attempt to reduce fear and anxiety and to feel that he is in control of the situation.

6 Aggression: Hostility is direct and intentional; physical expression takes precedence over verbal expression.

7 Denial and withdrawal: The child is able to ignore interruptions and disavow any thought or feeling that would result in a painful experience.

8 Fantasy: A mental activity to help the child to bridge the gap between reality and fantasy through imagination. The child has difficulty separating reality from fantasy because of lack of experience.

Nursing Intervention

1 Minimize stress of separation by providing for parental presence and participation in care. Strive to shorten the hospital stay. Help parents understand what hospitalization means to the child.

2 Identify defence mechanisms apparent in the child and help him through the

stressful situation by accepting him, showing him love and concern, and being alert to his readiness to relinquish them.

3   Set limits for child. Let him know that someone is there. Help child become master of something in the situation.

4   Provide opportunity and encouragement for child to verbalize.

5   Careful preparation should be made for all procedures done on the child's level of development and comprehension.

6   Be sure child has opportunities for play. Play is one important medium through which the child can overcome his fear and anxiety.

7   Provide consistency in nursing personnel and approach to care.

8   Allow child to wear own clothes whenever possible. Changing from day to night clothes as at home.

9   Ensure that each child's personal locker has sufficient space for storing own toys and 'precious' items.

School-age Child (5-12 years)

Concerns

1   Many fear loss of recently mastered skills.

2   Many worry about separation from school and peers. They may fear loss of former roles.

3   Castration anxieties and mutilation fantasies are common.

4   Some may believe that they or their parents magically caused the illness merely by thinking that the event would occur.

5   Often they have increased concerns related to modesty, privacy.

6   The imposed passivity may be interpreted as punishment.

7   Children may feel their body no longer is their own, but rather is controlled by doctors and nurses.

Reactions

(See 'Reactions' regarding the preschool child for a more complete description of these responses.)

1   Regression

2   Conscious attempts at mature behaviour

3   Suppression or denial of symptoms

4   Reaction formation

5   Repression

6   Depression

7   Obsessive-compulsive behaviour (common)

8   Sublimation

9   Tendency to be phobic (normal):

   a Fears include that of the dark, doctors, hospitals, medication, and death.

   b Unrealistic fears are commonly attached to needles, x-ray procedures, and blood.

Nursing Intervention

1   Obtain a thorough nursing history, including information regarding health and physical development, hospitalizations, social-cultural background, and normal daily activities. Utilize this information to plan care.
2   Provide for continuity of nursing personnel.
3   Provide order and consistency in the environment whenever possible.
4   Establish and enforce reasonable policies to protect the child and to increase his sense of security in his environment.
5   Arrange the environment to allow for as much mobility as possible (i.e.make sure articles are appropriately placed; move the bed if the child is immobilized). Ensure that bedside locker is available to store personal items, toys, and books.
6   Respect the child's need for privacy and respect modesty during examinations, bathing, etc. Allow child to wear his own clothes wherever possible. If ward clothes are worn, allow child to choose.
7   Utilize treatment rooms whenever possible if you are performing painful or intrusive procedures.
8   Help young children identify problems and questions (often through play). Then help them to find the answers.
9   Provide information about the illness and hospitalization based on assessment of what facts the child needs and wants and how this information can be made readily understandable to him.
10   View all nursing care activities as teaching situations. Explain the function of equipment and allow the child to handle it.
11   When explaining a procedure, make sure that the child knows its purpose, what will be done, and what will be expected of him. Reassure the child during the procedure by continuing the explanations and support.
12   Reassure the child having surgery; explain where the organ to be removed or repaired is located, and that no other body part will be removed.
13   Utilize play whenever appropriate to provide information about the hospital experience and to identify and decrease the child's fantasies and fears.
14   Reassure the child that he or his parents are not to blame for his illness.
15   Facilitate discharge of energy and aggression through appropriate play activities or through sharing in aspects of ward management.
16   Encourage the child's participation in his care and self-hygiene.
17   Support intellectual potential through the use of games, books, puzzles, school work, and drawings.
18   Assist the child's family to understand his reactions to illness and hospitalization so that family members can facilitate positive coping patterns.
19   Let the child know that his normal status as a family member remains intact during his hospitalization.
20   Help parents to deal with their own anxieties about hospitalization and assist them to help their child cope with the situation.
21   Encourage parental participation in the child's care when appropriate.
22   Encourage written communication with classmates, and allow friends to

visit when appropriate.

23   Begin discharge planning early, including plans for physical and emotional needs. Alert families to possible behavioural changes, including phobias, nightmares, regression, negativism, and disturbances in eating and learning.

Adolescent

Concerns

1   Physical illness, exposure, and lack of privacy may cause increased concern about body image and sexuality.
2   Separation from security of peers, family, and school may cause anxiety.
3   Interference with his struggle for independence and emancipation from his parents is a concern.
4   The adolescent may be very threatened by helplessness. He may see illness as a punishment for feelings not mastered or for breaking rules imposed by his parents or physician.

Reactions

1   May be anxious about or embarrassed by loss of control.
2   May be insecure.
3   May intellectualize about details of the disease to avoid addressing actual concerns.
4   May reject treatment measures, even if they had been previously accepted.
5   May be angry because goals are being thwarted. This anger may be directed toward staff.
6   Depression may occur.
7   Increased dependence on staff and parents may occur.
8   May show denial or withdrawal.

Nursing Intervention

1   Assess the impact of illness on the adolescent by considering factors such as timing, nature of illness, new experiences imposed, changes in body image, and expectations for the future.
2   Introduce the adolescent to the hospital staff and to regular routines soon after admission. Ensure that bedside locker is available to store personal items.
3   Obtain a thorough nursing history that includes information about hobbies, school, family, illness, hospitalization, food habits, and recreation.
4   Encourage adolescents to wear their own clothes, and allow them to decorate their beds or rooms to express themselves.
5   Allow the adolescent access to a telephone.
6   Allow adolescents control over appropriate matters, i.e. timing of bath,

selection of food, etc.

7   Respect their need for periodic isolation and privacy.

8   Have a well-supervised recreational and activites programme.

9   Accept adolescent's level of performance. Allow regression with expectation of growth.

10 Involve adolescent in planning his care so that he will be more accepting of restrictions and receptive to health teaching. He should be accepted as a vital member of the health care team.

11 Explain clearly all procedures, routines, expectations, and restrictions imposed by illness. If necessary, clarify interpretation of illness and hospitalization.

12 Facilitate verbal rejection of treatment measures to protect adolescent from harming himself physically by stopping treatment.

13 Assess the adolescent's intellectual skills and provide him with the necessary information to allow him to use problem-solving to deal with his illness and hospitalization.

14 Recognize positive and negative coping behaviours as attempts to adjust to a threatening situation. Attempt to deal with the feeling that caused the behaviour as well as with the behaviour itself.

15 Be a good listener.

16 Provide opportunities such as writing, art work, and recreational activities to allow nonverbal adolescents to express themselves.

17 Foster interaction with other hospitalized adolescents and continuation of peer relationships with outside friends.

18 Establish regular group meetings to allow patients to meet with staff members and with each other to comment and to ask questions about their hospital experiences.

19 Set necessary limits to foster independence and self-control.

20 Help adolescents work through sexual feelings. Avoid behaviour which could be interpreted as provocative or flirtatious. Masturbation, unless excessive, may be considered a psychologically healthy way to discharge sexual tension.

21 Interpret the needs and reactions of hospitalized adolescents to parents.

22 Assist parents to cope with the illness and hospitalization as well as to deal effectively with the adolescent's response to related stress.

23 Encourage continuation of education.

Family-centred Care

Family-centred care provides an opportunity for the family to care for the hospitalized child under nursing supervision.

The *goal* of family-centred care is to maintain or strengthen the roles and ties of the family with the hospitalized child in order to promote normality of the family unit.

Benefits for Parents and Child

1 Continued close family interactions during stress.
2 Absence of separation anxiety.
3 Reactions of protest, denial, and despair are decreased or nonexistent.
   a There is little inconsolable crying.
   b Sleep is more relaxed.
4 Greater sense of security for the child.
5 Opportunities for family to fulfil their needs to care for their child physically and emotionally.
6 Allows parents to feel useful and important rather than making them dependent and destroying their confidence.
7 Lessening of parental guilt feelings.
8 Opportunities for parents to increase their competence and confidence in caring for the sick child.
9 Comfort for the family provided by other families.
10 Greater absorption of staff teaching by the family.
11 Posthospitalization reactions are diminished.

General Principles of Family-centred Care

1 The nurse must be equipped with a broad knowledge base from the physical and behavioural sciences. Special emphasis is required in such areas as growth and development, family dynamics, socialization, and communication. Continuing education programmes must be designed to support and improve family-centred care.
2 Staff must realize that parents are not time savers for nurses when they are participating in their child's care. The parents are not there to relieve the nurse of her responsibility for care.
   Additional nursing time is necessary to answer questions, to orient parents to the unit, and to teach child care and comfort parents.
3 Family-centred care places a great deal of responsibility on the nurse and offers an opportunity to administer total patient care to the child and his family.
4 Family-centred care units should present a relaxed, comfortable atmosphere.
   a Do not require parents to stay, but allow them to stay if they desire:
      (1) Some mothers may feel too anxious or guilty to participate.
      (2) Outside responsibilities may prohibit parents staying.
   b Provide physical comfort for participating parents:
      (1) Folding chair or bed in child's room.
      (2) Comfortable sitting or waiting room.
      (3) Eating facilities.
   c Encourage parent(s) to take frequent breaks from attending to the child:
      (1)Provides rest for the parent.
      (2)Helps child learn parent(s) will return and not abandon him.

5   When parents are active participants in their child's care, they too have certain needs, because they are concerned about their ill child.
   a They want to care for their child as they would do at home.
   b They are interested in working with the staff and learning from the staff how they can help their child.
   c They like to keep busy and to have something to do. This lessens their feeling of helplessness.

6   If parents know what is expected of them and what they can expect of the staff, many problems can be avoided. It helps parents feel more comfortable.
   a Nursing and medical observations and care will be continued with or without the parents (or mother) present.
   b What can parents do for their child? Example: They can bathe, play with, and feed him.
   c What activities will the nurse do in caring for the child? Example: She will give medications and assist with procedures.
   d Parents should allow child to become involved with other children in the unit.
   e Parents should take care of their own needs and not ask for personal services.

7   Families of hospitalized children can offer a great deal of support to one another. Often they have similar problems.
   Allow families to gather in groups — informal or formally planned group meetings.

Role of Parents

1   To serve as the child's primary resource of security and support so that he will be better able to tolerate unfamiliarity and discomfort and will be able to emerge from the experience with less likelihood of posthospitalization reactions.
2   To serve as the child's advocate in order to ensure that his basic human rights will be respected.
3   To teach nurses specific ways in which they can support the child.
4   To serve as role models and to support other families who may be dealing with similar problems.

Role of Nurse

1   To create an environment conducive to maintaining family integrity and unity. The nurse should do each of the following:
   a Help to maintain healthy mother-child relationship. (Mother should not be threatened by the nurse.)
   b Help father establish or maintain his role of supporting mother and child, of keeping things going at home, and of relieving mother in the hospital.

c Include siblings in planning and intervention as appropriate.

d Supplement the family in the common goal of the child's welfare.

2　To assist parents to make decisions about when to stay with their child.

a Parents' presence is especially important if the child is 5 years or younger, is especially anxious or upset, or is in medical crisis.

b The parents' decision is influenced by needs of other family members, as well as by job and home responsibilities.

c The nurse should try to alleviate guilty feelings of parents who are unable to stay with their child.

3　To develop trusting, goal-directed relationship with families.

a Obtain a thorough nursing history that provides information to assess strengths, relationships, and concerns.

b Plan with the family toward mutual, realistic goals.

c Recognize good care that the child receives from parents.

4　To observe the parent-child relationship in order to do the following:

a Evaluate the degree of participation of the parents in physical and emotional care.

b Observe parents' attitudes, skills, and techniques and the child's behaviour and response to them.

c Assess what teaching needs to be done.

d Detect problems in parent-child relationships.

5　To teach parents knowledge, understanding, and skills necessary to function effectively with the hospitalized child. The nurse should do the following:

a Perform nursing techniques safely and efficiently.

b Interpret the behaviour of the hospitalized child to parents so that they can understand it and intervene appropriately (refer to the section, 'Impact of Hospitalization on the Child's Stage of Development').

c Interpret and reinforce what the paediatrician has told parents. Answer questions thoroughly and honestly as knowledge permits.

d Interpret medical procedures and diagnostic tests.

e Provide health education teaching as appropriate.

f Offer anticipatory guidance.

6　To help parents adapt to the situation and to develop their own feeling of value by coping with the child's illness.

a Be aware of common parental reactions to the stress experienced by families of children who have severe or chronic illness.

b Be aware that defence mechanisms, if employed in moderation, are constructive and may facilitate optimal coping.

c Help parents recognize their own feelings.

d Identify parental support systems as well as adaptive and maladaptive coping.

e Be perceptive of parents' physical and emotional needs and limitations.

　(1) Do not allow parents to become fatigued.

　(2) Allow parents to leave, take a break.

7   To assist families as appropriate in dealing with normal family developmental tasks.
    a Be aware that the child's hospitalization is often only one of many stresses a family experiences at a given time. Others frequently include:
       (1) Interpersonal problems
       (2) Debt, unemployment, job change
       (3) Recent changes in dwelling place and consequent disruption
       (4) Problems associated with child care and discipline
       (5) Concurrent illness of other family members.
8   To ensure continuity of family-centred care between the hospital and home.

Play Programmes

In the past decade there has been an increasing recognition of the importance of play for children in hospital throughout the United Kingdom. Many health authorities have now established play programmes in their children's wards, clinics, and departments.

Rationale for Play Programmes

1   Hospitalization separates a child from his home, family, and all that is familiar, and places him in an institution where he may experience intrusive, embarrassing, painful, and mutilating invasion of his body.
2   The short-term and long-term effects of illness and hospitalization on the intellectual, social, and emotional development of children has been documented by observations and research.

Goals of Play Programmes

1   **a** To prevent some of the emotional pain and fear associated with illness and hospitalization. Play staff may assume primary responsibility or a supportive role in the preparation of children and their parents for hospitalization, surgery, and/or particular procedures.
    b In some hospitals, nursing and play staff arrange for preadmission tours of the ward or department, puppet shows, and similar activities to which all children who are planned admissions to the department are invited.
2   To provide a comfortable, accepting, and non-threatening environment where the child may play and interact with other children and with an adult.
    a Ideally there should be a separate playroom in every unit. However, sometimes there may only be an open space at the end of the corridor or in the middle of the ward that is available for play activities.
3   To provide the child with an opportunity for choice.
    a The child may choose whether or not he wishes to come to the playroom. Once there, he may choose what he wants to do.
    b A variety of craft and play materials, including real and miniature medi-

cal equipment, should be available.

c Should the child choose just to sit and watch or be held and dropped, these activities are seen as acceptable choices.

d The child may be given the opportunity to play at whatever time he wishes to do so; play materials should be available during his waking hours.

4 Play can take place anywhere in the ward, either at the bedside or in the designated playroom or play space.

Guidelines to Play

1 The sick child tires easily so select a choice of activities within the child's capacity from which he can choose. Toys and occupation will need frequent changing.
2 Some children who are immobile will need playing with; for example, the child attached to a ventilator. Encourage parents also to do this for their children.
3 Big and complex toys tire a child more quickly than small, simple toys which can be easily changed. A toy enjoyed today may be boring tomorrow.
4 Toys given for the various age groups will please older or younger children.
5 The value of any of these toys will be quickly lost if they are lying around, neglected or broken. They should be tidied away and maintained regularly.
6 Supply a good steady surface such as a tray for a child confined to a bed or cot; protective covers will prevent undue soiling of the bed linen.

Story Telling

Books can be exciting to children of all ages. They can be used to gain rapport with a child who needs individual attention or can be used as a shared experience with a group of children in the play room.

Guidelines

1 Enjoy yourself, pick a book appropriate to the age of the child or children which you yourself like so that you can show your enthusiasm whilst reading it.
2 Sit at the child's level; hold the book at an angle so that the child can see the pages and the pictures.
3 If possible, know the story. Rather than memorizing word for word, learn the sequence of the events and specific phrases. If it is not possible to prepare beforehand, simply read the book through once yourself. Better to read it well than to tell it poorly.
4 Make noises of any of the characters or animals in the story real.
5 Tell the story quickly, build to the climax, using your voice and movements to provide contrast.

6　Occasionally involve children directly in the story, encourage some participation but do not overdo it — you may lose the plot in too much discussion.

7　After finishing the story allow the child or children to handle and look at the book.

Education in Hospital

Education has been provided for children in hospital for many years. The 1944 Education Act stated that all children should be educated according to 'age, ability, and aptitude' but also empowered education authorities to provide education 'other than at school', thus opening the way for the provision of home tuition and individual tuition in hospital.

It is extremely important that whenever the sick child's condition allows, education and school work should continue in hospital. The role of the teacher is valued by the child and parents by acting as a bridge between normal school experience and life in the hospital ward. The daily routine of going to school and the intellectual stimulus which regular teaching provides not only links the past and the future but introduces an element of normality into the hospital ward. It also provides a basis to the child for gaining a greater degree of security and of emotional order whilst in hospital. Parents also recognize the value of this continuity and the cooperation exhibited between parents and teachers enables the parents in turn to be of greater support to their child. Teachers of young children, particularly those under 5 years, should welcome the presence of mother during school hours in the hospital ward and include her in the school programme wherever possible.

The nature of the illness for the child, and the anxiety he feels, will all affect his span of concentration and ability to concentrate on school work. Individual assessments need to be made by the teacher. To make these, the nurse should ensure that the teacher is fully informed of the relevant nursing-medical information and treatment which might have influence upon the child's capacity and behaviour as a student. In the light of this knowledge, the teacher is able to plan a teaching programme that is suited to the development and condition of the individual child. The special circumstances in hospital schools demand an imaginative and flexible approach by its teachers in the development of these individual programmes.

The hospital schoolteacher can help to relieve some anxiety for the older child who may be worried about forthcoming examinations and end-of-term grades, by ensuring that work begun in the normal school is continued and developed.

Schooling in Hospital

Schooling in hospital provides:

1　Continuity of an important element of the child's normal life.

2　Intellectual stimulation and occupation.

3　An atmosphere of purpose which is emotionally, physically, and educationally beneficial to the child.

4   Relief of anxiety for those children who fear falling behind school peers during hospitalization by maintaining appropriate standards of work.
5   Opportunity for parents to cooperate with the teacher and thus provide encouragement and support for their child's progress.

Neonatal Intensive Care

Nurse's Role and Responsibilities in an Intensive Care Nursery

1   The nurse is an active, integral part of the essential nurse paediatrician or neonatologist team in caring for the sick newborn.
    a The nurse has a major responsibility in caring for the sick newborn. Much credibility is given to her observations because of continual contact with and care of the infant and past experience in making similar observations.
    b The nurse will need to use initiative (i.e. must employ independent nursing judgement) in evaluating the infant's condition and must make changes in therapy when there are signs of deterioration or be able to handle a medical emergency. Subtle changes in behaviour or condition of the infant detected early by the nurse and related to the paediatrician often result in treating the infant before he is critically ill or beyond the point where permanent damage may have occurred.
2   The nurse must have an understanding of pathogenesis of diseases of the newborn in order to programme nursing activities in caring for the infant. The nurse must be informed about the following:
    a Specific diseases of the newborn
    b The treatment of their problems
    c The uses of the equipment employed in caring for these infants.
3   In addition, the nurse must possess the following qualities:
    a Improved clinical awareness
    b Increased diagnostic skills
    c Ability to make nursing assessments
    d Skills in performing special procedures.
4   Working with the critically ill infant requires technical skills in several areas. Some of these include:
    a Infant feeding:
       (1) Tube feeding using a fine (3.5 FG) indwelling polyvinyl nasogastric tube.
       (2) Hyperalimentation, supplying essential nutrients intravenously as total parenteral nutrition.
       (3) Bottle feeding.
    b Oxygen administration and monitoring
    c Exchange transfusion and blood administration
    d Umbilical catheterization
    e Ventilator care

     f Laboratory and x-ray studies
     g Blood pressure monitoring
     h Phototherapy
     i Temperature control
     j Cardiac monitoring
     k Equipment control (i.e. equipment working properly).

5   The knowledge acquired in caring for the critically ill newborn will equip the nurse to compare signs such as respiration, fluctuating blood pressure, heart rate, subtle movement or lack of movement, and provide:

     a Cardiopulmonary support
     b Respiratory management
     c Fluid and nutritional assessment and management
     d Observation for complications and other illnesses.

6   Infection control is within the realm of nursing responsibilities. Constant surveillance and strict adherence to procedures directed toward preventing infection must be practised.

     a Good handwashing technique:
       (1) 2-3 min scrub using Hibiscrub (containing chlorhexidine) as the antiseptic lotion or whatever unit procedure demands, e.g. Betadine
       (2) Alcohol hand rub between infants providing hands already socially clean, or shorter hand wash using recommended antiseptic lotion
     b Consider contact with incubator or cot the same as contact with the infant himself
     c Nonhuman areas of contact and sources of possible contamination might be scales, examining table, and handbasins
     d Need for adequate and appropriate nurse-baby ratios
     e Surveillance of infant to recognize evidence of illness and source of infection to others
     f Removal from the area of staff experiencing viral or bacterial illness
     g Effective cord care of the newborn
     h If staphylococcal or streptococcal infection develops in the area, the following procedures should be followed:
       (1) Periodic bathing of infants using Infacare in the water
       (2) The incubator serves as effective isolation when good handwashing is practised.

7   The nurse must begin to help form a bond between infant and his mother as well as to build cohesiveness of the family immediately upon the infant's admission to the intensive care unit (see below).

8   Research indicates that to enhance the quality of the life saved and to provide the best chance for the child to achieve his potential, early environmental, emotional, and psychosocial stimulation is essential. By virtue of involvement, the nurse has a tremendous responsibility and opportunity in this area (see below).

9   It is vitally important that the nurse practise meticulous recording and documentation for the protection of the infant as well as the nurse:

a Always record routine procedures, i.e. hourly ventilator care.
b Never erase. Errors should be crossed out with a single line, marked 'error' and initialed, according to unit procedure
c Record events accurately, e.g. emergency treatment.

Caring for Parents of Infant in Intensive Care Nursery

Research has documented that infant-mother bonding is signficantly influenced by events before and immediately after delivery and may greatly influence later maternal behaviour and the infant-mother relationship. Mother's attachment to her infant is critical for his optimal growth and development, since he depends entirely upon his mother to satisfy his needs.

Barriers to Healthy Mother-Infant Bonding

1   Grief, guilt, anger, fear, and anxiety felt by mother at the birth of a child she expected to be perfect. Mother may mourn over loss of this perfect child.
2   Maternal background factors — socioeconomic status, educational training, own childhood experiences, emotional stability.
3   Expectations and attitudes of the mother toward her infant.
4   Separation of mother and her infant at a time when her sensitivity may be at a maximum for attachment to her infant.
5   Anticipatory grieving for possible loss of this infant and emotional withdrawal from infant.
6   Maternal attitude about herself— her lack of self-confidence in her ability to care for her infant; her negative feelings about her inability to carry her infant to term or to produce a normal child.
7   Disruption of care-eliciting behaviours by the infant; the infant serves as a stimulus for mother in helping her identify her offspring and promote her caretaking behaviours.
8   Stress elicited by physical presence of infant in intensive care nursery, i.e. realization of severity of illness of infant, emergency atmosphere, sensory deprivation — all tend to diminish her self-confidence — since she cannot give her own infant the special care he needs.

Nursing Intervention to Help Foster Mother-Infant Bonding as Well as Eventual Appropriate Parenting Behaviours

1   Wherever possible, get to know the mother and father before delivery, show them the neonatal intensive care unit with the prepared incubator
2   Allow mother to see and touch her infant immediately after delivery and again as soon and as often as possible.
3   Describe in detail all the equipment surrounding the infant in the intensive care nursery, prior to the mother's seeing the infant and again when she is near him.
4   Talk with mother on a personal basis; call her by name; make personal

comments. Encourage parents to name their baby and refer to him by that name.

5   Encourage mother to enter the intensive care nursery as soon as possible and allow unlimited visiting. If daily visits are not always possible, encourage phone contact with nursery staff. The nurse should also call the mother.

6   Carefully consider the mother's concerns and feelings. Being the parent of a critically ill infant is emotionally devastating. Communicate to her your caring concern. Teach by example, so that the mother can learn from the nurse's consideration of the baby as an individual.

7   Encourage mother to touch her infant.
   a This will help her to see him as real and will decrease some of her fears.
   b Touching is the first step in the mother's developing her own self-confidence.
   c Show mother how she can gradually assume more of baby's care and is better at mothering than the nurse.

8   Open communication channels with parents early:
   a Meet parents in hospital of origin. Provide parents with a Polaroid photograph of their child taken on admission to the unit.
   b Reinforce information given.
   c Share good news — first feeding, physical activity, less oxygen needed, etc.
   d Support them when discouraging news (e.g. discontinued feedings, increased apnoeic spells) is given.
   e Often there develops a closeness between the mother and nurse that allows her to participate knowledgeably and confidently with the nurse in evaluating the infant's progress.

9   Observe the intensive care nursery physical setting in terms of parental needs, i.e. need for rocking chairs, bright pictures on the walls, parents' visiting area inside the nursery, pictures of past intensive care nursed babies that are growing and thriving. A 'Know the Unit Staff' board displaying photographs of all the staff with their names is helpful to parents, especially during the first days following admission of their baby when they are often feeling confused and anxious. Such a board helps the parents to identify the many staff faces in the unit with a name and role in the unit.

10   Encourage active participation by the mother in the care of her infant (as the infant's condition permits). For example, instruct the mother on how to enter the incubator; encourage her to visit during feeding and to do something in connection with feeding.
   a Explain how her visits and contact will benefit the baby.
   b Assist her in touching and talking to her infant as necessary.
   c Show her that increasing her physical contact with infant will increase her involvement and confidence in caring for the child.
   d Continually assess the parents' (the mother's, in particular) ability to be involved; be sensitive to their tolerance for handling the infant and their degree of emotional tolerance.

e Remember that the father will need similar help and support to establish an early relationship with the new baby.

11 There should be continuous focus on the family. Parents and infant must be treated as a unit.

a Priorities for this are:

(1) Crisis intervention

(2) Continual parent contact

(3) Encouragement of parenting behaviours.

b Goals are:

(1) To develop mother's self-confidence and ability to rely on her own instincts and common sense in caring for her infant

(2) To assist the father in becoming involved emotionally and in developing competence in taking care of his family after discharge as well as in taking pleasure in his infant.

12 There is a necessity to decrease the social isolation that is often inherent in the birth of a critically ill baby.

a Inform the paediatric liaison health visitor who can then notify the family's own health visitor.

b Provide mother (parents) with an opportunity to talk with other mothers (or parents) of infants with similar conditions, thus affording them the opportunity to express their feelings and concerns and to realize that they are not alone in feelings of guilt, failure, and fear.

c Encourage visits to infant and parents by others who will be a support to them.

13 Provide some mechanism by which information concerning parents can be evaluated and trouble areas can be recognized early. Document information such as the following:

a Parental involvement (phone calls, visits, handling and caring for infant)

b Specific or special procedures observed by, taught to, and performed by parents

c Specific information discussed with parent — by whom and when

d Discharge teaching and plans.

Stimulation: the Infant in Intensive Care Nursery

Every infant has the emotional need and right to recognize his mother's face, touch, and voice. The sick or preterm infant is forced to accept less. Research has shown that problems can arise from early sensory deprivation. The intensive care nursery is devoid of much sensory and perceptual stimuli — a situation that is harmful to the infant, the mother, and the mother-infant interactions. To maximize the potential to which the infant can develop, an early stimulation programme should be planned.

1 Each stimulation programme should be individualized for the specific infant-parent unit, based upon:

		FAMILY — STAFF INFORMATION GUIDE			

NEONATAL UNIT

Date	Time	Telephoned	Viewed	Touched	Held	Breast Fed	Bottle Fed	Changed	Bathed		Signature	RECORD ALL VISITS — USE CODES AND INITIALS M = Mother F = Father S = Sibling GM = Grandmother GF = Grandfather O = Others (Give Names)				
												INFORMATION DISCUSSED	Nurse	Dr.	M.S.W.	C.N.
												Visiting and Phoning				
												Hand Washing				
												Photograph				
												Encouraged to visit after Mother's discharge				
												Medical Problems:				
												EXPLANATION OF NEED FOR:				
												Incubator				
												Monitors				
												I.V. Equipment				
												Intra Gastric Feeding				
												Headbox				
												Ventilation				
												C.P.A.P.				
												Phototherapy				
												DISCHARGE TEACHING:				
												Bath Demonstration				
												Cord Care				
												Feed Preparation				
												Management at Home				
												Follow Up Appointments				
												Other:				
												Name:		Hospital Number:		
												Time of Birth:				
												Date of Birth:				
												Birth Weight:		Sheet No.:		

Figure 1.1 Family-staff information guide.

a Familiarization with the baby's physical condition and limitations
b Assessment of the baby's behavioural skills and development status
c Assessment of the parents' abilities to be involved.

2 Some general guidelines for establishing a psychosocial stimulation environment to be adapted for each infant include:

a Provide for the continuity of the same caretaker each day, each shift. This will benefit both infant and parents.

b Make the baby as attractive as possible — clean, colourful linen, lotion on skin, ribbon in hair. The general appearance of a preterm or sick infant makes it difficult for mother to relate to her infant.

c Help infant establish a day/night cycle. Dim lights or cover infant's eyes.

d Place an active mobile or colourful object in baby's line of vision, and adjust as his vision accommodation changes with age — about 23 cm for newborn. This will increase visually directed reaching.

e Encourage personnel to talk to and touch infant when caring for him. Hold him at feedings as well as between feedings when infant's condition allows this. Have personnel attempt to have infant focus upon their face and follow their head movement with his eyes.

f Encourage personnel to follow specific procedure when feeding if infant is able to tolerate it.

(1) Hold infant in nursing position to aid in establishing enface.

(2) Rock, talk to, fondle, and pat infant before, during, and after feeding. Hold infant in upright position when burping to aid in this visual orientation.

g Encourage parent participation in this programme.

(1) Assist the parents so they become emotionally involved with the baby.

(2) Point out specific responses and behaviour of the infant they can look for. This will help them learn to pay attention to the baby's behaviour and to respond to his needs. Talk about this behaviour and the parents' feelings about it.

(3) Encourage parents to visit during feeding time and to participate in the procedure. Keep record of progress — see Figure 1.1. Even if nasogastric feedings are done, parents can hold infant, give him a dummy, fondle him, and relate to him in many ways.

h Be aware of specific sensory stimulation for the infant:

(1) Olfactory — mother's article of clothing near infant

(2) Visual — change position of infant; change location of incubator, use of mobiles or bright objects

(3) Auditory — music box, tape of mother's voice.

Discharge Planning Begins Early

1 Maternal behaviours are learned. In order to provide the mother with an opportunity to build self-confidence and to develop to her potential, active

participation with her infant during the infant's hospitalization is essential. Mother-infant bonding must be started and allowed to grow during this time for the well-being of both infant and mother.

2   Detailed preparation for home care is essential and must be given in advance:

   a Specific or special procedures and medications.

   b Information concerning routine baby care.

   c Crying pattern of the newborn.

3   Following referral to the paediatric liaison health visitor, arrange for the family's own health visitor to visit the unit if possible.

   a This provides parents with continual support by someone they know.

   b Initiating these referrals also gives the nurse feedback about the home situation and possible areas where problems can be averted.

   c Continual support by the health visitor is important. Follow-up care can be directed also at assessing family interaction and parenting behaviours as well as development of the baby.

4   Evaluate the parents' willingness and ability to accept the child into their total care.

   a Permit the mother a special nesting period when she can have close physical contact with her infant in privacy and can provide complete care for her infant. Nursing support and help are readily available for the mother to call on if needed.

   b Instructions, demonstrations, and practice of procedures should have occurred prior to this time.

   c It is possible that this period may enhance normal maternal attachment behaviours days or weeks after birth.

5   Encourage parents to continue psychosocial and intellectual stimulation of their infant at home.

Realities of Nursing in the Intensive Care Nursery

Nursing in an intensive care nursery can be an emotionally draining experience; it can be difficult and depressing as well as hopeful and rewarding. Nurses frequently become surrogate mothers, grieving and rejoicing as the infant's condition changes. To minimize the personal agony frequently encountered, certain areas should be explored and opened to discussion.

1   Each nurse working in the intensive care nursery setting must be completely and totally educated to work in the area.

2   Discussions on grief and grieving should be open and frequent to allow each nurse to explore her own feelings.

3   Patient-centred discussions should be part of the routine to allow the nurse to express feelings about a particular patient.

4   Parent-centred discussions should focus on the parents' coping behaviours and stages of grief.

5   Each nurse must explore and acknowledge her feelings about the work in which she is involved.

Paediatric Intensive Care Unit

Nursing Role and Responsibilities in a Paediatric Intensive Care Unit

1 To provide continuing, comprehensive physical care and supportive treatment required to maintain life and to aid recovery of acutely ill children.
2 To provide emotionally supportive care to acutely ill children.
3 To provide empathetic support to parents and families of children in the intensive care unit.
4 To act as an integral and essential member of the health care team by assessing patient needs as well as by planning care and evaluating its effectiveness.
5 To act as child advocate by ensuring that basic human rights are respected.
6 To serve as nursing care consultants when children who require some intensive care nursing skills are admitted to the children's ward.
7 To serve as members of appropriate committees (e.g. committees that decide policy on emergency care, protocol for admission to the paediatric intensive care unit, etc.).
8 To teach intensive care nursing principles and skills to appropriate groups.
9 To function effectively and safely, the intensive care unit nurse should demonstrate the following capabilities.
   a Good physical and emotional health required to withstand the strain of continually nursing critically ill children and supporting their families
   b Understanding of pathophysiology underlying disease
   c Knowledge and understanding of sophisticated monitoring equipment and special apparatus
   d Ability to reason objectively and to judge and be aware of rapidly changing situations
   e Ability to interpret data and to take rapid, decisive action
   f Ability to perform complex technical skills correctly and in an organized manner
   g Understanding of the impact of illness and hospitalization on the life of the child
   h Understanding of parental response and ways of coping with the stress of a critically ill child
   i Ability to record data concisely, accurately, and thoroughly.

Physical Care of the Child

1 Apply understanding of the pathogenesis of the disease in assessing patient needs and in planning care.
2 Perform complex technical skills to monitor and support the child (see text for specific procedures). These may include:
   a Cardiac, respiratory, and blood pressure monitoring
   b Basic interpreting of ECG tracing

    c Endotracheal suctioning
    d Oxygen administration and monitoring
    e Tracheostomy care
    f Ventilator management
    g Monitoring central venous pressure
    h Monitoring intracranial pressure
    i Measuring arterial pressure
    j Hyperalimentation
    k Collection of specimens
    l Chest drainage.

3 Perform nursing activities related to life support of the child (see text for specific procedures). These activities include the following:
    a Cardiopulmonary support
    b Respiratory management
    c Fluid and nutritional assessment and management
    d Observations for complications and changing status.

4 Apply general nursing measures for patient comfort and prevention of complications:
    a Positioning — to prevent contractures, to drain secretions from the lungs, and to minimize pressure effects on skin.
    b Controlling of body temperature.
    c Skin care — to prevent breakdown.
    d Eye care — to prevent conjunctivitis and injury to the cornea in unconscious children.
    e Fluid balance — record daily fluid intake by all routes and losses of urine, stool, vomit, blood, and other drainage. Be sensitive to weight loss and gain.
    f Care of bladder — to prevent infection. Urine should be expressed manually, or an indwelling catheter should be inserted to prevent retention.
    g Mouth care — to cleanse mouth of secretions, vomitus, especially in unconscious patient or patient with an endotracheal tube.
    h Control of infection.

5 Provide careful, continuous clinical observations of the child.

Emotional Support of Child

1 Refer to the section on the impact of hospitalization on the developmental stage of the child, pp. 58-66.
2 Provide immediate physical care that communicates strength and facilitates trust.
3 Be alert to behavioural changes that may indicate physical distress.
4 Question parents concerning the child's own way of responding to emotional stress. Utilize particular comforts that are most soothing to the child.
5 Support parents so that they will be best able to support their child.
6 Time activities; dim lights to allow for adequate sleep whenever possible.
7 Do everything possible to reduce the amount of pain that the child must endure.

8 Provide age-appropriate stimulation when indicated by the child's condition (TV, games, books, toys, etc.).

9 If possible, avoid exposing an alert child to the death or resuscitation of another child. If the child is exposed, provide adequate explanation. The child must also be helped to express and work through the experience.

10 Prepare the child for transfer from the intensive care unit by implementing a nursing care plan similar to that which the child will experience on the children's ward (e.g. decrease frequency of monitory of vital signs, encourage independence). Give a thorough report to the receiving nurse during transfer.

Emotional Support to Family

1 Assure parents that everything possible is being done for their child. Allow them to see child receiving treatment.

2 Provide opportunities for parents to talk with a person, e.g. the social worker or, for some people, an appropriate spiritual advisor, with whom they can share their concerns and fears.

3 Provide opportunities for parents to ask questions and have them answered.

4 Make certain that parents are informed of important changes in the child's clinical state. Reinforce medical interpretations.

5 Be sensitive to parents' additional commitments to family and home as well as to their need to remain with their child. Visiting should be unrestricted.

6 Explain special equipment and changes in nursing management.

7 Allow parents to participate in some aspects of care when appropriate. Support them in this endeavour.

8 In nursing care, communicate comfort, reassurance, and consideration for the child.

9 Refer to section on Family-centred Care (p. 66).

The Child Undergoing Surgery

Preoperative Care

1 Provide emotional support, psychological preparation, and preoperative teaching appropriate for the age of the child. Such preparation and support will minimize stress and will help the child cope with his fears.

   a Potential threats for the hospitalized child anticipating surgery are:

     (1) Physical harm — body injury, pain, mutilation, death

     (2) Separation from parents

     (3) The strange and unknown — possibility of surprise

     (4) Confusion and uncertainty about his limits and expected behaviour

     (5) Relative loss of control of his world, his autonomy.

   b All preparation and support must be based upon the child's age, developmental stage, and level; personality; past history and experience with health professionals and hospitals; background — including religion, socioeconomic group, culture, and family attitudes.

(1) Know what information the child has already received.

(2) Determine from the child what he knows or expects.

c Familiarize patient and family with the ward, location of playroom, operating theatre and recovery room and introduce them to other children, parents, and some of the personnel. Make arrangements for child to meet the anaesthetist.

d Allow and encourage questions. Give honest answers.

(1) Such questions will give the nurse a better understanding of the child's fears and perceptions of what is happening to him.

(2) Infants and young children need to form a trusting relationship with those who care for them.

(3) The older child tends to be reassured by the information he receives.

e Provide opportunity for child and parent to work out concerns and feelings with play, and talk. Such supportive care should result in less upset behaviour and more cooperation.

f Prepare child for what to expect postoperatively (i.e. equipment to be used or attached to child, different location, how he will feel, what he will be expected to do, diet).

2   Assist in physical preparation of patient for surgery.

a Assist with necessary laboratory studies. Explain to child what is going to happen prior to procedure and how he can respond. Give continual support during procedure.

b See that patient has nothing by mouth (NPO) (from Latin *nil per os*). Ensure that the parents and, if possible, the child know what this means. Babies and small children may be given a feed of dextrose or a glucose drink 2-3 hours before an anaesthetic to minimize the risk of hypoglycaemia in postoperative period.

c Assist with fever reduction.

(1) Fever will result from some surgical diseases, i.e. intestinal obstruction.

(2) Fever increases risk of anaesthesia and need for fluid and calories.

d Administer appropriate medications as ordered. Sedatives and drugs to dry the secretions are often given on the unit.

e Establish good hydration. Parenteral therapy may be necessary to hydrate the child, especially if he is receiving nil by mouth, is vomiting or is febrile.

3   Support parents during this time of crisis. The attitudes of the parents towards hospitalization and surgery largely determine the attitudes of their child.

a The experience may be emotionally distressing.

b Parents may have feelings of fear or guilt.

c The preparation and support should be integrated for parent and child.

d Give individual attention to parents; explore and clarify their feelings and thoughts; provide accurate information and appropriate reassurance.

e Stress parents' importance to the child. Help mother understand how she can care for her child.

Postoperative Care

Immediate

1 Maintain a patent airway and prevent aspiration.

    a Position child on his side or abdomen to allow secretions to drain and prevent tongue from obstructing pharynx.

    b Suction any secretions present.

2 Make frequent observations of general condition and vital signs.

    a Take vital signs every 15 minutes until child is wide awake and his condition stable.

    b Note respiratory rate and quality, pulse rate and quality, blood pressure, skin colour.

    c Watch for signs of shock.

        (1) All children in shock have signs of pallor, coldness, increased pulse and irregular respirations.

        (2) Older children have decreased blood pressure and perspiration.

    d Change in vital signs may indicate airway obstruction, haemorrhage or atelectasis.

    e Restlessness may indicate pain or hypoxia. Medication for pain is not usually given until anaesthesia has worn off.

    f Check dressings for drainage or constriction and pressure.

3 See that all drainage tubes are connected and functioning properly. Gastric decompression relieves abdominal distention and decreases the possibility of respiratory embarrassment.

4 Monitor parenteral fluids as ordered. (See p. 159.)

5 Be physically near the child as he awakens to offer soothing words and a gentle touch. Rejoin parents and child as soon as possible after child recovers from anaesthesia.

After Recovery from Anaesthesia

After undergoing simple surgery and receiving a small amount of anaesthesia, the child may be ready to play and eat in a few hours. More complicated and extensive surgery debilitates the child for a longer period of time.

1 Continue to make frequent and astute observations with regard to behaviour, vital signs, dressings or operative site and special apparatus (intravenous, chest tubes, oxygen).

    a Note signs of dehydration

        (1) Dry skin and membranes

        (2) Sunken eyes

(3) Poor skin turgor

(4) Sunken fontanelle in infant.

b Record any passage of flatus or stool.

c Record micturition time, amount, characteristics.

2   Record intake and output accurately.

a Parenteral fluids and oral intake.

b Drainage from gastric tubes or chest tubes, colostomy, wound, and urinary output. Dressing may need to be weighed for more accurate estimate of output.

c Parenteral fluid is evaluated and ordered by considering output and intake. Parenteral fluid is usually maintained until child is taking adequate oral fluids.

3   Advance diet as tolerated, according to child's age and the surgeon's or paediatrician's directions.

a First feedings are usually clear fluids; if tolerated, advance slowly to full diet for age. Note any vomiting or abdominal distention.

b Since anorexia may occur, offer child what he likes in small amounts and in an attractive manner.

4   Prevent infection.

a Keep child away from other children or personnel with respiratory or other infections.

b Change the child's position every 2-3 hours — prop infants with a towelling roll.

c Encourage patient to cough and breathe deeply — let infant cry for short periods of time.

d Keep operative site clean.

(1) Change dressing as needed.

(2) Keep nappy away from wound.

5   Provide good general hygiene.

a Good skin care will increase circulation and prevent pressure sores.

b Provide proper rest and sleep periods.

c Allow child exercise and movement out of bed when he feels better. Advance gradually.

d Allow diversional activity at intervals appropriate for age.

6   Offer the child measures of comfort.

a See that child is warm and changes position as needed.

b Provide mouth care.

c Allow child to have and hold favourite toy or object.

d Anticipate his needs.

e Holding and rocking the infant or young child may be comforting.

7   Provide emotional support and psychological security.

a Encourage child to talk about his operation.

b Allow child to play out his feelings.

c Return often to see and talk to the child.

d Reassure him that things are going well. Talk about going home, if appropriate.

8   Continue to offer support to the parents.
    a Help to maintain family relationships. (Encourage parents to care for their child.)
    b Encourage parents to talk about their concerns.
    c Begin early to prepare for discharge.
       (1) Teach any special procedures to be continued at home.
       (2) Arrange for referral to health visitor or district nurse as appropriate.
       (3) Determine limits of activity for the child.
       (4) Make follow-up appointments.
       (5) Anticipate reactions of the child as a result of the hospitalization.

TRANSCULTURAL KNOWLEDGE OF ETHNIC MINORITY GROUPS' HEALTH-ILLNESS BEHAVIOURS

General Principles

1   Comprehensive nursing should include being alert and responsive to the many cultural cues present in daily nursing situations. A conscious effort should be made to become knowledgeable about cultural diversity, and distinctiveness and similarities of the culture most likely to be served in nursing practice. Cues will then be more meaningful and can be incorporated into patient assessment and care.
2   The nurse should be aware that cultural beliefs affect how a family perceives, experiences, and copes with illness. Culture influences how a family communicates about its health problems, the manner in which the symptoms are presented, when and to whom members go for care, how long they remain in care, and how that care is evaluated.
3   It is possible that some health behaviours generated from cultural beliefs may be anxiety-producing and threatening to the nurse. Knowledge of and sensitivity to cultural diversity will decrease these anxieties, thus facilitating effective interaction and relationships with the child and his family.
4   The nurse should be aware of the beliefs of the popular (family, community) and folk (non-professional healers) domains of health care available to her patient's family as well as the accepted views of the medical profession so that discrepancies can be discussed and resolved.
5   Knowledge of the cultural beliefs of the patient's family will assist the nurse in understanding behaviours that may seem negative, confusing, illogical, or primitive and help in producing a response that is more appropriate for the child's condition.

Assessment

Cultural backgrounds determine issues nurses should be aware of when caring for a child and his family.

1 Areas to consider when involved in cultural assessment:
  a Patterns of lifestyle of an individual or cultural group
  b Specific cultural values, norms, and experiences of the child and family regarding health and illness
  c Cultural taboos and myths
  d The world view or ethnocentric tendencies
  e The extent of assimilation into the main stream cultural group
  f Health and child care rituals
  g Folk and professional approaches to healing
  h Objectives and methods of caring for self and others
  i Indicators of cultural change or adaptive behaviour.

2 In an attempt to become knowledgeable about cultural and ethnic beliefs relating to paediatric nursing, the nurse must determine the following:
  a What is the meaning of children in the culture?
  b Do cultural patterns determine infant or child care? What are these patterns?
  c Do cultural patterns determine parental responses to behaviour and appearance of the infant or the child?
  d What meaning does language or nonverbal communication have in the culture?

3 The acceptance of health care by a family or subculture may depend upon the nurse's knowledge of the cultural beliefs and her attempt to understand their values whilst working within given guidelines. It is essential to know how the family unit is culturally defined, the family's functions and the functions of the child in order to work effectively with that family.

4 The following questions may be helpful in eliciting the family's perceptions of the illness and related cultural beliefs:
  a What do you think caused the problem?
  b Why do you think it started when it did?
  c What do you think your child's illness does to him?
  d How severe is your child's illness? Will it have a short or long course?
  e What kind of treatment do you think your child should receive?
  f What results do you hope to receive from this treatment?
  g What are the major problems your child's illness has caused for you?
  h What do you fear most about your child's illness?

5 In addition to health care, cultural patterns and bereavement behaviour must also be understood in order to provide effective, psychological services and support for the child, his parents and his family whilst in hospital and at home.

THE DYING CHILD

Nursing Objectives

To work out one's own feelings about death and to develop a philosophy which enables the nurse to be a source of support to the dying child and his family.

1 Become familiar with literature in the area of death and dying and use as a resource in planning and developing nursing care.
2 Recognize that the goal is to assist the child and his family to cope with this pain and grief in such a way that the experience will promote growth rather than destroy family integrity and emotional well-being of the family.
3 Share personal feelings about death and dying with colleagues. It is not unusual for the nurse to experience personal feelings of anger, frustration, helplessness, and guilt.

To recognize the stages of dying as identified by E. Kübler-Ross and to utilize this knowledge in planning and implementing care (Table 1.5).

1 Be aware that dying children, their families, and the staff will all progress through these stages, not necessarily at the same time.
2 Children experience the stages with much variation. They tend to pass more quickly through the stages and may merge some of these stages.
3 The nursing goal is to be aware of one's own feelings and to accept the child and family wherever they are, not to push them through the stages.

To understand the meaning of illness and death to the child at the various stages of growth and development and to utilize this information in planning and implementing care.

1 Refer to Table 1.6 which identifies stages in the development of a child's concept of death.
2 Be aware of other factors that influence a child's personal concept of death. Of particular importance are:
   a The amount and type of direct exposure a child has had to death
   b Cultural values, beliefs, and patterns of bereavement
   c Religious beliefs about death and afterlife.

Table 1.5   Stages of dying as identified by Dr Elizabeth Kübler-Ross

Stage	Nursing implications
I. Denial; shock; disbelief	Accept denial, but function within a reality sphere. Do not tear down the child's (or family's) defences. Be aware that denial usually breaks down in the early morning when it may be dark and lonely. Be certain that it is the child or family who is using denial, not the staff.
II. Anger; rage; hostility	Accept anger and help child express it through positive channels. Be aware that anger may be expressed towards other family members, nursing staff, doctors, and other persons involved. Help families to recognize that it is normal for children to express anger for what they are losing.
III. Bargaining (from 'No, not me' to 'Yes, me, but . . .')	Recognize this period as a time for the child and family to regain strength. Encourage the family to finish any unfinished business with the child. This is the time to do such things as take the promised trip or buy the promised toy.
IV. Depression (the child and/or family experiences silent grief and mourns past the future losses)	Recognize this as a normal reaction and expression of strength. Help families to accept the child who does not want to talk and excludes help. This is a usual pattern of behaviour. Reassure the child that you can understand his feelings.
V. Acceptance	Assist families to provide significant loving human contact with their child.

Table 1.6 Stages in the development of a child's concept of death

Age of child	Stage of development
Child up to 3 years	At this stage the child cannot comprehend the relationship of life to death, since he has not developed the concept of infinite time. The child fears separation from protecting and comforting adults. The child perceives death as a reversible fact.
Preschool-age child	At this stage the child has no real understanding of the meaning of death; he feels safe and secure with his parents. The child may view death as something that happens to others. The child may interpret his illness as a type of punishment for real or imagined wrongdoing. The child may interpret the separation that occurs with hospitalization as punishment; the painful tests and procedures that he is subjected to support this idea. The child may become depressed because he is not able to correct these wrongdoings and regain the grace of adults. The concept may be connected with magical thoughts and mystery.

School-age child	The child at this age sees death as the cessation of life; he understands that he is alive and that he can become 'not alive'; he fears dying.
	The child differentiates death from sleep. Unlike sleep, the horror of death is in pain, progressive mutilation, and mystery.
	The child is vulnerable to guilt feelings related to death because of difficulty in differentiating between death wishes and the actual event.
	The child learns the meaning of death from his own personal experiences:
	    Pets
	    Death of family members, political figures, etc.
	Television and movies have contributed to his concepts of death and understanding of the meaning of illness:
	    Develops more knowledge in the meaning of diagnosis
	    Death may occur violently.

Adolescent	The adolescent comprehends the permanence of death much as the adult does, although he may not comprehend death as an event occurring to persons close to himself. He wants to live — he sees death as thwarting pursuit of his goals: independence, success, achievement, physical improvement, and self-image. He fears death before fulfilment. The adolescent may become depressed and resentful because of bodily changes which may occur, dependence, and the loss of his social environment. The adolescent may feel isolated and rejected, since his own adolescent friends may withdraw when faced with his impending death. The adolescent may express rage, bitterness, and resentment. He especially resents the fact that he is fated to die.

To utilize the knowledge about children's interpretation of the meaning of death at the various stages of growth and development in talking to the child about his illness and in answering questions concerning death.

1   Research indicates that children generally can cope with more than adults will allow, and that children appreciate the opportunity to know and understand what is happening to them.

2   It is important that the child's questions be answered simply, but truthfully, and that they be based on his particular level of understanding.

3   The following responses have been suggested by Eassom in *The Dying Child* and may be useful as a guide.

   a *Preschool-age child*

    (1) When the child at this age is comfortable enough to ask questions about his illness, he should be told what he asks. When death is anticipated at some future time and the child asks 'Am I going to die?' a response might be, 'We will all die someday, but you are not going to die today or tomorrow.'

    (2) When death is imminent and the child asks, 'Am I going to die?' the response might be, 'Yes, you are going to die, but we will take care of you and stay with you.'

    (3) The parents should be allowed to stay with the child to provide him with protection and support.

    (4) When the child asks 'Will it hurt?' the response should be truthful and factual. Death may be described as a form of sleep — a sleep where he will be secure in the love of those around him. (Some children may fear sleep as the result of this type of explanation.)

    (5) Parents can express to the child the fact that they do not want him to go and that they will miss him very much; they feel sad too that they are going to be separated.

   b *School-age child*

    (1) Responses to the school-age child's questions about death should be answered truthfully. The child looks for support from those he trusts.

    (2) The school-age child should be given a simple explanation of his diagnosis and its meaning; he should also receive an explanation of all treatments and procedures.

    (3) The child should be given no specific time in terms of days or months since each individual and each illness is different.

    (4) When the school-age child asks 'Am I going to die?' and death is inevitable, he should be told the truth. The school-age child does have the emotional ability to look to his parents and those he trusts for comfort and support.

    (5) The school-age child believes in his parents. He should be allowed to die in the comfort and security of his family.

    (6) The school-age child knows death means final separation and he knows what he will miss. He must be allowed to mourn this loss as he dies. He may be sad and bitter and demonstrate aggressive behaviour. He must

be allowed the opportunity to verbalize this if he is able to.

c *Adolescent*

(1) The adolescent should be given an explanation of his illness and all necessary treatment procedures.

(2) The adolescent feels deprived and reasonable resentment regarding his illness because he wants to live and reach fulfilment.

(3) As death approaches, the adolescent becomes emotionally closer to his family.

(4) The adolescent should be allowed to maintain his emotional defences — he may deny absolutely his obvious ill-health. The adolescent will indicate by his questions what kind of answer he wants.

(5) If the adolescent states 'I am not going to die' he is pleading for support. Be truthful and state 'No, you are not going to die right now.'

(6) The adolescent may ask 'How long do I have to live?' He is able to face reality more directly and can tolerate more direct answers. No absolute time should be given since that absolutely blocks all hope. If an adolescent has what is felt to be a prognosis of approximately 3 months, the response might be 'People with an illness like yours may die in 3 to 6 months, but some may live much longer.'

(7) The bitterness and resentment of the fact that he is fated to die may interrupt necessary procedures and treatments. This behaviour must be appropriately handled.

To confer with the parents regarding feelings about discussing the illness with the child and to give them information which will be helpful in allowing them to play a more supportive role.

1 Determine what information they have given the child about his illness, and how the child related to this information.

2 Determine what specific questions the child has asked about his illness and how the parents have responded.

3 Share with parents your assessment of what the child knows about his illness and what he wants to know.

4 Discuss with the parents how children of various age levels interpret the meaning of death and offer suggestions as to how children's questions regarding death may be answered.

5 Provide parents with helpful literature about explaining death to children.

6 Assist parents to explain the child's illness to siblings and to answer their questions. If appropriate, help parents to identify ways that siblings can share in the child's care.

To assist the parents in dealing with their adaptation to their child's illness and anticipated death.

1 Develop a plan of care that includes the following approach:

a The primary responsibility for communicating with the parents should be designated to one nurse.

b Information regarding the parents' concerns should be communicated to all staff members.

2   Accept parental feelings about the child's anticipated death and help parents
deal with these feelings.

a   It is not unusual for parents to reach the point of wishing the child dead
and to experience guilt and self-blame because of this thought.

b   Parents may withdraw emotional attachments to the child if the process
of dying is lengthy. This occurs because parents complete most of the
mourning process before the child reaches biological death. They may relate
to the child as if he were already dead.

3   Be aware of factors which affect the family's capacity to cope with fatal
illness, especially social and cultural features of the family system, previous
experiences with death, present stage of family development, and resources
available to them.

4   Recognize the various stages that the parents will go through during the
child's illness.

*To perform the nursing measures which provide the child with both physical and emotional care
during illness.*

1   Provide physical care that makes the child as comfortable as possible.
Deliver care in a calm, assured, gentle manner.

2   Talk to the child and answer his questions truthfully.

3   Provide an atmosphere that offers the child the greatest security (e.g. room
with another child, room near nurse's station, etc.).

4   Provide opportunities for play as the child's condition permits.

5   Plan for consistency of assignment so that the child can experience
continuity of contact with a few nurses who inspire confidence and trust.

6   Encourage active involvement in living to the extent that the child is able
(e.g. participation in activities of daily living, play, schooling, socialization).

7   Observe children carefully during play for clues to their symbolic language.
Watch carefully what they do and listen to what they say. Drawings and self-
portraits may also help the child to express his feelings.

8   Communicate caring through touch. The child is comforted by being held,
especially by his parents.

9   Allow the child opportunity to direct activities and to let his wishes be
known.

10   Set realistic limits for the child when necessary, and enforce them
consistently.

*To encourage the parents to spend as much time as possible with the child and allow the
opportunity to participate in the child's care* (refer to section on Family-centred care, pp. 66-
70).

1   Allow the parents to bathe the child and to do procedures within their ability
and desire. This allows the parents the feeling that they are doing something
for their child.

2   Provide the parents with the opportunity to learn how to care for the child
and assure them that he will be cared for in their absence.

3 Provide the parents with a place to stay and be comfortable. They should be told where they can find privacy when they want to be alone.

To utilize appropriate services and resources in planning the care of the child and family.

1 Team members often include:
   a Paediatrician
   b Nurse
   c Child
   d Family
   e Social worker
   f Psychiatrist
   g Clergyman
   h Health visitor
   i School nurse
   j Parent groups.
2 Teamwork is essential because:
   a Terminally ill children and their families may require different kinds of assistance at different points in time.
   b They face many problems that are nonmedical in nature.
   c The child's need for assistance may be very different from that required by his family.
   d Team members may support one another.
3 To be effective team members, nurses must:
   a Communicate, collaborate, and cooperate with other members of the team.
   b Accept responsibility for their contribution to the plan of care and be accountable for the outcome.

To provide emotional support for parents following the death of the child.

1 Allow families who wish it, the opportunity to spend some time alone with the child after death.
2 Provide privacy for parents to express their grief in whatever manner they choose.
3 If appropriate, compliment parents on the excellent care they gave their child.
4 Be aware that your compassionate silence may be more helpful to families than small talk.
5 Assist families to contact other relatives and funeral services as appropriate.
6 Make certain that families have a safe and comfortable means to get home.
7 Invite parents to call if they have lingering questions or concerns that they wish to discuss.

FURTHER READING

General

Books and Pamphlets

Brimblecombe F, Barltrop D, *Children in Health and Disease,* Baillière Tindall, 1978.
Chiswick M, *Neonatal Medicine,* Update Books, 1978.
Committee on Child Health Services, *Fit for the Future,* report of the Committee on Child Health Services, HMSO, 1976.
Consumers Association, *Caring for Teeth,* Which?, 1970.
Gallagher J R, Harris H I, *Emotional Problems of Adolescents,* Oxford University Press, 1976.
Klaus M H, Kennel J H, *Maternal and Infant Bonding,* Mosby, 1976.
MacKeith R, *et al., Infant Feeding and Feeding Difficulties,* 5th edn, Churchill Livingstone, 1977.
Petrillo M, Sanger S, *Emotional Care of Hospitalized Children,* Lippincott, 1980.
Present Day Practice in Infant Feeding, HMSO, 1980.
RoSPA, *Facts About Accidents,* Ref. SE62, published yearly.
Scowen P, Wells J (eds), *Feeding Children in the First Year, Edsall, 1979.*
Stone L J, Church J, *Childhood and Adolescence,* Random House, 1973.

Articles

Auerbock K G, The role of the nurse in support of breast feeding, *Journal of Advanced Nursing,* May 1979: 263-285.
Davies M, You've a lovely baby — what more do you want? *Midwife, Health Visitor and Community Nurse,* November 1979: 452-456.
Haws L J, Brook C, The influence of body fatness in childhood on factors in adult life, *British Medical Journal,* January 1979.
Illingworth C, Injuries and accidents to children in playgrounds, *Journal of Maternal and Child Health,* September 1978: 315-318.
Jones R, Davies P, Infant Feeding, *Midwife, Health Visitor and Community Nurse,* November 1979: 438-443.
Playground accidents, *Royal Society of Health Journal,* August 1978: 148.
Spira M, The problem of trimming the fat baby down to size, *Modern Medicine,* June 1979: 41-47.
The dental health of children, *British Dental Journal,* November 1979: 279-280.
Through the eyes of the child, *Nursing Mirror,* November 1979: 19-38.
Wilkinson P W, Davies D, When and why are babies weaned?, *British Medical Journal,* June 1978: 1682-1683.

For Parents

Fenwick P E, *The Baby Book for Fathers,* Angus & Robertson, 1978.
Rayner C, *Family Feelings,* Arrow Books, 1977.
Richards M, *Infancy — World of the Newborn,* Harper & Row, 1980
The First Years of Life, Open University/Health Education Council, Ward Lock, 1977.
Woodward J, *Has Your Child Been in Hospital?,* National Association for the Welfare of Children in Hospital, 1978.

For Children

Althea, *Going into Hospital,* Dinosaur Publications, 1974.

Bergman T *et al., Children in Hospital,* Kestrel, 1981.

Bruna Dick, *Miffy in Hospital,* Methuen, 1976.

Burton N, Burton M, *First Time in Hospital,* MacDonald Educational, 1980.

Peacock F, *The Hospital,* Franklin Watts, 1976.

Rey M, Rey H, *Zozo Goes to Hospital,* Chatto and Windus, 1967.

Simpson J, *Come and See Hospital,* Felix Gluck, 1976.

Starters Facts, *Going to Hospital,* Macdonald Educational, 1980.

Watts M A, *Crocodile Medicine,* André Deutsch, 1977.

The Hospitalized Child, The Dying Child, Play, Education in Hospital

Books

Adamson F, St J, Hull D, *Nursing Sick Children,* Churchill Livingstone, 1984.

Bowlby J, *Loss: Sadness and Depression,* Hogarth Press, 1980.

Brimblecombe F *et al.* (eds), *Separation and Special Care Baby Units,* Heinemann Medical Books, 1975.

Burton L, *Care of the Child Facing Death,* Routledge & Kegan Paul, 1974.

Cooks S *et al., Children and Dying: An Exploration and Selective Bibliographies,* Health Sciences Publishing Co., 1974.

Dearden R *et al., Hospitals, Children and Their Families,* Routledge & Kegan Paul, 1970.

Eassom W M, *The Dying Child: The Management of a Child or Adolescent Who is Dying,* Charles C Thomas, 1970.

Garvey C, *Play,* Fontana, 1977.

General Nursing Council, *Aspects of Sick Children's Nursing,* General Nursing Council 1982.

Gould J (ed.), *Prevention of Damaging Stress in Children,* Churchill Livingstone, 1968.

Hall D, Stacey M, *Beyond Separation,* Routledge & Kegan Paul, 1979.

Hawthorne P, *Nurse I want my Mummy,* RCN Publications, 1974.

Kalafatich A, *Approaches to the Care of Adolescents,* Appleton-Century-Crofts, 1975.

Kübler-Ross E, *On Death and Dying,* Macmillan, 1976.

Martinson I M, *Home Care of the Dying Child,* Prentice-Hall, 1978.

Newson J, *Toys and Playthings in Development and Remediation,* Allen & Unwin, 1979.

Petrillo M, Sanger S, *Emotional Care of the Hospitalized Child,* 2nd edn, Lippincott, 1980.

Piaget J, *Play, Dreams and Imitation in Childhood,* Routledge & Kegan Paul, 1951.

Robertson J, *Young Children in Hospital,* Tavistock, 1970.

Rowen R (ed.), *The Dying Patient,* Pitman Medical, 1975.

Schiff H S, *The Bereaved Parent,* Souvenir Press, 1977.

Weller B, *Helping Sick Children Play,* Baillière-Tindall, 1980.

Articles

Alberman E, Collingwood J, Separation at birth and the mother-child relationship, *Developmental Medicine and Child Neurology,* October 1979.

Association of British Paediatric Nurses, Spotlight on children, *Nursing Times,* March 1980.

Chapman J A, Goodall J, Helping a child to live whilst-dying, *Lancet,* April 1980: 753-756.
Chapman J A, Goodall J, Symptom control in ill and dying children, *Journal of Maternal and Child Health,* April 1980: 144-154.
Crow, R, Sensory deprivation in children, *Nursing Times,* February 1979: 229-233.
Davies, J, Death of a child, *World Medicine,* November 1979: 23-26.
DHSS, Children in hospital, maintenance of family links, HC(78)28.
Franklin A W, Telling the Parents, *Journal of Maternal Health,* January 1978 5-7.
Fredlund D J, A nurse looks at children's questions about death, in *ANA Clinical Sessions 1970,* Appleton-Century-Crofts, 1971.

Transcultural Knowledge

Books

Berg A, *The Nutrition Factor,* Brookings Institution, 1973.
DHSS, *Prevention and Health: Avoiding Heart Attacks,* HMSO, 1977.
Guillaume A, *Islam,* Penguin, 1954.
Henley A, *Asian Patients in Hospital and at Home,* King Edward's Hospital Fund, 1981.
Royal College of Physicians, *Smoking or Health, The Third Report from the Royal College of Physicians,* Pitman Medical, 1977.
Van der Bergs & Jurgens, *Asians in Britain: A Study of Their Dietary Patterns in Relation to Their Cultural and Religious Background,* Van der Bergs and Jurgens, 1982.
Wadsworth M E J *et al., Health and Sickness: The Choice of Treatment,* Tavistock, 1971.
Wilson A, *Finding a Voice: Asian Women in Britain,* Virago, 1978, Chap. 1.

Articles

Ali A R *et al.,* Surma and lead poisoning, *British Medical Journal,* 1978, ii: 915-916.
Aslam M *et al.,* Asian medicines: in the best of traditions? *Nursing Mirror,* 1981, 153 (4): 34-36.
Becker M, Maiman L, Sociobehavioural determinants of compliance with medical care recommendations, *Medical Care,* 1975, 1 (18): 10-24.
Becker M H *et al.,* Mothers' health beliefs and children's clinic visits: a prospective study, *Journal of Community Health,* 1977, 3: 125-135.
Evans N *et al.,* Lack of breast feeding and early weaning in infants of Asian immigrants to Wolverhampton, *Archives of Disease in Childhood,* 1976, 51: 608-612.
Godfrey M, While A, Health visitor knowledge of Asian cultures, *Health Visitor,* October 1984: 279-298.
Goel K M *et al.,* Infant feeding practices among immigrants in Glasgow, *British Medical Journal,* 1978, ii: 1181-1183.
Homans H, Satow A, We too are strangers, *Journal of Community Nursing,* 1981, 5 (5): 10-13.
Homans H, Satow A, The nuclear family rules, OK. *Journal of Community Nursing,* 1981, 5 (6): 6-8.
King J B, Attributions, health beliefs and behaviour, paper presented at the annual London conference of the British Psychological Society, London, December 1982.
King J B, Health beliefs in the consultation, in *Doctor's Patient Communication,* D A Pendleton and J C Hasler (eds), Academic Press, 1983.
King J B, The health belief model, *Nursing Times,* October 1984: 53-55.
Knight L, Eastern promise in the East End? *Nursing Mirror,* 1979, 149 (16): 35-37.
Webb P, Health problems of London's Asians and Afro-Carribeans, *Health Visitor,* 1981, 54 (4): 141-147.

2

PAEDIATRIC TECHNIQUES

MEASURING VITAL SIGNS IN CHILDREN

Normal Vital Sign Ranges in Children

Temperature

Oral: 36.4-37.4 °C
Rectal: 36.2-37.8 °C
Axillary: 35.9-36.7 °C

Pulse and Respiratory Rates

Age	Pulse	Respirations
Newborn	70-170	30-50
11 months	80-160	26-40
2 years	80-130	20-30
4 years	80-120	20-30
6 years	75-115	20-26
8 years	70-110	18-24
10 years	70-110	18-24
Adolescence	60-110	12-20

Blood Pressure* (mmHg)

Age	Mean systole	Range in 95% of normal children	Mean diastolic	Range of 95% of normal children
6 months-1 year	90	±25	61	±19
2-3 years	95	±24	61	±24
4-5 years	99	±21	65	±15
6 years	100	±15	56	± 8
8 years	105	±16	57	± 9
10 years	109	±16	58	±10
12 years	113	±18	59	±10
15 years	121	±19	61	±10

* Reproduced with permission from John Hopkins Hospital *The Harriet Lane Handbook*, 7th edition, Dennis L. Headings MD (Editor). Copyright © 1975 by Yearbook Medical Publications Ltd

General Considerations for Measuring Vital Signs

1   Vital sign values provide the nurse with only rough estimates of physiological activity. It is important to identify trends, sudden discrepancies, and wide deviations from normal.
2   Vital signs should be taken as often as the nurse thinks necessary. They should not be delayed until the next scheduled time if it is suspected that a trend is developing.

Temperature

1   Normal body temperature represents a balance between the body heat produced and body heat lost.
2   The mode for taking the temperature should be kept as constant as possible. (Refer to Table 2.1 for methods of measuring body temperature in infants and children.)
3   Never leave the child alone when taking his temperature.
4   For security, safety, and accuracy keep one hand on the thermometer when it is in place when the temperature is being taken rectally or in the axilla.
5   Record the temperature value and method used.
6   Report an elevated or subnormal temperature and initiate whatever nursing measures are indicated by the child's condition.

Pulse

1   Take apical rate on an infant.
   a Place stethoscope between left nipple and sternum.
   b Take heart rate for one full minute.
2   With an older child, the pulse rate may be obtained easily at the radial, temporal, or carotid locations. (The pulse may be taken for 30 seconds and multiplied by 2.)
3   Take pulse rate prior to taking temperature because child may cry when temperature is taken; this increases the pulse rate and makes it more difficult to hear the apical rate.
4   Record accurately the following:
   a Rate
   b Rhythm (regular or irregular)
   c Strength of beat (full, bounding, weak, faint)
   d Activity of child at time pulse is taken (sleeping, crying, etc.).
5   Report immediately any changes in pulse characteristics, and initiate whatever nursing measures are indicated by the child's condition.

Table 2.1   Methods of measuring body temperature in infants and children

Method	Advantages	Disadvantages	Length of time required for accurate measurement
Rectal	1 Safe for children who are unable to cooperate and may bite the thermometer 2 Not directly influenced by the ingestion of hot or cold fluids 3 Method of choice if: child has seizures or breathing difficulties; is receiving oxygen therapy; has had oral surgery	1 Values may be altered by the presence of stool 2 Emotional response may be negative 3 Damage to rectal mucosa may occur 4 Replication of thermometer placement is difficult 5 Contraindicated when child has diarrhoea and following rectal surgery	2 min
Oral	1 Easily accessible 2 Replication of thermometer placement is easy 3 Responds more quickly and regularly to changes in arterial temperature than does rectal method 4 More aesthetically pleasing	1 Value is readily influenced by ingestion of hot or cold fluids, oxygen therapy 2 Requires child's cooperation to keep mouth closed and not to bite the thermometer 3 Contraindicated if child has had oral injuries or surgery or is under the age of 5 years	2 min
Axillary	1 Safe and easily accessible 2 Avoids the danger of rectal or colon perforation 3 Avoids initiating the defecation stimulus 4 Often recommended for infants under one year	1 Value is more readily influenced by environmental temperature and airflow 2 Requires a relatively long period of time to obtain accurate reading	3 min

Respirations

1 Count respirations on an infant for one full minute. Observe chest movement as well as abdominal movements.
2 Respirations may be counted for 30 seconds and multiplied by 2 in the older child.
3 Obtain respiratory rate prior to taking temperature and pulse since child may cry during these procedures.
4 Note and record accurately the following:
   a Respiratory rate.
   b Depth of respirations.
      (1) Feel exhaled air to estimate adequacy of tidal volume.
      (2) Observe excursions of the chest and diaphragm.
   c Quality of respirations.
      (1) Determine if respirations are predominantly costal or abdominal. Dyspnoea should be suspected in an infant who is breathing costally or a school-age child who is breathing primarily with the abdomen.
      (2) Listen for unusual noises such as expiratory grunts, crowing noises, wheezing, or inspiratory stridor.
      (3) Observe for signs of dyspnoea:
         (a) Restlessness
         (b) Retractions-sternal or intercostal
         (c) Nasal flaring
         (d) Cyanosis.
   d Activity of the child during the procedure.
5 Report immediately any change in respiratory status. Initiate whatever nursing measures are indicated by the child's condition.

Blood Pressure

Generally, the technique for taking the blood pressure of a child is the same as for the adult. The following principles are important to observe when dealing with the paediatric patient.

General Considerations

1 The cuff should cover no less than one-half and no more than two-thirds the length of the upper arm or leg. Even small variations in cuff size may produce significant differences in blood pressure reading.
   a A cuff that is too narrow will produce an apparent increase in blood pressure.
   b A cuff that is too wide will produce an apparent decrease in blood pressure.

c Using a flexible blood pressure cuff that can be folded to the correct size is frequently easier and more effective for the nurse than choosing among several assorted premeasured cuffs.

d The cuff should be of consistent width each time that a child's blood pressure is measured during hospitalization.

2   If the child is excited or uncomfortable or if he distrusts the person taking the blood pressure, the systolic pressure may rise significantly.

a The blood pressure should be taken when the child is at rest and in a consistent position.

b The blood pressure should be explained to the child before it is done.

(1) He should know that it will not hurt.

(2) He should be allowed to handle the equipment, pump the cuff, etc.

(3) It may be helpful for the child to use the equipment on his parents, the nurse, or a doll in order for him to overcome his fears and understand its use.

Methods Used in Obtaining Blood Pressure Measurements in Paediatrics

1   *Auscultatory method* (method of choice whenever possible.)

a Centre the bladder of the cuff over the artery.

b Apply the cuff evenly and snugly over the bare arm with the lower edge about 1.25 cm above the antecubital space.

c Support the arm in a slightly flexed and abducted position at the level of the child's heart.

d Palpate the brachial artery and inflate the cuff until the palpated pulse is lost. Then pump for an additional 20-30 mmHg beyond that.

e Deflate the cuff slowly at a rate of about 5 mmHg/second.

f Deflate the cuff rapidly and completely when all sounds disappear.

g Record the reading and compare it with previous values. There continues to be a controversy as to what best indicates diastolic pressure. Therefore, it is good practice to record all three readings: (1) systolic-point at which pulse becomes audible; (2) diastolic-point of muffling of sound; and (3) point of disappearance of sounds.

h The blood pressure may be obtained by the same method in the leg, using the popliteal artery.

2   *Palpatory method* (This method provides only an approximate mean pressure which lies between the systolic and diastolic pressures obtained by the auscultatory method.)

a Follow steps 1-3 of the auscultatory method.

b Inflate the cuff to about 200 mmHg.

c Take the reading when the pulse distal to the cuff becomes palpable in the course of deflation.

3   *Flush method* (This method is especially useful with infants, but also has the disadvantage of providing only an approximate mean pressure.)

a The infant should be quiet and in the supine position.

b Apply a blood pressure cuff to the upper or lower extremity, just above the wrist or ankle.

c Squeeze the extremity distal to the cuff with a hand or with a firm wrapping.

d Simultaneously pump the manometer to 120-140 mmHg. This will blanch the child's arm or leg below the cuff.

e Release the hand or the wrapping at the same time that the cuff is deflated.

f Take the reading at the point at which blood re-enters the hand or foot, causing a sudden flushing.

4   *Electronic methods*

a Electronic equipment utilizes a tiny microphone within the cuff to amplify the Korotkoff sounds or to convert them to another type of signal such as a flashing light.

b More sophisticated equipment is available which can inflate and deflate the cuff and either hold or automatically record the measurement.

c Advantages of electronic methods:
(1) Observer bias is minimized as electronic circuitry rather than the human ear analyses the Korotkoff sounds. Therefore, blood pressure readings are more consistent.
(2) The child is subjected to minimal handling despite frequent monitoring of the blood pressure.

d Nursing considerations:
(1) Read specific instructions carefully before operating an electronic device since each unit has a slightly different operating procedure.
(2) Note whether the equipment measures muffling or silence, or both, as the diastolic pressure.

5   *Ultrasonic equipment*

a Utilizes an ultrasonic transducer in the cuff to detect and amplify blood pressure sounds.

b Some equipment is capable of measuring only systolic pressure, while other instruments can sense both systolic and diastolic sounds.

c Advantages of ultrasonic methods:
(1) Measurements correlate closely with intra-arterial pressures.
(2) Especially useful in infants when the Korotkoff sounds may be inaudible by ordinary methods.

d Nursing considerations:
(1) Read specific instructions carefully before operating an ultrasonic device.
(2) Note specifically what sounds are being measured and whether the equipment measures muffling or silence, or both as the diastolic pressure.

Principles Related to Paediatric Blood Pressure Values

1   The blood pressure varies with the age of the child and is closely related to his height and weight.
2   Variability of blood pressure among children of approximately the same age and body build is normal.
3   The pressure in the legs with the cuff technique is ordinarily 20 mmHg higher than in the arms in children over 1 year of age.

NURSING MANAGEMENT OF THE CHILD WITH FEVER

Fever is any abnormal elevation of body temperature. Prolonged elevation of temperature above 40°C may produce dehydration and harmful effects on the central nervous system.

Causes

1   Infection
2   Inflammatory disease
3   Dehydration
4   Tumours
5   Disturbance of temperature regulating centre
6   Extravasation of blood in the tissues
7   Drugs or toxins.

Assessment

1   Consider basic principles related to temperature regulation in paediatric patients.
    a Usually an infant's temperature does not stabilize before the first week of life. A newborn's temperature varies with the temperature of his environment.
    b The degree of fever does not always reflect the severity of the disease. A child may have a very serious illness with a normal or subnormal temperature.
    c Fever, itself, may cause convulsions in some children when the temperature goes very high, very fast.
    d The range for normal temperature varies widely in children. A common explanation for 'fever' is misinterpretation of a normal temperature reading. (Refer to Measuring Vital Signs in Children, p. 99.)
    e The child's temperature is influenced by activity and by time of day; temperatures are highest in late afternoon.

2   Be certain that accurate technique is used for temperature measurement. The mode should be appropriate for the child's age and condition, and the thermometer should be left in place for the required period of time. (Refer to Measuring Vital Signs in Children, p. 99.)

3   The following will be useful in ascertaining the cause of the fever:

   a *History* Information should be elicited regarding:
   (1) Age of the child
   (2) Pattern of the fever
   (3) Length of the illness
   (4) Change in normal patterns of eating, elimination, recreation, etc.
   (5) Other symptoms
   (6) Exposure to any illnesses
   (7) Recent immunizations or drugs
   (8) Treatment of the fever and effectiveness of treatment
   (9) Previous experiences with fever and its control.

   b *Physical examination* Of special significance are:
   (1) General appearance of the child
   (2) Inspection of the skin for rashes, sores, flushed appearance
   (3) Inspection of eyes, ears, nose, and throat for redness and/or drainage
   (4) Neurological observation for changes in state of consciousness, pupillary reaction, strength of grip, abnormal muscle movement or lack of movement
   (5) Inspection of the external genitals for redness and/or drainage
   (6) Presence of abdominal or flank pain.

   c *Laboratory tests* Initial tests frequently include: complete blood count, urinalysis, cultures of the throat, nasopharynx, urine, blood, and spinal fluid, and x-ray of the chest.

4   Attempt to identify the pattern of the fever. Take the child's temperature by the same method every hour until stable, then every 2 hours until normal, then every 4 hours for 24 hours.

Nursing Measures to Reduce Fever

Fever itself does not necessarily require treatment. The presence of fever should not be obscured by the indiscriminate use of antipyretic measures. However, if the child is uncomfortable or appears toxic because of fever, an attempt should be made to reduce it by any of the following nursing measures or by a combination of these measures.

Nursing Action	Rationale/Amplification
1 Increase the child's fluid intake to prevent dehydration.	1 Fever increases the child's fluid requirements by increasing the metabolic rate.
2 Expose the skin to the air by leaving the child lightly dressed in an absorbent material. Avoid warm, binding clothing and blankets. Utilize a protected cooling fan, positioned near the child but out of his reach.	2 Loss of heat from the skin by radiation is the main temperature regulating mechanism available to the infant or small child.
3 Administer a tepid sponge bath if ordered by the paediatrician. (See Guidelines: Adminstering a Tepid Water Sponge, below.)	3 The temperature is lowered by evaporation of water from the surface of the skin.
4 Administer antipyretic drugs, as prescribed.	4 Although effective in reducing fever, antipyretic drugs may obscure the clinical picture and cause numerous side effects including: diaphoresis, skin eruptions, nausea, vomiting, haematological changes, and fever. Paracetamol elixir is often recommended rather than aspirin for infants and small children because of its lower overall toxicity in therapeutic dosages.
5 Utilize ice bags for local comfort.	5 These should not be used for infants since they may produce chilling.

GUIDELINES: ADMINISTERING A TEPID WATER SPONGE FOR FEVER

A tepid water sponge is bathing of the body for a period of time to reduce fever.

Equipment

1 Basin of tepid water (21.1-27 °C)
2 Plastic sheet
3 Two bath blankets
4 Towels
5 Six washcloths.

Nursing Alert: Cold water or alcohol sponges must not be administered to children. Cold water may produce vasoconstriction and shivering, which raise central body temperature. Alcohol sponges may reduce the temperature too rapidly, leading to convulsions in small children. In addition, the fumes may be toxic.

Nursing Action	Rationale/Amplification
Preparatory Phase	
1 Secure the child's cooperation.	1 This helps to increase the effectiveness of the procedure.
a Explain the procedure to the child in language he can understand.	
b A small infant may be held during sponging.	
c Allow the child or his parent to participate in the procedure.	
d Discontinue sponging if the child is extremely upset and uncooperative.	
2 Take temperature, pulse, and respiration before starting the sponge.	2 This serves as a baseline for comparison to determine the effectiveness of treatment.
3 Give antipyretic medication as ordered 15-20 minutes before starting the sponge.	3 There is more rapid reduction of fever when sponging is combined with administration of antipyretic medication.
Method	
1 Place a plastic sheet covered with a bath blanket under the child.	
2 Place a bath blanket over the child, and remove top bedding.	
3 Place cold, moist cloths over the superficial blood vessels in the axillae and the groins.	3 This aids in lowering body temperature.
4 Expose the body area to be sponged. Place a towel under the area.	
5 Slowly stroke the extremities with long, soothing strokes of the washcloth.	
a Stroke each arm from the neck to the axilla and down to the palm of the hand.	
b Stroke each leg from the groin to the foot.	
c Bathe the back and buttocks.	
6 Use gentle friction to bring the blood to the surface.	6 This increases the effectiveness of the treatment and prevents chilling.
7 Change the water as often as necessary to maintain a water temperature of 21.1-27°C	
8 Continue this procedure until temperature is adequately reduced, more drastic measures are ordered, or the child's condition indicates that it should be discontinued.	8 Generally, the sponge should not last more than 30 minutes. Observe for shivering. If this occurs, cover the child and wait a few minutes before proceeding. Stop the sponge if

cyanosis, mottling, or chilling do not stop when friction is applied to the skin. These symptoms indicate a change in vasomotor tone.

9 Pat dry with towel.

Follow-up Phase

1 Remove bath blankets and plastic sheet. Place a dry gown on the child.
2 Record vital signs 30 minutes after the sponge is finished.

2 Postsponge values indicate whether or not treatment has been effective.

3 A cool drink may be appreciated.

ADMINISTERING MEDICATIONS TO CHILDREN

Purpose

To safely administer medications to the child as prescribed by the paediatrician.

Important Considerations

1 The nurse's manner of approach should indicate that she firmly expects the child to take the medication. This manner often convinces the child of the necessity of the procedure.
2 Explanation about the medication should appeal to the child's level of understanding (i.e. colour, comparison to something familiar).
3 The nurse must mask her own feelings regarding the medication.
4 Always be truthful when the child asks, 'Does it taste bad?' or 'Will it hurt?' Respond by saying, 'The medicine does not taste good, but I will give you some juice as soon as you swallow it,' or 'It will hurt for just a minute'.
5 It is often necessary to mix distasteful medications or crushed pills with a small amount of honey, jam, yoghurt, or apple sauce.
6 Never threaten a child with an injection if he refuses an oral medication.
7 Medications should not be mixed with large quantities of food or with any food that is taken regularly (e.g. milk).
8 Medications should not be given at mealtime unless specifically ordered.
9 The nurse must know the following about each medication she is administering: common usages and dosages, contraindications, side effects, and toxic effects.
10 When preparing intramuscular injections, draw in 0.2 ml of air after the correct amount of solution is in the syringe. This serves to clear all medication from the needle upon injection and prevents backflow and the depositing of medication in subcutaneous fat upon withdrawal of the needle.

Calculating the Paediatric Dosage

It is not the nurse's responsibility to determine the dosage of a drug.
1   Know what factors determine the amount of drug ordered.
   a Action of the drug, absorption, detoxification, excretion are related to the maturity and metabolic rate of the child.
   b Neonates and preterm infants require a reduced dosage because of:
      (1) Deficient or absent detoxifying enzymes
      (2) Decreased effective renal function
      (3) Altered blood-brain and protein binding capacity.
   c Dosages recommended according to age groups are not satisfactory since a child may be much smaller or larger than the average child in his age group.
   d Dosage calculations based on weight have limitations.
2   Be alert to a prescription that would be inappropriate for a child.
3   Consult drug literature for recommended dosage and other information.

Surface Area

The following formulas are used to estimate the paediatric dosage based on the child's body surface area:

1    $\dfrac{\text{Surface area of child in sq. metres}}{1.75} \times \text{adult dose} = \text{child dose}$

2    $\dfrac{\text{Surface area of child}}{\text{Surface area of adult}} \times \text{dose of adult} = \text{approximate child dose}$

3   Surface area in square metres x dose per square metre = approximate child dose

Identifying the Patient

Always check a child's identification bracelet before administering a medication. Ask the older child his name.

Oral Medications

Infants
1   Draw up medication in a plastic dropper or disposable syringe.
2   Whenever possible, hold the child comfortably on lap.
3   Medicines are best offered before a feed unless contraindicated.
4   Elevate infant's head and shoulders; depress chin with thumb to open mouth.
5   Place dropper or syringe on the middle of the tongue and slowly drop the medication on the tongue.
6   Release thumb and allow child to swallow.

Toddlers
1   Draw up medication in syringe or measure into medicine cup.
2   Elevate the child's head and shoulders.
3   Squeeze cup and put it to the child's lips; or place the measuring syringe (without the needle) or dropper in the child's mouth and slowly expel the medicine.
4   Allow the child time to swallow.
5   Allow the child to hold the medicine cup by himself, if he is able, and to drink it at his own pace. (This may be a more agreeable method.)
6   The small, safe, disposable medicine cups can be given to the child for play.

Note: In some instances, a young child may need some restraint when being held — to achieve good comfort control, wrap in blanket. Remember to praise afterwards and offer drink.

School-age children
1   When a child is old enough to take medicine in pill or capsule form, he should be taught to place the pill near the back of his tongue and immediately swallow fluid such as water or fruit juice. If the swallowing of the fluid is emphasized, the child will no longer think about the pill.
2   Always praise a child after he has taken his medication.
3   If the child finds it particularly difficult to take oral medications, the nurse must let him know that she understands some of his fear and displeasure and that she wants to help him.

Intramuscular Injections   (Figure 2.1)

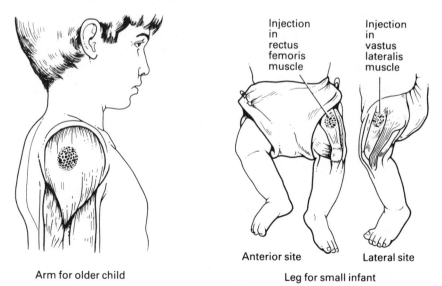

Figure 2.1   Sites for intramuscular injections in children.

Infants

1 Site selection
   Lateral and anterior aspect of the thigh — there are no major nerves in this area.
2 Administration
   a Nurse or mother to hold the child in a secure position to prevent movement of the extremity.
   b Do not use a needle longer than 2.5 cm.
   c Use upper outer quadrant of the thigh.
   d Insert needle at a 45° angle in a downward direction, towards the knee. Hold and cuddle the infant following the injection.
   f This site is also used on the older child who may be difficult to restrain.

Toddlers and School-age Children

1 Site selection
   a Buttocks — upper outer quadrant (dorsogluteal)
   (1) Gluteal muscles do not develop until the child begins to walk; they should be used only when the child has been walking for 1 year or more.
   (2) Upper outer quadrant of the young child's buttock is smaller in diameter than an adult's; thus accuracy in determining the area comprising the upper outer quadrant is essential.
   (3) Administration
     (a) Do not use a needle longer than 2.5 cm.
     (b) Position the child in a prone position.
     (c) Place thumb on the trochanter.
     (d) Place middle finger on the iliac crest.
     (e) Let index finger drop at a point midway between the thumb and middle finger to the upper outer quadrant of the buttock.
     (f) Insert needle perpendicular to the surface on which the child is lying, not perpendicular to the skin.

   b Ventrogluteal
   (1) This site provides a dense muscle mass which is relatively free of the danger of injuring the nervous and vascular systems.
   (2) The disadvantage is that the injection site is visible to the child.
   (3) Administration
     (a) Place child on his back.
     (b) Place index finger on the anterosuperior spine.
     (c) With the middle finger moving dorsally, locate the iliac crest; drop finger below the crest. The triangle formed by the iliac crest, index finger,
     and middle finger is the injection site.

   c Arm — upper outer aspect (deltoid)
   (1) May be used for older, larger children.
   (2) Determine injection site as with an adult.

d Lateral and anterior aspect of the thigh.
(1) Do not use a needle longer than 2.5 cm.
(2) Use the upper outer quadrant of the thigh.
(3) Insert needle at a 45° angle in a downward direction, towards the knee.

2 Nursing support
a Explain to the child where you are going to given him the injection (site) and why he must receive the injection.
b Allow the child to express his fears.
c Carry out procedure quickly and gently. Have needle and syringe completely prepared and ready prior to contact with child.
d Always secure the assistance of a second nurse or one of his parents to help immobilize the child and divert his attention as well as to offer him support and comfort.
e Praise the child for his behaviour after the injection. Often, allowing him to assist with applying an adhesive dressing will give him some feeling of comfort.
f Also encourage activity that will use the muscle site of injection — promotes dispersal of medication and decreases soreness.
g Record accurately the injection site to ensure proper site rotation.

ENEMA

An *enema* is the insertion of fluid into the rectum for the purpose of cleansing the lower bowel for therapeutic or diagnostic reasons. An enema for an infant or a young child is based on the same principles as for an adult and is essentially the same, except that *less fluid and pressure are used than in an adult.*

GUIDELINES: ADMINISTERING AN ENEMA TO A CHILD

Types
1 Cleansing — to evacuate the bowel; to soften hard faeces.
2 Therapeutic — to administer drugs or correct an early intussusception, e.g. barium enema by hydrostatic pressure.
3 Diagnostic — x-ray examination with barium.

Procedure

Nursing Action	Rationale/Amplification
Preparatory Phase	
1 Explain procedure to the child according to his level of understanding.	1 Even though the child may not fully understand, an explanation will soothe him and build his trust in you.
2 Position **a** *Older child;* Have him lie on his left side with his upper leg flexed. **b** *Infant* Place infant in a supine position, with a pillow under his head and back and a small bedpan under his buttocks. Gentle restraint may be needed — nappy placed under the bedpan, brought over thighs, and then pinned.	**a** This position places the descending colon at the lowest point. **b** Infants cannot retain enema fluid. Pillows provide the body alignment.
Method	
1 Insert lubricated rectal tube 3.7-10 cm into the rectum just within the anal sphincter.	
2 Hang solution reservoir no higher than 30-45 cm above the infant's hips.	2 This allows the solution to run slowly with minimum pressure.
3 Do not administer more than 300 ml of solution at 38°C to infant unless otherwise ordered.	3 Fluid volume may range from 30-300 ml depending on the size of the child.
4 Once the rectal tube is removed, the abdomen can be gently massaged, if there are no contraindications.	4 This gentle massage will help relax the infant and assist in expelling the solution.
5 If young child is 'potty trained', have a small potty chair available for his use.	5 The familiarity of a potty chair will provide great comfort for the child and eliminate the possible embarrassment of soiled bed or pants.
6 When a retention enema is administered, the buttocks may be held or taped together to assist retention of fluid. Keep child as quiet as possible.	

PROTECTIVE MEASURES TO LIMIT MOVEMENT (RESTRAINTS)

Protective measures to limit movement are mechanisms for restraining children (Figure 2.2).

Purpose

1   To maintain the child's safety and protect him from injury.
2   To facilitate examination and minimize the child's discomfort during special tests, procedures, and specimen collections.

Underlying Principles

1   Protective devices should be used only when necessary and as a deliberate decision by a qualified nurse or member of medical staff, and never as a substitute for careful observation of the child.
2   The reason for using the protective device should be explained to the child and his parents to prevent misinterpretation and to ensure their cooperation with the procedure. Restraints are often interpreted as punishment by children.
3   Any protective device should be checked frequently to make sure that it is effective. It should be removed periodically to prevent skin irritation or circulation impairment.
4   Protective devices should always be applied in a manner that maintains proper body alignment and ensures the child's comfort.
5   Any protective device that requires attachment to the child's bed should be secured to the bed springs or frame, *never* the mattress or side rails. This allows the side rails to be adjusted without removing the restraint or injuring the child's extremity.
6   Any knots that are required should be tied in a manner that permits their quick release. This is a safety precaution.
7   When a child must be immobilized, an attempt should be made to replace the lost activity with another form of motion. For example, even though restrained, a child can be moved in a stroller, wheelchair, or in his bed. When arms are restrained, the child may be allowed to play kicking games. Water play, mirrors, body games, and blowing bubbles are helpful replacements.
8   Improvised body restraint must never be used.

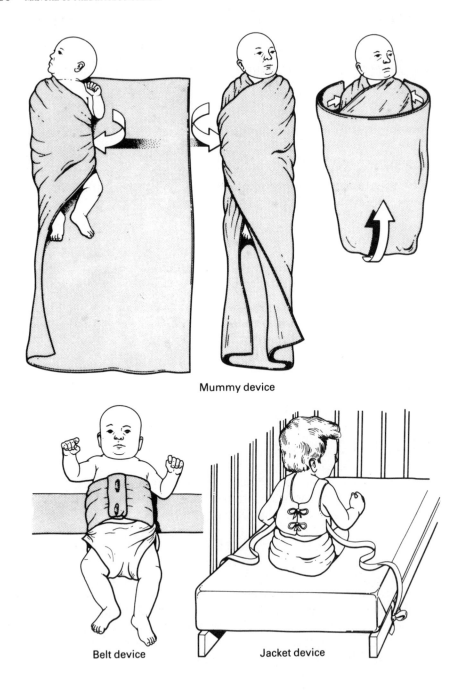

Mummy device

Belt device   Jacket device

Figure 2.2   Types of restraints.

Mummy Device

The *mummy device* involves securing a sheet or blanket around the child's body in such a way that his arms are held to his sides and his leg movement is restricted (Figure 2.2).

Purpose

To restrain infants and small children during treatments and examinations involving the head and neck.

Equipment

1   Small sheet or blanket.
2   Several large safety pins.

Nursing Action

1   Place the blanket or sheet flat on the bed.
2   Fold over one corner of the blanket.
3   Place the child on the blanket with his neck at the edge of the fold.
4   Pull the right side of the blanket firmly over the child's right shoulder.
5   Tuck the remainder of the right side of the blanket under the left side of the child's body.
6   Repeat the procedure with the left side of the blanket.
7   Separate the corners of the bottom portion of the sheet, and fold it up towards the child's neck.
8   Tuck both sides of the sheet under the infant's body.
9   Secure by crossing one side over the other in the back and tucking in the excess, or by pinning the blanket in place.

Special Precautions

Make certain that the child's extremities are in a comfortable position during this procedure.

Jacket Device

The *jacket device* is a piece of material that fits the child like a jacket or halter. Long tapes are attached to the sides of the jacket (Figure 2.2).

Purpose

To keep the child in his wheelchair, highchair, or cot.

Nursing Action

1   Put the jacket on the child so that the opening is in the back.
2   Tie the strings securely.

3   Position the child in his highchair, wheelchair, or cot.
4   Secure the long tapes appropriately:
  a Under the arm supports of a chair.
  b Around the back of the wheelchair or highchair.
  c To the springs or frame of the cot.

Special Precautions
The child in a cot must be observed frequently to make certain that he does not entangle himself in the long tapes of the jacket device.

Belt Device

The *belt device* is exactly like the jacket method of restraining, except that the material fits the child like a wide belt and buckles in the back (Figure 2.2).

Elbow Device

The *elbow device* consists of a piece of material into which tongue depressors have been inserted at regular intervals. It is especially useful for infants receiving scalp-vein infusion, those with eczema or cleft lip repair, and children having eye surgery.

Purpose
To prevent flexion of the elbow.

Equipment
1   Elbow cuff
2   Wooden tongue depressors
3   Safety pins, tapes, or string.

Nursing Action
1   Insert tongue depressors into the appropriate places in the elbow cuff.
2   Place the child's arm in the centre of the elbow cuff.
3   Wrap the cuff around the child's arm.
4   Secure the cuff with pins, tapes, or string.

Special Precautions
1   The tongue depressors should be cut to about 10 cm in length if the elbow cuff is to be used for an infant — for greatest comfort.
2   Additional security may be provided by dressing the child in a long-sleeved shirt prior to the application of the elbow cuff. The ends of the shirt can then be turned back over the cuff and pinned securely.

Devices to Limit Movement of the Extremities

There are many different kinds of devices to limit motion of one or more extremities. One commercial variety consists of a piece of material with tapes on both ends to be secured to the frame of the cot. The material also has two small flaps sewn to it for securing the child's ankles or wrists. Similar devices are available which utilize sheepskin flaps. These should be used when the device will be necessary over a prolonged period, or for children with very sensitive skin.

Purpose

To restrain infants and young children for such procedures as intravenous therapy and urine collection.

Equipment

1   Extremity restraint of appropriate size for the child (small, medium, or large)
2   Several safety pins
3   Cotton wadding covered with gauze.

Nursing Action

1   Secure the device to the cot frame.
2   Pad the extremities to be restrained with cotton wadding covered with gauze or other suitable material.
3   Pin the small flaps securely around the child's ankles or wrists.
4   Adjust the device by pinning a tuck in the centre of the material, if it is too large

Special Precautions

1   The infant's fingers or toes should be observed frequently for coldness or discoloration and the skin under the device checked for signs of irritation.
2   The device should be removed periodically to provide for skin care and range of motion exercises.

Abdominal Device

The abdominal device is used for restraining a small child in his cot. It operates exactly like the method described for limiting the movement of the extremities. However, the strip of material is wider and has only one wide flap sewn in the centre for fastening around the child's abdomen.

Clove-hitch Device

The *clove-hitch device* is a mechanism for restraining an extremity by tying crepe bandage or Tubegauz in a special way.

Equipment

Cotton wadding covered with gauze cut in lengths of 1.37m.

Nursing Action

1   Pad the extremity to be restrained with the cotton wadding covered with gauze or other suitable material.
2   Make a figure-8 loop in the centre of the bandage.
3   Place the child's wrist or ankle in the loop of the device.
4   Pull the ends of the device to the desired tightness.
5   Tie the ends to the cot springs or frame.
6   Check the device to make certain that it does not tighten when both ends are pulled taut or slip over the child's hand or foot.

Using Tubegauz

1   A short narrow length of Tubegauz is slipped over wrist.
2   Narrow adhesive tape is placed around the wrist over the end of the tubular bandage.
3   The length is drawn over the hand and tied to an immobile horizontal bar of the cot.

INFANT FEEDING AND NUTRITION

The best food for babies is undoubtedly human breast milk. Nurses and midwives should encourage and support mothers to breast feed even if it is only achieved for a few weeks. However, if a mother has decided, for whatever reason, to use a milk formula method of bottle feeding she should be given the same support, understanding, and help as the mother who breast feeds.

Good Reasons for Breast Feeding

1   Promotes 'bonding' between mother and child.
2   Many infections are far less common in breast-fed babies. Immunoglobulins are transferred in the colostrum, other antibodies are present in breast milk together with the iron building protein lactoferrin which inhibits the growth of pathogenic Escherichia coli. The acid stools of breast-fed babies also have a role to play in reducing the risk of gastrointestinal infarctions.
3   The fat in human milk is better absorbed than the fat in cows' milk.
4   The danger of giving an over-concentrated or a too diluted feed is avoided.
5   The risk of eczema, asthma, and other allergic disorders is considerably reduced.
6   Low birth weight and preterm infants thrive best on breast milk.

Preparation for Breast Feeding

Ideally preparation for breast feeding should be part of a health education programme for parentcraft to both boys and girls whilst in secondary schools. This early awareness should be expanded in antenatal sessions for both parents when a baby is expected. These sessions should include:

1 Knowledge of the physiology of breast feeding
2 Management and comfort of the breasts and nipples
3 The importance of a well-balanced diet during pregnancy and of the need of extra protein and calories whilst breast feeding
4 Practical demonstration and discussion with a breast feeding mother.

Management of Breast Feeding

Immediately after birth, whilst the mother is still in the delivery room, all mothers should have the opportunity to hold their baby for 10-15 minutes quietly and contently. If the mother intends to breast feed, she should suckle her infant for 1-2 minutes at each breast. Skin-to-skin contact and early suckling are important at this time in promoting 'bonding' and to encourage the release of prolactin and oxytocin hormones which stimulate milk secretion and help the uterus to contract.

GUIDELINES: TEACHING THE MOTHER BREAST FEEDING PROCEDURE

Purposes

1 To provide psychological and emotional satisfaction for the infant and the mother.
2 To feed the infant a natural and ideal food that will supply him with adequate nutrition.
3 To have milk always available, at the right temperature.
4 To prevent chance of gastrointestinal disturbances and development of allergies.
5 To provide physical closeness of baby to mother during feeding.

Procedure

Teaching Points	Rationale/Amplification
1 Wash hands before breast feeding.	1 Protects infant and breast from infection.
2 Prepare to nurse shortly after birth and at least every 4 hours; feeding later on demand.	2 Initially regular feeding (every 4 hours) establishes nursing pattern. Will fit in with family life.

3 Nurse infant at night feeding.

3 Prevents engorgement and helps bring in milk supply quickly.

Position of Mother

1 Lie on side with pillow under head. Position left arm above head *or*
2 Use a chair with back support. Place pillow on lap to hold infant.

1 The mother should be relaxed and comfortable.
2 The infant's head should be higher than his abdomen to prevent regurgitation.

Nursing Technique

1 With the right hand, press darkened area around nipple into infant's mouth.
2 If breast is full and firm, use one finger to press breast away from infant's nose.
3 Use both breasts at each feeding; 5 minutes on each breast, then increase nursing time to 10 minutes.
4 At each feeding alternate the breast that is used first. Pin a safety pin to the bra as a reminder of which breast to start with at the next feeding.
5 Break the suction by putting a finger into the corner of the infant's mouth.
6 'Burp' infant midway through the feeding. Pat gently on the back or hold in upright position.
7 Uterine cramps may occur.

1 This manoeuvre is necessary for adequate suction.

2 Prevents obstruction of airway; infant breathes mainly through his nose.

4 The infant will empty the first breast; nursing at the second breast will increase milk production.

5 Pulling the nipple abruptly away from the infant will result in sore nipples.
6 Helps infant to release air bubbles in stomach.
7 Nursing stimulates release of oxytocin hormone, causing uterine contractions.

Other Considerations for Mother

1 Drink water for two. Continue to eat a balanced, nutritious diet. (Nursing mother may require 1000 more calories (4200 kJ) and an additional 8-10 g of protein daily.)
2 Get adequate rest.
3 Avoid emotional stress and do not become discouraged.
4 Avoid taking medications and drugs.

3 It takes time to establish a good nursing routine.
4 Cold or allergy medication will limit fluid output. Birth control medication may suppress milk production.

GUIDELINES: BREAST FEEDING THE ILL OR HOSPITALIZED INFANT

Breast feeding is suckling of an infant at the mother's breast to provide him with nourishment.

Equipment

1 Clear water
2 Cotton balls.

Procedure

Nursing Action	Rationale/Amplification

Preparatory Phase

1 When an infant who is nursing is hospitalized, it is the nurse's responsibility to encourage the mother to continue breast feeding if the infant's condition does not contraindicate it. Explain to the mother that:
a Supplemental infant formula can be given to the infant if she is not available; *or*
b She can express her breasts by hand or by using a pump and bring in her milk to be given to the infant via bottle when she is not available.

1 Some mothers have very strong feelings about wanting to breast feed their baby. It gives them an emotional satisfaction that is vitally important to the mother-child relationship since it is an integral part of the total mothering process. The nurse must help to foster this relationship as much as she can.

2 When nursing is to be done in the hospital paediatric setting, the physical surroundings may need to be altered somewhat. Provide the mother and infant with a relatively quiet area that is as private as possible and free from interruption.

2 This will provide the mother and infant with an opportunity to continue to develop their relationship during the crisis of illness and hospitalization.

3 Provide the mother with a comfortable armchair or pillow so that she can assume a comfortable position during the feeding. A footstool should also be available so that she can support her feet and the infant.

3 Proper and comfortable position of the mother will enable her to hold the baby correctly and support him while he is at the breast.

4 The infant should be awake and dry before the feeding is started.

4 If the infant is comfortable he will settle down and feed better.

5 Dress the infant appropriately so that he is not too warm or too cool during the feeding. The infant should also be hungry.

5 If he is too warm, he may fall asleep after the first few sucks of milk. A sleepy baby will not nurse well. If he is too cool, he may be fussy and restless.

6 Have mother wash her hands. Then she should wash her nipples with clear water and cotton balls.

6 Washing the nipples will remove any old milk that may have leaked and dried on them, providing a good medium for the growth of bacteria that can cause gastrointestinal disturbance in the infant.

7 Position the baby at breast. Put him in a semi-sitting position with his face close to the breast and supported by one arm and hand. A pillow may be used under the baby to support him.
The breast may need to be supported by mother's hand.

7 Proper positioning will provide the infant with comfort and security and make it easier for him to suck and swallow.

This makes the nipple more easily accessible to the baby's mouth and prevents obstruction of nasal breathing.

Method

1 When the feeding is to start, let the breast touch the infant's cheek. Do not hold his cheek and try to help him find the nipple.

1 The rooting reflex will take over and the infant will turn his head towards the breast with his mouth open. If his cheek is touched with a hand, he will become confused, perhaps turning towards the hand.

2 The infant's lips should be out over the areola and not just around the nipple before he begins to suck.

2 Since the nipple is so small, suction cannot be achieved merely by grasping it. The areola must be in the infant's mouth in order to establish suction and make the suck effective.

3 Note the presence or absence of the 'letdown' reflex during the nursing period.

3 Milk flowing from the other breast during nursing is quite normal. It is not usually present when the mother is worried.

4 The length of feeding time may vary from 5 to 20 minutes. Let the infant feed until he is satisfied.

4 When the infant is satisfied and has nursed well, he is relaxed and usually falls asleep. He will stop sucking.

5 Instruct the mother to burp the baby during and at the end of the feeding.

5 When the infant is sucking he swallows some air. Burping will help prevent abdominal distension and discomfort as well as regurgitation.

6 One or both breasts may be used at each feeding. It makes no difference as long as (a) baby is satisfied at the end of the feeding and (b) one breast is completely emptied at the feeding.

6 Regular and complete emptying of the breast is the only stimulation for the production of milk.

7 Once the infant has stopped sucking, he likes to cling to the breast. To break this suction, instruct mother to put her finger to the corner of the baby's mouth and gently pull.

7 Gentle pulling will not hurt the mother or infant.

Follow-up Phase

1 When the infant has finished feeding, change his nappy if it is wet or soiled.

1 To provide comfort for a restful sleep and to prevent nappy rash.

2   Position infant on his right side or on his abdomen on his bed.

2   This facilitates emptying of the stomach and decreases the possibility of regurgitation.

3   Note if baby appears satisfied or still seems to be hungry.

3   Mother may not have enough milk to satisfy the baby. Supplemental infant formula may be necessary.

4   Record descriptively and accurately:
  a   How baby fed
  b   How baby went to breast
  c   Satiety or hunger after feeding
  d   Breast or breasts used; which breast was emptied and which breast was nursed from thereafter.

d   If both breasts were used, the second breast is not usually emptied and should be used first at the next feeding.

GUIDELINES: BOTTLE FEEDING

Modified milk formulas are acceptable substitutes for human breast milk. These preparations need no extra sugar and when used in the dried form need only the addition of boiled water. Modified milk formulas which are sometimes known as low solute milks can be used until the child is introduced to a mixed diet and changes to cows' milk at 8-12 months.

Purposes

1   To provide the baby adequate fluid and calorie intake for appropriate growth.
2   To supplement breast feeding with formula or water.
3   To provide additional fluid intake between feedings.

Calculation of Feeds

The aim is to feed the normal healthy infant according to expected weight. If over-weight or very underweight then take the average between actual and expected weight. Individual modification will be required for sick infants according to weight, specific condition, and clinical state.

Expected Weight Gain

Know infant's birth weight, he loses weight in first week, but regains birth weight by 10th-14th day. During the first year of life hereafter he gains approximately:
200 g per week for 3 months
150 g per week for next 3 months
100 g per week for third 3 months
50-75 g per week for final 3 months

Fluid Requirements Each 24 Hours per Kilogram Body Weight

Preterm infants (up to 1.4 kg): 250 ml
1.4 — 2.5 kg: 220 ml
Infants over 2.5 kg: 150 — 200 ml
These amounts will provide for the infant's total protein, energy, and fluid requirements to meet growth and development.

Suggested Fluid Volume for Weight

Baby's weight	Suggested milk feed in 24 hours divided into 5 or 6 feeds
2.7 kg	405 ml
3.6 kg	540 ml
4.5 kg	675 ml
5.5 kg	825 ml
6.4 kg	960 ml

The number of feeds given varies with age, weight, and condition, e.g. very small (under 1.4 kg) or very sick infants may require hourly or 2 hourly feeding. In some circumstances continuous feeding may be given by nasogastric (p. 117) or nasojejunal tube (p. 124).
As a general guide:
Infants over 2.5 kg give 4 hourly feeds × 6
Infants over 3.0 kg give 4 hourly feeds × 5 or 6

Energy Requirements in 24 Hours

Preterm infants under 2.5 kg, 540-750 kJ/kg wt/day (130-180 calories/kg wt/day)
Normal infants over 2.5 kg, 420-540 kJ/kg wt/day (100-130 calories/kg wt/day)

Education for Bottle Feeding

Preparation of Feeds

As with preparation for breast feeding this should be included in antenatal sessions on parentcraft. Teaching in the home should also be included as kitchens and equipment obviously varies from home to home.

Mothers choosing this method of feeding should be made aware of the need for scrupulous hygiene in the preparation of feeds. Some method of bottle and teat sterilizing will be required. The majority of mothers prefer to use a chemical method of sterilization by immersion of teats and bottles as being most convenient. This may be with either hypochlorite liquid or one of the proprietary makes of tablets containing, for example, potassium monopersulphate which can be obtained at High Street chemists. Alternatively teats and bottles can be boiled in a covered saucepan for 3 minutes but this is less satisfactory.

Mixing instructions on the packet or tin of the feed must be strictly adhered to, and the mother should know how to use the measuring scoop correctly.

Equipment

1 Sterile bottle and teat.
2 Sterile infant formula or feeding fluid.

Procedure

Nursing Action	Rationale/Amplification
Preparatory Phase	
1 Baby should be awake and hungry. Change wet or soiled nappy.	1 A sleepy baby will not feed well. A dry nappy will provide comfort so that the baby will settle down and eat more easily.
2 Check infant formula for correct type and amount.	2 To prevent error.
3 Sit in a comfortable chair. Cradle baby with one hand and arm, while supporting baby against your body or lap.	3 Proper position will provide the baby with comfort and security and will make it easier for him to suck and swallow.
4 The temperature of the feed is checked by allowing a drop of milk to fall on to back of wrist — if pleasantly warm (blood heat), feed suitable to give.	
5 Any medicines prescribed should be given before commencement of feed, from a 5 ml spoon, dropper, or disposable syringe.	
Method	
1 Let the baby root for the teat by touching the corner of his mouth with the teat. When he opens his mouth, insert the teat.	1 Place the teat on top of the tongue and far enough in his mouth so suction can be created when he sucks.
2 Hold the bottle at an angle to completely fill the teat with fluid.	2 This prevents the baby from sucking and swallowing excessive amounts of air.
3 NEVER prop the bottle or leave the baby unattended during feeding.	3 This is unsafe. Should vomiting occur, aspiration is more likely.
4 The bottle should be handled so as not to contaminate the teat or fluid.	4 Contamination will increase the chances of gastrointestinal disturbances.
5 Baby's feeding time will vary from 10 to 25 minutes.	5 The length of time will depend on the age of the baby and how vigorously he sucks.

6 Burp the baby at least once during the feeding and at the end of the feeding.

a Place the baby in sitting position in nurse's lap, tilt him slightly forward, and gently rub or pat his back.

b Place baby in prone position on nurse's shoulder and gently pat or rub his back.

c Place baby in prone position on nurse's lap and gently pat or rub his back.

7 Take teat out of mouth periodically.

6 Most babies swallow some air during feeding.

These positions aid in expelling air and thus prevent abdominal distension, discomfort, and regurgitation.

7 To allow the baby to rest and to let air into the bottle so that the teat does not collapse

Follow-up Phase

1 After final burping, change wet or soiled nappy and place baby in cot on his abdomen or right side.

2 Check baby in a few minutes. If he is restless, pick him up and burp him again. Note if any regurgitation has occurred.

3 Accurate and descriptive recording:

a What was fed and amount

b How feeding was tolerated

c Any regurgitation or emesis — amount and material

d Length of time and feeding

e How baby sucked and took the feeding.

1 This position aids in emptying the stomach and prevents regurgitation.

2 Some babies relieve themselves of air when in the cot and also bring up small amounts of formula at the same time.

Note: When feeding a preterm infant, the same principles apply. The preterm infant, however, will tire more easily and fall asleep. Allow him frequent rest periods and use a soft teat so that less energy is needed to suck. To stimulate this infant to suck, the nurse can brush the infant's cheek with her finger, place thumb or finger under the infant's chin or move the teat back and forth in his mouth. Feeding time should not exceed 45 minutes.

GUIDELINES: WEANING

The age at which solid foods can be introduced to the infant must depend upon individual family circumstances. Most authorities agree, however, that it should be sometime between 3 and 6 months of age for the normal healthy infant.

Principles of Weaning

Nursing Action	Rationale/Amplification
1 Start with one food at one feed time, offering a small quantity only.	1 Enables the infant to adjust to new texture and spoon feeding, thus becoming nutritionally less dependent on milk.
2 Introduce new foods one at a time at 3-4 day intervals.	2 To provide a variety of textures which will enable the infant to partake at family meals.
3 Decrease feed kilojoules (calories) and volumes as solids are introduced and increased in quantity. Do not add sugar to cereals or other dishes.	3 To prevent obesity.
4 Do not add salt to savoury foods.	4 To avoid stressing the relatively immature kidneys.
5 Introduce second meal after 3-4 weeks. Include iron-containing foods, e.g. liver, green vegetables.	5 After 5-6 months the inherited iron store from the mother is depleted and needs to be replaced in order to meet requirements for haemoglobin production.
6 As solid foods increased and milk volume reduced, remember to offer dilute fruit juice or water from a cup to infant at least twice a day particularly during hot weather.	6 Prevents dehydration and enables infant to become used to drinking from a cup.
7 Breast milk or milk formula can continue to be offered until 10 months-1 year, then replaced by cows' milk given from a cup.	7 Allows infant to retain comfort of breast or bottle especially for the evening feed whilst weaning is introduced.
8 About age of 7 months offer 'finger foods', e.g. rusks, peeled apple.	8 Promotes self-feeding and chewing.

Nursing Alert: Do not leave young infant alone with hard foods since there is a risk of choking due to immature chewing and swallowing mechanisms at this age. The transition from breast or bottle feeding to family meals is normally slow and may take several months. By about the age of 9-10 months most infants can share in some of the family meals.

Nursing Alert: Avoid giving peanuts, pistachio nuts, etc., to young children. These may be inhaled and, if not extracted, can break down and release oily toxins which cause the collapse of the alveoli by preventing gaseous exchange.

GUIDELINES: NASOGASTRIC FEEDING

Nasogastric feeding is a means of providing food via a catheter passed through the nares or mouth past the pharynx, and into the stomach, slightly beyond the cardiac sphincter.

Purposes

1   To provide a method of feeding or administering medications that requires minimal patient effort, when the infant is unable to suck or swallow.
2   To provide a route that allows adequate kilojoule (calorie) or fluid intake.
3   To prevent fatigue or cyanosis which is apt to occur from bottle feeding.
4   To provide a safe method of feeding an unconscious child or one who is too limp or weak to feed normally.

Equipment

1   Sterile catheter, rounded-tip, size 5-10 FG
2   Clear, calibrated reservoir for feeding fluid
3   Syringe 2-5 ml
4   Stethoscope
5   Water for lubrication
6   Tape/scissors
7   Feeding fluid
8   Dummy
9   Litmus paper.

Procedure

Nursing Action	Rationale/Amplification
Preparatory Phase	
1 The conscious child should be told about the procedure in language he understands.	
2 Position the infant on his side or back with his neck hyperflexed with a nappy roll placed under neck. A mummy restraint may be necessary to help maintain this position.	2 This position allows for easy passage of the catheter, facilitates observation, and helps avoid obstruction of the airway.
3 Measure feeding catheter and mark with tape. a *Preterm infant and neonate* Measure from bridge of nose to just	3 Premeasuring the catheter provides a guideline as to how far to insert catheter. Chilling catheter will stiffen it and facilitate insertion.

beyond tip of sternum.

b *Older child* Measure from tip of nose past ear, to tip of sternum.

Method

1 Lubricate catheter with water.

1 Do not use oil because of danger of aspiration.

2 Stabilize patient's head with one hand; use the other hand to insert the catheter.

a If necessary, nostrils should first be cleaned with moistened cotton wool, the nostrils should be used alternately where intubation is necessary.

b *Insertion through nares:* Slip the catheter into nostril and direct toward the occiput in a horizontal plane.

c *Insertion through the mouth:* Pass the catheter through the mouth towards the back of the throat.

b This direction will follow the nares passageway into the pharnyx. Do not direct the catheter upward.

3 If patient swallows, passage of the catheter may be synchronized with the swallowing.

3 Swallowing motions will cause oesophageal peristalsis, which opens the cardiac sphincter and facilitates passage of the catheter.

4 If there is no swallowing, insert the catheter smoothly and quickly.

4 Because of cardiac sphincter spasm, resistance may be met at this point. Pause a few seconds, then proceed.

5 In the infant, especially, observe for vagal stimulation, i.e. bradycardia (slow heart rate) and apnoea.

5 The vagus nerve pathway lies from the medulla through the neck and thorax to the abdomen. Above the stomach, the left and right branches unite to form the oesophageal plexus. Stimulation of these nerve branches with the catheter will directly affect the cardiac and pulmonary plexus.

6 Once the catheter has been inserted to the premeasured length, tape the catheter to the patient's face (Figure 2.3).

6 This prevents movement of catheter from the premeasured, pre-established correct position.

7 Test for correct position of the catheter in the stomach with one or more of the following ways:

a The syringe is attached to the tube and the piston of the syringe is gently withdrawn. If no fluid is withdrawn, pass tube a little more and repeat aspiration. Check aspirate with litmus paper; stomach juices are acid and will turn blue litmus red.

a Failure to obtain aspirate does not indicate improper placement; there may not be any stomach content or the catheter may not be in contact with the fluid.

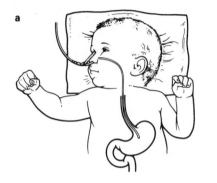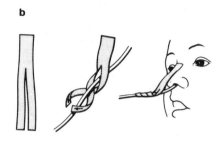

Figure 2.3 Nasogastric feeding: (a) nasogastric tube in jejunum; (b) steps in preparing adhesive tape to retain tube.

b Inject 0.5-1 ml air into the catheter and stomach. At the same time listen to the typical growling sound with a stethoscope placed over the epigastric region.
c Hold free end of tube under water. If the water flows into the tube on inspiration or air bubble through the water on expiration, the tube is in trachea. Remove tube immediately.

b Aspirate injected air from stomach to prevent abdominal distension.

Nursing Alert: Avoid inserting catheter into infant's trachea. (An infant's anatomy makes it relatively difficult to enter the trachea.) If improper placement occurs, and the catheter enters the trachea, the patient may cough, fight, and become cyanotic. Remove the catheter immediately and allow the patient to rest before attempting intubation again.

8 Using non-allergic tape, attach tube to face. The feeding position should be supine or sidelying, with head and chest slightly elevated. Attach reservoir to catheter and fill with feeding fluid. Allow infant to suck on dummy during feeding.
9 Aspirate tube before feeding begins.
a If over half the previous feeding is obtained, withhold the feeding.
b If a small residual of formula is obtained, return it to stomach and subtract that amount from the total amount of formula to be given.

8 This position allows the flow of fluid to be aided by gravity. The use of a dummy will relax the infant, allowing for easier flow of fluid as well as provide for normal sucking needs.

9 This is done to monitor for appropriate fluid intake, digestion time, and overfeeding that can cause distension.

10 The flow of the feeding should be slow. Do not apply pressure. Elevate reservoir 15-20 cm above the patient's head.

10 The rate of flow is controlled by the size of the feeding catheter: the smaller the size, the slower the flow. If the reservoir is too high, the pressure of the fluid itself increases the rate of flow.

11 Food taken too rapidly will interfere with peristalsis, causing abdominal distension and regurgitation.

11 The presence of food in the stomach stimulates peristalsis and causes the digestive process to begin.

12 Feeding time should last approximately as long as when a corresponding amount is given by bottle and teat.

13 When the feeding is completed, the catheter may be irrigated with clear water Spigot tube.

13 Clamp the catheter before air enters the stomach and causes abdominal distension. Clamping also prevents fluid from dripping from the catheter into the pharynx, causing patient to gag and aspirate when the tube is being removed.

Note: Frequent passage of a nasogastric tube is not advisable. A fine polyvinyl or other plastic tube with care can be kept in position for 1-2 weeks. Ensure that the tube does not cause pressure on the nares or nasal septum, otherwise necrosis could ensue. Tube changes should be recorded in nursing records.

Follow-up phase

1 Burp the child if necessary.

1 Adequate expulsion of air swallowing or ingested during feeding will decrease abdominal distension and allow for better tolerance of the feeding.

2 Place patient on right side or on abdomen.

2 To minimize regurgitation and aspiration.

3 Observe condition after feeding; bradycardia and apnoea may still occur.

3 Because of vagal stimulation as mentioned above.

4 Note any vomiting or abdominal distension.

4 Due to overfeeding or too rapid feeding.

5 Note infant's activity.

5 Fatigue or peaceful sleep.

6 Accurately describe and record procedure, including time of feeding, type and amount of feeding fluid given, amount retained or vomited, how patient tolerated feeding, and activity following feeding.

GUIDELINES: GASTROSTOMY FEEDING

Gastrostomy feeding is a means of providing nourishment and fluids via a tube that has been surgically inserted via a stab wound through the abdominal wall into the stomach.

Purposes

1   To provide a method of nutrition and fluids that requires minimal effort when the patient is unable to suck or swallow for long periods of time.
2   To allow for better decompression of stomach (because of large tube size) following a surgical procedure.
3   To provide a safe method of feeding a child with oesophageal stricture or one who cannot tolerate alternative methods.
4   To provide a route that allows adequate kilojoule (calorie) and/or fluid intake in a child and chronic lung disease or in one who does not have continuity of the gastrointestinal tract, i.e. oesophageal atresia.

Equipment

1   Warm feeding fluid, 38 °C
2   Dummy
3   Reservoir syringe or funnel
4   Syringe for aspirating.

Procedure

Nursing Action	Rationale/Amplification
Preparatory Phase	
1 Gastrostomy tube may be in one of three positions between feedings: **a** Lowered and open to start drainage. **b** Open, connected to reservoir (funnel, syringe) that is elevated 10-12 cm **c** Clamped.	**a** Constant decompression **b** To serve as safety valve outlet to prevent oesophageal reflux and increased stomach pressure. **c** Most 'normal' physiological setup: preparation for home care or tube removal.
2 The nurse may be directed to check residual stomach contents prior to any feeding.	2 This is done to monitor for appropriate fluid intake, digestion time, and over-feeding that can cause distension.

a Attach syringe and aspirate stomach contents.

b Measure.

c Residual fluid may be returned to stomach or discarded depending on amount.

3 A Y-tube which is connected at the point where reservoir and gastrostomy tube join may be used during feeding.

4 When feeding is about to begin, infant/child should be placed in comfortable position in bed — either flat or with head slightly elevated. If condition permits, the nurse should hold infant. A dummy can be given to him.

3 To provide simultaneous decompression during feeding.

4 When infant/child is comfortable and relaxed, feeding fluid will flow more easily into stomach. Dummy will satisfy normal sucking activity, provide exercise for jaw muscles, and relax musculature as well as provide pleasure normally associated with feeding.

Procedure

1 Attach reservoir syringe to tube (if not already open to continuous elevation) and fill reservoir with feeding fluid prior to unclamping tube.

2 Elevate tube and reservoir to 10-12 cm above abdominal wall. Do not apply any pressure to start flow.

3 Feed slowly, taking 20-45 minutes. Fill reservoir with remaining fluid before it is empty to avoid instillation of air.

4 Continue to provide infant with pleasant feelings associated with feeding.

5 When feeding is completed:

a Instill clear water (10-30 ml) if tube is to be clamped. Apply clamp before water level reaches end of reservoir.

b Leave tube unclamped and open to continuous elevation.

1 Prevents air from entering tube (and then stomach), which may cause distension.

2 This elevation level will allow for slow, gravity-induced flow. Pressure may cause a backflow of fluid into the oesophagus.

3 Too rapid a feeding will interfere with normal peristalsis and will cause abdominal distension and backflow into reservoir or oesophagus.

a This rinses tubing and will prevent clogging.

b Feeding fluid is allowed to return to reservoir if infant cries or changes position, and thus decreases pressure on the stomach.

Follow-up Phase

1 Check dressing and skin around point of tube entry for wetness. Clean skin and apply skin barrier preparation or ointment. See that there is no pull on tube.

1 Skin breakdown is caused by continued exposure to stomach contents that may be leaking out around tube. Constant pulling on tube can cause widening of skin opening and subsequent leakage.

2 Leave infant dry and comfortable. If unable to hold him during feeding, this may be a good time to hold, fondle, and provide him with warmth and love.

2 To promote relaxation and improved digestion of feeding.

3 Accurately describe and record procedure, including time of feeding, fluid given, amount and characteristics of residual (if any) and what was done with it, how patient tolerated feeding, any abdominal distension, and activity following feeding.

Note: Should infant pull gastrostomy tube out, cover ostomy site with sterile dressing and tape, notify the surgeon, and accurately record events.

GUIDELINES: NASOJEJUNAL FEEDING

Nasojejunal feeding is a means of providing full enteral feeding via a catheter passed through the nares, past the pharynx, down the oesophagus, bypassing the stomach through the pylorus into the jejunum.

Purposes

1 To provide a method of feeding that requires minimal patient effort when the infant is unable to tolerate alternative feeding methods.
2 To provide a route that allows for adequate kilojoule (calorie) or fluid intake (full enteral feeding) via intermittent or continuous drip.
3 To provide a method of feeding a critically ill infant that minimizes regurgitation, aspiration, and gastric distension.
4 To provide a route for administration of oral medications.

Equipment

1 Sterile radio-opaque silicone or polyvinyl nasojejunal tube, 1m
2 Tape
3 Litmus paper
4 Reservoir for feeding
5 Three-way stopcock
6 Syringe — 0.5 ml normal saline or sterile water
7 Equipment for insertion of nasogastric tube.

Procedure

Nursing Action	Rationale/Amplification

Preparatory Phase

1 Attach cardiac monitor to infant.

1 To allow for continuous monitoring of heart rate and rhythm. The vagus nerve pathway lies from the medulla through the neck and thorax to the abdomen. Above the stomach, the left and right branches unite to form the oesophageal plexus. Stimulation of these nerve branches with the catheter will directly affect the cardiac and pulmonary plexus.

2 **a** Measure from glabella (prominent point between eyebrows) to the heel for estimated length.
b Measure and mark the remaining length of tubing and record.

b This serves as a double check to ensure that tube has not advanced farther than intended.

3 Place infant on his right side with hips slightly elevated. Gentle restraint or soft mittens may have to be applied.

3 Facilitates passage of the tube. Restraints prevent infant from pulling out tube before the tip passes the pylorus

4 Tube is inserted through a nostril into the stomach — allowing adequate length so that it can pass the pylorus into the jejunum. Securely tape tube in place so as not to block nasal canal or cause pressure necrosis or irritation.

5 Check intestinal aspirate for pH every 1-2 hours. Infant may be positioned on right side, back, or abdomen. Once the tube is past the pylorus, abdominal posteroanterior and lateral x-rays are taken to confirm that tip of catheter is at the ligament of Treitz.

6 If gastric residual is significant, it will interfere with ordered feeding. Notify paediatrician. A reflux of 4 ml/kg in stomach is tolerated. Do not remove nasogastric tube since it will adhere to nasojejunal tube during withdrawal and pull out nasojejunal tube also.

7 Feeding schedules vary from unit to unit, but are usually based on the following:

a Sterile water for first feeding, 2-3 ml/kg.

b Expressed human breast milk (when available) or infant formula, e.g. SMA 1-3 ml/kg per feed hourly. After 24 hours, increase to 4 ml/kg.

c Continued daily increments of 1-2 ml until 10 ml/kg per feed is attained.

d Medications may be given via the nasojejunal tube if ordered. A three-way stopcock will have to be placed at the connection of the nasojejunal tube and the line from the feeding fluid using a syringe pump or constant infusion pump.

d Flush tubing with 0.5 ml normal saline or sterile water after medication is administered to ensure that infant receives entire dosage prescribed and to prevent any sediment from remaining in tubing.

Note: In the event of diarrhoea or of gastric aspiration exceeding previous input, it will be necessary to reduce the rate of daily progression of total amount of fluid and kilojoules (calories).

Method

1 Nasojejunal feedings can be given as follows:

a Intermittently — i.e. every 1-3 hours, *or*

b In a continuous slow drip.

b Generally the preferred method to minimize the satiety-hunger cycle.

2 If intermittent feeding is the method used, the feeding techniques are the same as for nasogastric feeding.

2 Feeding is given at room temperature. Avoid cold fluid, which may cause infant discomfort.

3 If slow continuous drip method is used, the setup used is similar to the paediatric intravenous infusion using an infusion pump and small (100-250ml) closed chamber for reservoir.

a Reservoir chamber and tubing should be changed every 8-24 hours.

a To prevent growth of bacteria.

b Record input to hour. Fill reservoir as needed.

b To ensure a constant flow and minimize overinfusion directly into the jejunum.

Follow-up Phase

1 Be constantly alert for mechanical problems.

1 Tube clogging due to inadequate rinsing. Tube advancing too far into jejunum. Check protruding tube measurement. Fluid overload causing aspiration.

2 Observe infant closely to avoid potential dangers as tube passes the

2 Diarrhoea — as the tube passes through the pylorus it (the tube)

pylorus.

a Close attention to amount, type, concentration, and osmolality of feeding fluid is stressed.

3 Hold, fondle, and give positive stimulation to the infant if conditions permit. (See Preterm Infant, p.240.)

4 Accurately describe and record condition of infant and procedure, including type and amount of feeding given, amount of residual and characteristics, any signs of impending infant distress or problems.

becomes stiff due to the change in pH. A stiff tube has been reported to cause intestinal perforation. If tube becomes clogged or dislodged, it must be removed.

3 This procedure limits the normal pleasure associated with feeding. Infant needs some attention to his psychological needs in order to thrive.

SPECIMEN COLLECTION

GUIDELINES ASSISTING WITH BLOOD COLLECTION

Blood collection from a venous puncture in the extremity of an infant or young child is the same as for an adult, with the following exceptions or additions.

Equipment

1 No. 23-19 gauge short needle or scalp-vein needle
2 Smaller volume or micro blood-collecting tubes
3 Smaller tourniquet (rubber band may be used).

Procedure

Nursing Action	Rationale/Amplification
Preparatory Phase	
1 Whenever possible, involve the mother's participation in the procedure. Explain the need for test. Ask her to hold the child during the test. If necessary, immobilize the child by placing him in a mummy restraint (see p.117).	1 Infants and young children squirm. The mother's cooperation will help reassure and comfort the child. Immobilizing them allows easier access to the venipuncture site. It also helps keep infant warm.
2 Position the patient **a** *Femoral venepuncture:* Place child on his back with legs in frog-like	2 These positions allow for optimum visualization and stabilization of the patient.

position. Nurse places her hands on child's knees. (See position for bladder puncture, p. 143).

b *External jugular venepuncture:* Place child in mummy restraint and lower his head over the side of the bed or table. Stabilize his head. Crying will make external jugular vein visible and causes blood to flow more readily. This procedure is only used when superficial veins in an infant are inaccessible.

c *Antecubital fossa venepuncture:* Place the child in a supine position. The nurse stands on the side opposite the site to be used (across from the person drawing the specimen). The nurse positions her right arm across the upper part of the child's chest and grasps the shoulder at the axilla position. Her left arm is placed across the lower part of the child's chest and is used to extend the child's arm at the wrist (p. 156).

Method

1 After the specimen is collected and the needle is removed, apply pressure to the site with dry gauze for 3-5 minutes.
   a *Jugular venepuncture:* While applying pressure to the site, place the patient in an upright sitting position.
2 When the bleeding has been stopped, soothe and comfort the child before leaving him.

1 Both the femoral and jugular veins are large vessels. Since respiratory pressure is great, bleeding, oozing, and haematoma formation may result. External pressure prevents this from happening.
2 Crying and thrashing about may initiate bleeding.

Follow-up Phase

1 Check patient frequently for an hour after the procedure for oozing, bleeding, or evidence of a haematoma.
2 Record carefully and accurately:
   a Site of venepuncture
   b How patient tolerated procedure
   c Bleeding stopped or continued and for how long
   d What test the specimen was collected for.

1 Reapply pressure and report if oozing continues.

GUIDELINES: COLLECTING URINE SPECIMEN FROM THE INFANT AND YOUNG CHILD USING A STERILE URINE COLLECTING BAG

Urine collection is a safe method of obtaining urine for a specified purpose.

Purposes

1 To check urine for presence of sugar, acetone, bacteria, and other urinary products.
2 To aid in diagnosis.
3 To determine the condition of the patient.
4 To determine effectiveness of therapy.

Equipment

1 Collecting device — plastic, disposable urine bag or collector
2 Wiping material — sterile cotton balls
3 Sterile water (warm)
4 Receptacle for used swabs
5 Sterile laboratory container together with appropriate form and label.

Procedure

Nursing Action	Rationale/Amplification
Preparatory Phase	
1 Position patient so that genitalia are exposed by placing him on his back with legs in frog-like position. Assistance may be needed to hold the legs of the young child in proper position.	1 Proper positioning will facilitate cleansing and allow for proper placement of collection device.
Procedure	
1 Ensure that buttocks and external genitalia are clean. Wash with soap and water and dry thoroughly. **a** *Female:* Using cotton balls, moistened with warm sterile water, wipe labia majora from top to bottom (clitoris to anus) only once with each cotton ball. Repeat this once more.	1 This method of cleansing the female will prevent contamination of the genitalia from the anus, and will prevent contamination of the urine specimen obtained. During the cleansing, be gentle to avoid any injury or possible stimulation of urination.

Then spread labia apart with one hand wiping the labia minora in the same manner with other hand. Wipe area dry.

b *Male:* Wipe tip of penis using cotton wall balls moistened with warm sterile water, using each swab once only, in circular motion down towards the scrotum. Be certain to retract foreskin, if present. Dry the area.

2 Apply collecting bag firmly so that the opening is exposed to receive urine.

2 If collecting bag is properly and securely placed, the procedure will not have to be repeated.

3 Change nappy and comfort child; possibly give him additional clear fluids.

4 Check the patient frequently (30-45 minutes) to see if he has micturated. When patient has micturated, remove bag gently. Clean area and apply a fresh nappy.

If child has not voided within 45 minutes, procedure must be repeated.

4 The adhesive on the collecting bag may tend to be sticky. Careful removal of the bag will prevent skin injury on and around genitalia. Also avoid spilling urine out of the bag during removal.

Reapplication of bag will decrease the possibility of unreliable test results.

Follow-up Phase

1 Pour specimen into proper collecting container. Send specimen to the laboratory within 30 minutes or refrigerate.

1 Prompt delivery of specimen to the laboratory will prevent growth of organisms is an uncontrolled environment and distortion of the test results.

2 Accurately chart and describe the following in the nurse's notes:
a Time specimen collection was started and ended
b Amount of urine micturated
c Colour of urine (cloudy, clear, any sediment)
d Type of test to be done
e Condition of skin of perineal area.

GUIDELINES: ASSISTING WITH A PERCUTANEOUS SUPRAPUBIC BLADDER ASPIRATION

Percutaneous bladder aspiration is an aseptic method of entering the bladder in the suprapubic location with a needle to obtain a urine specimen.

Purposes

1 To obtain urine in an aseptic manner for culture.
2 To aid in diagnostic workup.
3 To determine condition of the patient and aid in treatment.

Equipment

1 Skin cleansing solution
2 Sterile swabs
3 Sterile gloves
4 Sterile needle, No. 21 gauge, 3.7 cm long
5 Sterile syringe, 20 ml
6 Sterile specimen container
7 Band-Aid/adhesive tape and gauze dressing.

Procedure

Nursing Action	Rationale/Amplification
Preparatory Phase	
1 Discuss need for test with mother. If possible, enable her to hold child for procedure or stand beside child and talk to him.	1 The presence of the mother will help to comfort and reassure the child.
2 Check nappy for wetness. If child has just passed urine, report this to the paediatrician or report last micturition time. In some instances a single dose of frusemide may be prescribed.	2 In order to perform a successful bladder aspiration, enough urine must be present to distend the bladder up above the pubic symphysis, so that the bladder is accessible. Frusemide causes a diuresis and results in bladder filling.
3 Position child on his back on the examining table. His head should be towards nurse, his feet towards the paediatrician. Spread his legs apart in a frog-like position. Place hands on his knees and thumbs along his side at the hip level.	3 This position allows the nurse to stabilize the child. It also gives a full view of the child, making it easier to observe him, talk to him, and soothe him.
4 Ensure that the skin over the puncture site is cleansed in an antiseptic manner.	4 To prevent infection from being introduced into the bladder by inserting the needle through unclean skin which would contaminate the specimen.
Method	
1 While the procedure is being performed, note the condition of the patient and any signs of distress.	1 Report any changes in colour or respiration rate or other signs. Soothing the child will help him to

Comfort him by talking to him and smiling at him.

2 When urine has been obtained or the procedure is discontinued and the needle is removed, apply pressure over the puncture site with a 10cm × 10cm dressing and fingers.

3 Apply dressing or Band-Aid. Apply a fresh nappy to child. Hold and comfort him for a few minutes.

Follow-up Phase

1 Check child periodically for 1 hour after procedure to see that bleeding or oozing has not occurred.

2 Note time of first micturition after procedure. Note colour of urine (it may be pink). Bloody urine should be reported to the paediatrician.

3 Accurately describe and chart the procedure, including:
a Time of procedure
b Whether or not a specimen was obtained
c How the child tolerated the procedure
d Description and amount of urine obtained
e Child's condition and activity following the procedure.

relax so that he will not move about so much. Crying increases the muscle tone of the lower abdomen, making it more difficult to insert the needle.

2 This prevents any bleeding from occurring either internally or externally. Pressure should be maintained about 3 minutes or until oozing ceases and coagulation has taken place.

3 Holding the child will help to restore and maintain a good nurse-patient relationship and will help the child to relax after a frightening and painful procedure.

1 This is not likely if pressure was applied properly after procedure and patient was left quiet.

2 It is important to note any changes in micturition pattern following the procedure, since change might indicate injury. The first micturated urine may be bloody due to a small amount of local capillary bleeding at the time of the procedure.

GUIDELINES: 24 HOUR URINE COLLECTION FROM SMALL CHILDREN

Continuous urine collection is an accurate collection of urine excreted over a specific time. (Continuous urine collection in the older child is based on the same principles and is essentially the same as for the adult patient. The importance of saving all the urine passed during the time period and keeping it separate from faeces must be stressed.)

Purposes

1   To determine accurately the rate of urine production.
2   To measure the excretion of specific chemicals produced by the body.

Methods

1   Using a urine collecting bag.
2   Using a Hollister U Bag with attached nonkink tubing.
3   Using Paul's tubing (boys only).

Nursing Action	Rationale/Amplification
Preparatory Phase	
1 Agree on urine collection period and record.	1 Necessary for accurate collection.
2 First urine passed is discarded. At the end of 24 hour period retain last specimen which overlaps into next 24 hours.	
3 Legs may need restraining. If child is sitting in chair, legs may need supporting.	3 To avoid dislodging bag or tubing and prevent oedema.
4 Offer child play activities appropriate to age. Encourage parents to continue to give physical contact.	

Note: The exact time span chosen for small children is immaterial, but it must be accurately recorded on nursing records and on laboratory forms and bottles.

Equipment (Method 1, see above)

1   10 ml syringe
2   Catheter and spigot
3   Laboratory bottle and forms.

Method

1   Proceed as on p. 141.
2   A catheter is inserted through a small opening made in top corner of bag. Secure in position with adhesive tape. Spigot catheter.
3   Inspect bag 1-2 hourly, aspirate urine micturated using syringe. Place in laboratory collection bottle.

	3 Enables each specimen to be collected without loss.

Equipment (Method 2, see p.145)

1   Hollister U Bag with attached nonkink tubing
2   Laboratory bottle and forms.

Method

1   Proceed as on p. 141.
2   Secure into neck of collecting bottle on floor free end of tubing. Collecting bag must be dependent to allow drainage of urine.

             2   Enables urine to be collected without loss.

Equipment (Method 3, see p. 145)

1   Paul's tubing of sufficient width and length.

Method

1   Proceed as on p. 141.
2   Instead of attaching bag, attach Paul's tubing which should be sufficient width to fit over penis and scrotum. Secure with adhesive tape.
3   Distal end of tubing is secured into neck of bottle attached to side of cot or bed.
4   Ensure child is nursed is semi-recumbent position and that tubing is kept free.

             4   Provides for good drainage of urine, to ensure that all specimens are collected.

Follow-up Phase

1   At end of time for collection collect last micturation which may overlap into next 24 hours.
2   Remove bag or tubing. Wash genital area. Alternatively give bath.

3   Record accurately in nursing notes end of collection. Ensure that the urine collection is sent to the laboratory immediately, appropriately labelled with completed forms.

             1   This will ensure an accurate output of the collection specimen.

             2   Will make the child comfortable whilst enabling the genital area to be examined for any irritation.

GUIDELINES: COLLECTING A STOOL SPECIMEN

Stool collection is a method of obtaining a single stool specimen from the patient.

Purposes

1 To check stool for presence of specific material, i.e. blood, ova, and parasites or bacteria
2 To aid in diagnosis
3 To determine condition or status of the patient
4 To determine effectiveness of therapy.

Equipment

1 Nappy
2 Cellophane or plastic liner (used when stool is loose or watery)
3 Tongue blade/wooden spatula
4 Specimen container.

Note: Collecting a stool specimen from an older child who is toilet-trained is the same as collecting such a specimen from an adult.

Nursing Action	Rationale/Amplification
Preparatory Phase	
1 If a specimen is needed from a patient whose stools are loose or watery enough to be absorbed in the nappy, line the nappy with a piece of Cellophane or plastic. Place this liner between the nappy and the skin. Then apply nappy to the child and position him so that his head is slightly elevated. If stools are soft or formed, simply place a fresh nappy on the child.	1 The liner and position will allow the loose stool specimen to collect in the liner and not be absorbed by the nappy.
Method	
1 Check child frequently.	1 A fresh specimen should be obtained so that test results will not be distorted by timelapse. This will also decrease the chance of contamination of the stool with urine and will prevent skin irritation from the stool.
2 Remove soiled nappy from child. Clean perineal area, apply clean nappy, and leave child comfortable.	
3 Remove small amount of stool from nappy with the tongue blade and place it in the specimen container.	
4 Ensure that labelled specimen is sent promptly to the laboratory.	4 Prompt delivery to the laboratory will prevent changes from taking place in

the specimen that could alter the test results.

Follow-up Phase

1 Accurately describe and record the following:
   a Time specimen was collected
   b Colour, amount, and consistency of stool (note any foul smell)
   c Type of specimen collected
   d Nature of test for which the specimen was collected.
   e Condition of the skin.

GUIDELINES: ASSISTING WITH A SPINAL TAP—LUMBAR PUNCTURE

A spinal tap in an infant or young child is based on the same principles and is essentially the same as for an adult, with the following exceptions.

Equipment

1   No. 21-20 gauge, 3.5 cm long spinal needle

Procedure

Nursing Action	Rationale/Amplification
Preparatory Phase	
1 In language the child understands, he should be told about the procedure and why he needs to lie in such an awkward position. The parents cooperation too should be sought and, where possible, they should be encouraged to stay during the procedure and comfort their child.	1 This understanding will help to reassure both parents and child and ensure their cooperation.
2 Position the patient. **a** *Side position* (similar to the adult): Wrap the lower extremities in a sheet, if an older child; place the patient on his side facing the nurse; flex knees and neck by placing one hand on his shoulders and head and the other on buttocks and upper thigh.	2 In either position the patient may squirm. Hold him securely to prevent him from moving and causing injury to himself or causing the spinal needle to be inserted too far resulting in a traumatic tap.

b *Sitting position:* This position is primarily used with small infants. Place infant in sitting position; extend legs and arms in front of the infant; flex his neck so chin is almost resting on chest; back is rounded by placing thumbs on his shoulders and hands along side of his hips.

Nursing Alert: Observe for signs of respiratory distress. Because the trachea in the infant is so soft, it can kink very easily when the neck is flexed. If this happens and the airway is obstructed, the infant will stop breathing. This is an emergency situation.

Follow-up Phase
1   It is not usually necessary to keep the infant or young child flat in bed following the procedure unless there are contraindications to his being up. It will help to provide play activity and offer fluids to the child.

FLUID AND ELECTROLYTE BALANCE IN CHILDREN

Basic Principles

1   Infants and small children have different proportions of body water and body fat than do adults (Table 2.2).
    a The body water of a newborn infant approaches 80% of his body weight, compared to that of an average adult male, which approaches 60%.
    b The normal infant demonstrates a rapid physiological decline in the ratio of body weight to body water during the immediate postpartum period.
    c Proportion of body water declines more slowly throughout infancy and reaches the characteristic value for adults by approximately 2 years of age.

2   Compared to adults, a greater percentage of the body water of infants and small children is contained in the extracellular compartment.
    a Infants — approximately half of the body water is contained in the cell.
    b Adults — approximately two-thirds of the body water is contained in the cell.

3   Compared to adults, the water turnover rate per unit of body weight is three or more times greater in infants and small children.
    a The child's metabolic rate is about three times that of an adult.
    b The child has more body surface in relation to weight.
    c The immaturity of kidney function in infants may impair their ability to conserve water.

Table 2.2.   Body fluids expressed as percent of body weight

Fluid	Adult		Infant
	Male	Female	
Total body fluids	60%	54%	75%
Intracellular	40%	36%	48%
Extracellular	20%	18%	27%

4   Electrolyte balance is dependent on fluid balance and cardiovascular, renal, adrenal, pituitary, parathyroid, and pulmonary regulatory mechanisms.

5   Infants and children are more vulnerable to disorders of hydration than are adults.

   a The basic principles relating to fluid balance in children make the magnitude of fluid losses considerably greater in children than in adults.

   b Children are prone to severe disturbances of the gastrointestinal tract that result in diarrhoea and vomiting.

   c Young children cannot independently respond to increased losses by increased intake. They depend on others to provide them with adequate fluid.

Common Fluid and Electrolyte Abnormalities

See Table 2.3.

General Goals of Fluid and Electrolyte Therapy

1   Repair of pre-existing deficits which may occur with prolonged or severe diarrhoea or vomiting:

   a Deficits are estimated and corrected as soon and as safely as possible.

   (1) Initial therapy is aimed at restoring blood and extracellular fluid volume in order to relieve or prevent shock and restore renal function.

   (2) Intracellular deficits are replaced slowly over 8-12 hour period after the circulatory status is improved.

2   Provision of maintenance requirements:

   a Maintenance requirements occur as a result of normal expenditures of water and electrolytes due to metabolism.

   b Maintenance requirements bear a close relationship to metabolic rate and are ideally formulated in terms of caloric expenditure.

3   Correction of concurrent losses which may occur via the gastrointestinal tract by vomiting, diarrhoea, or drainage of secretions:

Replacement should be similar in type and amount to the fluid being lost. Replacement is usually formulated as millilitres of fluid and millimoles of electrolyte replaced per millilitre of fluid and millimole of electrolyte lost.

Determining Maintenance Fluid and Electrolyte Requirements for Infants and Children

Action	Rationale
1 Determine the child's weight or surface area. Example: child weighs 5 kg.	1 Surface area is estimated from a nomogram using the child's height and weight.
2 Determine the kilojoule (caloric) expenditure per 24 hours. Example: basal kilojoules = 1134.	2 This is done by using a table such as Table 2.4, which reflects the decreased metabolic rate with increasing body weight. Similar tables are also available utilizing surface area.
3 Adjust the basal kilojoule (caloric) expenditure for temperature and activity. **a** Add 12% for each degree Celsius above a rectal temperature of 37.8 °C **b** Add 0-30% (as above) according to activity, i.e. comatose, very active Example: Temperature = 39°C $1134 \times 0.12 = 136.08$ $1134 + 136.08 = 1270.08\,kJ/24\,hours$ Child moderately active $1134 \times 0.15 = 170.1$ $1270 + 170.1 = 1440.18\,kJ/24\,hours.$	
4 Determine the average water expenditure per 100 kJ metabolized in 24 hours. **a** The usual basal water requirement is actually 1.2-3.5 ml less than is indicated by Table 2.5 because of the production of endogenous water by oxidation (i.e. the usual water requirement per 100 kJ metabolized is 26.2-28.5 ml). Example: 26.2 ml/100kJ.	4 This is done by utilizing a table such as Table 2.5. It is important to measure urine, estimate diarrhoea and perspiration so that adjustments for contemporary losses may be made if necessary.
5 Determine the maintenance fluid requirement for 24 hours. **a** Divide the total kilojoules expended in 24 hours (obtained by steps 2 and 3)	

Table 2.3   Common abnormalities of fluid and electrolyte metabolism

Substance	Major function	Abnormality	Cause	Clinical Manifestation	Laboratory Data
Water	Medium of body fluids, chemical changes, body temperature, lubricant	Volume deficit	1 Primary — inadequate water intake 2 Secondary — loss following vomiting, diarrhoea, excessive gastrointestinal obstruction, etc.	Oliguria, weight loss, signs of dehydration including: dry skin and mucous membranes, lassitude, sunken fontanelles, lack of tear formation, increased pulse, decreased blood pressure	Concentrated urine azotaemia, elevated haematocrit, haemoglobin and erythrocyte count
		Volume excess	1 Isotonic — due to clinical oedematous states such as congestive heart failure, renal disease 2 Hypotonic — due to retention of water in excess sodium	Weight gain, peripheral oedema, signs of pulmonary congestion	Oliguria, concentrated urine with reduced sodium chloride
Potassium	Intracellular fluid balance, regular heart rhythm, muscle and nerve irritability	Potassium deficit	1 Excessive loss of potassium due to vomiting, diarrhoea; prolonged cortisone, ACTH or diuretic therapy; diabetic acidosis 2 Shift of potassium into the cells such as occurs with the healing phase of burns, recovery from diabetic acidosis	Signs and symptoms variable, including weakness, lethargy, irritability, abdominal distension, and eventually cardiac arrhythmias	Low plasma K$^+$ level (may be normal in some situations); polyuria very dilute urine; hypochloraemic alkalosis
		Potassium excess	Excessive administration of potassium-containing solutions, excessive release of potassium	Variable, including: listlessness, confusion, heaviness of the legs, nausea, diarrhoea,	Elevated potassium plasma level

Element	Function	Disturbance	Causes	Signs and symptoms	Laboratory findings
			due to burns, severe kidney disease, adrenal insufficiency	ECG changes, ultimately paralysis and cardiac arrest	
Sodium	Osmotic pressure, muscle and nerve irritability	Sodium deficit	Water intake in excess of excretory capacity; replacement of fluid loss without sufficient sodium; adrenal insufficiency; malnutrition	Headache, nausea, abdominal cramps, confusion alternating with stupour, diarrhoea, lacrimation, salivation, later hypotension; early polyuria, later oliguria	Low sodium plasma level, oliguria with concentrated urine of except in severe K^+ depletion or simple overhydration
		Sodium excess	Inadequate water intake especially in the presence of fever or sweating; severe, watery diarrhoea; hyperventilation in warm, dry air, diabetes insipidus	Thirst, oliguria, weakness, muscular pain, excitement, dry mucous membranes, hypotension, tachycardia, fever	Elavated Na^+ plasma level, high specific gravity of urine
Bicarbonate balance	Acid-base	Primary bicarbonate deficit	Diarrhoea (especially in infants); diabetes mellitus; starvation; infectious disease; shock or congestive heart failure producing tissue anoxia	Progressively increasing rate and depth of respiration — ultimately becoming Kussmaul respiration: flushed, warm skin, weakness, disorientation progressing to coma	Urine pH usually less than 6; plasma bicarbonate less than 20 mmol/l; plasma pH less than 7.35
		Primary bicarbonate excess	Loss of chloride through vomiting, gastric suction, or the use of excessive diuretics; excessive ingestion of alkali	Depressed respiration, muscle hypertonicity, hyperactive reflexes, tentany, and some times convulsions	Urine pH usually above 7.0; plasma bicarbonate above 25 mmol/l (30 mmol/l in adults; plasma pH above 7.45

by 100.

Example: 1440.18 ÷ 100 = 14.14018 or 14.4

b Multiply this figure by the water expenditure per 100 kJ metabolized per 24 hours (obtained in step 4). Example: 26.2 × 14.4 = 377.28/24 hours.

6 Determine the infusion rate per hour.
a Divide the total number of millilitres to be infused by 24.
Example: 377.28 ÷ 24 = 15.72 or 16 ml/hour.

7 Electrolyte maintenance requirements are met by utilizing solutions containing:
Na+ and Cl :30 mmol/l(30 mEl)
K+ 20 mmol/l(20 mEl)

7 This is provided by:
a 5 or 10% glucose in H_2O: 800 ml
Isotonic saline: 200 ml
Potassium chloride concentrate: 5 ml
b Dextrose 4% in 0.18% of NaCl (0.18g/100ml) + 20 mmol/l of potassium chloride

8 Other electrolytes are generally not needed in the intravenous solution.

8 Calcium, magnesium, and phosphate can be mobilized from body stores to maintain stable blood levels. However, they must be provided in prolonged parenteral fluid therapy and in some clinical conditions.

9 Parenteral fluids cannot generally provide the child with his normal energy requirements.

9 Five per cent dextrose is added to normal parenteral fluids to provide energy. This minimizes the breakdown of the child's fat stores.

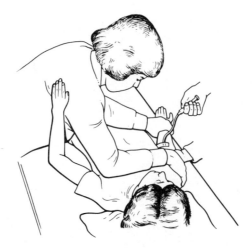

Figure 2.4 Positioning for antecubital fossa venipuncture. Mother assisting by holding child.

Table 2.4   Standard basal kilojoules and calories

Weight (kg)	Kilojoules (kJ)/24 hours Male and Female		Calories/24 hours Male and Female	
3		588		140
5		1134		270
7		1680		400
9		2100		500
11		2520		600
13		2730		650
15		2982		710
17		3276		780
19		3486		830
21		3696		880
25	4284	4032	1020	960
29	4704	4368	1120	1040
33	5082	4704	1210	1120
37	5460	4998	1300	1190
41	5670	5250	1350	1250
45	5922	5544	1410	1320

Table 2.5   Average water and electrolyte expenditure per 100 kilojoules metabolized per 100 calories metabolized per 24 hours are given in parentheses)

Route	H_2O(ml)	Na (mmol/l)	K (mmol/l)
Lungs	3.5 (15)	0 (0)	0 (0)
Skin	9.5 (40)	0.024 (0.1)	0.048 (0.2)
Stool	1.2 (5)	0.024 (0.1)	0.048 (0.2)
Urine	15.5 (65)	0.71 (3.0)	0.48 (2.0)

GUIDELINES: INTRAVENOUS FLUID THERAPY

Intravenous therapy refers to the infusion of fluids directly into the venous system. This may be accomplished through the use of a needle or by venous cut-down and insertion of a small catheter directly into the vein.

Purpose

To restore and maintain the child's fluid and electrolyte balance and body homeostasis when his oral intake is inadequate to serve this purpose.

Equipment

Needle Method

1 Intravenous solution
     The kind of solution is prescribed by the paediatrician.
2 Intravenous stand
3 Intravenous administration set
     The set should include a closed reservoir with a minidropper to ensure that the child will not receive an excessive amount of fluid in a brief period of time.
4 Syringe, 5 or 10 ml — approximately one-half to two-thirds filled with normal saline
5 Butterfly needle or catheter of appropriate gauge
     The size of the needle depends on the age and size of the child and the type of fluid to be administered.
6 Swabs — wool and gauze
7 Skin cleansing solution
8 Normal saline
9 Small tourniquet or rubber band
10 Adhesive tape, 1.2 cm, 2.5 cm, 5 cm
11 Padded armboard or polystyrene bean bag
12 Bandage for securing the extremity to the armboard
13 Restraining devices — bath blanket, extremity restraint, covered sandbags
     The type of restraint depends on the child's age, his level of cooperation, and the kind of intravenous infusion to be started.
14 Safety razor (if scalp vein is to be used).

Cutdown Method

1 Intravenous solution, intravenous stand, intravenous administration set
2 Swabs — wool and gauze
3 Adhesive tape, 1.2 cm, 2.5 cm, 5 cm
4 Padded armboard
5 Dry sponges
6 Bandage
7 Sterile cutdown tray
     The tray should include the following equipment: medicine cups, dressing towels, wound towel, syringe, No. 1-25 gauge 1.5 cm needle, No. 1-20 gauge 2.5 cm needle, knife handle and No. 15 blade, forceps, scissors, gauze sponges, 4-0 black silk suture, needle holder.
8 Assorted sizes of sterile polyethylene tubing and Luer adapters
9 5-0 black silk suture with a straight eye needle
10 1% lignocaine
11 2 ml syringe   } for local anaesthetic
12 No. 17 and 12 needles

13   Normal saline
14   Tourniquet
15   Sterile gloves
16   Restraining devices.

Procedure

Nursing Action	Rationale/Amplification
Preparatory Phase	
1 Obtain the intravenous solution.	1 Although the type of solution and the rate of flow are prescribed by the paediatrician, the nurse should be aware of the composition of common parenteral solutions and should know how to calculate maintenance therapy. (Refer to Tables 2.4 and 2.5, p. 155.)
2 Check the fluid for sediment or contaminant by holding the solution up to the light.	2 If sediment is observed, the solution should be discarded.
3 Insert the end of the administration set into the solution container's opening. Use aseptic technique.	
4 Hang solution from the intravenous stand and allow fluid to fill the tubing. Make sure that there are no air bubbles present.	4 Filling the drip chamber halfway by compressing the chamber will prevent air from entering the tubing.
5 When small quantities of intravenous fluids are to be given, the infant's giving set incorporating a graduated burette gives an accurate guide to the volume of fluid being given.	5 The danger of overloading the infant's circulatory system with fluid is lessened.
a For older children requiring larger amounts of intravenous fluids at a greater rate per hour the markings on the solution bag give a reasonably accurate guide.	
b An infusion pump impelling infusion fluid through the set at a constant preset rate is invaluable, especially in small infants. The injection site must be checked hourly to ensure that extravasation has not occurred.	**b** This helps to maintain the patency of the vein. The infusion pump is designed to function against resistance; leakage may occur through a dislodged cannula.

Nursing Alert: Because of the risk of tissue damage due to extravasation of hypertonic solutions, some paediatric units will not use infusion pumps on peripheral lines.

6 Shut off the fluid flow and keep the end of the tubing sterile until ready to connect it to the needle.

7 Promote the cooperation of the child.
a Explain procedure to mother. If possible ask her to participate and hold and comfort the child.
b Infant: Provide with a dummy if he is used to one.
c Older child: Explain the procedure and its purpose.
d Ensure that child's own assigned nurse is present.

8 Position the child so he is comfortable.

9 Restrain the child as necessary.
a Infant or young child: Restraints may include mummy wrappings, jacket or elbow restraints, small sandbags or polystyrene beanbags.

b Older child: The extremity to be used should be comfortably restrained on the armboard. Free extremities may also require light restraints to remind the child not to move.

7 The procedure will be least traumatic for the child if he is able to cooperate and is not frightened or resistant.

9 Protective devices may be necessary to prevent the child from dislodging the intravenous needle. The type and size of such devices should be appropriate for the child's age and position of the intravenous infusion.
b Toes and fingers should be visible to prevent the child from dislodging the intravenous needle. The restraint board must be padded, and the main pressure points (heel, palm) padded with gauze. Before strapping an extremity to the armboard back the adhesive with tape or gauze, wherever it touches the skin (Figure 2.5).

Method

1 Assist the paediatrician as necessary. This may involve holding the child, cutting tape, regulating fluid flow, applying the tourniquet, etc.

2 A simple method is to apply a rubber band tourniquet before inserting a scalp vein infusion.
a When applying the tourniquet, a second tourniquet is placed cross wise under it.
b To remove the tourniquet, grasp the unstretched rubber band, pull up and cut the tourniquet.

3 Check the restraints at intervals and adjust them as necessary.

3 The restraints may become loose after a period of time and must be secured to ensure the child's safety. They may also become too tight and require loosening to maintain adequate circulation.

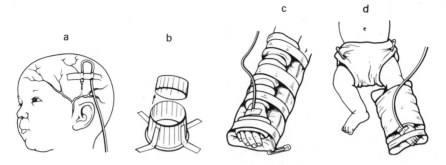

Figure 2.5 Intravenous fluid therapy: (a) venepuncture of scalp; (b) paper cup taped over venepuncture site for protection; (c) restraint of arm when hand is site of infusion; (d) infant's leg taped to sandbag or immobilization.

4 Comfort and reassure the child.

4 The procedure is usually disturbing for the child. This should be acknowledged. If crying and upset, the child should be reassured that his behaviour is acceptable.

5 Regulate the intravenous flow at the designated rate. Set infusion pump at prescribed rate.

6 Record:
   Type of solution being used
   Reading on the burette and infusion pump
   Rate of flow
   Time that the infusion began
   Site of administration
   Reaction of the child to the procedure.

Follow-up Phase

1 Check the child at least hourly.
   a Note the location of the intravenous flow.
   b Note the colour of the skin at the needle point.
   c Check for swelling of the skin at the needle point.
   (1) If in hand or foot, compare with the opposite extremity.
   (2) If in the head, look at the face to determine asymmetry.
   d Feel the area around the intravenous site for sponginess or leakage.

1 The child must be observed frequently to make certain that the intravenous flow is not infiltrating into the tissues and is functioning properly. Report any swelling, discoloration, or leakage.

e Make certain that the child is adequately restrained.

2 Observe closely for complications.

a *Local reactions:*
(1) Compromised circulation
(2) Pressure sores
(3) Thrombophlebitis.

b *Fluid and/or electrolyte disturbances:*
(1) Maintain an accurate record of intake and output.
(a) Total the intake and output every 8 or 12 hours.
(b) Describe carefully the amount and consistency of all stools and vomiting.
(c) Collect all urine and weigh soiled nappies if more accurate measurement of the child's output is necessary.
(2) Weigh the child at regular intervals, using the same scales each time.
Record the amount of clothes the child is wearing, etc.
(3) Report:
(a) Decreased skin turgor
(b) Marked increase or decrease in urination
(c) Fever
(d) Sunken or bulging fontanelles in an infant
(e) Sudden change in weight or vital signs
(f) Diarrhoea
(g) Weakness, apathy, or lethargy.

c *Pyrogenic reactions*

3 Record essential information:
a Reading on the bottle or reservoir
b Amount of fluid absorbed in the hour
c Total amount of fluid absorbed (compare with the total amount of fluid intended to have been absorbed)
d Rate of flow
e Apparent condition of the child.

2 Complications associated with the administration of intravenous fluids to infants and children are very serious and may have fatal consequences. Any signs of complications must be reported immediately.
b Refer to Table 2.3, p. 152.

(2) An increase or decrease of 5% within a relatively brief period of time is usually significant and should be reported.

c If severe, the intravenous flow should be discontinued. The solution should be saved for possible analysis.

4 Regulate the rate of flow as necessary by any of the following methods:
a Raising the height of the infusion
b Adjusting the flow regulator
c Adjusting the position of the extremity
d Removing excess tubing or coiling it on the bed

e Adjusting the restraint

d If excess tubing falls below the level of the bed, the flow is slowed because the fluid must run uphill.
e If an extremity is restrained too snugly, the restraint acts as a tourniquet and the flow of solution will be slowed or stopped.

5 Change the infusion bottle and tubing.
a Every 24 hours.

5 **a** The infusion setup should be changed daily to maintain sterility and prevent contamination of the intravenous fluid during intravenous therapy.
b To prevent clots forming in tubing.

b Following a blood transfusion.
c If blood is to follow a dextrose solution.
d If a saline solution is to be given or after the administration of Intralipid.

d To prevent particles of fat being precipitated.

6 If a catheter is used, change the dressing to the insertion side at least once every 24 hours.

6 This reduces the incidence of infection and other local complications.

7 Disconnect the intravenous flow when ordered or if it is obviously infiltrated.
a Gather equipment.
(1) Scissors.
(2) Sterile gauze swab.
(3) Elastoplast dressing or Band-Aid.
b Explain the procedure to the child, depending on his age.
c Clamp off the flow of the intravenous fluid.
d Determine the location of the needle.
e Loosen the tape around the needle, holding the needle firmly in position so that it does not slip out.
f Hold the swab lightly over the insertion site and remove the needle quickly and carefully.

f Inspect an intracath or plastic needle to ensure that no portion has been left in the vein. If this is suspected, notify the paediatrician. Alcohol-impregnated swabs should not be used for removing intravenous needles because the stinging of alcohol on the puncture site causes unnecessary discomfort.

g Apply pressure to the site immediately and hold until bleeding stops.

h Apply Elastoplast dressing or Band-Aid.

h The Band-Aid should not be applied until all bleeding has stopped to minimize the possibility of prolonged or unnoticed bleeding.

i Remove the tape and armboard from the extremity.

j Comfort the child as required.

k Note the fluid level on the infusion container or burette and complete recordings.

l Record that the intravenous flow was discontinued.

GUIDELINES: TOTAL PARENTERAL NUTRITION (HYPERALIMENTATION)

Hyperalimentation is a method of providing complete nutrition entirely by the intravenous route. It involves the infusion of hypertonic solutions of glucose, a nitrogen source, water, vitamins, minerals, and electrolytes at a constant rate through an indwelling catheter placed in a central vein, usually the superior vena cava.

The procedure has been used successfully in children with gastrointestinal diseases such as chronic diarrhoea, malabsorption syndrome, bowel fistulas, oesophageal atresia or obstruction, and omphalocele.

It is also useful when a child's condition produces excessive nutritional needs, as in the case of burns, neurosurgical procedures, major trauma, large wound infections, and cancer.

Hyperalimentation has been successful in the treatment of preterm infants of very low weights and infants with malnutrition or failure to thrive.

Purpose

To sustain life and promote growth in patients when oral or gastrointestinal tube intake is either impossible, potentially hazardous, or insufficient for an extended period of time.

Equipment

1   Hyperalimentation solution

The type, amount, and composition of the solution is ordered by the paediatrician. The concentration of glucose in the solution may be gradually increased to 20% according to the child's tolerance.

2   Micropore filter

3 Intravenous extension tubing
4 Silastic catheter of appropriate size
5 Constant infusion pump
6 Acetone
7 Betadine
8 Benzoin.

All of the equipment listed in the procedure for intravenous fluid therapy by cutdown method: see Intravenous Fluid Therapy, cutdown method, p. 156. The administration set may be a special V or W type to connect two or three solutions to one line; or if separate administration sets are used for each hyperalimentation solution, then a three-way tap or a four-way 'traffic lights' junction will be required.

Procedure

Nursing activities for all phases of the administration of hyperalimentation solution are the same as those specified in the procedure for intravenous fluid therapy, with the following additions:

Nursing Action	Rationale/Amplification
Preparatory Phase	
1 Mix the components of the hyperalimentation solution under strict aseptic conditions. Culture each bottle to assure the adequacy of the technique.	1 It is essential to prevent microbial contamination of the infusate in order to protect the child from septicaemia.
a Mixing should be done in the pharmacy, using a closed system such as a laminar flow filtered air hood.	
b In hospitals without a laminar flow system, a closed system for mixing the glucose and protein should be used.	**b** This can be done safely by carefully following package directions and using the cleanest area possible for mixing.
Procedure	
1 Assist the paediatrician with the insertion of the hyperalimentation catheter. This may involve obtaining equipment, positioning and restraining the child, etc.	
a The hyperalimentation catheter should be inserted under sterile conditions.	**a** Violation of aseptic techniques at the time of insertion can result in overwhelming septicaemia and death.
b In infants and small children the vena cava is usually approached through one of the common facial,	**b** This prevents catheter displacement by the child's movements, and allows asepsis to be maintained away

internal jugular, or (usually) external jugular veins. The free end of the catheter is passed through a subcutaneous tunnel and is anchored in place at the parietal scalp (Figure 2.6).

from the child's oral and nasal secretions.

Follow-up Phase

1 Until x-ray confirmation of the location of the catheter tip, infuse only isotonic solutions at a slow, 'keep open' rate.

1 A chest x-ray confirms proper placement of the line and rules out complications such as pneumothorax or haemothorax which may be associated with catheter insertion. Infusing an isotonic solution minimizes the possibility of complications arising from the infusion of solution through a misplaced catheter.

2 Do not use the catheter for the administration of medications or for blood sampling.

2 This increases the risk of infections and the possibility of dislodging the catheter.

3 Check the infusion rate every $\frac{1}{2}$-1 hour to make certain that the solution is infused continuously and at a constant rate.

a Use a constant-infusion pump.

b Reset the rate to that prescribed by the paediatrician as necessary, but do not slow or increase the drip to make up for an excess or deficit without consulting the paediatrician.

3 Continuous infusion is necessary to prevent such metabolic complications as osmotic diuresis, hypoglycaemia, and pulmonary oedema.

b Increasing the rate may cause hyperglycaemia with osmotic diuresis. Slowing the rate may cause hypoglycaemia.

4 Change the bottles, tubing, and filter at least once each day, wearing masks and sterile gloves.

a Remove the tape which secures the filter to the dressing.

b Attach new infusion set to the new bottles.

c Prime tubing and tap the end gently.

d Connect the infusion set to the new filter housing carefully.

e Hang the new bottle on the infusion stand.

f Remove the protective covering from the distal end of the filter and discard.

g Hold the filter parallel to the floor and run solution through the entire line.

h Gently tap the filter housing to dispel air and tap the end to free

4 This is another attempt to prevent contamination and reduce the possibility that the child will develop infection.

c This dislodges any glucose droplets.

d Avoid contamination of the filter.

g This position allows for complete filling of the filter housing.

h Air bubbles will cause difficulty in maintaining constant flow.

glucose droplets. Be careful not to contaminate the end of the filter. If a volumetric infusion pump is being used, a new cassette should be incorporated into the intravenous line at the same time.

i The patient's end is swabbed with 70% isopropyl alcohol prior to insertion into end of new intravenous line.

i Helps to reduce the possibility of introducing infection.

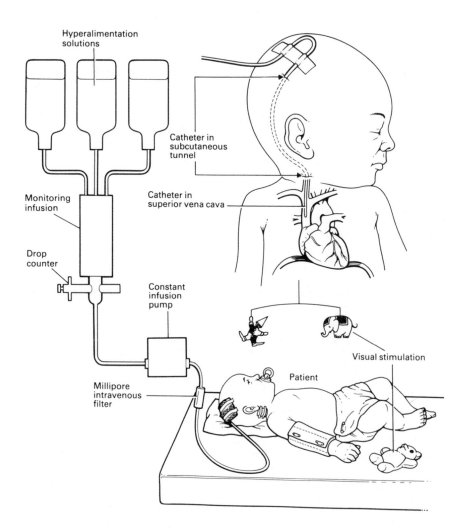

Figure 2.6 Hyperalimentation.

j Change the intravenous line at the catheter union rapidly with the patient flat in bed or in low Fowler's position. Use sterile artery forceps to grasp the catheter hub for leverage during the tubing change.

k Anchor the filter to the dressing.

l Secure all intravenous tubing joints with adhesive tape.

m Readjust flow rate.

n Write time and date on new tubing.

o Culture the filter each time it is changed.

5 Change the dressing around the catheter at least three times each week, using strict aseptic technique. Face masks should be worn by all persons at the head of the bed to prevent airborne contamination of the insertion site by nasopharyngeal organisms. If possible, the child should also wear a mask and turn his head away from the dressing.

a Remove the dressing carefully.

b Swab of site should be taken for laboratory culture.

c Using acetone or ether on a sterile 10 cm x 10 cm gauze square, scrub a large area surrounding the insertion site.

d Paint the skin with Betadine solution.

e Apply a small dressing around the catheter.
  Using sterile scissors, cut a slit in the lower piece of a small nonadhering dressing, enabling it to fit around the catheter at the insertion site.

f Apply benzoin to the area where tape will be applied.

j This technique minimizes the danger of air embolism. Using a Kelly clamp help reduce traction on the catheter and the chance of dislocation.

k This prevents tension on the catheter.

l This prevents accidental separation of the tubing from the catheter and prevents air embolus.

n It is possible, by culturing the filter to detect microbial contamination prior to the development of clinical signs.

o Cultures should include fungal studies since a special danger of hyperalimentation is fungal septicaemia.

5 This reduces the possibility of infection at the catheter site.

a Extreme care is necessary to avoid dislodging the catheter.

b For early detection of infection.

c This removes surface skin fats that might harbour organisms and removes remaining traces of adhesive tape that have adhered to the skin.

f Even nonirritating tape may produce damage to the underlying skin with prolonged use.

g Apply sterile dressings.

g In infants and small children, the catheter is coiled to reduce tension on the site, and a small, sterile gauze sponge is applied. A generous length of the catheter is left to facilitate head and body movements without undue tension on the catheter. In older children, the entire catheter is included in the dressing.

h Cover the entire sterile dressing and the union of the catheter and tubing with 5 cm adhesive tape.

i If the dressing is exposed to moisture such as tracheal secretions or humidified oxygen, protect it with a plastic adhesive.

j Record the dressing change, how the child tolerated the procedure, and any relevant condition.

h This provides a totally occlusive dressing. Neither the sterile dressing nor the tubing union is exposed to air.

i In this situation, use paper tape to secure all tubing connections and anchor the filter, because adhesive will tear holes in plastic.

j Consider condition of the skin, drainage, catheter placement, placement of needle guard, and presence of suture.

6 In infants with a cutdown site on the neck, change the dressing as needed, using aseptic technique. Discontinue the dressing when the wound is healed.

7 Test urine daily for glucose and acetone. Report any glycosuria.

6 Since this site is closest to the vascular bed, it should be observed closely for signs of infection. Wound sepsis can easily lead to bacteraemia.

7 Some children require supplemental parenteral insulin to utilize the required amount of infused glucose. Children receiving certain drugs may show false positive results. Positive urine sugars are confirmed by blood glucose levels.

8 Keep an accurate record of the child's total intake and output, including bowel movements, emesis, and gastric drainage. If the child is allowed oral intake, a calorie count should be kept.

9 Monitor the child's weight daily. Weigh at the same time each day, with the same amount of clothing, and on the same scales.

10 In infants, measure length and head circumference weekly.

11 Observe for signs of complications resulting from therapy.

    a Complications related to the catheter:
    (1) Septicaemia
    (2) Thrombosis of a major blood vessel

8 This helps to provide a clear picture of the child's fluid and electrolyte balance.

9 Weight gain is one of the most reliable indications of a positive response to therapy. It also indicates any hidden retention of fluid.

10 Hyperalimentation promotes growth in these dimensions.

    a Three-quarters of the major complications of therapy are of this variety. Sepsis accounts for more than half of these problems.

(3) Plugging or dislodging of the catheter

(4) Local skin infection

(5) Cardiac arrhythmia

(6) Leak around catheter or hole in catheter

(7) Air embolism.

b Metabolic complications:

(1) Hyperglycaemia

(2) Hypoglycaemia

(3) Dehydration

(4) Metabolic acidosis

(5) Electrolyte imbalances

(6) Amino acid imbalance

(7) Postinfusion hypoglycaemia.

b Careful clinical and chemical monitoring, especially during the initial period of hyperalimentation, can greatly reduce the incidence of these types of complications.

12 Frequent mouth care, should be given.

a If allowed use a variety of mouthwashes to provide some change in taste.

b Sips of iced water if allowed.

c Offer favourite iced lollies to suck if allowed.

12 For those patients who are not allowed anything by mouth, the tongue, throat and mouth tend to become dry, inflamed, and uncomfortable. The total absence of taste is unpleasant for older children, and for those only being given small amounts by mouth.

13 Provide the infant with a dummy.

13 It is especially important to meet the sucking needs of the infant since hyperalimentation therapy may be necessary for several weeks or months.

14 Discontinue the infusion when ordered.

a Turn the flow rate off.

b Remove the dressings.

c Cut and remove the stay suture.

d Pull the catheter out.

e Apply pressure with a 10cm x 10cm sterile gauze for a minute or two.

f Cover the site with a Band-Aid or Elastoplast dressing.

g Record time and date procedure was discontinued, by whom, cultures sent, and child's condition.

h Send the tip of the catheter, the filter, and the fluid in the tubing for culture.

14 The child is gradually tapered off from hyperalimentation to allow for adjustment to decreased levels of glucose. Final cessation is often followed by isotonic glucose infusion for at least 12 hours to protect against rebound hypoglycaemia from still high insulin levels. During the weaning process, the child's oral intake is gradually increased as the hyperalimentation solution is proportionally decreased.

GUIDELINES: ASSISTING WITH EXCHANGE TRANSFUSION

Exchange transfusion is replacement of circulating blood by withdrawing blood and injecting donor's blood in equal amounts.

Purposes

1　To prevent accumulation of bilirubin in the blood above a dangerous level.
2　To prevent kernicterus (brain damage — occurs when there is yellow staining of brain tissue from deposits of indirect bilirubin).
3　To prevent accumulation of other by-products of haemolysis from haemolytic disease, i.e. ABO incompatibility.
4　To raise a very low haemoglobin at birth when haemoglobin level is 15 g/dl or less.
5　To replace red blood cells which have poor oxygen releasing capacity and poor carbonic anhydrase activity, i.e. as in a preterm infant.
6　To remove toxic metabolites.

Equipment

1　Fresh donor blood
2　Monitoring equipment
3　Sterile disposable exchange transfusion
　　set containing:
　　Instruments
　　Stopcock with extension tubing
　　Extra extension tubing
　　Umbilical catheters of varying sizes
　　Two 20 ml syringes
　　One 5 ml syringe and No. 23 gauge needle
　　Waste-blood container
　　Blood administration set
　　Gauze sponges
4　Transfusion record
5　Cleansing solution
6　Means of warming infant
7　Blood warming apparatus set at 35°C
8　10% calcium gluconate
9　50% glucose solution in 10 ml syringe
10　Sodium bicarbonate in 10 ml syringe
11　Sterile gown and gloves for paediatrician
12　Resuscitative equipment
13　Appropriate laboratory forms and specimen bottles for bilirubin and haemoglobin estimation.

Procedure

Note: This procedure is a lengthy one of at least 2 hours and preferably longer when jaundice is severe. Staff participating should check that everything is available before commencement. They should have stools to sit on comfortably during the procedure. Two nurses are needed, one to observe, care, and comfort the infant, the other to maintain accurate records and to assist the doctor as required.

Nursing Action	Rationale/Amplification
Preparatory Phase	
1 Place infant under heat lamps or radiant heating unit to keep his temperature within the thermoneutral zone. Environment temperature of 32°C will usually maintain correct infant body temperature, depending on size of infant.	1 Chilling of the infant during the procedure can result in apnoea and in increased caloric need and oxygen consumption, which can be exhausting to a baby with already limited amount of energy. Abnormal decrease in blood pH leading to acidosis can result from the stress of prolonged chilling.
2 If the infant has been fed during the previous 3-4 hours it may be necessary to empty stomach content via stomach tube.	2 To prevent aspiration, should vomiting occur during the procedure.
3 Urine collection bag may be placed in position (see p.141.)	3 To avoid possible contamination of site and equipment.
4 Attach electronic cardiac monitoring device to infant if available. Otherwise place stethoscope over apex of heart. Also attach temperature monitoring device.	4 Apnoea, bradycardia, and cardiac arrest are complications of an exchange transfusion. Close monitoring will allow for immediate observation of signs of trouble.
5 Place infant on his back. Restrain all four extremities.	5 This will prevent the infant from moving and inadvertently pulling out the exchange catheter.
6 Have resuscitative equipment ready for immediate use: oxygen supply, mask, intubation equipment, laryngoscope, breathing bag, suction, sodium bicarbonate, and 50% glucose solution.	6 Should the infant develop bradycardia, hypoglycaemia, or cyanosis during procedure, these items will be necessary for immediate and supportive treatment.
7 Check donor blood for type, age and other identifying data.	7 Freshly donated blood — group O Rhesus negative or the ABO group of the infant and compatible with the mother's serum is used to avoid incompatibility problems.
8 Assist the paediatrician in setting up blood and exchange equipment. Blood should be run through a coil of tubing through a water bath at 38°C.	8 Although hypothermia, i.e. rapid chilling of the infant, is a primary concern, increased blood viscosity and ventricular fibrillation can also result from administering cold blood.

Method

1 The infant's skin is cleansed with soap and water followed by an antiseptic solution. Sterile towels are applied by the paediatrician who is gowned and gloved. Strict attention should be paid to maintaining aseptic technique.

1 To prevent infection or sepsis. A foreign body introduced into the blood vessel is always a potential for infection due to an infected cord stump or contaminated equipment.

The umbilicus can be grossly contaminated and is impossible to sterilize.

2 Once the umbilical catheter is in place in the umbilical vein, the initial venous pressure is measured (although it is not usually accurate) and the exchange is begun. (Preferred site is the umbilical artery; jugular or femoral vessels may be used.)

2 Record the venous pressure. This will be maintained at about 10-12 cm by equal volume exchanges. An increase in pressure during the procedure is an indication to stop and assess the infant.

3 Note and record the time the exchange started. Record each successive withdrawal and infusion of blood stating exact amount and time. Report to the paediatrician when each 100 ml of blood is exchanged. (see Figure 2.7, p.172).

This will prevent system overload from excessive infusion — resulting in cardiac failure and shock from too-rapid removal of infant's blood.

3 Blood is exchanged slowly in amounts of 5-20 ml, depending on the infant's size and condition. The total amount exchanged is about 170 ml of blood per kilogram of body weight. About 75-85% of the infant's total blood volume is exchanged.

The exchange should never take less than 2 hours. Rapid exchange can aggravate cardiovascular changes.

4 After each 100 ml of blood is exchanged, 1 ml of 10% calcium gluconate is cautiously injected. Monitor cardiac rate very carefully during the injection.

4 Calcium decreases the irritability and irregularity of the heart. Too rapid an injection will cause bradycardia.

5 Constant monitoring of the cardiac rate is imperative. Also note respirations, skin colour, and colour of withdrawn blood.

Keep transfusion lines tightly secured to prevent air embolus or exsanguination.

5 Observation and monitoring will allow immediate treatment if untoward signs appear. Bradycardia may occur at any time during the procedure due to a low pH of donor blood or if old blood is given.

6 Protamine sulphate may be given after the transfusion is completed.

6 Because heparinized blood will affect the coagulation potential of the infant from 4-6 hours postexchange.

Follow-up Phase

1 When transfusion is completed, umbilical catheter may be:
a Left in place with an umbilical obturator or intravenous infusion

1 If catheter is left in place, it is usually done for the future exchange transfusions, easy withdrawal of blood for blood studies, administration of intra-

NEONATAL UNIT **EXCHANGE TRANSFUSION RECORD** Date					No. XYZ 1234 Surname SMITH First Names David Russell D. of B. 11/12/80　　　Sex　M	
Time	In	Out	Total In	Total Out	H.A.B.	Observations
10·25					140	Temp 36⁸ B/P ⁸⁵/45 C.V.P. +4
10·30		10		10	142	Pre-exchange specimen saved.
10·34	10		10		138	Baby quiet, colour good. C.V.P.+3
10·35		10		20	140	Dextrostix 90 in gms %
10·39	10		20		160	Baby restless
10·41		10		30	146	Quieter now.
10·45	10		30		142	
10·47		10		40	140	B/P ⁸⁰/50
10·51	10		40		138	
10·52		10		50	138	Settled.
10·56	10		50		140	
10·58		10		60	142	
11·03	10		60		144	Temp 36² Incubator temperature raised.
		Continue with cycles of 10 ml in / 10 ml out at 4-5 minute intervals. Regular observations of vital signs maintained. finally :—				
12·50	10			320	144	Specimen saved for laboratory
12·54		10	320		148	B/P ⁸⁵/40　　C.V.P. +4 Dextrostix 45.90 in — %
			Baby left comfortably settled. Mother will come from post-natal ward shortly to sit with David.			

Figure 2.7　Exchange transfusion record.

b Removed.

c A dry dressing is secured in position.

2 Finish charting by recording accurately:

    a Time transfusion was completed

    b Total amount blood withdrawn and infused

    c Any changes in vital signs

    d Medications administered during exchange

    e Infant's colour and current vital signs

    f Catheter removed or left indwelling

    g How infant tolerated the procedure

    h Any blood samples taken before or after exchange.

3 Observe infant closely after the procedure: respirations, pulse (heart rate), temperature, evidence of lethargy or jitteriness, increasing jaundice, pigmentation of urine, cyanosis, oedema, or convulsions. Report any of these signs immediately.

    Change infant's position frequently, but handle gently and minimally following procedure.

venous fluids and medications. Keep infant restrained. If catheter is removed, apply small pressure dressing and observe for any bleeding. Check the area every hour for 3 hours, then every 3 hours for 24 hours.

3 The complications associated with an exchange transfusion can be: heart failure, hypocalcaemia, hypoglycaemia, sepsis, acidosis, shock, hyperkalaemia (from old blood), transfusion reaction, and necrotizing enterocolitis.

CHEST PHYSIOTHERAPY

GUIDELINES: PROMOTING POSTURAL DRAINAGE

Physiotherapy is a specialty, using treatment by natural forces, and demands special training and qualifications. However, in certain situations a nurse may be called upon to carry out the following physiotherapy exercises in the absence of the physiotherapist. It is important that the nurse and the physiotherapist consult and plan together the programme of suitable exercises for each child.

Postural drainage is the positioning of the patient so that gravity will assist in the movement of secretions from the smaller bronchial airways to the main bronchus and trachea, from which the secretions can be removed by coughing or suctioning.

Procedure

Nursing Action	Rationale/Amplification
Preparatory Phase	
1 Assess the child's respiratory status. **a** Obtain a baseline respiratory rate. **b** Observe for respiratory distress, retractions, nasal flaring, etc.	1 This is necessary in order to evaluate the effectiveness of the therapy.
2 Identify the involved portion(s) of the lung on consultation with the physiotherapist.	2 The positions selected for drainage will depend on what portion of the lung is involved.
3 Explain the procedure to the child and/or the parent.	3 This allays anxiety and helps to secure the child's cooperation.
4 Make the child comfortable. **a** Remove constricting clothes. **b** Flex the child's knees and hips.	**b** To assist in relaxing and decreasing strain on the abdominal muscles during coughing.
c Have tissues and a vomit bowl available.	**c** To collect mucus.
d Have several pillows available.	**d** To facilitate positioning.
5 Provide bronchodilator and/or nebulization therapy if indicated.	5 It is easier to raise mucus mechanically after the bronchi are dilated and the secretions are thinned.

Nursing Alert: Postural drainage should not be done immediately after meals because it may induce vomiting.

Table 2.6   Postural drainage positions

Area of lung to be drained	Position	Area of percussion
Upper lobes, left and right anterior apical segments	Child sitting, leaning slightly backward	Percuss over the top of shoulder and anterior thorax. Hand, in cupped position, should be over the clavicle
Upper lobes, left and right posterior apical segments	Child sitting, leaning slightly forward	Percuss over the upper posterior thorax. Fingers should be contoured over the top of the child's shoulders
Upper lobes, left posterior segment	Child sitting, slightly reclined and rotated to the right. (Infant may be positioned on stomach with left shoulder elevated on nurse's arm)	Percuss over the left scapula
Upper lobes, right posterior segment	Child lying flat and rotated on to the left side. (Infant may be positioned on stomach with right shoulder elevated on nurse's arm)	Percuss over the right scapula
Upper lobes, left and right anterior segments	Child lying flat on back	Percuss the anterior chest directly under the clavicles. Avoid direct pressure on the sternum
Upper lobe, lingular segment	Child lying on right side, rotated back one-quarter turn and tilted 30°	Percuss over the left breast
Right middle lobe	Child rotated one-quarter turn from supine position on to the left side and tilted 30°	Percuss over the right breast
Lower lobes, left and right apical segments	Child lying flat in prone position	Percuss below the inferior angle of the scapula
Lower lobes, left and right anterior basal segments	Child lying on back, tilted about 45°	Percuss slightly above the lower ribs
Lower lobe, left lateral basal segment	Child lying on right side, tilted about 45°	Percuss the left lateral thorax at the level of the 8th rib
Lower lobe, right lateral basal segment	Child lying on left side, tilted about 45°	Percuss the right lateral thorax at the level of the 8th rib
Lower lobes, left and right posterior basal segment	Child lying on stomach, tilted about 45°	Percuss just above the 11th and 12th ribs

Method

1 Place the child in a series of appropriate positions.

   a The area to be drained should be elevated and its respective bronchus placed in a vertical position. (Specific drainage positions are described in Table 2.6, p. 165.)

   b The spine should be as straight as possible to permit optimal expansion of the rib cage.

2 Unless contraindicated, cup the chest wall for 1-2 minutes.

3 Have the child inhale deeply; then as he exhales, vibrate the chest wall during three to five exhalations.

4 Encourage the child to cough.

5 Allow the child to rest for a minute, then repeat cupping, vibration, and coughing until no more mucus is produced or the child's condition indicates that the procedure should be stopped.

6 Provide for patient safety.

---

1 The positions are selected and modified according to the lung area involved, the child's age and general condition, and equipment such as intravenous infusion, tracheostomies, monitors, ventilators, etc.

   b Infants are positioned on the nurse's lap; older children may be treated on a tilt board or in bed.

2 More secretions can be raised in a shorter period of time when cupping and vibration are added to posturing.

4 Infants and young children may require suctioning.

5 Total treatment time should generally not exceed 20-30 minutes.

   a In acute conditions such as atelectasis, postural drainage may be done for 5 minutes out of every hour.

   b In chronic conditions such as cystic fibrosis, postural drainage may be done between two and five times per day for 15-30 minutes.

6 Stay with the child during the procedure, especially when he is in a head-down position.

Follow-up Phase

1 Assist the child slowly to resume a normal position.
2 Provide a mouthwash or mouth care.

3 Assess and record the effectiveness of the procedure and how well it was tolerated by the child.

---

1 It may take a few minutes for the child to regain his equilibrium.
2 This removes residual mucus from the child's mouth and promotes comfort.

Cupping and Vibrating the Paediatric Patient

1   Cupping, or percussion, should be performed with a cupped hand, contoured to the thorax. For infants, it may be more effective to use cupped fingers or a small face mask from a self-inflating bag. (If this method is used, the rim should be filled with air so that it is firm.) In some infant units a

battery-operated toothbrush is used — a separate head for each child. This method has the advantage of giving even and controlled chest vibration.

2   Light clothing or a single thickness nappy may be used between the therapist's hand and the child's chest to minimize discomfort during the procedure.

3   A hollow sound should be produced by the trapped air between the cupped hand and the patient. A slapping sound indicates that the hand is not cupped enough.

4   Cupping should not be performed directly over recent incisions, open wounds, or drainage tubes.

5   Cupping should be discontinued immediately if the percussion site is noted to be reddened.

GUIDELINES: ASSISTING THE PATIENT TO COUGH

Coughing is the process of expelling air suddenly and noisily from the lungs through the glottis.

Purpose

To clear secretions from the airways.

Procedure

Nursing Action	Rationale/Amplification
Preparatory Phase	
1 Position the child to help loosen and drain secretions.	1 **a** Turn side to side. **b** Position for postural drainage as indicated. (See p. 175.)
2 Administer appropriate medications and allow time for them to take effect.	2 Medications may be utilized to loosen secretions or decrease pain awareness.
3 Explain the procedure to the child and/or parents.	3 This helps to secure the child's cooperation.
4 Position the child for optimal chest expansion.	4 The head should be elevated as high as possible.
Method	
1 If the child has had surgery, splint the operative area with a pillow or by placing your hands on either side of the operative site.	1 This decreases the pain associated with the procedure by decreasing movement in the area.
2 Have the child take three or four deep breaths with emphasis on complete exhalation. Have him attempt to cough at the end of a series of deep breaths.	2 This helps to stimulate the cough reflex. Full exhalation causes secretions to be moved into the larger airways where mechanical cough receptors are present.

3 Repeat the procedure according to the child's tolerance until the airways are cleared.

4 Additional techniques for stimulating a cough in paediatric patients:

a Offer cold fluids or ice chips.

b Have the child swallow several times in sequence.

c Apply manual pressure by using an up-and-down movement of the finger with firm steady pressure over the trachea above the manubrial arch.

3 Suctioning may be indicated if the child is unable to produce an effective cough.

4 These techniques cause an irritating sensation in the trachea, triggering the cough reflex.

Follow-up Phase

1 Provide mouth care.

2 Assess and record the effectiveness of the cough, the amount and nature of the secretions, and successful techniques for stimulating the child to cough.

1 This removes residual mucus from the child's mouth and promotes comfort.

Assisting the Paediatric Patient with Breathing Exercises

Nursing Considerations

1 Breathing exercises must be performed routinely and diligently to be effective. Whenever possible, the same nurse should instruct and work with the child.

2 The respiratory tract should be free of secretions. If indicated, aerosol treatments, postural drainage, coughing, or suctioning should be done prior to deep breathing exercises.

3 The child should be relatively free of pain. If necessary, pain medication should be administered and time allowed for it to take effect before breathing exercises are initiated.

Operative incisions should be splinted.

4 The nurse should be relaxed and unhurried. Her tone of voice, approach, and mannerisms affect the child's ability to relax.

5 The child should be positioned to eliminate excessive muscular activity.

a Flexion of the hips and knees reduces tension of the abdominal muscles, aiding inspiration.

b Supporting the upper extremities on pillows relieves the thorax of this additional weight during inspiration.

c The position for breathing exercises depends on the specific pulmonary problem and its severity as well as on the child's age and general condition.

6   Techniques to facilitate diaphragmatic breathing:
Have the child place a book or favourite small toy on his abdomen. Instruct him to make the book fall off as he takes air in and makes his abdomen round. Have him watch his abdomen get flat as he blows all the air out. The chest should move as little as possible.

7   Techniques to facilitate pursed-lip breathing:
a Blow cotton balls or ping-pong balls across a bedside table.
b Blow bubbles.
c Blow a harmonica or party favour.
d Blow a pinwheel.
e Suspend a ping-pong ball on a string from an overhead bar or doorframe. Have the patient see how long he can keep it propelled away before he needs to inhale. He should attempt to increase his time.

8   Techniques to facilitate deep breathing:
a Rebreathing tube.
b Blowing up balloons or examining surgical gloves.
c Blowing bubbles.

GUIDELINES: SUCTIONING

Suctioning is a method for removing excessive secretions from the airway. Suction may be applied to the oral, nasopharyngeal, or tracheal passages.

Procedure

To provide a patent airway by keeping it clear of excessive secretions.

Equipment

1   Suction source
2   Suction catheter with vent
3   Connecting tube
4   Sterile basin (for tracheal and tracheostomy suctioning)
5   Sterile distilled water
6   Tissues
7   Sterile towel
8   Sterile gloves (for tracheal and tracheostomy suctioning)
9   Collection bottle
10 Tongue blades

Procedure

Nursing Action	Rationale/Amplification

Oral Suctioning

Preparatory Phase

1 Gather equipment, including extra catheters of the appropriate size. Connect collection bottle and tubing to vacuum source.

2 Establish the need for suctioning by observing respirations.

3 Wash hands thoroughly.

4 Turn on suction to check system and regulate pressure if indicated and if equipment makes it possible.

5 Fill basin with sterile distilled water.

6 Position child on his side, with his head slightly lowered. If necessary, seek an assistant or the parent to help maintain the child in this position.

7 Attach catheter to suction tubing; use a glove when handling catheter.

8 Place catheter tip in the basin and draw sterile distilled water through it.

Method

1 Use padded tongue blades to separate the teeth, if necessary.

2 Leave vent open to air and introduce catheter into the area to be suctioned.

---

1 Since suctioning is often done on an emergency basis, it is mandatory that the nurse keep the necessary equipment at the bedside.

2 The frequency of suctioning will vary with each patient. The need will be evidenced by noisy, moist respirations in a child who is unable to cough adequately.

4 Recommendations for *negative pressure*

	Portable Suction
Infants	7.5-12.5 cm Hg
Children	12.5-25 cm Hg

	Wall Suction
Infants	102-152 cm Hg
Children	152-290 cm Hg

With excessive suction, catheter may adhere to the mucosa and cause trauma as it is withdrawn.

6 This position aids in pooling and draining secretions.

7 Wear a glove to keep the catheter clean and to keep the nurse's hand clean.

8 This checks the patency of the system, lubricates catheter, and allows some water in the collection bottle which will prevent aspirated secretions from sticking to it.

1 This prevents the child from biting the catheter.

2 Area may include cheeks, beneath the tongue, and back of mouth. Avoid overstimulation of the gag reflex to prevent vomiting.

3 Occlude vent with thumb and slowly withdraw catheter while rotating it between the thumb and finger. If catheter 'grabs' remove thumb to stop suction.

4 Dip catheter in and out of the basin, drawing sterile distilled water through it to clean it.

5 Repeat steps 1-4 as necessary, suctioning no longer than 10 seconds at a time and allowing 1-3 minutes between suctioning periods (unless abundance of secretions makes this impossible).

3 If catheter is allowed to remain in one place, the mucous membrane will be drawn against it. This will occlude the catheter and injure the tissues.

4 Use 50-100 ml of water to clean catheter adequately. The bubbles created by the interrupted flow of water through the catheter increase the mechanical cleansing action.

5 Prolonged suctioning can produce laryngospasm, profound bradycardia and/or cardiac arrhythmias from vagal stimulation and loss of oxygen.

Follow-up Phase

1 Turn off suction source, detach catheter from tubing, and wrap tubing in sterile towel. Discard disposable catheter.

2 Make child comfortable and give mouth care.

3 Assess effectiveness by observing respirations and auscultating lungs.

4 Record the following:
   a Amount, colour, and consistency of secretions
   b Coughing
   c Dyspnoea
   d Cyanosis
   e Frequency of suctioning
   f Any bleeding
   g Response of child to suctioning.

5 The suction jar should be emptied as necessary. The jar and tubing should be replaced with further sterilized ones at least daily.

1 Ideally, a new catheter is used each time suctioning is required. The connecting tube should be changed at the end of each tour of duty, or more often if necessary.

3 Respirations should be quiet and occur with less effort.

Nasopharyngeal Suctioning

Preparatory Phase

This is the same as for oral suctioning. In addition, the nurse should:

1 Measure the distance between the tip of the child's nose and the tragus of the

1 The catheter tip will reach the naso-pharynx.

ear to determine how far to insert catheter.

Method

1 Leaving the vent in the catheter open, elevate the tip of the nose and introduce the catheter along the floor of the nose (with the patient facing straight ahead).

1 This position will facilitate introduction of the catheter.

2 If obstruction is encountered, do not force, but remove and insert at another angle or try the other nostril.

2 Some resistance should be expected when the catheter reaches the nasopharynx.

3 Follow steps 3-5 of the procedure for oral suctioning. Alternate nostrils when introducing the catheter.

3 Alternating nostrils will ensure cleaning of both nasal passages and will minimize trauma to either side.

Follow-up Phase

This is the same as for oral suctioning.

Nasotracheal Suctioning

Preparatory Phase

1 Follow steps 1-4 of the Guidelines for oral suctioning

2 Make certain that an oxygen source is available.

2 This procedure may produce hypoxia and necessitate oxygen therapy.

3 Using aseptic technique, fill a sterile basin with sterile distilled water.

3 Tracheal suctioning should be done with sterile equipment to minimize the danger of infection.

4 Position child facing straight ahead with his neck slightly hyperextended.

4 This position facilitates introduction of the catheter.

5 Open the package containing the sterile catheter. Wear a sterile glove on the hand that will handle the catheter. Attach the catheter to the suction tubing.

5 From now until termination of the procedure, this hand should touch only the catheter.

6 Place catheter tip in the basin and draw sterile distilled water through it.

6 This checks the patency of the system, lubricates catheter, and allows some water in the collection bottle which will prevent aspirated secretions from sticking to it.

Method

1 Leaving the vent in the catheter open, elevate the tip of the nose and introduce the catheter along the floor of the nose (with the patient facing straight ahead).

1 This position will facilitate introduction of the catheter.

2 If obstruction is encountered, do not force, but remove and insert at another angle or try the other nostril.

2 Some resistance should be expected when the catheter reaches the nasopharynx.

3 Move catheter forward slowly until it enters the trachea — when the following may happen:
  a Child may cough.
  b Air will be felt from vent in catheter on expiration.
  c Voice or cry may change.
  d Child may show marked anxiety.
4 When catheter is in the trachea, occlude vent with the thumb of the ungloved hand and slowly withdraw catheter while rotating it between the thumb and finger.
5 Remove thumb from vent for several seconds between inspirations.

6 Dip catheter in and out of the basin, drawing sterile distilled water through it to clean it.

7 If necessary repeat steps 1-6 as required with another sterile catheter and glove suctioning no longer than 5 seconds at one time and allowing 1-3 minutes between suctioning periods (unless the secretions are too abundant).

3 Pulling the tongue forward (using a gauze swab) and having the patient take several deep breaths may help in advancing the catheter into the trachea.

4 If catheter grabs, remove thumb from vent to stop suction.

5 Suctioning must be stopped at intervals to prevent hypoxia. During normal suctioning, 4 litres of air will be pulled out of the lungs in 15 seconds.
6 Use 50-100 ml of water to clean catheter adequately. The bubbles created by the interrupted flow of water through the catheter increase the mechanical cleansing action.
7 If child is receiving oxygen, provide oxygen, during these rest periods.

Nursing Alert: Tracheal suction can result in laryngospasm. This may be recognized as obstructed respiration (rapid and laboured with inspiratory stridor) and may rapidly progress to complete apnoea. The nurse should call for assistance; she should straighten the airway by hyperextending the patient's neck and pulling his jaw forward and should administer oxygen.

Follow-up Phase

1 Follow the same procedure as for oral suctioning.
2 Administer oxygen if it is required by the patient's condition.

GUIDELINES: CARE OF A CHILD WITH A TRACHEOSTOMY

Kinds of Tracheostomy Tubes for Paediatric Patients

1 Plastic (polyvinyl chloride ot Silastic) tubes, usually without an inner cannula
2 Silver tubes consisting of three parts: obturator, inner cannula, and outer cannula
3 An inflatable cuffed tube may be used to achieve an airtight seal when prolonged positive ventilation is required to maintain life.

Common Reasons for Performing Tracheostomies

1 Laryngotracheal bronchitis
2 Congenital abnormalities such as laryngeal stenosis, choanal atresia, and various anomalies of the heart and lung
3 Foreign bodies lodged in the hypopharynx or larynx
4 Severe chest trauma
5 Burns of the head and neck
6 Laryngeal oedema from prolonged intubation
7 Management of secretions and provision of assisted ventilation post-operatively.

Nursing Management

Nursing Action	Rationale/Amplification
Physical Care of Patient	
1 Provide adequate humidity, usually via a ventilator, humidifier, or tent.	1 The natural humidifying pathway of the oropharynx is no longer used. Mist will loosen mucus and secretions and reduce the chances of a mucus plug.
2 Aspirate secretions (using sterile technique) whenever indicated by noisy respiration, retractions, poor colour, or change in vital signs.	2 It takes a very small amount of secretions to obstruct a small tube.
3 Suction the child after he has had nebulization therapy, chest therapy, and postural drainage.	3 The secretions will be more liquid, more copious, and more easily removed following these procedures.
4 Observe closely for rising pulse rate and restlessness.	4 These are the first clinical signs of respiratory insufficiency and should be followed by careful tracheobronchial toilet.

5 Monitor respirations frequently and observe for unequal chest expansion.

5 This might indicate the development of a pneumothorax.

6 Keep the area around the tube clean and dry:

a Cleanse area with an applicator dipped in hydrogen peroxide.

b Observe the site for bleeding and irritation.

c Place an unfrayed sterile dressing around the tube and under the tapes that hold the tube in position.

6 To minimize irritation and the risk of infection.

7 Observe the child closely to prevent accidental removal of the tube. Arm restraints may be necessary.

a Have necessary equipment available at the bedside:

(1) Duplicate tracheostomy tubes with tapes attached

(2) Tracheostomy set for emergency tracheostomy including a tracheal dilator

(3) Materials for suctioning and cleansing tubes

(4) Materials for cleansing stomal site.

b Never immerse the child in a full bath.

7 These are safety precautions.

b To prevent water from entering the airway.

8 Make certain that the tapes which hold the tube in place are tied securely with the proper amount of tension.

8 This prevents the tube from slipping out of place as the child becomes distressed or frightened or moves about.

Special Considerations for the Infant

1 Position the infant with his neck extended by placing a small roll under his shoulders.

1 An infant has a tendency to occlude the tube with his chin when his neck is flexed.

2 Support the infant's head when moving him.

2 Sudden movements of the head and neck can cause the tube to slip out.

3 When feeding, cover the tracheostomy. A bib may be used for older infants and young children.

3 This prevents food particles from dropping into the tube.

Psychosocial Care of Patients

1 Explain, at the level of the child's understanding, the reasons for the tracheostomy and for all procedures and treatments.

1 The child's fantasies about what is happening and why may be more frightening than the truth.

2 Allay fears and anxieties of parents by explanations and support.

2 Parental attitudes are conveyed to the child.

3 Provide some means of communication such as gesture, lip reading, magic slate, pad and pencil. An older child may enjoy alphabet letters or a word board.

3 The child is unable to communicate verbally.

4 Make sure that a call bell is within easy reach of the child, and answer it promptly.

4 The child is dependent on others to meet even his most basic needs. Prompt attention to his needs will help the child build trust in the nursing personnel.

5 Whenever possible, assign one nurse to meet child's total nursing care needs.

5 It takes time for a child to develop trust in strangers. He will be frightened by constantly changing personnel.

6 Provide an environment that will support the child's developmental potentials.

6 The child's developing sense of identity is threatened. He may be deprived of the ability to perform tasks that he has recently mastered.

Nursing Considerations if the Child is Discharged with a Tracheostomy Tube in Place

1   Involve the parents with the child's care as soon as possible. First, explain procedures and their rationale, and have them observe. Gradually turn more of the procedure over to them under nursing supervision.
2   Teach at the parent's level and pace of understanding.
3   Help parents to obtain necessary equipment. Make sure that they have a very specific list of the equipment (and the amounts needed).
4   Make certain that parents know what to do and where to go in an emergency.
5   If possible, put parents in contact with other families who have managed children at home with tracheostomies.
6   Refer to community nursing services before discharge. Enable the district nurse to visit child in ward prior to return home.
7   Provide the parents with a written procedure to study and take home.
8   Assist parents to appreciate the normality of their child and to recognize his needs for an environment that will support developmental potentials.
9   Refer to social worker if appropriate.

GUIDELINES: OXYGEN THERAPY FOR CHILDREN

General Nursing Responsibilities

Nursing Action	Rationale/Amplification
1 Explain the procedure to the child and allow him to feel the equipment and the oxygen flowing through the tube, mask, etc.	1 The child will be reassured if he understands the procedure and knows what to expect.

2 Maintain a clear airway by suctioning, if necessary.
3 Provide a source of humidification.

4 Measure oxygen concentrations every 1-2 hours when a child is receiving oxygen via incubator hood, tent, or Croupette.
a Measure when the oxygen environment is closed.
b Measure the concentration close to the child's airway.
c Record oxygen concentrations and simultaneous measurements of the pulse and respirations.

d Flushing the tent with up to 10 litres of oxygen per minute (dependent upon tent size) is required at commencement of therapy and again whenever tent apertures are opened.
5 Observe the child's response to oxygen.

6 Organize nursing care so that interruption of therapy is minimal.

7 Periodically check all equipment during each tour of duty.

8 Clean equipment daily and change it at least once a week. (Tubing and nebulizer jars should be changed daily.) Take cultures of oxygen tubing, water, nebulizers, and the interior of incubators at least every 3 days.
9 Keep combustible materials and potential sources of fire away from oxygen equipment.
a Avoid using oil or grease around oxygen connections.

2 The delivery of oxygen requires a clear airway.
3 Oxygen is a dry gas and requires the addition of moisture to prevent drying of the tracheobronchial tree and thickening and consolidation of secretions.
4 It is desirable to keep the oxygen concentration as low as possible while still providing for physiological requirements. This minimizes the danger of the child's developing retrolental fibroplasia or pulmonary oxygen toxicity. (Desired oxygen concentrations are determined by the arterial oxygen tension measurement.)
The concentration of oxygen within the space is determined by the litre flow, the efficiency of the equipment, and the frequency with which it is opened to the external environment.
d Necessary to provide oxygen concentration.

5 Desired response includes:
a Decreased restlessness
b Decreased respiratory distress
c Improved colour
d Improved vital sign values.
6 Interruption of therapy may result in the return of anoxia and defeat the goals of therapy.
7 For optimum functioning, the equipment should be clean, undamaged, and in good working order.
8 Unclean equipment may be a source of contamination.

9 Oxygen supports combustion.

b Do not use alcohol or oils on a child in an oxygen tent.

c Do not permit any electrical devices in or near an oxygen tent.

d Avoid the use of wool blankets and those made from some synthetic fibres because of the hazards resulting from static electricity.

e Prohibit smoking in areas where oxygen is being used.

f Know where the nearest fire extinguisher is available.

10 Terminate oxygen therapy gradually.
a Slowly reduce litre flow.
b Open air vents in incubators.
c Open zips or flip a section of the canopy over the top of the tent.

10 This allows the child to adjust to normal atmospheric oxygen concentrations.

11 Continually monitor the child's response during weaning. Observe for: restlessness, increased pulse rate, respiratory distress, cyanosis.

11 These are indications that the child is unable to tolerate reduced oxygen concentration.

Specific Methods for Administering Oxygen to Paediatric Patients

Nursing Action

Rationale/Amplification

Oxygen by Nasal Cannula or Catheter

Infants and small children rarely tolerate administration of oxygen by these methods.

Oxygen by Mask

1 Choose an appropriate size mask that covers the mouth and nose but not the eyes.

1 Extra space under the mask and around the face is added dead space and decreases the effectiveness of the therapy.

2 Using a mask that is capable of delivering the desired oxygen concentration.

2 Venturi masks, available for use in paediatrics, deliver low to moderate concentrations of oxygen: 24%, 28%, 35%, or 40%.

3 Place the mask over the child's mouth and nose so that it fits securely. Secure the mask with an elastic head grip.

3 Make sure that the mask is adjusted properly over the mouth and nose. Do not allow the oxygen to blow in child's eyes.

Small pieces of cotton may be placed above the ears to help relieve pressure and discomfort caused by the head strap.

4 Remove the oxygen mask at hourly intervals; wash the face and apply a cream to area where mask contacts the face.

4 Makes the patient feel more comfortable.

Oxygen Tent

1 This is the preferred method of administering moderate concentrations of oxygen to paediatric patients.
2 Select the smallest tent and canopy which will achieve the desired concentrations of oxygen and maintain patient comfort.
3 Ensure that the pillows supporting the child in a comfortable position do not occlude oxygen outlet.
4 Maintain the tent temperature at 17.8-21.1°C.

5 Analyse and record the tent atmosphere every 1-2 hours. Concentrations of 30-50% can be achieved in well maintained tents.

6 Maintain a tight-fitting canopy.

   a Whenever possible, provide nursing care through the sleeves or pockets of the tent.
   b Show a parent how to hold the child's hand through a small opening in one of the zips of the canopy.
7 Make certain that the cot sides are up.

8 Select toys that retard absorption, are washable, and will not produce static electricity.

1 Tents also provide for control of humidity and temperature and allow the child some mobility.
2 This increases the efficiency of the unit.

4 This is done by placing the ice in a trough on the back of the tent. It should be checked periodically and replaced as needed.
5 The concentration varies with the efficiency of the tent, the rate of flow of oxygen, and the frequency with which the tent is opened to the outside environment.
6 This prevents oxygen leakage and disruption of the tent atmosphere.
   a Fastening the canopy to the bedsprings with clothespegs may be helpful.
   b This will help to comfort a restless child.
7 The canopy, when tucked into the mattress, often gives the illusion of a safe, confined environment.
8 The child needs toys for stimulation and diversion. They should be safe and practical.

Croupette

1 This is an oxygen tent equipped with a high humidification system. (Refer to procedure under oxygen tent.)
2 Change the child's clothing and bed linen when damp. Cover the child with a cotton blanket.
3 Check the child frequently. Wipe inside of canopy frequently.

1 If the child's condition requires high humidity but not oxygen, the unit can be operated with compressed air.
2 This prevents chilling in an environment of cooled, supersaturated, aerated mist.
3 Condensation on the canopy may make it difficult to observe the child.

4 If possible, remove the child from the mist periodically.

4 This prevents maceration of the skin. Mist may be delivered via nebulizer tubing or mask during these periods.

5 Promote postural drainage and suction the child as necessary.

5 Rapid mobilization of secretions may follow initiation of mist tent therapy.

6 Observe the small infant for signs of overhydration.

6 This occasionally results from intensive use of an ultrasonic nebulizer, especially if a saline solution is nebulized.

Incubator with Oxygen

1 The incubator is used to provide a controlled environment for the neonate.

1 The unit is able to provide precise environmental control of temperature, oxygen, humidity, and isolation.

2 Adjust the oxygen flow to achieve the desired oxygen concentration.
a An oxygen limiter prevents the oxygen concentration inside the incubator from exceeding 35-40%.
b If extra oxygen is required to relieve cyanosis, the amount should be ordered by the paediatrician and administered by free mask or into any oxygen concentrator

a This is desirable since it reduces the hazard of the child developing retrolental fibroplasia.

3 Secure a nebulizer to the inside wall of the incubator if mist therapy is desired.

3 This should be cleaned and autoclaved daily. Sterile solutions are used to keep the bacteria count at a minimum.

4 Keep sleeves or portholes of incubator closed to prevent loss of oxygen.

4 When incubator portholes or sleeves are opened, supply supplemental oxygen with oxygen mask to face and nose.

5 Periodically analyse the incubator atmosphere.

5 To be certain that the child is receiving the desired concentration of oxygen.

Oxygen Hood

1 Warmed, humidified oxygen is supplied via a plastic container that fits over the child's head.

1 This is especially useful when high concentrations of oxygen are desired. The hood may be used in an incubator or with a warming unit.

2 Continuously monitor the oxygen concentration, temperature, and humidity inside the hood.

2 Oxygen should be warmed to 31-34°C to prevent a neonatal response to cold stress — including oxygen deprivation, metabolic acidosis, rapid depletion of glycogen stores, and reduction of blood glucose levels.

3 Open the hood or remove the baby from it as infrequently as possible.

3 This prevents fluctuations of heat and oxygen which may further debilitate the young infant.

GUIDELINES: CPAP (CONTINUOUS POSITIVE AIRWAY PRESSURE)

Continuous positive airway pressure (CPAP) is a system of applying a constant distending or gas pressure which is greater than atmospheric pressure to the airway during spontaneous breathing. The real mechanisms of action are unknown.

Purposes

1   To prevent alveolar collapse during expiration by keeping the alveoli open with pressure.
2   To prevent intrapulmonary right-to-left shunting.
3   To increase the oxygenation of the lungs, which in turn decreases potential for hypoxia, brachycardia or apnoea.
4   To decrease the work of breathing on the part of the infant.
5   To increase the functional residual capacity.

Equipment

1   A source of air and oxygen; warmth and humidity. A device for varying pressure in the system.
2   Means of connecting the system to the infant's airway:
Orotracheal tube
Face mask
Nasal tube
Nasal CPAP attachment.
3   Mechanical ventilator of a continuous flow, pressure controlled, time cycled type, with facilities for intermittent mandatory ventilation (IMV) and continuous positive airway pressure (CPAP).
Note: Commencing CPAP often produces a startling rise in arterial oxygen tension. Repeated and frequent blood gas estimations are essential initially and during CPAP to determine the optimal inspired oxygen concentrations.

Nursing Care of the Child Requiring Mechanical Ventilation

Characteristics of the Ventilator

Available ventilators have a wide range of capabilities, versatility, and clinical application. Some are more suitable for use with infants, others with children. It is wise for the nurse to be well acquainted with the characteristics of the machine that is being used and to be able to answer the following questions.

Rate Control
1   How is the rate controlled?

2 Can the patient initiate the cycle? (assisted ventilation).
3 What is the response time? (time elapsed between the initiation of respiration and response of the ventilator). This must be rapid in infants.
4 Is there a sensitivity control which allows the machine to be more or less sensitive to the patient's efforts to initiate respiration?

Volume Control
1 How is the volume controlled?
   a Automatically preset, *or*
   b Variable, with a preset pressure.
2 What is the range of inspiratory flow rate capability?
   A very low flow rate is required by neonates; the rate will increase with the size of the child.

Cycling
1 What controls the cycle of the machine?
   a *Time cycle*: Inspiration is terminated at the end of a preset period that is controlled by a timing device. The volume delivered is usually a function of flow per unit of time.
   b *Volume cycle*: The inspiratory phase is terminated after the predetermined volume of gas has been delivered. The pressure generated is dependent on the characteristics of the lung.
   c *Pressure cycle*: The inspiratory phase ceases when a preset pressure is achieved. The volume of gas delivered and the time required to achieve the preset pressure are dependent on the characteristics of the lungs.
   d *Mixed cycle*: Many ventilators have two or more cycling modes.

Humidification
1 How is moisture added to the inspired air?
   a Humidification
   b Nebulization.
2 Is there a means of controlling the temperature of the inspired air?
   Many models provide an adjustable thermostat on the humidifier controls.

Oxygen Control
1 What is the oxygen source?
2 How is the oxygen concentration controlled?

Pressure Control
1 How is the pressure controlled?
   a Automatically preset, *or*
   b Variable, with a preset volume
2 What do the pressure gauges indicate and how are they read?

   a Airway pressure indicator
   b Machine pressure indicator.
3   What is the peak effective pressure capability?

Ratio of Inspiration to Expiration (I/E Ratio)

1   Is this variable?
2   How is it controlled?

PEEP (Positive End Expiratory Pressure)

Does the ventilator have this feature? How is it controlled?

1   Involves exhalation against a threshold resistance.
2   Inspiratory pressure is increased by PEEP; in addition, back pressure remains throughout the expiratory phase.
3   This keeps the lungs in an expanded state and elevates the lung's resting volume, which prevents excessive alveolar collapse.

Sigh

Does the ventilator have this feature? How is it regulated?

1   Works by adding additional volume to the established tidal volume.
2   Has the effect of taking a deep breath and may expand alveoli, which tend to be collapsed at low volume ventilation.

Alarm Systems

What are the alarm systems to warn of possible problems?

1   Low pressure or disconnect alarm system
2   High pressure alarm system to indicate rising pressures within the lung
3   Electrical failure alarm system
4   Volume and rate monitor:
     a Acceptable low and high rates and tidal volumes are set for the alarm.
     b If either rate or tidal volume are outside acceptable parameters, an alarm sounds.

Nursing Management

The following general considerations should be kept in mind by the nurse who is caring for a child requiring mechanical ventilation.

Setting Controls

In setting controls, inspiratory flow rate will be less, and the respiratory rate will be greater than in the adult patient. These depend on the patient's size and condition and are determined by the paediatrician and/or respiratory therapist.

Humidification

1   Because of their small diameters, paediatric endotracheal tubes easily become obstructed by thickened secretions. Therefore, adequate humidification must be maintained to keep secretions loose.
2   During ventilation of an infant in an incubator, the amount of ventilator tubing outside the incubator should be kept to a minimum. The warm temperature inside the incubator helps decrease the amount of condensation in the tubing and thus provides higher water content in the inspired gas.

Oxygen Concentration

1   Inspired concentrations of oxygen should always be kept as low as possible (while still providing for physiological requirements), to prevent the development of retrolental fibroplasia or pulmonary oxygen toxicity.
2   The oxygen concentration should be checked periodically with an analyser.

Blood Gases

1   The arterialized capillary sample method is inaccurate for infants in respiratory distress because the constricted peripheral circulation may not reflect the arterial blood gases accurately.
2   An umbilical artery catheter is most frequently used to obtain arterial blood samples.

Sterile Precautions

The newborn has only those antibodies transferred across the placenta from the mother. Therefore sterile precautions are essential.

1   Ventilator tubing should be changed every 24 hours.
2   Routine cultures should be taken after intubation; there should be daily Gram staining of secretions.
3   Suctioning requires aseptic technique.

Tubing Support

1   Special frames are available to support ventilator tubing; this helps to prevent accidental decannulation in infants and small children.
2   Infants may require folded nappies or padding on either side and at the top of their heads to decrease mobility and take up space between the head and the frame.

Monitoring the Ventilator

1   Pressure gauges should be checked at frequent intervals since this gives an indication of changing compliance or increased airway resistance.

2   Volume measurements are difficult to obtain in infants since most spirometers incorporated into ventilators and meters (such as the Wright respirometer) do not read accurately at low volumes and flows. However, they are helpful with older children.
3   Measure respiratory rates of the machine and the child at least every hour.

Fluid Balance

1   Record intake and output precisely and obtain an accurate daily weight.

1   Positive fluid balance resulting in increase in body weight and interstitial pulmonary oedema is a frequent problem in patients requiring mechanical ventilation. Prevention requires early recognition of fluid accumulation

Abdominal Complications

1   Test all the stools and gastric drainage for occult blood.

1   About 25% of all patients requiring mechanical ventilation develop gastrointestinal bleeding; many of these patients require blood transfusions.

2   Measure abdominal girth daily.

2   Abdominal distension occurs frequently with respiratory failure and further hinders respiration by elevation of the diaphragm. Measurement of abdominal girth provides objective assessment of the degree of distension.

Communication

1   Provide writing paper and pad. A patient on mechanical ventilation with tracheostomy is unable to talk.
2   Establish some form of nonverbal communication if child is too sick to write.
3   Provide with suitable toys and play activities. Develop a regular routine of care to avoid undue exertion. Encourage parents to touch, fondle, and communicate with their child and participate in care.

Recording

1   Maintain a flow sheet to record ventilation patterns, arterial blood studies, venous chemical determinations, haematocrit, status of fluid balance, weight, and assessment of child's condition.

Weaning the Paediatric Patient from the Ventilator

Method I

Permits the patient to breathe spontaneously for short periods of time.

1 Often used when ventilation has been solely for apnoea.
2 The length of time without ventilator assistance is gradually increased, while ensuring that the infant does not become fatigued.
3 This method is often facilitated by applying continuous positive pressure to the airway when the infant is off the ventilator.
4 The CPAP can then be gradually decreased until the infant can breathe without assistance. (See p.188.)
5 Humidified gas is provided during the weaning process.

Method II

Switches from the 'control' to the 'assist' mode to permit the child to trigger respiration by his own effort.

1 This method is preferred for children with lung disease.
2 The ventilator is switched to the 'assist' mode.
3 The trigger sensitivity is gradually decreased as the patient is encouraged to provide greater effort until he is able to ventilate adequately without the assistance of the machine.
4 The patient is then taken off the ventilator for progressively longer periods until use of the ventilator can be discontinued completely.
5 CPAP can be used with this method during the periods that the patient is off the ventilator.

Nursing Management

1 Weaning children from a ventilator is frequently a long and tedious process. The child and his parents may need a lot of support and encouragement.
2 Frequent blood gas determinations are necessary to determine if the child is maintaining adequate oxygenation.
3 The child should be observed closely for signs of respiratory difficulty including fatigue, nasal flaring, increased pulse, sweating, facial pallor and cyanosis, and rising blood pressure.
4 A calm atmosphere should be maintained.
5 Whenever possible, the ventilator should remain at the bedside until the child is satisfied that he can breathe without it.

CARDIAC AND RESPIRATORY MONITORING

Cardiac and respiratory monitoring refers to electrical surveillance of the heart and respiratory rates and patterns. It is indicated for all those children whose condition is unstable or potentially unstable.

Nursing Management

1   Select a monitor that is appropriate for the child's needs. This will depend upon the child's age, ability to cooperate, purpose for monitoring, information desired and equipment available.

2   Stabilize the device to reduce the amount of mechanical noise for safety considerations.

3   Reduce the child's anxiety.
   a Provide language-and-age-appropriate explanations of the equipment.
   b When possible involve the child or his parents in care, including change of electrodes.

4   Select lead placement sites according to equipment specifications:
   a Cardiac monitors frequently employ three leads located at:
      (1) Upper right laterial chest wall below clavicle
      (2) Lower left chest wall in the interior axilliary line
      (3) Left upper chest wall.
   b Respiratory monitors frequently employ three electrodes located:
      (1) On either side of the chest (anterior axilliary line in fourth or fifth intercostal space)
      (2) At a reference electrode placed on the manubrium or other suitable distal point.

5   Apply electrodes by:
   a Clearing the appropriate areas on the chest with alcohol
   b Placing a small amount of conductive gel on each area of contact — unless pre-gelled disposable electrodes are used.
   c Apply the electrode firmly to completely dry skin.

6   Plug the leads into the lead cable at appropriate insertion points.

7   Be certain that the monitor alarms are in the 'on' position. High and low alarm limits should be set according to the child's age and condition so that apnoea, tachypnoea, bradycardia, and tachycardia can be readily detected.

8   Avoid skin breakdown by changing lead placement sites as needed. Clean and dry old sites. Expose them to fresh air to assist healing.

9   Check integrity of the entire system at least twice in 24 hours.
   a Carefully inspect lead wires and cable for breaks and proper attachment.
   b If malfunction is suspected, change equipment and report problem to nurse in charge.

10   Continue to count respiratory and apical rates at frequent intervals.
   a Compare with monitor rates to verify accuracy of equipment.
   b It must be remembered that monitors cannot substitute for close observation of the child.

11   Apnoea mattresses or pads that employ sensing devices may be used for infants, eliminating the need for electrodes, But note:
   a Although less susceptible to cardiovascular artefact, these devices may record physical impact, vibrations or body movements as breaths
   b In addition older infants can easily roll or crawl off the pad.

CARDIOPULMONARY RESUSCITATION

Cardiopulmonary resuscitation involves measures instituted to provide effective ventilation and circulation when the patient's respiration and heart have ceased to function.

Underlying Considerations

Cardiac Arrest

1   Signs — absence of heartbeat and absence of carotid and femoral pulses.
2   Causes — asystole, ventricular fibrillation, or cardiovascular collapse related to arterial hypotension.

Respiratory Arrest

1   Signs — apnoea and cyanosis.
2   Causes — obstructed airway, depression of the central nervous system, neuromuscular paralysis.

Emergency Preparation

1   Every hospital should have a well-defined and organized plan to be carried out in the event of cardiac or respiratory arrest.

Equipment

1   Emergency trolley or box — assembled and ready for use
Positive pressure breathing bag with nonrebreathing valve and universal 15 mm adaptor.
Masks (preterm infant, infant, child, adult sizes)
Oropharyngeal airways (Guedel sizes 0, 1, 2, 3, 4)
Laryngeal handle and blades of various sizes
Extra batteries and light bulbs for laryngoscope
Endotracheal tubes with connectors (complete sterile set, 2.5-8.0 mm i.d.)
Portable suction equipment and sterile catheters of various sizes
Sterile mucus extractor
Oxygen source — portable supply, guage and tubing, masks of various sizes
Cardiac board
Emergency drugs

Sodium bicarbonate	Atropine
Adrenaline	Phenytoin
Isoprenaline	Phenobarbitone
Calcium chloride	Propranolol
Dextrose	Digoxin

Saline (for dilution)   Naxolone
Lignocaine (xylocaine)
Intracardiac needles, 20 and 22 gauge, 6-8 cm long
Intravenous infusion equipment

Fluids   Longdwell catheters of various
Infusion set   sizes
Tourniquet   Three-way stopcock
Armboards   Cutdown set
Tape   Intravenous infusion stand
Scalp vein needles of various sizes Labels
Nasogastric tubes of various sizes

Equipment

Syringes of various sizes   Sterile gauze (10 cm x 10 cm)
Needles of various sizes   Sterile scissors
Mediswabs   Blood specimen tubes
Tongue blades

2   Electrocardiograph and monitor
3   D.C. defibrillator and paddles (paediatric and adult).

Artificial Respiration

Technique for Artificial Respiration

Mouth to Mouth
1   *Preterm infants, newborns, infants*
    a Clear mouth of mucus or vomitus with finger or suction.
    b Extend neck by placing a rolled towel or nappy under the infant's shoulders, or use one hand to support the neck in an extended position. Do not hyperextend the neck since this narrows the airway.
    c Take a breath.
    d Make a tight seal with your mouth over the infant's mouth and nose.
    e Gently blow air from the cheeks and observe for chest expansion.
    f Remove your mouth from infant's mouth and nose and allow the infant to exhale passively.
    g Repeat approximately 40 times per minute.
2   *Older children and adolescents*
    a Clear mouth of mucus or vomitus with finger or suction.
    b Hyperextend neck with one hand or a rolled towel.
    c Clamp the nostrils with the fingers of one hand which also continues to exert pressure on the forehead to maintain the neck extension.
    d Take a deep breath.
    e Make a tight seal with your mouth over the child's mouth.
    f Force air into the lungs until chest expansion is observed.

g Release your mouth from the child's mouth and release nostrils to allow the child to exhale passively.

h Repeat approximately 15-20 times per minute.

Hand-operated Ventilation Devices

1   Remove secretions from mouth and throat and move mandible forward.
2   Appropriately extend the neck with one hand or a nappy roll.
3   Select an appropriate size mask to obtain an adequate seal, and connect mask to the bag.
4   Hold the mask snugly over the mouth and nose, holding the chin forward and the neck in extension.
5   Squeeze the bag, noting inflation of the lungs by chest expansion.
6   Release the bag, which will expand spontaneously. The child will exhale and the chest will fall.
7   Repeat 20-40 times a minute (depending on size of the child).
8   Since this technique is often difficult to master, it should be practised in advance, under supervision.

Indications of Effective Technique

1   Child's chest rises and falls.
2   Nurse can feel in her own airway the resistance and compliance of the child's lungs as they expand.
3   Nurse can hear and feel the air escape during exhalation.
4   Child's colour improves.

Management of Complications

1   Gastric distension (occurs frequently if excessive pressures are used for inflation).
   a Turn victim's head and shoulders to one side.
   b Exert moderate pressure over the epigastrium between the umbilicus and the rib cage.
   c A nasogastric tube may be used to decompress the stomach.
2   If vomiting occurs:
   a Turn patient on side for drainage.
   b Clear the airway with fingers or suction.
   c Resume ventilations.

External Cardiac Massage

General Principles

(Technique of external cardiac massage; see Figure 2.8, Table 2.7)

1   A backward tilt of the head lifts the back in infants and small children. A firm support beneath the back is therefore essential if external cardiac compression is to be effective.
2   A supine position on a firm surface, e.g. table or floor, is mandatory. Only in this position can chest compression squeeze the heart against the immobile spine enough to force blood into the systemic circulation.
3   External cardiac compression must always be accompanied by artifical ventilation for adequate oxygenation of the blood.

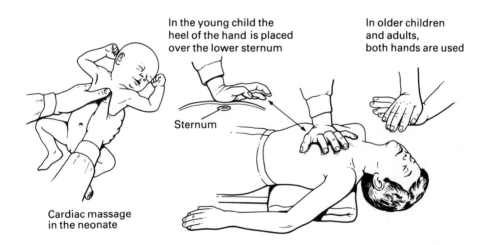

In the young child the heel of the hand is placed over the lower sternum

In older children and adults, both hands are used

Sternum

Cardiac massage in the neonate

Figure 2.8   External cardiac massage.

Table 2.7 Technique of external cardiac massage

Size of child	Preparatory phase	Action phase	Distance of compression	Rate	Ratio compressions ventilations
Neonate, preterm or small infant	1 Place in supine position	1 Compress mid-sternum with both thumbs, gently but firmly	Two thirds of the distance to the spine or 1.3-1.8 cm	100-120 per minute	3:1
	2 Encircle the chest with the hands, with thumbs over the midsternum				
	or				
	Use method for a larger infant, at a rate of 100-120 per minute				
Larger infant	1 Place on a firm, flat surface	1 Compress the midsternum with the tips of the index and middle fingers	1.3-1.8 cm	80-100 per minute	3:1
	2 Support the back with one hand or use a small blanket under the shoulders				
	3 Place the tips of index and middle fingers of one hand over the mid-sternum				

Small child	1 Place on a firm, flat surface	1 Apply a rapid downward thrust	1.8-3.8 cm	80-100 per minute to the mid-sternum, keeping the elbow straight	4-5:1
	2 Support the back by slipping one hand beneath it, or use a small blanket under the shoulders	2 Hold for approximately 0.4 second			
	3 Place the heel of one hand over the midsternum, parallel with the long axis of the body	3 Instantly and completely release the pressure so the chest wall can recoil			
		4 Do not remove the heel of the hand from the chest			
Larger child	1 Place on a flat, firm surface or place a board under the thorax	1 Exert pressure vertically down-wards to depress lower sternum, keeping elbows straight	2.5-5.0 cm	60-80 per minute	5:1

Table 2.7 Techniques of external cardiac massage (*continued*)

Size of child	Preparatory phase	Action phase	Distance of compression	Rate	Ratio compressions ventilations
	2 Place the heel of one hand on the lower half of the sternum about 2.5-3.8 cm from the tip of the xiphoid process and parallel with the long axis of the body	2 Hold for approximately 0.4 second			
	3 Place the other hand on top of the first one (may interlock fingers)	3 Instantly and completely release the pressure so the chest wall can recoil			
	4 Place shoulders directly over child's sternum, in order to use own weight in application of pressure	4 Do not remove the hands from the chest			

4   Compressions must be regular, smooth, and uninterrupted. Avoid sudden or jerking movements.

5   Relaxation must immediately follow compression; relaxation and compression must be of equal duration.

6   Between compressions, the fingers or heel of the hand must completely release their pressure but should remain in constant contact with the chest.

7   Fingers should not rest on the patient's ribs during compression. Pressure with fingers on the ribs or lateral pressure increases the possibility of fractured ribs and costochondral separation.

8   Never compress the xiphoid process at the tip of the sternum. Pressure on it may cause laceration of the liver.

9   Indications of effective technique include: (1) a palpable femoral or carotid pulse; (2) decrease in size of pupils; (3) improvement in patient's colour.

Nursing Care in Cardiopulmonary Resuscitation

1   Recognize cardiac and/or respiratory arrest.

2   Send for assistance and note time (screen bed if possible).

3   If alone:

a First ventilate the child's lungs rapidly two or three times, using appropriate technique (p. 202), and then proceed with external cardiac compression, using appropriate technique (p. 203).

b After each series of 15 cardiac compressions, reventilate the lungs rapidly two or three times. Then proceed with external cardiac compression.

c Continue repeating this cycle until additional help arrives.

4   When help arrives:

a One operator performs mouth-to-mouth resuscitation or institutes bag breathing according to the proper ratio of compressions to ventilations.

b Other operator performs cardiac massage.

5   Anticipate and assist with emergency procedures and medications.

a Assist with intubation, monitoring, placement of cutdown, administration of intravenous fluids, defibrillation, and other definitive measures.

b Prepare and administer emergency medications as prescribed. Record dose and time.

6   After resuscitation:

a Care for the child as required.

b Determine whether family members have been notified and are being cared for.

c Record all events.

d Restock emergency trolley as appropriate.

THE CHILD UNDERGOING DIALYSIS

Dialysis refers to the process of separating substances in solution by the differences in their rates of diffusion through a semipermeable membrane. Dialysis is used in the treatment of renal failure to remove uraemic toxins from the body fluids by allowing blood to equilibrate across a semipermeable membrane with fluids lacking these toxins.

Purpose

To preserve life by acting as a substitute for kidney function during renal failure.

1 Aids in the removal of toxic substances and metabolic wastes.
2 Removes excessive body fluid.
3 Assists in regulating the body's fluid and electrolyte balance.

Types of Dialysis

Peritoneal Dialysis

1 Mechanism
   a The peritoneal lining is used as the semipermeable membrane.
   b A catheter is inserted through the anterior abdominal wall and the dialysate is instilled into the abdominal cavity.
   c After an equilibration time (about 30 minutes), the fluid is drained by gravity and fresh dialysate is instilled.
2 Major uses
   a Acute, reversible uraemic episodes such as those due to sudden illness, trauma, poisoning, or drug intoxication.
   b In terminal illness, to keep the child comfortable for as long as possible.
   c Prior to acceptance in a long-term haemodialysis and transplantation programme.
   d In selected cases of chronic renal failure.
      The child is dialysed at night through a semipermanently implanted abdominal cannula by an automatic, continually recycling, machine.
3 Advantage
   a Relatively safe and readily available.
   b A particularly efficient method in infancy as the surface area of the peritoneal cavity is relatively large.
4 Disadvantages
   a Long periods of time required to effectively remove waste products.
   b May cause abdominal pain and discomfort.
   c Sterile dialysate is required.
   d Complications:
      (1) Peritonitis
      (2) Bowel perforation during insertion of the catheter

(3) Respiratory distress caused by upward displacement of the diaphragm by fluid in the peritoneal cavity

(4) Shock due to excessive fluid loss

(5) Protein loss because serum proteins pass through the peritoneal membrane during dialysis

(6) Bleeding and leakage at the catheter insertion site

(7) Inadequate fluid return

(8) Nausea, vomiting, diarrhoea.

Haemodialysis

1   Mechanism

   a The semipermeable membrane is located in a machine through which the child's blood is directed.

   b Access to the circulation is provided via a Teflon — Silastic arteriovenous shunt or a subcutaneously implanted arteriovenous fistula.

   c The child's blood is diverted through the machine adjacent to the semipermeable membrane to equilibrate with dialysate on the other side of the membrane.

   d Selection of the dialyser depends on the size of the child. Considerations include:

   (1) Amount of blood the machine holds relative to the amount that the child can safely spare from the body at one time

   (2) Efficiency of the machine relative to the child's weight

   (3) Speed with which fluid can be removed by the machine.

Note: Dialysis can be dangerous if it is too rapid

2   Major uses

   a Long-term therapy for chronic renal failure

   b Holding procedure prior to kidney transplant.

3   Advantages

   a Shorter period of time than peritoneal dialysis required to effectively remove waste products (about four times more efficient)

   b Does not require sterile dialysate

   c Is less traumatic to initiate once access to the circulation is made

   d Home dialysis is available in selected situations.

4   Disadvantages

   a Is costly

   b There are inherent moral, legal, logistical, and technical problems.

   c Complications:

   (1) Clotting, infection, accidental separation of shunt

   (2) Anaemia — because a small amount of blood remains behind in the machine with each run

   (3) Malaise, headache, nausea, and vomiting during dialysis

   (4) Hepatitis due to transfusions necessitated by uraemic anaemia

   (5) Rickets, growth failure, and delayed or absent sexual maturation

   (6) Long-term emotional problems.

GUIDELINES: CARING FOR THE CHILD UNDERGOING DIALYSIS

Nursing Care

Nursing Action	Rationale/Amplification
1 Prepare the child for the procedure. **a** Explain the procedure to the child in terms that he can understand. (1) Allow the child to handle equipment similar to that which will be used during dialysis. (2) Encourage the child to express his fears so that misinterpretations can be corrected. (3) Provide simple pictures and diagrams, if appropriate. (4) Allow the child to talk with peers who have undergone dialysis. **b** Explain the procedure to the family and answer questions so that they will be in the best position to support their child.	1 Dialysis is threatening to most children and may evoke fears of pain, mutilation, immobilization, helplessness, and dependence. Many children have fears of losing all of their blood in this process. A child who is well prepared will be less frightened and better able to cooperate during the procedure.
2 Protect the child from infection. **a** Keep the dressings and area around the catheter or shunt clean and dry. **b** Use aseptic technique throughout the dialysis procedure. **c** Avoid exposure to children or adults with infection. **d** Provide supplemental vitamins since a protein-restricted diet is poor in vitamins. **e** Provide meticulous daily hygiene.	2 These children are prone to infection because of their general debilitated state and because of protein loss and anaemia.
3 Provide a high energy diet which is low sodium and protein. Since the child often experiences anorexia, it may be helpful to allow him to choose foods from his allowances and offer small, frequent meals.	3 Energy intake (in kilojoules) is increased since growth failure is observed in children while on dialysis. Sodium and protein are limited to prevent the blood pressure and blood urea from going too high between dialyses. The child may see dietary restrictions as punishment and must be helped to realize the purpose of the restrictions.
4 Maintain careful records of intake and output, vital signs, blood pressure, and daily weights.	4 These provide valuable information about the effectiveness of the therapy.
5 Support the child during the dialysis procedure.	5 These provide valuable information about the effectiveness of the therapy.

a Provide symptomatic relief of nausea, vomiting, malaise, or headache.

Notify the paediatrician if these symptoms are severe.

b Be alert to clues from the child for helpful methods of offering support.

(1) Young children often cling to stuffed toys or blankets or depend on parent's presence at the bedside.

(2) Older children may benefit from radio, television, magazines, or contact with peers.

6 Provide an environment that is as normal as possible.

a Encourage the family to bring in articles that will make the child's room appear more homelike, i.e. pictures, posters, etc.

b Encourage the child to be as independent as possible in his daily care.

c Provide for age appropriate support recreation and/or diversion.

d Help the child to keep up with his school work.

7 Offer appropriate support to the family.

a Provide opportunity for family members to discuss their feelings, fears, and frustrations and to ask questions.

b Allow family members to become involved in the child's care to the extent that they wish and that is helpful for the child and family.

c Provide for continuity of personnel.

d Initiate appropriate referrals. These may include referrals to a social worker and community nursing service, other families who are coping with dialysis.

8 Teach the child and family about all of the important aspects of renal failure and dialysis, including:

a Signs and symptoms of uraemia

b Shunt care and protection

c Protection from infection

d Dietary restrictions and recommendations; ways of incorporating the special diet into the family meal plan

6 Although life is preserved, it is by no means normal during the time on dialysis or between dialysis. These measures may increase the child's feeling of self-esteem and diminish regression and social isolation. By serving as role models, health professionals may encourage parents to recognize and foster the normal, healthy aspects of the child's daily life.

7 Families often need extensive support. Attention must be focussed on siblings as well as parents since siblings relationships are often strained and difficult.

8 The family should be prepared to care for the child at home well before the day of discharge. Learning about the child's care also helps restore some sense of control in a frightening situation.

     e Dialysis schedule
     f Medications
     g Emergency procedures.

Peritoneal Dialysis: Specific Nursing Responsibilities

Peritoneal dialysis is a simple and relatively safe method of achieving the exchange of basic substances in solution through the peritoneum which acts as a semipermeable membrane. It is a particularly efficient method in infancy as the surface area of the peritoneal cavity is relatively large.

GUIDELINES: CARING FOR THE CHILD UNDERGOING PERITONEAL DIALYSIS

Purposes

1   To aid in the removal of toxic substances and metabolic wastes
2   To remove excessive body fluid
3   To assist in regulating the fluid balance of the body
4   To control blood pressure.

Equipment

Dialysis administration set (disposable, closed system)
Peritoneal dialysis solution as ordered
Supplemental drugs as ordered
Local anaesthesia
Central venous pressure monitoring equipment
ECG
Suture set
Sterile gloves
Skin antiseptic.

Procedure   (Figure 2.9)

Nursing Action	Rationale/Amplification
Preparatory Phase	
1 Prepare the child emotionally and physically for the procedure. Explain in a language that he understands. Explain procedure to parents.	1 Nursing support is offered by explaining procedure mechanics, providing opportunities for the patient to ask questions, allowing him to verbalize his feelings, and giving expert physical care.
2 See the consent form has been signed.	
3 Weigh the patient before dialysis and every 24 hours thereafter, preferably on an in-bed scale.	3 The weight at the beginning of the procedure serves as a baseline of information. Daily weight is helpful in assessing the state of hydration.

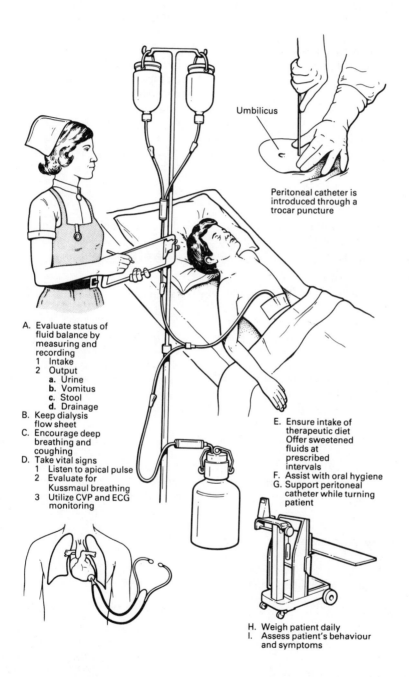

Umbilicus

Peritoneal catheter is
introduced through a
trocar puncture

A. Evaluate status of
   fluid balance by
   measuring and
   recording
   1 Intake
   2 Output
      a. Urine
      b. Vomitus
      c. Stool
      d. Drainage
B. Keep dialysis
   flow sheet
C. Encourage deep
   breathing and
   coughing
D. Take vital signs
   1 Listen to apical pulse
   2 Evaluate for
      Kussmaul breathing
   3 Utilize CVP and ECG
      monitoring

E. Ensure intake of
   therapeutic diet
   Offer sweetened
   fluids at
   prescribed
   intervals
F. Assist with oral hygiene
G. Support peritoneal
   catheter while turning
   patient

H. Weigh patient daily
I. Assess patient's behaviour
   and symptoms

Figure 2.9 Nursing management of patient undergoing peritoneal dialysis.

4 Take temperature, pulse, respiration, and blood pressure readings prior to dialysis.

4 A knowledge of vital signs at the beginning of dialysis is necessary for comparing subsequent changes in vital signs.

5 Have the patient empty his bladder. If necessary catheterize.

5 If the bladder is empty there is less likelihood of perforating it when the trocar is introduced into the peritoneum.

6 Assist with insertion of central venous pressure catheter. ECG monitoring may also be employed.

6 Central venous pressure measurements may be carried out to assess fluid volume changes. Cardiac arrhythmias may occur due to serum potassium changes and vagal stimulation.

7 Make the patient comfortable in a supine position.

8 Check dialysis fluid for sediment or contaminant by holding the solution up to the light.

8 If sediment is observed, fluid should be discarded (returned to pharmacy for analysis).

Method (by the paediatrician)

The following is a brief résumé of the method of insertion of the peritoneal catheter (done under strict asepsis).

1 The abdomen is prepared surgically and the skin and subcutaneous tissues are infiltrated with a local anaesthetic.

1 Surgical preparation of the skin minimizes or eliminates surface bacteria and decreases the possibility of wound contamination and infection.

2 A small midline stab wound is made 3-5 cm below the umbilicus.

2 The midline area is relatively avascular.

3 The trocar is inserted through the incision with the stylet in place, or a thin stylet cannula may be inserted percutaneously.

4 The patient is requested to raise his head from the pillow after the trocar is introduced.

4 This manoeuvre tightens the abdominal muscles and permits easier penetration of the trocar without danger of injury to the intra-abdominal organs.

5 When the peritoneum is punctured, the trocar is directed towards the left side of the pelvis. The stylet is removed, and the catheter is inserted through the trocar and manoeuvred into position.

  Dialysis fluid is allowed to run through the catheter while it is being positioned.

  This prevents the omentum from adhering to the catheter, impending its advancement or occluding its opening.

6 After the trocar is removed, the skin may be closed with a purse-string suture. (This is not always done.) A sterile dressing is placed around the catheter.

6 The catheter is attached to the skin in the abdomen.

7 Flush the tubing with dialysis solution.

7 The tubing is flushed to prevent air from entering the peritoneal cavity. Air causes abdominal discomfort and drainage difficulties.

8 Attach the catheter connector to the administration set which has been previously connected to the container of dialysis solution (warmed to body temperature, 37°C).

8 The solution is warmed to body temperature for patient comfort and to prevent abdominal pain. Heating also causes dilation of the peritoneal vessels and increases urea clearance.

9 Dry the dialysate bottles before inverting.

10 Drugs (heparin, etc.) are added in advance.

10 The addition of heparin prevents fibrin clots from occluding the catheter. Potassium chloride may be added on order unless the patient has hyperkalaemia.

11 Permit the dialysing solution to flow unrestricted into the peritoneal cavity (about 15-25 ml/kg of body weight). Usually takes 5-10 minutes for completion.

11 The inflow solution should flow in a steady stream. If the fluid flows in too slowly the catheter may need to be repositioned since its tip may be buried in the omentum, or it may be occluded by a blood clot.

12 Allow the fluid to remain in peritoneal cavity for the prescribed time period (15-30 minutes). Prepare the next exchange while the fluid is in the peritoneal cavity.

12 In order for potassium, urea, and other waste material to be removed, the solution must remain in the peritoneal cavity for the prescribed time. The maximum concentration gradient takes place in the first 5-10 minutes and this is the most effective dwell time.

13 Unclamp the outflow tube. Drainage should take approximately 10 minutes or more, although the time varies with each patient.

13 The abdomen is drained by a siphon effect through the closed system. Gravity drainage should occur fairly rapidly, and steady streams of fluid should be observed entering the drainage container. The drainage is usually straw coloured.

14 If the fluid is not draining properly, move the patient from side to side to facilitate the removal of peritoneal drainage. The head of the bed may also be elevated.

Ascertain whether the catheter is patent.

14 If the drainage stops, or starts to drip before the dialysing fluid has run out, it may indicate that the catheter tip is buried in the omentum. Rotating the patient may be helpful (or it may be necessary for the paediatrician to reposition the catheter).

15 When the outflow drainage ceases to run, clamp off the drainage tube and infuse the next exchange, using strict aspetic technique.

16 Take blood pressure and pulse every 15 minutes during the first exchange and every hour thereafter.

Monitor the heart rate for signs of arrhythmia.

16 A drop in blood pressure may indicate excessive fluid loss from the glucose level concentrations of the dialysing solutions. Changes in vital signs may indicate impending shock or over-hydration.

17 Take patient's temperature every 4 hours (especially after catheter removal).

17 An infection is more apt to become evident after dialysis has been discontinued.

18 The procedure is repeated until the blood chemistry levels improve. The usual time is 12-36 hours; depending on the patient's condition, he will receive 24-48 exchanges.

18 The duration of dialysis depends on the severity of the condition and on the size and weight of the patient. Patients requiring only a few peritoneal dialysis treatments may have a plastic T-shaped button placed in catheter tract between dialyses to avoid need to repuncture the abdomen for catheter insertion. Patients requiring pro-longed peritoneal dialysis should have implanted Silastic catheters used with closed automated dialysis systems.

19 Specimens of dialysate should be sent for culture and biochemical analysis.

19 For early detection of infection and electrolyte imbalance.

20 Keep an exact record of the patient's fluid balance during treatment.

a Know the status of the patient's loss or gain of fluid at the end of each exchange.

b The fluid balance should be about even or should show slight fluid loss.

20 Complications (circulatory overload, hypertension, congestive heart failure) may occur if most of the fluid is not recovered.

21 Promote patient comfort during dialysis.

a Frequent back care and massage of pressure areas.

b Rotate from side to side.

c Elevate head of bed at intervals.

d Allow patient to sit in chair for brief periods if condition permits.

e Provide frequent mouthwashes as oral fluids may be restricted.

f Provide suitable play activities.

e To prevent the mouth from becoming sore and dry.

f This will help the child to have some normality in his life during the dialysis.

22 Observe for the following:

a Respiratory difficulty

(1) Slow the inflow rate.

(2) Make sure tubing is not kinked.

a This is caused by pressure from the fluid in the peritoneal cavity and the upward displacement of the dia-praghm — producing shallow respir-ations.

(3) Prevent air from entering peritoneum by keeping drip chamber of tubing three-quarters full of fluid.

(4) Elevate head of bed; encourage coughing and breathing exercises.
(5) Turn patient from side to side.
b Abdominal pain
(1) Encourage the patient to move about.

c Leakage

(3) In severe respiratory difficulty, the fluid from the peritoneal cavity should be drained immediately and the paediatrician notified.

b Pain may be caused by the dialysing solution's not being at body temperature, incomplete drainage of the solution, chemical predisposes to peritonitis.
c Leakage around the catheter predisposes to peritonitis.
(1) Change the dressings frequently.
(2) Use sterile plastic drapes to prevent contamination.

23 Keep accurate records:
   a Exact time of beginning and ending of each exchange; starting and finishing time of drainage
   b Amount of solution infused and recovered
   c Fluid balance
   d Number of exchanges
   e Medications added to dialysing solution
   f Pre- and post-dialysis weight and as often as required by the paediatrician
   g Level of responsiveness at beginning, throughout, and at the end of treatment
   h Assessment of vital signs and patient's condition.

Note: During dialysis the child may be unable to hold still and some restraint may be necessary.

Complications

1 Peritonitis
   a Watch for abdominal pain, tenderness, rigidity, cloudy dialysate return.
   b Send specimen of dialysate for smear and culture.

1 Peritonitis is the most common complication. Antibiotics may be added to dialysate and also given systemically.

2 Bleeding	2 A small amount of bleeding around the catheter is not significant if it does not persist. During the first few exchanges, blood-tinged fluid from subcutaneous bleeding is not uncommon. Small amounts of heparin may be added to inflow solution to prevent the catheter from becoming clogged.
3 Shock	3 Symptoms of shock may occur due to excessive fluid loss.
4 Protein loss	4 There may be a significant protein loss, because most serum proteins pass through the peritoneal membrane during dialysis. Serum albumin determinations are made throughout the treatment.

Haemodialysis: Specific Nursing Responsibilities

1 Care for the arteriovenous shunt (refer to Guidelines, below).
2 Assist in teaching the child and family proper care and protection of the shunt.
3 When possible, avoid giving subcutaneous or intramuscular injections because the child is anticoagulated with heparin at least twice weekly during dialysis and extensive bleeding occurs as a result of such injections.
4 Care for the child during dialysis. (This aspect of nursing care is not presented since it is generally provided by specially trained personnel in dialysis unit.)

GUIDELINES: CARE OF THE ARTERIOVENOUS SHUNT

Purpose
To preserve shunt function and prevent separation of the cannulas.

Equipment
1 Two shunt clips
2 Dressing tray with:
    Sterile plastic bowls
    Sterile 5 cm x 5 cm sponges
    Sterile 10 cm x 7.5 cm sponges
    Kling bandage
    Hydrogen peroxide
    Recommended skin cleansing lotion

Sterile water
Antibiotic ointment if prescribed
Sterile applicators
Sterile scissors
Mask
Sterile gloves.

Note: The Silastic tubing should never be punctured since it will not seal.

Procedure

Nursing Action	Rationale/Amplification
1 Place shunt clip in the dressing and stay with the child at all times.	1 The clamps are used to close the shunt in case it separates at its connection.
2 Use another extremity for:	2 Disturbing the shunt in any way can encourage clotting and infection.
a Taking blood pressure	**a** Inflation of blood pressure cuff may precipitate clotting by slowing the flow of blood through the tubing.
b Giving injections **c** Giving infusions	**b, c** Injections in the extremity increase the possibility of thrombosis of the vein.
d Taking blood samples.	**d** A rubber puncture site may be added to the shunt. This can be punctured with a needle to obtain blood specimens.
3 Cleanse the area around the shunt and change the dressing daily or as required. **a** Remove old dressing. **b** Observe the shunt for malalignment or kinks	**b** These factors increase the possibility of clot formation and must be corrected.
c Observe the area around the cannula insertion sites for signs of inflammation (redness, swelling, drainage).	**c** If noted, report signs of inflammation, and take culture before cleansing the area.
d Using aseptic technique, carefully wash area around the cannula insertion sites and the entire circumference of the extremity in the area of the shunt using hydrogen peroxide followed by recommended skin cleansing lotion and sterile water. Rinse well and dry.	**d** Avoid leaving cleansing lotion on the cannulas as this may make the connections slippery.

e Apply dry sterile dressing to the areas of cannula insertion.

f Wrap arm with compression bandage firmly, but not tightly, leaving a small section of the shunt in view.

f Leave a section small enough that it cannot be pulled out by the child. If protective devices to limit movement are indicated, apply below the shunt.

g Retape shunt clips to outer dressing in full view.

4 Check frequently for shunt obstruction.

a Use stethoscope or place fingertips on area between cannula insertion points to detect bruit.

a Presence of bruit indicates free flow of blood through shunt.

b Observe child for signs of pain in the extremity.

c Observe colour of blood in tubing.

c Blood should appear smooth and should be of uniform colour. Fibrin may appear as white specks along the cannula wall.

d Report clotting immediately to the paediatrician.

d Clotting is indicated by separation of blood, i.e. presence of a darkened clot and clear serum. The shunt feels cool rather than warm to the touch. Delay in declotting may necessitate replacement of the entire shunt.

5 Be prepared for emergency action if the shunt should separate or the cannula should become dislodged.

a Identify source of bleeding by unwrapping bandage.

b Separation of shunt:
  (1) Clamp tubes with shunt clips and rejoin shunt *or*
  (2) Pinch of tubes with fingers and rejoin shunt.

c Dislodgement of arterial or venous cannula:
  (1) Apply firm pressure over bleeding cannula site and clamp remaining cannula.
  (2) Notify physician.

5 These are emergency situations which may result in severe haemorrhage and possible exsanguination.

6 Teach the child and parents how to care for the shunt.

a Dressing changes and cleansing of area around the shunt

b Observation for signs of inflammation, infection, obstruction

c Bathing

(1) Some children are permitted to bathe the shunted extremity, soaping the area at the beginning and at the end of the shower or bath.

(2) Swimming may be permitted if the extremity is completely protected with a waterproof covering.

d Prevention of clotting.

(1) Avoid constricting clothing which may impair blood flow through the shunt.

(2) Avoid keeping the extremity acutely flexed for long periods of time.

(3) Avoid sleeping on the shunted arm.

e Emergency measures in case of accidental separation or dislodging of the cannula.

c These activities are allowed at the discretion of the individual paediatrician.

TRACTION

Traction refers to the extension of an injured extremity in the direction and position which will promote healing and optimal functioning. It is accomplished by the use of weights which pull a part in the desired direction in the presence of countertraction.

Purpose

1   To maintain the approximation of fractured segments of a bone until union occurs.
2   To prevent deformities from resulting in the presence of injury or inflammation:
    a Fractures
    b Arthritis
    c Trauma.
3   To correct existing deformities:
    a Congenital dislocation of the hip
    b Flexion contractures of the knees.
4   To lessen muscle spasm.
5   To immobilize a part.
6   To reduce dislocation.

Types of Traction

1   Skin traction
    a Used for younger children when the condition of the skin is good and mild forces of traction are sufficient.
    b Traction is applied to the skin of the affected body part:
    (1) Elastoplast extension plaster or Ventfoam material are applied.
    (2) Crepe bandages are applied to hold them in place.
    (3) Weights are attached to the extensions by cords which pass over one or more pulleys.

2   Skeletal traction
    a Used in older children when greater traction force is required or if the skin is damaged.
    b Force is exerted against the bone by means of a metallic device such as a pin, wire, or Crutchfield tongs.
3   Traction may be continuous or intermittent, depending on its purpose
    a Continuous traction cannot be interrupted for dressing or other activities.
    b Intermittent traction may be temporarily disconnected as specified by the surgeon.

GUIDELINES: CARE OF A CHILD IN TRACTION

Equipment

1   Strips of Elastoplast extension plaster or ventfoam
2   Adhesive tape
3   Crepe bandages
4   Wooden spreaders and extension cord
5   Ropes, weights, pulleys
6   Traction bars
7   Slings.

Procedure

Nursing Action	Rationale/Amplification
1 Explain the procedure to the child and his parents.	1 If the traction is to be effective, it is essential that the parents understand the procedure and cooperate while the child is in traction.
2 Maintain even, constant traction: **a** Do not add or remove weights.	

b Allow the weights to hang free at all times. Do not allow them to touch the floor or bed.

c Be certain that the ropes are in the wheel grooves of the pulleys.

d Keep the weights out of the child's reach.

e Wrap knotted areas of the ropes with adhesive tape to prevent slipping.

f Do not elevate the head or foot of the bed without consulting the ortho-paedic surgeon.

g Supervise the child's position so that the purpose of the traction is accomplished.

2 Traction must be kept constant in order to achieve the desired results. Any change in the amount of weights or counteraction will affect the entire traction system.

3 Check for disturbance of circulation by observing:

a Skin colour — for redness, pallor, cyanosis

b Joint motion

c Skin temperature

d Tingling, numbness

e Swelling.

3 Compare the affected limb with the unaffected one.

4 Provide skin care

4 Immobilized children readily develop areas of pressure unless meticulous skin care is provided.

a Pad bony prominences (ankles) with strips of felt.

a Protects skin from injury.

b Wash and dry all exposed areas thoroughly.

c Massage the child's back and sacral area at least two to three times daily.

d Inspect the heels, ankles, popliteal space, and top of the foot for signs of pressure

d These are the areas most prone to breakdown.

e Keep the bed linen clean, dry, and free from wrinkles and crumbs.

e Making up a 'divided' bed facilitates changing the bed and makes the proce-dure less uncomfortable for the child.

f Do not allow any traction cords to dig into the child's skin.

5 Plan for short periods of muscle exercise every day.
  a Encourage the child to move and exercise his unaffected extremities.
  Provide diversional therapy which requires the use of these muscles.
  b Assist the child to exercise his toes.
6 Have the child breathe deeply at intervals.
  Provide him with soap bubbles, whistles, or party favours to make this more fun. An older child may use blow bottles.
7 Keep a record of the child's intake and output and do periodic urinalyses.

8 Provide a diet high in roughage and fluids (especially fruit juices) and low in calcium.
9 Provide daily diversion and encourage the child's family to visit frequently.

  a Attempt to replace the lost activity with another form of motion.

  b Suspend toys over the child's head so he can reach them. (Punching bag can help child relieve hostility.)
  c Provide continuing education for the school-age child.
  d Encourage projects that will allow child a feeling of accomplishment: painting, puzzles, knitting, ceramics.
  e Patients who are immobilized in traction or casts should be grouped together.
10 If not contraindicated, supply the child with an overhead trapeze.
11 Record:
  a Colour, temperature, and appearance of the affected extremity
  b Skin condition
  c Evidence of local oedema
  d Body alignment
  e Functioning of traction ropes, weights, and pulley
  f Response of the child to therapy.

5 Disuse of muscles can result in atrophy and deformities.

6 Prolonged periods of immobilization may cause the child to develop hypostatic pneumonia.

7 Immobilization renders the child prone to developing urinary retention and renal calculi.
8 This helps to prevent constipation and the development of renal calculi.
9 Enforced bed rest makes time pass very slowly and can be very traumatic for a small child.
  a Water play, mirrors, body games are helpful replacements. Often the child can be moved in his bed into the playroom or hall.

10 This will facilitate movement and self-help.

12 Make certain that countertraction is provided.

a The foot of the child's bed may have to be raised or placed on shock blocks to counteract the traction weight and prevent the child from being pulled to the end of the bed.

13 Never disturb the traction device.

14 Avoid jarring the bed or swinging the weights.

15 Do not allow the weights to hang directly over the child's body.

12 Usually, the patient's body acts as the counterweight which keeps the limb aligned and immobilized.

a The child's weight is often insufficient to provide countertraction.

13 If it appears to need adjustment, notify the surgeon.

14 This may cause pain and is upsetting to the child.

15 This is a safety precaution.

Skin Traction

1 Shave the area if hair is present and paint the skin with tincture of benzoin.

1 This allows the adhesive to grasp the skin more firmly. Benzoin also disinfects the skin, allays itching, and prevents skin breakdown under the tape.

Skeletal Traction

1 Treat all entry sites for pins, wires, or tongs as surgical wounds.
a Wipe the insertion site with Betadine. Cover with a sterile 10cm x 10cm gauze *or*

b Dress the insertion site with a 10 cm x 10 cm sterile gauze treated with an antiseptic prescribed by the surgeon.
c Check the entry site regularly for any signs of infection and to be certain that the pin has not slipped through the bone.

2 Place corks or plastic guards over the exposed ends of the pins.

a This is an attempt to reduce the hazard of infection along the track of the pin. Some surgeons prefer to let these areas crust over or cover them with plaster.

c Notify the surgeon of either of these conditions.

2 This is a safety precaution to prevent injury to the nurse, child or parent.

Gallows Traction

Purpose

1 Used to reduce fractured femurs in small children.
2 To allow burns on buttocks to heal.
3 To aid reduction of incarcerated inguinal hernia.

Mechanism of Action

Involves bilateral, vertical extension of the child's legs. The child's weight serves as countertraction to the vertical pull of the weights. Skin traction is applied to both legs in order to minimize potential trauma to the affected leg and maintain the stability of the position.

Nursing Action	Rationale/Amplification
1 Maintain the child in the appropriate position. **a** The legs are extended at right angles to the body. **b** The hips are elevated slightly from the bed. **c** The buttocks are elevated and clear of the bed. **d** The heels and ankles are free from pressure. **e** The child is flat in bed and unable to turn from side to side. 2 Check the position of the bandages and rewrap as necessary.	1 This position is essential in order to achieve the desired results. **e** A jacket or abdominal restraint is sometimes necessary. 2 The bandages should be wrapped snugly around the legs without compromising circulation. They should not slip and cause pressure on the dorsa of the feet.

Russell Hamilton Traction

Purpose

Used to reduce fractures of the femoral shaft and to treat knee injuries and hip fractures.

Mechanism of Action

Force is exerted on the long axis of the lower leg and the knee sling is used under the distal thigh to provide flexion of the knee and hip.

Nursing Action	Rationale/Amplification
1 Application of crepe bandages. **a** Wrap bandages from the ankle to the thigh on patients under 18 months of age. **b** Wrap bandages from the ankle to the knee on patients over 18 months of age.	 **a** The length of the leg from the knee to the foot is usually not long enough to maintain traction. **b** This length in an older child is sufficient to maintain traction.

2 Place foot supports against the soles of both feet.

2 Prevents foot drop.

3 If necessary, place a small pillow under the thigh to maintain hip flexion at approximately 20°.

3 Prevents hip contractures.

4 Keep the heel free of the bed.

4 Prevents pressure sore of the heel.

5 Carefully check the popliteal space for pressure sores. Make certain that the knee sling is positioned so that it does not exert pressure on the space.

5 Line the knee sling with a piece of felt or sheepskin for additional protection against sores.

6 Make certain that the bandages do not exert pressure over the dorsalis pedis artery (inside top of foot) or the Achilles tendon (back of heel).

6 Prevents discomfort, pressure sores, and circulatory complications.

7 Make certain that the footplate or spreader is wide enough to prevent irritation of the skin but not so wide that the tapes tend to pull from the skin.

Cervical Traction

Purpose

Used for children with spinal fractures, muscle spasms, or spinal injuries to provide immobilization in a neutral position which causes the least pressure on the spinal cord.

Mechanism of Action

Applied directly to the skull bone by a device such as the Crutchfield tong, or indirectly by using a head halter.

Cervical Skin (Head Halter) Traction

1 Check the position of the head halter frequently:
a The halter should not press on the ears.
b The rope should not rest against the skin.
c The chin piece should not press on the throat.
d Protect the chin halter when feeding the child.

1 It is important to prevent continuous pressure and rubbing on these areas in order to avoid skin breakdown.

2 Keep the position of the bed flat unless otherwise prescribed by the surgeon. Avoid lifting the child's head or flexing the neck.

2 Raising the head increases countertraction, which may be undesirable.

3 Keep the child flat on his back.
4 Diversion.
   a Position an adjustable mirror at the head of the bed so that the child can see around the ward.
   b Encourage companionship:
   (1) Place the child with other children of his own age.
   (2) Encourage visiting by parents, older siblings, and friends.
   c Place colourful objects, cards, pictures, etc., within sight of the child.
   d Utilize audiovisual stimulation — records, radio, television, etc.
   e Provide for continuing education for the child of school age.

Cotrel's Traction

Purpose

To provide distraction of the spine prior to surgery or to the application of a scoliotic brace.

Mechanism of Action

Traction is applied primarily to the occipital bone by means of a head harness which fits on to the chin and reaches around to the occiput. Pelvic straps maintain the pelvis in a fixed position.

Nursing Action	Rationale/Amplification
1 Check the head halter for proper placement. **a** The chin pad should not compress the child's throat. **b** The hair should be free from entanglement. **c** The halter should not pinch the ears.	1 This helps to ensure effectiveness of the treatment and prevents skin breakdown.
2 Check the facial skin, chin, occiput, and iliac crests for possible irritation and breakdown.	
3 Check the child frequently for maintenance of alignment.	3 It is relatively easy for the child to become malaligned in this type of traction.

Halo-femoral Traction

Purpose

Utilized to correct severe and resistant spinal curvatures.

Mechanism of Action

An aluminium halo is fixed to the cranium with four threaded pins and Steinman pins are placed in the distal ends of the femur. Upward traction is applied to the halo and downward traction to the femurs to pull the spine into alignment. Frequently, a suspension assembly is attached to the halo by threaded traction rods, the entire assembly being supported by a hoop attached to the pelvic pins. This apparatus allows control of position in all three planes plus progressive traction application. Femoral pins may be removed and countertraction applied by securing the halo device to a body jacket cast. This allows the child to be ambulatory.

Nursing Action	Rationale/Amplification
1 Prepare the child and the parents for the procedure.	1 The appearance of the apparatus may be overwhelming and frightening. Diagrams and visual aids will enhance comprehension and allay fear.
a Explain the purpose, method of application, and approximate time required for the therapy. The child should know that the treatment is relatively pain-free and that the device does not penetrate the brain.	
b If possible, introduce the child to other patients in the apparatus or those who have previously experienced it.	
c Emphasize that this will provide optimal correction of the deformity and allow the child to appear more normal.	**c** These children are often very sensitive about their body image, and will develop a more positive attitude once they realize that the deformity is being improved.
2 Observe the child carefully while traction is being increased for: **a** Neck pain **b** Respiratory distress **c** Nerve injury.	2 Alteration of neurological or respiratory status is regarded as a warning sign and a release of several turns on the extension bars may be carried out by the surgeon as an emergency measure. Neck pain is a less serious sign. The amount of traction is usually not increased until the pain disappears.

3 *Symptoms of injury*
  a Spinal cord
    (1) Weakness, numbness in legs
    (2) Loss of bladder function
    (3) Up- or down-turning of toes
    (4) Clonus of ankles or knees
  b Cranial nerves
    (1) Double vision
    (2) Difficulty in swallowing
    (3) Difficulty in coughing
    (4) Voice changes
    (5) Tongue weakness
  c Upper extremities
    (1) Difficulty in moving hand, shoulder, or arm
    (2) Numbness or weakness in hand (check grip).

4 Make certain that all of the fixtures on the apparatus are tightened.

4 Looseness and excessive movement of the apparatus may cause pain and infection. The surgeon should be notified.

5 Report complaints of pain or drainage at the pin sites.

5 Most children have mild pain and headache for the first few days. Thereafter, pain at the pin site usually means that the pin is loose or infected, and it may be necessary to change the pin.

CASTS

A *cast* is an immobilizing device made up of layers of plaster bandages, glass-fibre or resin-impregnated plaster of Paris bandages. Plaster of Paris is manufactured from calcium sulphate dihydrate (gypsum).

Purposes

1 To immobilize and hold bone fragments in reduction.
2 To apply uniform compression of soft tissues.
3 To permit early weight-bearing activities.
4 To correct chronic deformities with wedging or special hinges, or by serial cast changes.

Types of Casts

1 *Short-arm cast* — extends from below the elbow to the proximal palmar crease.

2   *Gauntlet cast* — extends from below the elbow to the proximal palmar crease, including the thumb (thumb spica).

3   *Long-arm cast* — extends from upper level of axillary fold to proximal palmar crease; elbow usually immobilized at right angle.

4   *Short-leg cast* — extends from below knee to base of toes.

5   *Long-leg cast* — extends from junction of the upper and middle third of thigh to the base of toes; foot is at right angle in a neutral position.

6   *Spica or body cast* — incorporates the trunk and an extremity.

Nursing Considerations

1   The child is usually more troubled by immobilization than the adult. A special attempt should be made to ensure that his activities are as normal as possible and that full use is made of his unaffected joints and muscles.

2   The younger child may not be able to understand why the cast is necessary. He may attempt to remove it, put pieces of toys or food under it, etc.
   a An attempt should be made to allow the child to work through his questions and feelings via play (e.g. give him a doll with a cast).
   b Close supervision is necessary to prevent the child from destroying the cast or injuring himself.

3   There is a danger of soiling a long-leg or hip-spica cast with faeces or urine. (The area of the cast near the buttocks and genitalia should be protected with waterproof material.)

Complications

Constriction of Circulation

Trauma or surgery affecting an extremity will produce swelling due to haemorrhage from bone and surrounding tissue and to tissue oedema. Vascular insufficiency due to unrelieved swelling can cause a reduction in or obliteration of blood supply to an extremity.

1   *Symptoms and signs*
   a Unrelieved or increasing pain.
   b Swelling.
   c Blanching or discoloration
      (1) Test nail beds and pulp of digits of injured extremity for prompt capillary return. A rapid return of colour should appear on release of pressure.
      (2) The colour should be pink; blueness suggests venous obstruction.
      (3) Whiteness and cold fingers or toes suggest arterial obstruction.
      (4) Compare uninjured with injured extremity.

   d Tingling or numbness.

e No pulse or diminished pulse.
Compare pulse on uninjured extremity with that of injured extremity.
f Inability to move fingers or toes; pain on extension of foot or hand may indicate ischaemia.
g Temperature change of skin — cold extremity may indicate ischaemia.

2 *Nursing Management*
    a Inform surgeon.
    b Bivalve the cast; split cast on each side over its full length into halves.
    c Cut the underlying padding — blood soaked padding may shrink and cause constriction of circulation.
    d Spread cast sufficiently to relieve constriction.

Pressure of Cast on Tissues, Especially on Bony Parts

1 Causes necrosis, pressure sores, nerve palsies from prolonged pressure on nerve trunk.
2 *Symptoms*
Severe initial pain over bony prominences; this is a warning symptom of an impending pressure sore. *Pain decreases when ulceration occurs.*
3 *Pressure sites*
    a *Lower extremity*— heel, malleoli, dorsum of foot, head of fibula, anterior surface of patella.
    b *Upper extremity* — medial epicondyle of humerus, ulnar styloid.
    c When plaster jackets or body spica casts are used — sacrum, anterior and superior iliac spines, vertebral borders of scapulae.
4 *Nursing management*
    a Examine the skin over the area by creating a 'window' in the plaster at the pain point (over bony prominence) *or*
    b Bivalve the cast but do not disturb the alignment; keep extremity in one portion of bivalved cast.

Nursing Alert: Do not ignore the complaint of pain, restlessness, or pyrexia of the patient in a cast. Suspect circulatory complications or a pressure sore.

Care of Patient While Cast Dries

1 Explain to the patient that he will experience the feeling of heat under the plaster; however, plaster application is not painful.
2 Leave area enclosed in cast *uncovered* until the cast is dry — covers restrict escape of heat, especially in large casts.
3 Elevate extremity on pillow *after the cast has cooled* and started to harden (above level of heart).
4 Avoid resting cast on hard surfaces or sharp edges that can cause denting of the cast and consequent pressure sores.

5   Avoid weight bearing or stress on cast for 48 hours.
6   Avoid handling cast while it is drying out in first 48 hours. Lift cast using palms of the hands and avoid digging fingers in.

Observation of the Patient in a Cast

1   Listen to the patient's complaints (see complications). Ask the patient to localize the exact site of pain, if this is possible.
2   Avoid giving analgesics for pain. Do not mask the pain until the cause has been determined.
3   Watch for signs of pressure and constriction of circulation
4   Notify surgeon if symptoms persist. Cast may have to be removed.

Care of Patient after Cast Dries

Leg Cast

1   Prevent or reduce swelling.
    a Elevate the extremity in the cast.
    b After patient begins ambulation, encourage him to elevate the cast when he is seated.
2   Prevent irritation at cast edge — pad edges.
3   Examine toes and foot for:
    a Blanching or cyanosis
    b Swelling
    c Inability to move toes.
4   Ascertain whether patient is experiencing sensory disturbances to foot (numbness, tingling, burning, cold) — peroneal nerve injury from pressure at the head of the fibula is a common cause of footdrop; may be initial finding in vascular compromise.
5   Encourage the patient to move about as normally as possible.
    a Do prescribed exercises faithfully.
    b Do not cover a leg cast with plastic or rubber boots since this causes condensation and wetting of the cast. Avoid walking on wet floors.
    c Report to the surgeon if the cast cracks or breaks; instruct the parents not to try to fix it.

Arm Cast

1   Watch for symptoms of circulatory disturbance in hand (blueness or cyanosis, swelling, inability to move fingers, forearm pain on extension of fingers).
2   Reduce and control swelling.
    Elevate arm with each joint positioned higher than preceding joint (i.e. elbow higher than shoulder, hand higher than the elbow).

Nursing Alert: Guard against Volkmann's contracture — a severe fibrosis with resulting contracture of muscles which have become ischaemic by obstruction of the arterial flow to the forearm and hand. This complication is prevented by proper care; if allowed to develop, the results are disastrous.

Exercising the Patient in the Cast: Health Teaching

1   Teach the patient to perform isometric exercises — contracting the muscles without moving the joint to maintain muscle strength and prevent atrophy (performed hourly when awake).
2   Leg cast — 'Push down on the popliteal (knee) space, hold it, relax, repeat'.
3   Arm cast — 'Make a fist, hold it, relax, repeat'.
4   Actively exercise joints that do not move bone fragments.
5   Exercise every joint that is not immobilized. Move the rest of the body.

On Discharge Home: Advice to Parents

1   Allow plaster cast to dry naturally, if a new plaster. Keep dry.
2   Seek medical help immediately if fingers or toes become discoloured, painful or swollen.
3   Return for earlier outpatient appointment if cast becomes soft or cracked.
Note: Should be given as written instructions to parents as it is easy to forget verbal advice in the excitement of taking their child home.

Reading for Parents

Greenwood A Greenwood D, *Your Child in an Immobilizing Plaster,* NAWCH Publications, 1984.

Reading for Children

Watts M A, *Crocodile Plaster,* Andre Deutsch, 1978.

GUIDELINES: CARE OF A CHILD IN A SPICA CAST

Procedure

Nursing Action	Rationale/Amplification
1 If possible, prepare the child for the application of the cast.	1 This can best be accomplished by allowing the child to put a cast on a doll. Older children should see a picture of the cast that is going to be

2 Facilitate drying and accurate moulding of the cast.

   a Place a bedboard under the mattress.
   b Support the curves of the cast with small, plastic-covered pillows.
   c Avoid placing a pillow under the head and shoulders.
   d Keep the cast uncovered and turn the child every 1-2 hours.
   e Handle moist cast with the palms of hands.

3 Observe for complications resulting from pressure of the cast.
   a Impaired circulation to the toes
   (1) Discoloration or cyanosis
   (2) Impaired movement
   (3) Loss of sensation
   (4) Oedema
   (5) Temperature change
   (6) Absent pedal pulses.
   b Complaints of pain or pressure in any areas where the cast fits closely over the body.

4 Provide good skin care.

   a Bathe accessible skin and massage with suitable skin cream or lotion. Pay special attention to the buttocks and genital area.
   b Inspect the skin for signs of irritation:
   (1) Around cast edge
   (2) Under the cast — pull skin taut and inspect under the cast, using a flashlight for illumination.
   c Investigate complaints of pain or burning or an offensive odour from inside the cast.

   d Relieve itching by blowing cool air through the cast with a hair dryer.

applied and receive an explanation of the method of application.

2 About 24-48 hours are required for a cast to dry completely. A cast dries from the outside to the inside. It may feel dry to the touch but still be wet on the inside.
   a Prevents sagging of the bed from pressure of the cast.
   b Prevents cracking while the cast is drying.
   c Causes pressure on the chest by thrusting it forward in the cast.
   d Allows moisture to evaporate from the surface.
   e Fingers may cause indentations in the moist plaster. To avoid dents, use palms of hands when touching wet or drying plaster of Paris.

3 Vascular insufficiency due to unrelieved swelling can cause necrosis and pressure sores. It may be necessary to bivalve the cast.

4 Prevents the development of pressure sores.

   c These may indicate that a pressure sore is forming or has become infected. It may be necessary to create a 'window' in the cast.
   d Some surgeons insert a strip of gauze through the cast which can be

e Do not allow a small child to put objects inside his cast.

(1) Keep small toys away from the child.

(2) Pad the edges of the cast with cotton padding or cover it with a towel to prevent food particles and foreign objects from being inserted by the child.

5 Prevent the skin around the edge of the cast from becoming excoriated.

a Smooth the edges of the cast and cover it with waterproof adhesive tape.

b Do not lift infants by their legs to change nappies.

6 Prevent urine and faeces from soiling the cast.

a Offer the bedpan frequently.

(1) Elevate the child's head slightly higher than his feet to prevent urine from running under the cast.

b Keep the perineum clean.

(1) Wash the skin under the edge of the cast whenever necessary and dry it thoroughly.

(2) Change nappies immediately after they become soiled.

7 Plan for short period of muscle exercise every day.

a Encourage the child to move and exercise his unaffected extremities. Provide diversional therapy which requires the use of these muscles.

b Exercise the child's toes.

8 Have the child breathe deeply at intervals. Provide him with soap bubbles, whistles, or party favours to make this more fun. An older child may use blow bottles.

9 Turn the child at least every 4 hours.

a Move the child to the side of the bed, using a steady, pulling motion.

b Place one hand under the head and back and one hand under the leg

used to gently massage the skin. Do not use sharp objects such as coat hangers or knitting needles.

e A small hand vacuum cleaner may be used to remove crumbs from inside the cast.

a This prevents flakes of plaster from breaking off and slipping under the cast. It also facilitates cleansing of the cast.

6 A soiled cast will cause skin irritation, become malodorous, and may mildew or partially disintegrate.

7 Disuse of muscles can result in atrophy and deformities.

8 Prolonged periods of immobilization may cause the child to develop hypostatic pneumonia.

9 Do not use the supporting bar between the legs as a lever when turning the child.

portion of the cast, and turn the child on his side.

c Second nurse accepts the support of the child and cast as he is turned completely.

10 Assess the child's bowel and bladder function.

a Provide an adequate fluid intake, especially fruit juices.

b Check the urine for signs of infection.

10 Immobilization may cause constipation and poor urinary drainage. Suppositories or mild laxatives may be necessary for the constipated child.

11 Maintain correct position of the cast. Support the contour of the cast with pillows. Allow the heel to extend beyond the pillow to avoid pressure sores.

11 This prevents cracking or flattening of the cast.

12 Provide as normal an environment as possible.

a Place the child on a cart or a stretcher so that he may leave his room. The child may be taken outdoors if the weather is suitable.

b Allow the child to be dressed. (Wide, flared trousers are especially suitable.)

c Encourage contact with peers.

d Provide for play activities.

(1) Provide the young child with large toys which he cannot put into his cast.

(2) Television is a good method of diversion if used with discretion.

(3) Older children often enjoy draughts, sewing, art work, building models, etc.

e Provide for education.

12 Enforced immobility is often traumatic for the child and may cause regression.

13 Evaluate the home situation for feasibility of home care. Consider:

a The child's place in the family and the number of siblings

b Additional needs of the parents, such as pursuing their vocations

c Physical setup of the home:

(1) Number of stairs

(2) Sleeping arrangements (type of bed, etc.)

d Ability of the family to keep follow-up appointments:

14 Assist the family in caring for the child after discharge:

a Initiate the appropriate referrals.
(1) Community nursing service
(2) Social worker if necessary.
b Begin teaching early.
(1) Instruct the parent on all aspects of the child's care.

(1) Teach only a few aspects of care each day. Have the parent(s) participate in the child's care until capable of providing total nursing care under supervision.

(2) Emphasize safety measures such as elevating the child's head during meals to prevent choking; preventing the small child from dropping objects into his cast; using good body mechanics when lifting and transporting the child, etc.
(3) Provide with detailed, written instructions.

15 Assist with cast removal.
a Prepare the child for the procedure.
(1) Describe the sensations that the child will feel (warmth, vibration, etc.) as well as the procedure itself.
(2) Allow the child to observe as the saw is lightly touched to the operator's palm.
b Immobilize the child as necessary so that the procedure can be carried out quickly and safely.

15 Children often believe that the saw will cut off a limb, and are frightened by the loud noise.

16 Care for the child after cast removal.
a Support the part with pillows.

b Move the extremity gently.
c Wash the skin gently with mild soap and apply oil or lanolin.

a Maintain the same position that existed in the cast.
b It will be very weak and stiff.
c An accumulation of sebaceous material and dead skin causes the skin to appear brown and flaky. Vigorous rubbing will cause skin trauma.

d Encourage the child to do prescribed exercises.
e Elevate the limb when sitting.

d These will strengthen muscles and relieve joint stiffness.
e Minimizes the development of oedema.

FURTHER READING

Paediatric Procedures

Books

Adamson E. F. St J Hull D, *Nursing Sick Children*, Churchill Livingstone, 1984.
Avery G B, *Neonatology*, J B Lippincott, 1981.
Brown R J K Valman H B, *Practical Neonatal Paediatrics*, Blackwell Scientific, 1979.
King E *et al.* (Adapted for the UK by B F Weller), *Paediatric Nursing Practice and Techniques*, Harper & Row, 1986.
Rickham P, *Neonatal Surgery*, Butterworth, 1978.
Young D Martin E, *Baby Surgery*, HM&M, 1979.

Articles

Anagnostakis D *et al.*, Risk of infection associated with umbilical vein catheterization, *Journal of Pediatrics*, 1975, 86: 759-765.
Boxall J, Measuring and passing a duodenal/jejunal feeding tube, *Nursing Times*, August 1979: 1459-1460.
Chambers T, When a child's kidneys fail, *Nursing Mirror*, December 1979: 995-999.
Hott J, The rule of Ws, *Nursing Update*, 1975, 6:14-16.
Luciano K Shumsky C, Pediatric procedures; the explanation should always come first, *Nursing*, January 1975, 5: 49-52.
Nicholson A, Chronic renal failure in a child, *Nursing Times*, June 1979: 995-999.
Szur R Earnshaw A, Experiences with newborn and very young infants, *Nursing Times*, August 1979: 1497-1500.
Wolfer J A Visitainer M A, Paediatric surgical patients' and parents' stress responses and adjustment, *Nursing Research*, 1975,24: 244-255.

Nursing Care of the Child Undergoing Dialysis

Articles

Caring for children in renal failure, King's Fund Conference Report, November 1979.
Chantler C, Should we treat children with kidney failure? *World Medicine*, April 1980: 37.
Dialysis and transplantation in young children, *Lancet*, January 1978: 26.
Dialysis and transplantation in young children, *British Medical Journal*, April 1979: 1033-1934.
Kershaw H C, Continuous ambulatory peritoneal dialysis in childhood, *Maternal and Child Health*, November 1983: 454-460.
Donaldson M D *et al.*, Peritoneal dialysis in infants, *British Medical Journal*, March 1983: 759-760.
Wheeler D, Teaching home dialysis for an 8-year-old boy, *American Journal of Nursing*, February 1977, 77: 273-274.
Winder E, Children on haemodialysis, *Nursing Times*, December 1978: 2011-2014.

Principles of Fluid and Electrolyte Balance in Children; Intravenous Fluid Therapy

Books

Burgess A, *The Nurses's Guide to Fluid and Electrolyte Balance*, McGraw-Hill, 1979.
Roberts K D Edwards J M, *Paediatric Intensive Care: A Manual for Resident Medical Officers and Senior Nurses*, Blackwell Scientific, 1976.
Winters R W (ed.), *The Body Fluids in Pediatrics*, Little Brown, 1973.

Articles

Abbott P Schlacht K, Paediatric IVs: a special challenge, *The Canadian Nurse*, November 1984: 24-26.
Kurdi W J, Refining your IV therapy techniques, *Nursing*, November 1975, 75: 41-47.
Miller V, Intravenous alimentation in paediatric practice, *Nursing Times*, December 1977, 1874-1877.

Protective Devices to Limit Movement

Books

Barlow S Weller B, *Paediatric Nursing*, Baillière Tindall, 1983.

Articles

Kukuk H, Safety precautions: protecting your patients and yourself, Part 2, *Nursing*, June 1976, 6: 49-52.
Kukuk H, Safety precautions: protecting your patients and yourself, Part 3, *Nursing*, July 1976, 6: 45-50.

Respiratory Procedures

Books

Petty T (ed.), *Intensive and Rehabilitation Respiratory Care*, Lea & Febiger, 1974.
Roberts K D Edwards J M, *Paediatric Intensive Care*, Blackwell Scientific, 1976.
Scipien G *et al.*, *Comprehensive Pediatric Nursing*, McGraw-Hill, 1979.

Articles

Affonso D Harris T, Continuous positive airways pressure, *American Journal of Nursing*, 1979, 6: 570-573.
Allan D, Nursing aspects of artificial ventilation, *Nursing Times*, June 1982: 1006-1009.
Beaumont E, Up to date survey of tracheal tubes, *Nursing*, November 1976: 66-72.
Ellis H, Top priority-the child with stridor, *Modern Medicine*, June 1979: 14-17.
Nethercott S G Price J F, Management of chronically ventilated infants, *Nursing Times*, July 1978: 1130-1135.

Total Parenteral Nutrition

Books

Fischer J E (ed.), *Total Parenteral Nutrition*, Little Brown, 1976.
Scipien G *et al.*, *Comprehensive Pediatric Nursing*, McGraw-Hill, 1979.

Traction and Casts

Books

Blockley N J, *Children's Orthopaedics: Practical Problems*, Butterworth, 1976.
Farrell J, *Illustrated Guide to Orthopaedic Nursing*, J B Lippincott, 1977.
Hilt N Schmitt W, *Pediatric Orthopedic Nursing*, C V Mosby, 1975.
Lloyd-Roberts G, *Orthopaedics in Infancy and Childhood*, Butterworth, 1978.
Powell M, *Orthopaedic Nursing*, Churchill Livingstone, 1982.

Articles

Hilt N, Care of the child in a hip spica cast, *Registered Nurse*, April 1976, 39: 27-31.
Johnson J *et al.*, Altering children's distress behaviour during orthopedic cast removal, *Nursing Research*, 1975, 24: 404-411.

Vital Signs

Books

Apley J *et el.*, *The Child and Symptoms*, Blackwell Scientific, 1978.
Illingworth R S, *Common Symptoms of Disease in Children*, Blackwell Scientific, 1984.

Articles

Barmes N D Robertson N R C, PUO in children, *Update*, April 1979: 1009-1016.
Earley A *et al.*, Problems of hypertension in childhood, *Practitioner*, August 1979: 203-208.
Jarvis C, Vital signs-how to take them more accurately and understand them more fully, *Nursing*, April 1976, 6: 31.
McKenzie S, Examination of children, *Journal of Maternal and Child Health*, March-April 1979: 100-102.
Meadow S R, Hypertension in childhood, *Journal of the Royal College of General Practitioners*, September 1978: 635-636.
O'Brian E T O'Malley K, ABC of blood pressure measurement, *British Medical Journal*, October 1979, 1048-1049.
Warren F M, Blood pressure readings: getting them quickly on an infant, *Nursing*, April 1975, 5: 13.

3

PROBLEMS OF INFANTS

MANAGEMENT OF THE PRETERM INFANT

The *preterm infant* is a viable infant born before the end of the 37th week of gestation.

Aetiology

1　Unknown
2　Maternal factors:
　　a　Chronic poor nutrition
　　b　Diabetes
　　c　Multiple births
　　d　Drug abuse
　　e　IUD in gravid uterus
　　f　Chronic disease
　　　　(1) Heart disease
　　　　(2) Kidney disease
　　　　(3) Infection

　　g　Complications of pregnancy
　　　　(1) Toxaemia
　　　　(2) Bleeding
　　　　(3) Placenta previa or abruptio placentae
　　　　(4) Incompetent cervix
　　　　(5) Preterm rupture of membranes
　　　　(6) Polyhydramnios
3　Fetal factors:
　　a　Chromosomal abnormalities
　　b　Anatomic abnormalities
　　　　(1) Tracheo-oesophageal atresia or fistula
　　　　(2) Intestinal obstruction
　　c　Fetoplacental dysfunction.

Clinical Manifestations

1   Physical appearance
   Hair — lanugo, fluffy
   Poor ear cartilage
   Skin — very thin; capillaries are visible (may be red and wrinkled)
   Lack of subcutaneous fat
   Sole of foot is smooth
      (36 weeks gestation — one-third of foot is creased)
      (38 weeks gestation — two-thirds of foot is creased)
   Breast buds 5 mm
      (36 weeks gestation — none)
      (38 weeks gestation — 3 mm)
   Testes — undescended
   Labia minora — undeveloped
   Rugae of scrotum — very fine
   Fingernails — softer
   Abdomen — relatively large
   Thorax — relatively small
   Head — appears disproportionately large
   Face resembles 'an old man'
   Muscle tone poor — reflexes weak
2   Generally, maturation and growth rate increase after birth.

Pathophysiology

The preterm infant has altered physiology due to immature and often poorly developed systems. The severity of any problem that occurs depends upon the gestational age of the infant.

Respiratory System*

1   Alveoli begin to form 26-28 weeks' gestation; therefore, lungs are poorly developed.
2   Respiratory muscles are poorly developed.
3   Chest wall lacks stability.
4   Production of surfactant is reduced.
5   There is reduced compliance and low functional residual capacity.
6   Breathing may be laboured and irregular with periods of apnoea and cyanosis.
7   Infant is prone to atelectasis.
8   Vomit and cough reflexes are poor; thus, aspiration is a problem.

Digestive System*

1   Stomach is small, vomiting is likely to occur. It is difficult to provide caloric requirement in early days.

*Systems and situations that are most likely to cause problems in the preterm.

2   Tolerance is decreased and therefore is impaired to absorb fat, vitamin D, and all fat soluble vitamins.

Poor Thermal Stability*

1   Has very little subcutaneous fat, thus, there is no heat storage or insulation.
2   Cannot shiver; has poor vasomotor control of blood flow to skin capillaries.
3   There is a relatively large surface area in comparison to body weight.
4   Sweat glands are decreased; infant cannot perspire.
5   Has reduced muscle and fat deposits that restrict metabolic rate and heat production.
6   Usually is less active.

Renal Function

1   Sodium excretion is probably increased, which may lead to hyponatraemia; there is difficulty in excreting potassium.
2   Ability to concentrate urine decreases; thus, when vomiting or diarrhoea occur, dehydration is likely to follow.
3   Ability to acidify urine decreases.
4   Glomerular tubular imbalance accounts for sugar, protein, amino acids, and sodium present in urine.

Nervous System

1   Response to stimulation is slow.
2   Suck, swallow, and vomit reflexes are poor; feeding and aspiration therefore are problems.
3   Cough reflex is weak or absent.
4   Centres that control respirations, temperature, and other vital functions are poorly developed.

Infection* (see p. 286, Septicaemia Neonatorum)

1   Actively formed antibodies are absent at birth (active immunity).
2   No IgM is present at birth (passive immunity).
3   Limited chemotaxis (reaction of cell to chemical stimuli).
4   Decreased opsonization (preparation of cells for phagocytosis).
5   Limited phagocytosis (digestion of bacteria by cells).

Liver Function

1   Does not have ability to handle and conjugate bilirubin.
2   Does not store or release sugar well; thus, there is a tendency toward hypoglycaemia.
3   There is a steady decrease in haemoglobin after birth and in the production of blood; therefore, anaemia may occur.
4   Does not make or store vitamin K; thus, infant is susceptible to haemorrhagic disease.

*Systems and situations that are most likely to cause problems in the preterm.

Eyes

1 Oxygen given beyond the point of infant need will cause retinal arteries to constrict, resulting in anoxic damage.
2 The retinae detach from the surface of posterior chambers and a fibrous mass forms, resulting in an inability to receive visual stimulation. This is retrolental fibroplasia (RLF).
3 There are many stages of RLF.
4 The exact amount and level of oxygen needed to produce RLF is unknown.

Complications in Preterm Infants

The severity of any problem that occurs in the preterm infant depends upon the gestational age of that infant.

1 Hyaline membrane disease (respiratory distress syndrome)
2 Aspiration
3 Infection
4 Hypoglycaemia
5 Hypocalcaemia
6 Patent ductus arteriosus
7 Impaired thermal haemostasis
8 Feeding problems
9 Functional intestinal obstruction
10 Necrotizing enterocolitis
11 Intraventricular or subarachnoid haemorrhage.

Diagnostic Evaluation

Neurological Assessment of Gestational Age

1 Maturation of the nervous system progresses at its own pace and is not increased by birth.
2 The value of a neurological evaluation increases after 48 hours of life. False results may be obtained if examination is made within a few hours of birth or when the baby is sleeping.
3 This examination is used primarily to estimate the infant's gestational age.
4 The examination should be done when the infant is awake and quiet.
5 Examination includes evaluation of muscle tone and evaluation of reflexes and reactions.

Techniques of Assessment of Neurological Criteria (see Figure 3.1)

Posture

Observed with infant quiet and in supine position. Score 0: arms and legs extended; 1: beginning of flexion of hips and knees, arms extended; 2: stronger flexion of legs, arms extended; 3: arms slightly flexed, legs flexed and abducted; 4: full flexion of arms and legs.

Square Window

The hand is flexed on the forearm between the thumb and index finger of the examiner. Enough pressure is applied to get as full a flexion as possible, and the angle between the hypothenar eminence and the ventral aspect of the forearm is measured and graded according to Figure 3.1 (Care is taken not to rotate the infant's wrist while doing this manoeuvre.)

Ankle Dorsiflexion

The foot is dorsiflexed on to the anterior aspect of the leg, with the examiner's thumb on the sole of the foot and other fingers behind the leg. Enough pressure is applied to get as full flexion as possible and the angle between the dorsum of the foot and the anterior aspect of the leg is measured.

Arm Recoil

With the infant in the supine position the forearms are first flexed for 5 seconds, then fully extended by pulling on the hands, and then released. The sign is fully positive if the arms return briskly to full flexion (score 2). If the arms return to incomplete flexion or the response is sluggish, it is graded as score 1. If they remain extended or are only followed by random movements, score 0.

Leg Recoil

With the infant supine, the hips and knees are fully flexed for 5 seconds, then extended by traction on the feet, and released. A maximal response is one of full flexion of the hips and knees (score 2). A partial flexion scores 1, and minimal or no movement scores 0.

Popliteal Angle

With the infant supine and his pelvis flat on the examining couch, the thigh is held in the knee-chest position by examiner's left index finger and thumb supporting the knee. The leg is then extended by gentle pressure from the examiner's right index finger behind the ankle and the popliteal angle is measured.

Heel to Ear Manoeuvre

With the baby supine, draw the baby's foot as near to the head as it will go without forcing it. Observe the distance between the foot and the head as well as the degree of extension of the knee. Grade according to Figure 3.1. Note that the knee is left free and may draw down alongside the abdomen.

Scarf Sign

With the baby supine, take the infant's hand and try to put it around the neck and as far posteriorly as possible around the opposite shoulder. Assist this manoeuvre by lifting the elbow across the body. See how far the elbow will go across and grade according to Figure 3.1. Score 0: elbow reaches opposite axillary line; 1: elbow.

To observe for any gross abnormalities and to pay special attention to respirations, heart rate, muscle tone, and activity.

Head Lag

With the baby supine, grasp the hands (or the arms if a very small infant) and pull him slowly towards the sitting position. Observe the position of the head in relation to the trunk and grade accordingly. In a small infant the head may initially be supported by one hand. Score 0: complete lag; 1: partial head control; 2: able to maintain head in line with body; 3: brings head anterior to body.

Ventral Suspension

The infant is suspended in the prone position, with examiner's hand under the infant's chest (one hand in a small infant, two in a large infant). Observe the degree of extension of the back and head to the trunk. Grade according to Figure 3.1.
Note: If score differs on the two sides, take the mean.

Nursing Objectives — Admission to the Nursery

To observe for any gross abnormalities, and to pay special attention to respirations, heart rate, muscle tone, and activity.

1   Respirations above 40 per minute over a period of time may be indicative of respiratory difficulty.
    a Expiratory grunting, retractions, or nasal flaring should be reported immediately.
    b Cyanosis (other than acrocyanosis — coldness and cyanosis of hands and feet) should be watched for along with other signs of respiratory distress.
2   Increased (above 120 per minute) or irregular heart rate may indicate cardiac or circulatory difficulties.
3   Muscle tone and activity can be a good guide to degree of prematurity.

To maintain a patent airway.

1   Have oxygen, suction, and resuscitation equipment readily available.

Scoring scheme for development assessment

Neurological

External (superficial) criteria

EXTERNAL SIGN	0	1	SCORE 2	3	4
OEDEMA	Obvious oedema hands and feet, pitting over tibia	No obvious oedema hands and feet; pitting ober tibia	No oedema		
SKIN TEXTURE	Very thin, gelatinous	Thin and smooth	Smooth; medium thickness. Rash or superficial peeling	Slight thickening. Superficial cracking and peeling esp. hands and feet	Thick and parchment like; superficial or deep cracking
SKIN COLOUR (Infant not crying)	Dark red	Uniformly pink	Pale pink; variable over body	Pale. Only pink over ears, lips, palms or soles	
SKIN OPACITY (trunk)	Numerous veins and venules clearly seen, especially over abdomen	Veins and tributaries seen	A few large vessels clearly seen over abdomen	A few large vessels seen indistinctly over abdomen	No blood vessels seen
LANUGO (over back)	No lanugo	Abundant; long and thick over whole back	Hair thinning especially over lower back	Small amount of lanugo and bald areas	At least half of back devoid of lanugo
PLANTAR CREASES	No skin creases	Faint red marks over anterior half of sole	Definite red marks over more than anterior half; indentations over less than anterior third	Indentations over more than anterior third	Definite deep indentations over more than anterior third
NIPPLE FORMATION	Nipple barely visible; no areola	Nipple well defined; areola smooth and flat; diameter 0.75 cm	Areola stippled, edge not raised; diameter 0.75 cm	Areola stippled, edge raised; diameter 0.75 cm	
BREAST SIZE	No breast tissue palpable	Breast tissue on one or both sides 0.5 cm diameter	Breast tissue both sides; one or both 0.5-1.0 cm	Breast tissue both sides; one or both 1 cm	
EAR FORM	Pinna flat and shapeless, little or no incurving of edge	Incurving of part of edge of pinna	Partial incurving whole of upper pinna	Well-defined incurving whole of upper pinna	
EAR FIRMNESS	Pinna soft, easily folded, no recoil	Pinna soft, easily folded, slow recoil	Cartilage to edge of pinna, but soft in places, ready recoil	Pinna firm, cartilage to edge, instant recoil	
GENTALIA MALE	Neither testis in scrotum	At least one testis high in scrotum	At least one testis right down		
FEMALES (With hips half abducted)	Labia majora widely separated, labia minora protruding	Labia majora almost cover labia minora	Labia majora completely cover labia minora		

NEURO-LOGICAL SIGN	0	SCORE 1	2
POSTURE			
SQUARE WINDOW		90°	60°	45°
ANKLE DORSI-FLEXION	90°	75°	45°
ARM RECOIL	180°	90–180°	<90°
LEG RECOIL	180°	90–180°	<90°
POPLITEAL ANGLE	180°	160°	130°
HEEL TO EAR			
SCARF SIGN			
HEAD LAG			
VENTRAL SUSPENSION			

Figure 3.1 Scoring scheme for developmental assessment. (From Dubowitz V, *Journal of Pediatrics*, 1970, 77: 1-10. Published by C.V. Mosby Company, with permission.)

criteria

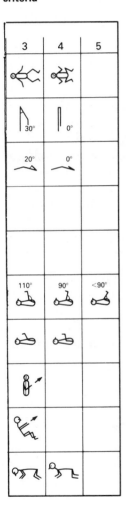

Graph for reading gestational age from total score

The total score for the neurological criteria (see opposite) and the external criteria (see p. 216) are added together and the gestational age is read on the graph below.

see opposite
see p. 216

$$y = 0.2642x + 24.595$$

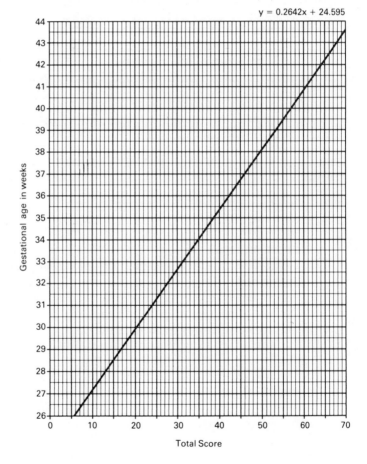

2   Suction mouth and pharynx if mucus is present — to prevent aspiration. Preterm infants often have an excess amount of mucus as well as poor cough, swallow, and gag reflexes.

3   Position infant in incubator or under radiant heater to allow for easy drainage of mucus from his mouth.

   a Very small preterm infant — place on side.

   b Larger preterm infant — place on abdomen.

   c Head may be tilted down — this may be contraindicated because of increased intracranial pressure or increased respiratory distress due to liver pushing against diaphragm decreasing lung expansion.

4   Administer emergency oxygen to just barely relieve cyanosis.

To provide and maintain thermal neutrality of the premature infant.

1   Obtain weight and temperature; then attach cardiac monitor leads quickly and place infant in warm environment (incubator, radiant heater). Omit bath until infant's temperature has stabilized.

2   The preterm infant's ability to control his own body temperature is inhibited by many factors related to his immaturity (see p. 242).

To ensure that prophylactic measures have been administered against ophthalmia neonatorum and that vitamin K_1 has been administered.

Since the preterm infant is frequently taken from the delivery room as soon as possible after birth, prophylactic measures may have been omitted.

To be aware of early complications that may arise as a result of complications of the pregnancy or delivery.

1   *Maternal medication*

   a Drugs pass quickly from mother's blood, across the placenta into the infant's blood.

   b Infant may be drowsy and have slowed respirations.

   c Because of poor development, respiratory difficulty may occur.

2   *Blood incompatibility of mother and infant.*

   a Preterm infant is more susceptible to jaundice, even without incompatibilities.

   b Observe closely for early signs of jaundice (see p. 275, hyperbilirubinaemia).

3   *Maternal conditions that may predispose to infant problems*

   a Infection or illness.

   b Diabetes.

   c Drugs.

4   *Neonatal asphyxia*

   a Apgar score of less than 5 at 1 minute and less than 7 at 5 minutes.

   b Asphyxia may be defined as any of the following:

(1) Hypoxia (reduced oxygen available)
(2) Anoxia (total lack of oxygen)
(3) Hypercapnia (inability to eliminate CO_2)
(4) Acidosis.
c Causes of asphyxia or hypoxia can originate in the mother, the placenta, the infant, or may be a result of the delivery.

The First 24-28 Hours of Life

This period after birth is the most critical time for the preterm infant.

To be constantly aware of the infant's condition and to make frequent observations.

1   This poorly developed, immature infant is prone to sudden changes in condition.
2   Early recognition of symptoms and reporting observations to paediatrician are the most valuable contributions the nurse can make in caring for and saving the preterm infant's life.
3   Note bleeding from the umbilical cord.
    a Should bleeding occur, apply pressure.
    b Estimate amount of bleeding and record.
    c Notify the paediatrician immediately — replacement transfusion may be necessary.
4   Note first micturition.
    a This may occur up to 36 hours after birth, but it usually occurs within the first 24 hours. Report any 4- to 6-hour period when micturition does not occur.
    b Note amount, colour, and frequency of micturitions.
    c Absence of micturition may indicate renal system anomalies, shock, or poor circulation.
5   Note stools.
    a Note when first stool occurred and its characteristics.
    b Abdominal distension and lack of stool may indicate intestinal obstruction or other intestinal tract anomalies.
6   Note activity and behaviour.
    a Note amount of lethargy or activity or need for stimulation.
    b Look for sucking movement, hand-to-mouth manoeuvre. This can help to determine oral feeding initiation.
    c Note quality of cry.
7   Observe for a tense and bulging fontanelle.
    a Full fontanelle may indicate hydrocephalus or intracranial haemorrhage.
    b Be alert to twitching and seizures.
8   Note colour of skin.
    a Cyanosis
        (1) Circulatory or cardiac difficulties may be present.

(2) Respiratory effort may be ineffective.
b Jaundice
(1) May indicate infection.
(2) Erythroblastosis fetalis is another possible difficulty.
9   Carefully monitor, record, and report vital signs.

To maintain respirations.

1   Immediate emergency support may be necessary, since respiratory system is poorly developed and ability to control respirations is often barely sufficient.
2   Have available resuscitative equipment, oxygen, and suction apparatus.
a Mucus may not be handled well, because of poor gag, cough, and swallowing reflexes.
(1) Clearing the airway is of major importance.
(2) A rubber ear bulb syringe or sterile mucus extractor is often all that is necessary for clearing the mouth.
(3) Frequent suctioning of the pharynx may not be necessary.

3   Position infant to allow for easy ventilation.
a Supine position permits free expansion of the thoracic cage (infant's body weight is on the chest and abdomen when he is prone).
b Elevate head and trunk to decrease pressure on diaphragm from abdominal organs.
c Slight neck extension affords opening of trachea; place small roll under shoulders.
d Do not constrict abdominal area, since abdominal muscles are used to aid respiratory effort.
e Flex and abduct arms to enhance chest expansion.
f Change position from side to side. Perform postural drainage with chest vibration (see p. 175) every 2 hours to aid in draining fluid accumulation in thoracic cavity.
4   Use only the percentage of oxygen necessary to relieve cyanosis or maintain colour.
a Oxygen is used with moisture to prevent mucous membranes from drying and becoming irritated.
b Monitor oxygen with analyser every hour to ensure consistency in percentage use.

5   Note any changes in respiratory effort and report these to paediatrician.
a Note quality and rate particularly.
b Hyaline membrane disease or respiratory distress syndrome occurs during the first 24-28 hours of life. Observe for and report immediately any signs and symptoms of respiratory difficulty:
(1) Increased respiratory rate (usually above 60 per minute)
(2) Thoracic retractions

(3) Nasal flaring
(4) Cyanosis
(5) Expiratory grunting
(6) Developing exhaustion
(7) Periods of apnoea.

6   Hypoxaemia is associated with birth asphyxia and recurrent apnoeic episodes. Serum P_aO_2 less than 5.3 kPa (40 mmHg).

7   Hypoventilation — tendency to retain CO_2 due to irregular breathing, poor respiratory muscle activity, and flexible thoracic cage. PCO_2 greater than 6.7 kPa (50 mmHg).

8   Identify periodic breathing versus apnoeic episodes.

    a *Periodic breathing*—cessation of breathing for short periods (5-10 seconds) followed by ventilation for 10-15 seconds at an increased rate.

    b *Apnoeic episodes*—nonbreathing periods of more than 20 seconds duration may be accompanied by bradycardia and cyanosis. Infant is hypotonic and unresponsive. Stimulation or resuscitation is required to restart breathing and increase heart rate. Provocative conditions that increase apnoeic spells include:

    (1) Hyperthermia
    (2) Hypoglycaemia
    (3) Hypocalcaemia
    (4) Acidosis
    (5) Hypobilirubinaemia
    (6) CNS disease — intraventricular haemorrhage
    (7) Pulmonary insufficiency
    (8) Infection
    (9) PDA (patent ductus arteriosus)
    (10) Sodium disturbances
    (11) Hypoxaemia.

To conserve the infant's energy while providing necessary care.

1   Be organized in caring for the infant.
    Collect all equipment before starting care, do what needs to be done, and then let the infant rest. Infant's position will affect his ability to rest.

2   Small infants tire very easily.
    a Any activity increases oxygen need, thus increasing respiratory rate, taxing already limited energy.
    b Adjust infant's environment so that rest and sleep are not hindered.
    c Interventions must be evaluated for their relative value versus the trauma they entail.

To provide and maintain thermal neutrality of the preterm infant.

1   Maintain infant's temperature at the thermoneutral zone, i.e. at the environmental temperature in which the resting infant maintains normal body

temperature and still utilizes minimum energy-oxygen consumption and calories.

a Infant's core temperature (rectal temperature) should be maintained at 37°C.

b Keep environmental (ambient) temperature range between 32 and 35°C. Smaller preterm infants may need higher temperature, 35°C; larger infants, around 32°C.

2 Be aware that the infant loses heat by radiation, conduction, convection, and evaporation; thus, the nurse must be alert to conditions that influence heat loss or gain by the infant.

a Note location of warming unit in relation to air conditioners, direct sunlight, and draughts. Move the unit, if necessary.

b Minimize porthole entrance activities into incubator; keep portholes tightly closed when they are not in use or tightly fitting around arm when entering incubator.

c If it is decided to nurse the infant naked to improve observation, excessive heat loss by radiation can be minimized by using a heat shield made of Perspex placed over the infant.

3 Avoid constant or drastic changing of temperature control dial.

4 Skin temperature probe should be placed on trunk of infant rather than extremities which are more susceptible to changes in peripheral circulation. Prevent infant from lying on thermistor.

5 Monitor both infant's temperature and incubator temperature. Temperature control centres are poorly developed in the preterm infant, and his temperature is easily influenced by his environment.

6 When assessing temperature regulation of the preterm infant, consider the following:

a Note if infant's body or extremities are cool to touch — possibly due to underheated incubator or heat loss due to radiation.

b Note activity — restlessness or hyperactivity may indicate inappropriate temperature for comfort.

c Be aware of reasons for increased temperature of infant — overheated incubator or early sign of illness.

d Be aware of causes for drop in temperature of infant — underheated incubator, or infection.

7 When humidity is increased in the incubator, it will reduce infant heat loss and insensible water loss.

To prevent infection of this very susceptible preterm infant.

1 The preterm infant is particularly susceptible to viral, fungal, and gram-negative bacterial infections. Septicaemia, meningitis and urinary tract infections are a constant hazard postnatally.

2 Specific techniques should be employed to ensure the control of infection (see p. 74).

a Scrupulous handwashing by all personnel handling the infant and entering the nursery must be practised.

b Use gown technique as required by unit practice. Short-sleeved gowns allow for proper handwashing up to the elbows.

c Minimize infant's contact with unsterile equipment; equipment should be individualized.

d Minimize number of persons who come in contact with infant.

e Exclude from nursery any person who is febrile, has draining lesions, or has acute respiratory or gastrointestinal infections.

Nursing Alert: Routine use of hexachlorophene for infant bathing is to be avoided. Data indicate a marked association between its use and neuropathological lesions.

3   Early symptoms of infection may include (see p. 286):
   a Hypothermia or hyperthermia
   b Jaundice
   c Lethargy
   d Poor eating
   e Apnoeic spells.
4   Predisposing factors of infection:
   a Maternal infection
   b Difficult and prolonged labour
   c Prolonged rupture of membranes
   d Manipulative measures — resuscitation, umbilical catheterization, surgery.

To be aware of complications that occur in the preterm infant and to be alert for early signs indicating a change in condition.

1   *Hypoglycaemia*
   a Hypoglycaemia — serum sugar levels are less than 1.4 mmol/l (25 mg/100 ml).
   b Hypoglycaemia is most likely to occur in first 12 hours after birth and as late as 48 hours after birth.
   c Hypoglycaemia is likely to occur in the preterm infant because of the reduced glycogen storage he has at birth and his limited carbohydrate tolerance.
   d Symptoms are nonspecific:
      (1) Jitteriness
      (2) Sweating
      (3) Tachypnoea or apnoea
      (4) Lethargy
      (5) Convulsions
      (6) Cyanosis.
   e Predisposing factors:
      (1) Infant of a diabetic mother

(2) Erythroblastosis fetalis
(3) Sepsis
(4) Intrauterine malnutrition
(5) Developmental defects
(6) Asphyxia.

f Dextrostix screening should be done by the nurse. If the Dextrostix test result is below 1.4 mmol/1 (25 mg/100 ml), blood glucose should be checked immediately.

g Treatment is to increase blood sugar intake by continuous intragastric milk or jejunal feeding. Intravenous glucose is also given, but if given too rapidly, it will stimulate insulin production, resulting in a rebound hypoglycaemia. Maintain blood sugar at greater than 2.5 mmol/ml (45 mg/100 ml).

Note: Volume of milk given should be raised by 25% to increase blood glucose levels.

2 *Hypocalcaemia*
   a Hypocalcaemia — serum calcium levels are less than 1.75 mmol/1 (7 mg/100 ml).
   b Low blood calcium is reached on the first day of life.
   c Symptoms are nonspecific:
      (1) Twitching
      (2) Convulsions (late sign)
      (3) Hypotonia
      (4) Lethargy
      (5) High-pitched cry
      (6) Increased apnoeic spells
      (7) Abdominal distension with ileus.
   d Hypocalcaemia occurs in the preterm infant because of reduced calcium storage at birth and because of total serum proteins.
   e Predisposing factors:
      (1) Hypoglycaemia
      (2) Previous maternal abortion
      (3) Low infant Apgar rating
      (4) Hyaline membrane disease
      (5) Lack of intake.
   f Try to maintain serum calcium about 2.0 mmol/1 (8 mg/100 ml).
   g Treatment includes (1) human milk or modified infant formula (low solute) feeds or (2) calcium intravenously or orally.

Note: Intravenous calcium given too rapidly will cause bradycardia.

3 *Hypoxia* or anoxia at birth
   a The degree of asphyxia is judged immediately after delivery by Apgar scores and blood gas changes.
   b Specific problems to be anticipated include:
      (1) Hyaline membrane disease
      (2) Profound acidosis

(3) Hypoglycaemia

(4) Abnormal clotting function

(5) Hyperbilirubinaemia

(6) Apnoeic episodes

(7) Poor temperature control

(8) Intracranial haemorrhage

(9) Cardiac failure.

4 Patent ductus arteriosus (PDA)

a PDA occurs occasionally in preterm infants with respiratory distress syndrome and in less mature infants (24-30 weeks' gestation) with associated congestive pulmonary failure.

b Clinical signs include:

(1) Bounding peripheral pulses

(2) Chest retractions with mild cyanosis

(3) Diminished breath sounds on auscultation

(4) Moist râles

(5) Elevated PCO_2

(6) Apnoeic periods

(7) Systolic murmur — clicking sound.

c Treatment:

(1) Medical — fluid restriction, maintenance of normal blood pH, oxygen as needed, maintenance of adequate haemoglobin levels.

(2) Surgical — ligation of ductus arteriosus.

d Spontaneous closure of the PDA in the preterm infant is likely to occur 2-6 weeks after birth.

5 *Sodium disturbances*

a Hypernatraemia — serum sodium level about 150 mmol/l (150 mEq/l); generally occurs because of inadequate hydration or when infant formula feeds are incorrectly reconstituted so that the concentration is too high.

b Hyponatraemia — serum sodium level below 125-130 mmol/l (125-130 mEq/l) is generally secondary to administration of hypotonic intravenous solutions.

6 *Intracranial haemorrhage* (most likely to occur in sick preterm infants)

a Intracranial haemorrhage is a common cause of death in extremely preterm infants.

b Factors predisposing infant to intracranial haemorrhage:

(1) Immaturity

(2) Respiratory distress syndrome

(3) Hypoxia in fetus or neonate.

c Clinical signs:

(1) Laboured respirations

(2) Hypoventilation

(3) Cyanosis

(4) Apnoea

(5) High-pitched cry

(6) Convulsions

(7) Bulging fontanelle

(8) Clinical deterioration; shocklike appearance.

d Prevention of intraventricular haemorrhage is the best treatment, because once bleeding begins, it is difficult to control.

(1) Keep infant adequately oxygenated. Prevents asphyxia and hypercapnia.

(2) Maintain thermoneutral environment.

(3) Maintain normal acid-base balance.

To offer support to the parents of the preterm infant during this crucial period

1   Most parents, particularly mothers, are physically and emotionally unprepared for the early arrival of their baby.

2   Allow parents to see their infant and touch him if this is feasible, and they are able to cope with doing so.

3   Listen to parents talk and express their concerns. Encourage them, but do not give them false hope. Assess where they are in their grief, in coping, and in accepting their infant.

The Growing or Older Preterm Infant

After the first few days have passed without any complications, the preterm infant is very busy growing. During this time, however, it must be remembered that other complications can occur. The areas of concern mentioned above are still important, along with the following:

To be constantly alert to signs and symptoms of complications.

1   Aspiration

a The growing preterm infant may still have poor gag and cough and may show signs of respiratory distress.

Action: Suction mouth and pharynx immediately and get medical assistance.

2   Neonatal tetany (see hypocalcaemia, p. 254)

a Onset is between 5 and 10 days and occurs in those units where infants are still receiving full cream milk preparations. Human or low solute milk should be given as cow's milk formulae have a high phosphorus content and the immature kidneys cannot handle the high phosphorus load that results when calcium levels are low in the infant.

b Treatment:

(1) The addition of 10% calcium gluconate, not to exceed 12 ml in 24 hours. All feeds to be low solute or breast milk.

3   Fluid retention

a Abnormal fluid retention results from infant's inability to excrete solutes or to excrete water.

b Symptoms include:

(1) Excessive weight gain

(2) Pitting oedema of feet, then body

(3) Chest retractions

(4) Inspired air diminished on auscultation with possible râles

(5) Increase in oxygen need; increase in PCO_2.

c Treatment consists of giving diuretic agent and possibly decreasing fluid intake.

d Predisposing factors that lead to fluid retention include:

(1) Patent ductus arteriosus with borderline heart failure

(2) Bronchopulmonary dysplasia

(3) Postventilator therapy

(4) Low total serum proteins.

4 Hyperbilirubinaemia/jaundice (see p. 275)

a Bilirubin concentrations are generally higher in the preterm infant because of the impaired ability to conjugate bile in the liver.

b If infant is bruised from delivery or is plethoric, the risk of hyperbilirubinaemia is increased.

c Hypoproteinaemia and acidaemia increase risk of low bilirubin kernicterus.

5 Necrotizing enterocolitis

a Iatrogenic disease of the intestine of uncertain aetiology; the bowel has patches of necrotic mucosa, with intramural gas (pneumatosis intestinalis).

b Predisposing factors:

(1) Prematurity

(2) Shock of any type

(3) Perinatal or neonatal asphyxia, low Apgar score

(4) Exchange transfusion

(5) Association with postnatal infection

(6) Mother having had prolonged ruptured membranes or fever at delivery

(7) Nasojejunal tube feeding

(8) Respiratory distress

(9) Polycythaemia

(10) Patent ductus arteriosus

(11) Umbilical artery catheterization

(12) Early milk feeding.

c Signs and symptoms — the onset of symptoms occurs suddenly between 1 and 14 days of life, most often between 4 and 7 days of life: infant has generally been tolerating feedings:

(1) Abdominal distension; delayed gastric emptying; vomiting

(2) Jaundice

(3) Apnoea

(4) Gastrointestinal bleeding; bloody diarrhoea

(5) Toxic-looking

(6) X-ray findings show distended, thickened bowl loops; they may show streaks of intramural gas in bowel wall and sometimes peritoneal air from perforation.

d Supportive treatment:

(1) Gastric decompression with nasogastric tube

(2) Antibiotic therapy — intravenously and orally

(3) Intravenous hyperalimentation

(4) Surgery — resection of gangrenous bowel.

e Nursing responsibilities:

(1) Acute, constant observations — place child in incubator or under radiant warmer.

(2) Close monitoring of vital signs and general condition; report even minute changes in infant.

(a) Abdominal measurement; note distension or rigidity, redness, or shininess.

(b) Check bowel sounds with stethoscope with minimal abdominal palpation.

(c) Check stools for occult blood; save specimen as appropriate for examination by paediatrician.

(3) Prevent additional stress to infant by maintaining stability in environment, intravenous intake, and gastric decompression.

(4) Minimize handling and trauma to abdomen.

(5) Do not take rectal temperatures.

(6) Provide meticulous skin care when diarrhoea and vomiting are present.

To provide and maintain adequate nutrition to allow for growth and development.

1   The growth rate of the preterm infant should parallel the expected in utero growth rate: about 20 g/24 hours after 30 weeks' gestation and 30 g/24 hours as the infant approaches term.

From birth to 5-10 days of age there will be 5-10% weight loss; the infant should begin to gain weight.

2   The preterm infant has a small gastric capacity but a great need for kilojoules (calories).

a Generally the preterm infant has adequate gastric capacity, intestinal motility, and absorption to tolerate small, frequent feedings.

b The gastric capacity expands during the first few weeks of life; this enables the infant to tolerate larger feedings.

c Overfeeding increases the risk of vomiting.

Vomiting can lead to dehydration, loss of hydrochloric acid, and alkalosis.

d Burp infant frequently during feeding.

e Infant formula should be adequate in kilojoules (calories), fluid electrolytes, iron, and vitamins to meet the needs of the infant.

3   Inappropriate weight gain in relation to intake can indicate problems.

a Unusually large weight gain for kilojoule (calorie) intake may indicate excessive fluid retention.

b No weight gain or loss with adequate kilojoule (calorie) intake may indicate acidosis, sepsis or malabsorption.

4   Allow the infant to rest prior to feeding. The small infant tires easily from procedures and will eat better if rested.

5   Feed appropriately for individual infant.
    a Nasogastric feeding is indicated for very small preterm infant who does not demonstrate good sucking or synchronized sucking and swallowing. Diarrhoea may result from malabsorption if feeding is advanced too rapidly.
    b Bottle feeding with a teat is indicated for a vigorous preterm infant with good suck, vomit, and swallowing reflexes.
6   Anaemia, although not a significant problem, does occur.
    a Preterm infants develop anaemia (haemoglobin less than 80-100 g/l). Reasons for the development of anaemia include the following:
       (1) Total body iron content is less.
       (2) There is a proportionately larger blood loss from sampling.
       (3) Relative body growth is more rapid and there is an expanding blood volume.
    b Supplemental iron is needed to supply new iron stores. Eventually haemoglobin is needed for the increasing blood volume during growth. The iron is generally started when the infant is 1.5-2 times birth weight.
    c Blood transfusions are indicated to replace sampling blood. Keep accurate records of blood output.

To meet the psychological needs of the preterm infant who is an individual in his own right.

1   At first, even though handling is minimal, the nurse should talk to and caress the infant while performing procedures.
    a Stroking and gentle handling will provide necessary sensory stimulation.
    b A soft musical sound may also be comforting.
2   Once the preterm infant is able to leave the incubator, even for short periods of time, he should be held for feedings.
    a While holding him, stroke him and talk to him.
    b Keep him warmly wrapped — this will also give him a feeling of security.
3   If the infant is restless in his incubator, he may be calmed by propping him against a blanket or nappy roll.
       The freedom of movement, restrained only by the mattress, cannot offer much security to the infant.
4   Remember that the infant's ability to hear, see, smell, and touch are intact. Give him the opportunities to develop these capabilities and encourage the development of his interaction potential by providing sensory input.
    a Physical contact is important for a sense of security.
    b Arrange environment so eye-to-eye contact can be established between nurse or mother and infant.
    c Allow infant freedom of movement for self-stimulation.
    d Change infant's position and location of incubator or cot to encourage him to see his environment.
5   Include parents in this activity to help them get to know their infant and incorporate these activities into their behaviour so they will continue this at home.

To provide the preterm infant with an environment that will help him to emerge successfully into a state of well-being and into a healthy growing baby.

1 Conserve his energy.
   a Promote rest and sleep by the following:
   (1) Appropriate handling
   (2) Organizing and controlling interruptions
   (3) Proper positioning of infant.
   b Support physiological functions and provide assistance as necessary — i.e. monitor respiration, temperature, and nutrition.
2 Change position every 2 hours. This does the following:
   a Stimulates circulation
   b Facilitates respirations
   c Prevents stasis of accumulated secretions
   d Minimizes skin irritation
   e Provides infant with opportunity for different stimulation input.
3 Provide for physical safety and comfort.
   a Bathing — gives nurse opportunity to observe infant thoroughly.
   b Protect infant from injury self-inflicted by own random movements.
   c Protect from injury by equipment.
   d Use protective devices as necessary but allow infant some unrestricted self-stimulation.
   e Keep portholes of incubator closed.

To foster healthy family relationships with the preterm baby.

1 Encourage parents to make frequent visits to the nursery so they can become familiar with all aspects of care of their infant.
   a When they visit, explain the equipment and procedures that may be foreign to them.
   b Help them to feel comfortable and confident in handling their infant.
   c Parents may lose interest in the infant if the hospitalization is long. If parents cannot visit daily, encourage them to telephone or telephone them at predetermined times.
2 Help mother to see infant as an individual and to develop mothering behaviours based on the infant's behaviour.
   a The infant's size and physical characteristics are generally unexpected and are different from those of the expected term baby.
   b The preterm infant's reflexes and responses to his environment are immature. Mother's expectations of his responses are based on those of a full-term baby.
   c Explain these discrepancies between expectations and reality. Mother may associate infant's responses with her inadequacies rather than the baby's.
   d Be aware of what reflexes and responses may elicit reactions in the mother. For example:

(1) Uncoordinated sucking and swallowing — mother experiences disappointment in not being able to feed, especially if she wanted to breast-feed her infant.

(2) Gag reflex — mother fears choking her infant.

(3) Respiratory immaturity — periodic breathing frightens her.

(4) Grasp reflex — mother is disappointed if infant does not grasp her finger.

(5) Moro reflex — exaggerated Moro reflex may make mother feel she has frightened her infant.

e Reassure mother that as the infant matures, he will change his response and reflex behaviour.

3 The support and help given to parents during hospitalization will make home care easier.

a Teach mother how to care for her infant. Thorough and careful preparation of the mother in feeding and caring for her infant often means earlier discharge.

b The small size of the infant often is the single factor that frightens parents the most.

4 Inform family health visitor of infant's admission to the unit. Keep the health visitor informed of subsequent progress.

5 Encourage parents to talk about their feelings or fears concerning their infant and how they will care for him.

a By listening, the nurse can gain some insight as to what to talk about or to teach the parents.

b Parents' feelings can frequently interfere with appropriate home care.

c Parents often treat the small infant as if he were fragile and more prone to illness. Over-concern is potentially harmful.

d Parents worry about how to feed and protect the infant.

6 Help the family prepare for the time when their new baby will arrive home.

a Because of the early, unexpected arrival of the infant, things such as clothing, cot, and feeding bottles may not be ready.

b If there are other children at home they need to be prepared for the homecoming of the preterm infant. This preparation should begin early — using, for example, pictures of infant and conversations about him. Encourage parents to bring siblings to visit the new family member in the unit.

c The readiness for the preterm infant to go home is evaluated and assessed in terms of the following:

(1) The infant's weight and progress

(2) Maternal attachment to the infant

(3) Maternal competence in caring for the infant.

Parental (Family) Teaching

1 Help the family to understand that caring for the preterm infant at home should not be any different from caring for a full-term infant.

a Special treatment may lead to behaviour problems later.

b At first a little extra caution should be practised. Cyanotic spells and severe infection are major concerns for preterm infant during first few weeks at home.

(1) Keep room temperature fairly constant: 20-22°C.

(2) When bathing infant, ensure he is kept warm during procedure.

(3) Feed him the recommended amount of infant formula to be certain he receives the necessary kilojoules for continual growth. Maintain iron therapy.

(4) Keep him away from crowds and people who have colds.

2 Spend enough time with the mother teaching her how to feed and care for her infant.

Show her how, then watch her and help her improve and gain confidence.

(1) Infant needs gentle, firm handling.

(2) He needs to be mothered and kept comfortable with minimal tension.

(3) A soothing voice can be comforting.

(4) Sucking provides a pleasant experience.

3 Stress the importance of medical follow-up for the baby after discharge from the hospital.

Anaemia and failure to thrive are common long-term side effects of 'prematurity'.

4 Help mother understand the importance of good, early antenatal care for subsequent pregnancies.

Once a woman has had one preterm infant, this classifies her as high-risk for another preterm delivery with future pregnancies.

SMALL FOR GESTATIONAL AGE (LIGHT FOR DATES) INFANT

The 'small for gestational age infant' (SGA) is a newborn who shows a discrepancy between growth and gestational age or whose weight is 2 standard deviations below expected weight for duration of gestation. *Intrauterine growth retarded* (IUGR) is used often interchangeably with small for gestational age (light for dates).

Aetiology

Intrauterine growth retardation may be due to reduction of total number of cells in the body, to a reduction in cell size, or both. While the aetiological factors are unknown in many cases, other cases may be due to the following causes.

Maternal Factors

1 Undernutrition

2 Diminished uterine blood flow

    a Pre-eclampsia
    b Toxaemia
    c Chronic hypertensive vascular disease
    d Diabetes mellitus
3   Small stature
4   Smoking
5   Inadequate antenatal care
6   Low socioeconomic class
7   Heart disease
8   Low maternal age
9   Primiparity
10 Grand multiparity
11 Low prepregnant weight
12 Narcotic usage
13 Haemoglobinopathy
14 Phenylketonuria.

Environmental Factors

1   High altitude
2   Teratogens
3   Irradiation.

Placental Lesions

1   Infarcts
2   Preterm placental separation
3   Haemangiomas
4   Thrombosis of fetal vessels
5   Single umbilical artery
6   Avascular terminal villi.

Fetal Causes

1   Genetic dwarfism
2   Anencephaly
3   Infections (rubella, cytomegalovirus, toxoplasmosis, herpes simplex)
4   Chromosomal aberrations
    a Turner's syndrome
    b Down's syndrome
    c Trisomy syndromes
    d Cri-du-chat syndrome
5   Congenital anomalies
    a Osteogenesis imperfecta
    b De Lange's syndrome
    c Cystic fibrosis
    d Galactosaemia.

Clinical Manifestations

Clinical manifestations of the small for gestational age (light for dates) infant are related to the duration, intensity, and time of onset of the influence (factors) causing intrauterine growth retardation.

Chronic Intrauterine Growth Retardation

Growth of fetus has been curtailed by insult for weeks or months prior to birth. Note the following characteristics:

1   Body proportions remain unaltered — weight, length, and possibly head circumference are below normal for gestational age
2   Creases on soles of feet
3   Coarse, straight, silky hair
4   Well-developed ear cartilage
5   Firm skull bones.

Subacute Intrauterine Growth Retardation

Growth of fetus has been curtailed by insult only a few days or weeks prior to birth, producing subacute retardation of intrauterine growth.

1   Weight is diminished; length of body and head circumference may be normal
2   Wasted look with loose, thin skin
3   Long, thin appearance
4   Face has look of 'worried little old man'
5   Scaphoid abdomen
6   Skin dry, cracked, and peeling
7   Thin umbilical cord that dries and hardens rapidly
8   Widened skull sutures.

Pathophysiology

Although in general, the physiological maturity of fetal organs develops according to gestational age, there are exceptions to organ maturation being consistent with gestational age that result in problems (conditions) associated with intrauterine growth retardation.

1   Poor glucose control.
   a Hyperglycaemia may occur immediately after delivery or following intravenous glucose administration.
   b Hypoglycaemia is probably due to rapid depletion of hepatic glycogen stores and to ineffective functioning of hepatic enzyme system responsible for glyconeogenesis.
2   Limited temperature control.
   a Infant has relatively large surface area per unit of body weight.
   b He lacks energy stores and subcutaneous fat insulation.
   c Infant can assume position of flexion of extemities — reduces surface area

exposed to environment and decreases heat loss by radiation and convection.

d Has vasomotor control over peripheral circulation to dilate or constrict capillaries as needed.

e Sweating mechanism is intact.

3 High haemoglobin, increased plasma volume, and enlarged extracellular fluid volume per kilogram of body weight.

4 Minimal weight loss with rapid initial weight gain.

a Weight gain is not maintained throughout first year.

b Rapid initial weight gain may suggest rehydration as well as tissue growth.

5 Late anaemia.

Secondary to rapid weight gain and poor iron stores present at birth, especially in the preterm infant.

6 Elevated immunoglobulin (IgM) in infants with intrauterine infection.

7 High nonprotein nitrogen levels, possibly due to:

a Increase in fetal catabolism *or*

b Impaired placental excretion of fetal waste products.

8 Prone to postasphyxial problems.

a The asphyxia process of normal labour is associated with metabolic acidosis.

b Fetal malnutrition, in addition to birth process, predisposes infant to asphyxia neonatorum.

9 X-ray findings:

a Atrophy of thymus

b Thin ribs.

Diagnostic Evaluation

1 Evaluate general appearance of infant.

2 Determine gestational age using physical characteristics and neurological examination (see p. 243).

3 Infant can be small for gestational age and preterm or small for gestational age and born at term.

4 Measure weight, length, and head circumference; plot on percentile chart.

5 Determine blood sugar.

6 Obtain haematocrit (HCT) and haemoglobin to determine polycythaemia and hyperviscosity venous haematocrit over 65%.

Complications

1 Problems associated with asphyxia neonatorum

2 Hypoglycaemia

3 Polycythaemia

4 Pulmonary haemorrhage

5   Prematurity with intrauterine growth retardation
6   Infection associated with maternal conditions
7   Hypothermia
8   Congenital infection
9   Late anaemia
10   Future growth retardation.

Nursing Objectives

The nursing management of the small for gestational age infant in many aspects is similar to that for the preterm infant (see p. 249). The following are major objectives of the nurse caring for the small gestational age neonate:

To observe for any gross and less obvious congenital anomalies as in the case of the full-term infant upon admission to the nursery.

1   Congenital anomalies are often associated with intrauterine growth retardation.
     Genitourinary and cardiovascular complications are the most common problems.
2   Certain types of intrauterine infection account for intrauterine growth retardation and may present signs of skin rash, petechiae and ecchymoses, hepatomegaly, splenomegaly, early onset of obstructive jaundice, chorioretinitis, lethargy, and irritability.
3   Report any suspicious findings and observations to the paediatrician immediately.

To observe for problems associated with asphyxia neonatorum.

The small for gestational age neonate has an increased incidence of asphyxia neonatorum. His lessened metabolic stores of carbohydrates lower his ability to handle the stresses of delivery. Acidosis may develop quickly.

1   Be aware of the Apgar scores which will help in determining degree of asphyxia (Apgar less than 5 at 1 minute or less than 7 at 5 minutes).
2   See that blood gas studies are done to confirm adequate oxygenation and acidosis. Frequent monitoring should be continued.
3   Observe for signs of respiratory distress.
     a Adequate oxygenation is imperative for improving prognosis.
     b Suction and oxygen equipment should be available and ready for immediate use.
     c Aspiration pneumonia and pulmonary haemorrhage are postasphyxiation problems.
4   Check vital signs frequently and note behaviour, i.e. reflex responses, irritability; cardiac function can be affected and central nervous system damage can occur with severe asphyxia.
5   Check and record intake and output. Renal damage is a common sequel of severe asphyxia.

6   Observe for abnormal clotting function and hyperbilirubinaemia — liver damage from severe asphyxia may be manifested by postasphyxial hypoglycaemia.
7   Postasphyxial hypocalcaemia may occur.
8   Record and report all observations appropriately.

To screen for hypoglycaemia, beginning soon after birth.

1   The small for gestational age infant has reduced carbohydrate stores at birth. Glycogen reserves are depleted almost immediately after birth. Gluconeogenesis is inadequate because of reduced stores of muscle protein and fat tissue, as well as because of reduced hyperglycaemic response to noradrenalin and glucagon, which activate the gluconeogenic process.
2   Hypoglycaemia is most likely to occur from 12 to 48 hours after birth.
      Severely hypoxic, hypothermic, small for gestational age infants can become hypoglycaemic as early as 6 hours after birth.
3   Blood sugars should be monitored frequently (every 30-60 minutes) by Dextrostix during the critical time after birth and during intravenous glucose therapy.
      a If Dextrostix is below 2.5 mmol/l (45 mg/100 ml) or above 14 mmol/l (250 mg/100 ml) report these findings to paediatrician immediately as measurement of serum glucose most likely will be done.
      b Keep Dextrostix bottle tightly covered and out of direct sunlight to avoid false reading on Dextrostix.
4   When intravenous infusion of glucose is used to treat hypoglycaemia, particular care must be given to prevent infiltration and subsequent slough and necrosis of tissue.
5   Oral feeding should be started as early as 2 hours after birth with the infant at risk for hypoglycaemia — if there are no contraindications.
6   Signs of hypoglycaemia include:
      a 'Jitteriness'
      b Sweating
      c Tachypnoea or apnoea
      d Cyanosis
      e Convulsions
      f Respiratory distress.
7   Report all observations to the paediatrician and record accurately.

To prevent hypothermia and maintain thermal stability of the small for gestational age neonate (see p. 242).

1   Ensure that adequate environmental heat is provided to maintain infant's abdominal skin temperature at 36.0-36.5°C.
2   Prevent infant from lying on thermistor.

To take measures to combat polycythaemia.

Polycythaemia, which is increased red blood cell volume, is frequently seen in small for gestational age infants when growth retardation is due to placental insufficiency.

1　Polycythaemia is identified by a high haematocrit or haemoglobin level, i.e. venous blood haematocrit over 65%; haemoglobin of 200-220 g/l (20-22 g/100 ml). Hyperviscosity can result from this condition.

2　Signs and symptoms of viscosity include:
   a Plethora
   b Jaundice
   c Tachypnoea
   d Tachycardia
   e Peripheral cyanosis
   f Grunting
   g Nasal flaring, intercostal retractions
   h Scrotal oedema
   i Priapism (persistent, abnormal erection of penis)
   j Tremors, irritability, possibly seizures.

3　Ensure that the haematocrit or haemoglobin is monitored during the first 6-12 hours after birth in the high-risk infant.

4　Treatment for haematocrit above 70% usually consists of partial exchange transfusion. The nurse must be prepared to assist with this by using plasma or whole blood.

To accurately measure and record daily weights and to monitor length and head circumference.

Rapid weight gain is expected the first few days and weeks.

To support the parents of the infant (see Preterm Infant, p. 260).

1　The long-term outcome of the small for gestational age infant often represents an increase in long-range sequelae frequently manifested in lowered intellectual achievement resulting from malnutrition during peak intrauterine brain growth.

2　Long-term prognosis depends upon adequate treatment of problems encountered immediately after birth, aetiology of problems, and subsequent home environment.

POSTMATURE INFANT

The *postmature infant* is one whose gestation is 42 weeks or longer and who may show signs of weight loss with placental insufficiency.

Aetiology

1 Not known in many cases
2 Maternal factors associated with postmaturity:
   a Primigravida and high-parity mother at any given age
   b Prolonged gestation in preceding pregnancies.

Clinical Manifestations

Physical appearance — the following characteristics are most often seen in infants of 44 weeks' gestation or more:

1 Reduced subcutaneous tissue — loose skin, especially buttocks and thighs
2 Long, curved fingernails and toenails
3 Reduced amount of vernix caseosa
4 Abundant scalp hair
5 Wrinkled, macerated skin; possibly pale, cracked, parchment-like skin
6 Having the alert appearance of a 2- to 3-week-old infant following delivery
7 Greenish-yellow staining of skin, indicating fetal distress.

Pathophysiology

1 The postmature infant appears to have suffered from intrauterine malnutrition and hypoxia.
   Before the termination of the pregnancy, but at the point when birth should have occurred, the placental function begins to diminish, resulting in impaired oxygen exchange and inadequate nutrient transfer to the fetus.
2 There are stages of postmaturity — severity of associated problems is determined by length of gestation, i.e. the longer the gestation, the more severe the problems.

Diagnostic Evaluation

1 Evaluate general appearance.
2 Determine gestational age — give neurological examination.
3 Measure weight, length, and head circumference.
4 Determine blood sugar. In hypoglycaemia the blood sugar level is below 1.7 mmol/l (30 mg/100 ml).
5 Assessment of asphyxia neonatorum.
   a Apgar score
   b Blood gas analysis.

Complications

1 Meconium aspiration
2 Hypoglycaemia and hypocalcaemia

3   Polycythaemia
4   Pulmonary haemorrhage
5   Problems associated with asphyxia neonatorum
6   Pneumonia
7   Pneumothorax.

Nursing Objectives

Problems and nursing care encountered in the postmature infant may include the metabolic disturbances of the small for gestational age infant and complications of asphyxia neonatorum as well as polycythaemia (see p. 262, small for gestational age). Massive meconium aspiration causes specific problems for the postmature infant. (Refer to nursing objectives for the preterm infant, p. 245, and small for gestational age, p. 266).

To be alert for respiratory distress that may indicate meconium aspiration.

1   The stage is set for meconium aspiration when placental function diminishes and oxygen transport to the fetus decreases, leading to cerebral hypoxia.
    a The anal sphincter relaxes and meconium passes into the surrounding amniotic fluid.
    b The asphyxiated fetus gasps and aspiration occurs.
2   Signs and symptoms of meconium aspiraton.
    a Tachypnoea, increasing signs of cyanosis; difficult breathing, with need for ventilation
    b Tachycardia
    c Inspiratory nasal flaring and retraction of chest
    d Expiratory grunting
    e Increased anteroposterior diameter of the chest
    f Palpable liver
    g Râles and rhonchi on chest auscultation.
3   Mainly supportive treatment.
    a Warmth — maintain thermally neutral environment so infant uses less energy and less oxygen.
    b Adequate oxygenation and humidification
    (1) Be aware that metabolic disturbances often accompany respiratory problems.
    (2) Ensure that monitoring of blood gases and pH is done.
    (3) Carefully record blood sampling.
    c Adequate administration of kilojoules (calories) and fluid
    Accurately record intake and output.
    d Antibiotics
    (1) Prophylactically — meconium can lead to a chemical pneumonia and the growth of gram-negative bacteria. Therefore antibiotics specifically for gram-negative bacteria may be used.
    (2) Treatment — antibiotics used only when clinical evidence indicates infection.

e Corticosteroids may be given to minimize irritating effects of meconium on respiratory epithelium, although clinical evidence for this is nonconclusive.

f Chest physiotherapy

(1) Postural drainage (p. 175).

(2) Pulmonary lavage — using nonirritating solution and immediate suctioning of mouth, pharynx, and trachea; bag ventilate using high concentrations of oxygen between lavage procedures.

(3) Change position from side to side frequently and elevate or lower head by adjusting the mattress to a 20° angle.

(4) Complications of meconium aspiration

(a) Pneumothorax and/or pneumomediastinum

(b) Secondary pneumonia

(c) Respiratory failure

(d) Death.

(5) Prevention

Most cases of meconium aspiration can be prevented if meconium is removed from the mouth and trachea by proper suctioning, prior to infant's taking his first breath.

Note: If ventilator management is indicated, treatment is similar to that of infant with hyaline membrane disease (p. 327).

To be aware that the postmature infant is particularly prone to hypoglycaemia within hours after birth (see Small for Gestational Age, p. 262).

1   Oral feeding or intravenous glucose is generally initiated soon after birth. If oral feedings are not contraindicated they can begin 1-2 hours after birth.

2   Close and careful monitoring of blood sugar should be done with Dextrostix every hour until condition stabilizes.

3   Persistent hypoglycaemia may contribute to central nervous system problems.

4   Be alert to signs and symptoms of hypoglycaemia and report to paediatrician.

To support the parents of the infant (see Preterm Infant, p. 260 and Intensive Care Nursing, p. 75).

The long-term sequelae common in the postmature infant are associated with central nervous system (neurological) problems.

INFANT OF A DIABETIC MOTHER

The *infant of a diabetic mother* (IDM) is the infant born to a mother with diabetes. The mother may be a diabetic or gestational diabetic. The severity of infant problems depends on classification of the maternal diabetes.

Clinical Manifestations

1　Macrosomia (gigantism)
2　Cardiomegaly
3　Hepatomegaly
4　Large umbilical cord and placenta
5　Plethora
6　Full-face
7　Tendency to be large for gestational age; some may be normal weight or small for gestational age
8　Abundant fat, hair, and vernix caseosa.

Pathophysiology

1　Increased amount of body fat, not oedema.
　　a Total body water is somewhat reduced at birth.
　　b High urinary output during first 2 days of life, probably due to freeing of intracellular water.
2　Hypoglycaemia
　　a Occurs within first 6-12 hours of life; may occur within minutes after birth.
　　b Infant's response to glucose is excessive, i.e. insulin blood level will have a slight elevation, will drop and then peak within 1 hour. This is probably due to maternal hyperglycaemia.
　　c Infant's cord insulin levels may not be higher than in a normal infant unless a large amount of glucose is given.
　　d Infant of a diabetic mother may be symptomatic of asymptomatic with blood sugars below 1.12 mmol/l (20 mg/100 ml).
3　Hypocalcaemia
　　a Associated with prematurity, difficult labour and delivery, and/or asphyxia at birth.
　　b Generally occurs during first 48 hours of life.
4　Hyperbilirubinaemia
　　a Most likely to occur within 48-72 hours after birth.
　　b Immature liver results in inability to conjugate bilirubin.
　　c Haematocrit is higher on the third day after birth and extracellular volume is decreased.
　　d Because of large size, birth trauma may increase risk of enclosed haemorrhage.
5　Maturity
　　a May be preterm or small for gestational age (light for dates) when associated with placental insufficiency.
　　b Respiratory function is similar to that of other preterm infants — thus infant is prone to hyaline membrane disease.
6　Polycythaemia

a Venous haematocrit greater than 65% or venous haemoglobin 220 g/l (22 g/100 ml).

b Polycythaemia increases the risks of occurrence of renal vein thrombosis, respiratory distress, hypoglycaemia, and hypocalcaemia.

7   Congenital anomalies

    a Increased incidence of congenital anomalies may be due to:

       (1) Divergent gene pattern

       (2) Abnormal intrauterine environment.

    b Most common anomalies are skeletal and cardiac.

8   Infection

    a Prematurity and lowered passive immunity

    b Possible maternal urinary tract infection and bacteria crossing the placenta.

Diagnostic Evaluation

1   Maternal history of diabetes
2   Physical assessment of infant and determination of gestational age
3   Blood studies

    a Glucose

    b Calcium

    c Haematocrit and haemoglobin levels

    d Blood gas analysis

    e Magnesium (if indicated).

Complications

1   Hypoglycaemia
2   Hypocalcaemia
3   Hyaline membrane disease
4   Polycythaemia and renal vein thrombosis
5   Infection
6   Hyperbilirubinaemia
7   Hypermagnesium or hypomagnesium
8   Congenital anomalies
9   Birth injuries — cephalohaematomas, facial nerve paralysis, fractured clavicles, brachial nerve plexus
10   Prematurity
11   Congestive heart failure.

Nursing Objectives

Except for specific considerations discussed below, the nursing care of the infant of a diabetic mother (IDM) is the same as for the preterm infant (p. 245).

To observe closely for hypoglycaemia.

Report any irregularities immediately to paediatrician.

1   Monitor by Dextrostix every 30-60 minutes beginning immediately after birth for 24 hours or until stabilized.
2   The infant with hypoglycaemia (blood sugar below 1.12 mmol/1 or 20 mg/ 100 ml) may be symptomatic or asymptomatic. Signs include:
    a Jitteriness
    b Tremors
    c Convulsions
    d Sweating
    e Cyanosis
    f Weak or high-pitched cry
    g Refusal to suck
    h Hypotonia (reduced muscle tone).
3   Hypoglycaemia may be prevented or treated by early oral feedings if asymptomatic (1-2 hours after birth) or with intravenous glucose if symptomatic.
        Intravenous glucose must not be stopped abruptly, as a rebound effect may occur causing insulin levels to increase and hypoglycaemia to reappear.

To monitor infant closely for changes in acid-base status, respiratory distress, temperature, hypocalcaemia, and sepsis.

To observe for hyperbilirubinaemia.

1   Infants of diabetic mothers have a higher incidence of hyperbilirubinaemia.
        Other predisposing factors include prematurity and polycythaemia, which increases the load of bilirubin from the natural process of red blood cell breakdown to be cleared.
2   The infant may need an exchange transfusion at relatively lower bilirubin levels (as in the preterm infant) to prevent kernicterus.
3   The blood sugar must be monitored during and following exchange transfusion.
        ACD (acid citrate dextrose) and CPD (citrate phosphate dextrose) contain large amounts of dextrose which may subsequently cause rebound hypoglycaemia.

To be aware of the infant who is predisposed to hypomagnesaemia or hypermagnesaemia and observe for signs and symptoms of each.

1   Hypermagnesaemia may occur when the pre-eclamptic mother was treated with magnesium sulphate insulin.
    a Signs and symptoms may include:
        (1) Hypotonia
        (2) Weak or absent cry
        (3) Severe respiratory distress with apnoea or cyanosis.

b Treatment is an exchange transfusion.
2 Hypomagnesaemia may accompany hypocalcaemia or follow an exchange transfusion.
   a Severe neuromuscular excitability may be the presenting symptom.
   b Replacement therapy with magnesium sulphate is required.

To be alert for development of renal vein thrombosis in the infant during the first few days of life.

1 Polycythaemia, transient dehydration, and decreased extracellular fluid may be causes.
2 Observe for haematuria and proteinuria.
3 Flank masses may be palpable.

To observe the infant for possible cardiac anomalies (see p. 367).

Monitor cardiac and respiratory rates.

To support the mother who may have feelings of severe guilt or inadequacy, since she is directly related to the problems her infant may be having.

1 Encourage and allow mother to talk about these feelings.
2 Encourage her, when appropriate, to have close obstetrical care for subsequent pregnancies.
3 Stress importance of a periodic evaluation for diabetes in her child.

JAUNDICE IN THE NEWBORN (HYPERBILIRUBINAEMIA)

Hyperbilirubinaemia (jaundice) in the newborn is an accumulation of serum bilirubin above normal levels.

Aetiology

1 Increased bilirubin load
   a Haemolytic disease — Rh and ABO incompatibility
   b Morphological abnormalities of red blood cells
   c Red blood cell enzyme defects
   d Physiological jaundice (see later discussion of 'physiological jaundice')
2 Extravascular blood
   a Cephalohaematoma
   b Pulmonary or cerebral haemorrhage
   c Any enclosed occult blood
3 Decrease or inhibition of bilirubin conjugation
   a Inherited bilirubin conjugation defect: Crigler-Najjar syndrome
   b Acquired bilirubin conjugation defect: breast-milk jaundice, Lucey-Driscoll syndrome, infant of diabetic mother, asphyxiated infant with respiratory distress.

4 Increased extrahepatic circulation
   Intestinal obstruction
5 Polycythaemia
   a Infant of diabetic mother
   b Small for gestational age infant
6 Mixed jaundice — increased bilirubin load and decreased clearance resulting in elevated indirect and direct bilirubin levels
   a Sepsis
   b Chronic intrauterine injections
   c Galactosaemia
   d Biliary artesia — absence of extrahepatic ducts or presence of cord-like structures without a lumen
7 Hypothyroidism
8 Unknown.

Clinical Manifestations

1 Onset of clinical jaundice seen when serum bilirubin levels are less than 85-120 mmol/l (5-7 mg/100 ml)
   a Physiological jaundice — occurs 3-5 days after birth
      (1) Increase in unconjugated bilirubin levels; levels must not exceed 85 mmol/l (5 mg/100 ml) per day.
      (2) Peak bilirubin levels not to exceed 205 mmol/l (12 mg/100 ml) in full-term infant and 225 mmol/l (15 mg/100 ml) in preterm infant.
      (3) Full-term peak levels 102 mmol/l (6 mg/100 ml) are reached by 48-72 hours after birth; clinical jaundice declines in 1 week and normal bilirubin levels are reached in 2 weeks.
      (4) Preterm peak levels of 170-205 mmol/l (10-12g/100ml) are reached by 4-5 days of age; clinical jaundice declines in 2 weeks and normal bilirubin levels are reached in 3-4 weeks.
   b Erythroblastosis — may occur within 24 hours after birth.
2 Signs and symptoms may include:
   a Sclerae appearing yellow before skin appears yellow
   b Skin appearing light to bright yellow
   c Lethargy
   d Dark amber, concentrated urine
   e Poor feeding
   f Dark stools.

Pathophysiology

Bilirubin Production

1 About 75% of the bilirubin present in the newborn is from red blood cell breakdown.

a The red blood cell is broken down into protein and globin combined with haem, which is an iron-porphyrin complex.

b In the presence of the enzyme called haem oxygenase:

(1) Globin is reduced to amino acids.

(2) Iron is broken off and stored.

(3) Porphyrin moiety is broken into biliverdin, which is reduced to bilirubin.

c This bilirubin is unconjugated or indirect and is fat soluble.

d Indirect bilirubin, bound to albumin, is present in circulating blood and tissues.

e The liver selectively removes this albumin-bound bilirubin from the blood.

f Once the unconjugated bilirubin is in the liver, it is converted to direct or conjugated water-soluble bilirubin with the aid of enzymes, one of which is glucuronyl transferase.

g From the liver, conjugated bilirubin is excreted via the bile into the intestines and is excreted in the stool or is hydrolysed to unconjugated bilirubin in the intestine and reabsorbed across the intestinal mucosa into the circulation.

2   The remaining bilirubin present in the newborn is from non-erythrocyte-containing haem proteins.

Physiological Jaundice

1   Increased load of bilirubin on liver cells.

a Increased bilirubin production — more rapid haemolysis because of higher level of circulating red blood cells per kilogram of body weight and a shorter red blood cell lifespan.

b Enterohepatic circulation — reabsorption of unconjugated bilirubin.

2   Decreased clearance of bilirubin from plasma.

a Predominant bilirubin-binding protein in liver cells may be deficient the first days of life.

b Glucuronyl transferase enzyme activity may be decreased, resulting in impaired conjugation of bilirubin.

c Liver may show decreased ability to excrete conjugated bilirubin.

d Poor portal blood supply may decrease the liver's capacity to act effectively.

e Open ductus venosus may allow blood to bypass liver.

Haemolytic Disease

1   Erythroblastosis fetalis

a Immune haemolysis or Rh/ABO blood group incompatibility; mother's and infant's blood are different

Rh factor; different ABO blood groups (see Coombs' test).

b Mother produces antibodies against the antigen of baby's blood. Fetal cells frequently cross placenta

c Antibodies of mother's blood are present in baby's blood at birth, causing the following conditions:

(1) There is haemolysis of infant's red blood cells

(2) Haemolysis leads to rising level of indirect bilirubin

2   Glucose-6-phosphate dehydrogenase deficiency (G-6-PD) — nonimmune haemolytic disease

a Deficiency results in reduced stability to oxidative destruction from substances that act as oxidizing agents (i.e. vitamin K, salicylates)

b X-linked recessive disease that affects primarily Negro, Mediterranean, Oriental groups

c Screen maternal blood for carrier state and screen infant's blood in high risk groups.

Other Considerations

1   Each gram of haemoglobin breakdown forms 60 mmol (35 mg) of bilirubin.

2   An unmeasurable amount of bilirubin does not bind to albumin. Free indirect bilirubin is very toxic to the cells of the central nervous system.

3   The enzyme system responsible for conjugation of bilirubin is oxygen dependent and altered by infant's pH, temperature, etc. Thus infants who are acidotic, hypoxic or hypothermic tend to present with higher levels of bilirubin.

Diagnostic Evaluation

1   All infants who have clinical signs of jaundice should have the following investigations made:

a Total bilirubin levels — indirect and direct

b Peripheral smear — for evidence of red blood cell immaturity or abnormality

c Reticulocyte count — to determine rate of haemolysis

d Coombs' test — to check for Rh and ABO group incompatibility between mother and baby

e Blood typing of mother and infant

f Total serum protein — to measure binding capacity

g Haematocrit or haemoglobin

h Acid-based status

i Albumin-binding test — to measure reserve binding sites (if available).

2   Measuring the bilirubin-albumin binding capacity of the plasma can be valuable in determining the risk of kernicterus (see below) and the need for an exchange transfusion. This test defines the upper limits to which serum bilirubin is allowed to rise when an exchange transfusion is done.

a $\dfrac{\text{Total bilirubin}}{\text{Total serum protein}} =$ (1) if less than 3.7 — no danger of kernicterus

(2) if greater than 3.7 — treatment by exchange transfusion is indicated.

b Total serum protein $\times$ 3.7 = level of bilirubin at which to do exchange transfusion.

3   The level of bilirubin at which the infant is at risk for brain damage depends upon the degree of prematurity, presence of acidosis, hypoxia, or drugs which bind albumin.
4   Appropriate cultures when infection suspected.

Complications — Kernicterus

Kernicterus is a yellow discoloration of specific areas of brain tissue by unconjugated bilirubin. (Bear in mind that neurological signs may not show up until later.)
1   Early signs of kernicterus
   a Poor feeding
   b Vomiting
   c Lethargy
   d High-pitched cry
   e Hypotonia
   f Decrease of normal reflexes, Moro reflex.
2   Later signs
   a Opisthotonus
   b Apnoea
   c Irritability
   d Seizures
   e Deafness to high-pitched sounds.
3   Occurrence of kernicterus at low levels of bilirubin may be seen in infants with
   a Previous asphyxia (acidosis)
   b Respiratory distress
   c Sepsis
   d Hypothermia
   e Prematurity
   f Hypoglycaemia.
4   Bilirubin is nephrotoxic and especially compromises renal concentrating capacity.
5   Bilirubin increases affinity of red blood cells for oxygen.

Treatment

1   Exchange transfusion — to mechanically remove bilirubin
2   Phototherapy — to allow for utilization of alternate pathways for bilirubin excretion.

Nursing Objectives

To observe infant's skin for appearance of or increase in jaundice.

1   Make observation in daylight, sunlight, or white fluorescent light.
2   Blanch the skin during the observation to clear away capillary coloration: forehead, cheeks, and clavical sites allow for clear view.
3   Be aware of any blood incompatibility between infant's and mother's blood.
4   Be alert to the infant's age in connection with the appearance of jaundice.

To note any changes in urine pigmentation and frequency of urination.

Careful notation of frequency, amount, and colour of urine should be made so changes will be noticed immediately.

To maintain adequate fluid intake.

1   Be aware of feeding history and amount of fluid taken.
2   If infant is a slow eater, feed small amounts frequently.
3   The amount of fluid intake determines the amount of hydration and in turn determines the excretion of bilirubin. Early feeding is a good preventive prescription for hyperbilirubinaemia.
4   If infant is receiving intravenous fluid, keep an accurate hourly record of fluid intake. Do not allow intake to fall behind ordered rate. Observe intravenous site for infiltration. If necessary, intravenous feed can be discontinued and restarted in another site.

To be alert to any behaviour changes.

Note particularly: increasing lethargy, change in sucking activity or quality of vomiting.

To be alert to signs of kernicterus.

Observe for signs of: decreased muscle tone, no sucking, no hand grasp, or regurgitation of feedings not previously observed. In time, the infant becomes opisthotonic and irritable.

To administer the treatment of phototherapy safely and properly, should it be ordered.

1   The shining of daylight fluorescent bulbs directly on the exposed skin of the infant reduces tissue bilirubin, which in turn reduces serum bilirubin by:
    a Photo-oxidizing tissue bilirubin to biliverdin, to secondary yellow pigments, to colourless, nontoxic compounds.

b Causing tissue-serum bilirubin equilibrium, or as the bilirubin decreases in tissue, pulling bilirubin from the serum into the tissue to maintain this equilibrium.

2 The paediatricain will determine the length of time the infant is to be under the lights based on serum bilirubin levels and clinical condition of the infant.

3 Nursing care peculiar to phototherapy;

a Have infant completely undressed so entire skin surface is exposed to light. Cover scrotum to protect testes.

b Keep infant's eyes covered to protect them from the constant exposure to high intensity light which may cause retinal injury. Do not apply pressure when the eyes are covered as this may cause corneal ulceration. Be certain both eyes are occluded with protective cover and that eyelids are closed. Change protective covers routinely and check for conjunctivitis. Make sure nose is not occluded.

c Develop a systematic schedule of turning infant so all surfaces are exposed.

d Maintain thermoneutrality — measure incubator temperature as well as infant's. Infants over 3 kg are nursed naked lying on a protected electrical blanket in a cot. Light affects the ambient temperature. Do not expose the thermistor probe to the lights without the probe's being covered with an opaque tape.

e Adequate fluid intake should be provided either orally or intravenously. Extra fluid as plain water should be given between milk feeds. Vasodilatation increases the insensible water loss and there is excess stool loss from occasional diarrhoea.

f Some infants require an additional Perspex heat shield to maintain normal temperature.

g Ensure that serum bilirubin levels are obtained as prescribed. The diminishing icterus, i.e. the lowering of unconjugated bilirubin from cutaneous tissue, does not reflect the serum bilirubin concentration. Lights should be turned off when blood is being collected to eliminate false bilirubin levels.

h Side effects of phototherapy
   (1) Lethargy
   (2) Loose green stools
   (3) Dark urine
   (4) Temperature elevation
   (5) Skin changes — greenish colour; rash due to capillary dilatation
   (6) Priapism — turn infant on abdomen for short periods of time and this will cease
   (7) Dehydration from increased skin evaporation.

i If possible, remove infant from under the lights, remove eye covers, and hold infant for feedings. This will allow for some human contact and pleasure during feeding, a chance to open his eyes and look around and perhaps encourage parental involvement in the infant's care.

j   Note sleeping and eating patterns. The feeding schedule may need to be adjusted to the infant's pattern for better feeding.

k   Develop a schedule for changing light bulbs according to manufacturer's instructions.

To assist in the treatment of exchange transfusion (see p. 168).

To foster a healthy family-child relationship

1   Encourage parents to visit infant as much as possible during hospitalization.
2   Allow parents to fondle, care for, hold, and feed infant as much as possible or as his condition permits.
3   Ensure that family health visitor is informed prior to infant's discharge.

Parental Teaching

1   Help family to understand what is wrong with their baby. Explain in simple terms what the doctor has already told them. Allow them to ask questions about the baby and treatment.
2   If the baby has erythroblastosis fetalis, help parents understand the importance of antenatal care and monitoring should another pregnancy occur.
3   Stress the importance of close follow-up of the baby after hospital discharge. Anaemia is a common long-term side effect of red blood cell haemolysis and exchange transfusion. The baby's haemoglobin level should be monitored for some time after illness so appropriate treatment can be initiated if necessary.

FAILURE TO THRIVE

'Failure to thrive' syndrome is a term used to identify infants characterized by growth and developmental failure along with psychosocial disruption.

Aetiology

1   Unknown.
2   Organic
   a   Central nervous system
   b   Cardiovascular
   c   Renal
   d   Gastrointestinal
   e   Respiratory
   f   Endocrine
   g   Metabolic.

3 Nonorganic
   a Inadequate kilojoule (calorie) intake; disturbed feeding patterns
   b Maternal deprivation or faulty mother-child relationship
   c Family problems (socioeconomic problems).

Clinical Manifestations

1 Weight measurement falls below 2 standard deviations from mean for age (weight and length fall below that expected for gestational and postnatal age).
2 Infant fails to gain weight or loses subcutaneous fat and muscle.
3 Possible presenting manifestations that are associated with maternal deprivation:
   a Developmental retardation
   b Disturbed psychosocial development
      (1) Inappropriate response for age to strangers
      (2) Avoidance of eye contact with another person
      (3) Exaggerated self-comfort measures
      (4) Withdrawn — no interest in environment.
4 Somatic manifestations
   a Gastrointestinal
      (1) Anorexia
      (2) Vomiting
      (3) Diarrhoea
      (4) Rumination
      (5) Dehydration
   b Respiratory — coughing.

Diagnostic Evaluation

1 Detailed history — including dietary and family
2 Physical examination — accurate measurements of length, weight, and head circumference — general condition
3 Laboratory data — preliminary tests should be minimal, unless history or examination indicates a specific line of inquiry. Include the following tests:
   a Complete blood count
   b Urinalysis and culture
   c Bone age
   d Stool for fat, occult blood, O + P (ovum and parasites), pH, trypsin
   e Levels of serum sodium, potassium, CO_2, chlorides, creatinine, calcium
4 Cessation of somatic clinical manifestations
5 Weight gain.

Treatment
(When no abnormalities have been identified)

1   Adequate energy intake for weight gain (550-630 kJ/kg/day; 130-150 cal/kg/day; based on appropriate weight for gestational and postnatal age).
2   Appropriate 'mothering' — nurturing activities and environmental stimulation. Investigation has suggested that weight gain will occur when adequate nutrition is taken independent of nurturing activities; however, one is also dealing with a hospitalized child who is subjected to parental separation or deprivation.
3   If after a trial of adequate caloric ingestion, the infant does not gain weight, intensive investigation is done. Trial period may have to be 7-10 days in some instances.

Prognosis

1   Prognosis generally depends upon the aetiology, severity, and duration of the condition, as well as on the home situation into which the child returns.
2   Long-term — continued impaired growth rate and failure to thrive, lowered intelligence, and emotional disorders.

Nursing Objectives

To make an assessment of the infant's general condition, level of development, coping mechanisms, and behaviour.

1   Carefully note what behaviours need attention and/or modifying.
2   Accurately record findings in nursing notes.
3   Obtain and record accurate height, weight, and head circumference.

To develop a detailed nursing care plan that is workable based upon:

1   Infant's physical condition and limitations
2   Medical management
3   Nursing history
4   Input from other multidisciplinary team members.

To understand that the reason for this child's condition may not totally be the mother's fault.

1   Disturbed feeding patterns may have continued despite attempts by mother to correct them.
2   Disturbed mother-infant relationship resulting from separation at neonatal period.

To provide and maintain nutritional intake that will allow for weight gain.

1   Determine if a feeding problem does exist.
2   Infant may need to be taught to eat appropriately for his age, i.e. cup, solids,

spoon, finger food.

3 If child vomits, then smaller, more frequent feedings may be necessary; prop up in sitting position for feeding. Assess what effect environment, position, and other factors have on vomiting and feeding behaviour.

Daily weights and accurate input and output are necessary to evaluate progress.

To gently and warmly provide nurturing to this infant.

1 Assess what the infant can tolerate and base nursing care on this.
2 Encourage the development of a trusting relationship between one or two persons and the infant.
3 Use each opportunity presented by daily care to develop the relationship, help infant become interested and enjoy his environment and eventually reach out to explore himself, people, and things around him.
4 Part of nurturing activities include the therapeutic use of tactile, visual, and auditory stimulation through play. Do not force this upon child if he is unable to tolerate it. Have items within reach, occasionally showing infant how they operate.
5 Talk to infant, use his name; slowly help him to tolerate eye-to-eye contact.
6 Document infant's reactions and responses to handling, playing, etc. Note mother's reaction and interaction with her baby.

To establish a relationship with the mother (parents) that will allow for open communication and cooperative efforts.

1 Accept the mother as a person, one who may have problems with which she cannot cope. She may be young and inexperienced or have doubts about her ability to be a mother, as well as other socioeconomic problems.
2 A trusting relationship between the nurse and mother will enhance identifying infant care problems the mother may be experiencing as well as make her more receptive to any teaching or information the nurse may pass on to her.
3 The mother (parents) must be allowed to express her (their) feelings.

To work as a contributing integral part of the multidisciplinary team caring for this infant and family.

1 The paediatrician — responsible for overall diagnosis and management of the family.
2 The social worker and health visitor — help parents handle the stress that prevents them from assuming their parenting roles.
3 The nurse — coordinates infant care and participates in teaching infant care to the mother.
4 The parents — they must be included in the team as the plan of approach must be acceptable and understood in order to be used by them.
5 Other members of the team may include psychiatrist and family practitioner.

To help mother and infant establish a healthy relationship that will continue to grow when the infant is discharged (see also Intensive Care Nursing, p. 73).

1   Encourage the mother to be active in the plan of treatment. Identify areas of involvement in nursing care plan.
2   Praise her positive efforts, gradually redirect negative aspects.
3   Identify and interpret for the mother the infant's behaviour pattern. Help her to understand the discrepancies between her expectations and reality.
4   Help her to understand her importance to the infant and that the relationship is based on reciprocal needs and responses between mother and infant.

To inform family health visitor before discharge.

1   Provides parents with continual support by someone they know.
2   Gives feedback as to the home situation and possible areas where problems can be avoided.

To help the mother (parents) understand and accept the need for continual follow-up care of her (their) infant.

1   Be certain mother knows where and when to obtain this care. Give outpatient appointment card. Ensure that date and time is convenient to the family.
2   Encourage her to seek support from appropriate resources as necessary.

SEPTICAEMIA NEONATORUM

Septicaemia neonatorum (sepsis) is a generalized infection which may occur in the neonate and is characterized by the proliferation of bacteria in the bloodstream and frequently involves the meninges (as distinguished from simple bacteraemia, congenital infection, septicaemia following major diseases or surgery, or major congenital anomalies).

Aetiology

1   The distribution of the main causative organisms varies from year to year and from one unit to another.
2   Gram-negative organisms:
    Escherichia coli
    Klebsiella (Enterobacteriaceae)
    Pseudomonas
    Proteus
    Salmonella
    Haemophilus influenzae.

3   Gram-positive organisms:
      Group B beta-haemolytic *Streptococcus*
      Staphylococcus aureus — coagulase negative and coagulase positive
      Listeria monocytogenes
      Staphylococcus epidermidis
      Streptococcus pneumoniae
      Streptococcus faecalis

4   Predisposing factors
    a Sex — male predominance
    b Perinatal factors
       (1) Maternal complications
       Prolonged rupture of membranes
       Prolonged and difficult labour; precipitous delivery
       Chorioamnionitis
       Endometritis
       Urinary tract infection
       Toxaemia
       Abruptio placentae
       Maternal illness
       (2) Infant complications
       Prematurity or low birth weight
       Congenital heart disease
       Intracranial bleeding
       Cardiovascular disease
       Colonization of organisms in genital tract
       Respiratory distress syndrome
       Skin infections
       Difficult/traumatic delivery
    c Iatrogenic or environmental factors
       (1) Related to type of equipment used in caring for infant
       Catheters
       Oxygen and humidity
       Resuscitative
       (2) Defective or unclean equipment
       (3) Obstetric and nursery practices.

5   Mode of entry
    a Infection may gain access into the amniotic sac either prior to or after rupture of the membranes; the fetus may aspirate some of this infected fluid.
    b Bacteria may enter the fetal circulation following invasion of the decidua from the amniotic cavity.
    c After birth, bacteria may enter the infant's circulation by a variety of routes. Infection may originate in the skin, umbilical stump, or mucous membranes of the eyes, nose, pharynx, and ear as well as the respiratory, gastrointestinal, and renal tracts.
    d Iatrogenic — equipment resuscitation.

Clinical Manifestations

1 The early signs of sepsis are usually vague and subtle. The infant is often described as not doing well. The signs often include:
   a Poor feeding
   b Lethargy, limpness
   c May have a subnormal, normal or raised body temperature.
2 Later signs and symptoms may include any of the following:
   a Pallor, cyanosis or apnoeic episodes, respiratory distress
   b Jaundice
   c Abdominal distension
   d Vomiting and/or diarrhoea
   e Paronychia
   f Petechiae or purpura
   g Vesicles or pustules
   h Hepatosplenomegaly
   i Irritability, convulsion
   j Bulging fontanelles
   k Hypoglycaemia.

Pathophysiology

1 Temporary breakdown or depression of infant defence mechanisms for unknown reason
   a Possibly due to stress of labour and delivery
   b Predisposing factors (see under Aetiology)
2 The defence systems of the newborn, especially the low birth weight infant, are ineffective with regard to:
   a Active immunity
      (1) Significant formation of IgG (immunoglobulin G) begins at 1-3 months of age
      (2) Significant formation of IgM (immunoglobulin M) begins at birth to 7 days
   b Passive immunity
      Born without IgM antibodies and bactericidal protection against Gram-negative organisms
   c Phagocytosis and minimal inflammatory response
      Neutrophils are less active in response to chemotactic stimuli and migrate more slowly to areas of inflammation
   d Unknown factors.

Diagnostic Evaluation

1 History of predisposing factors
2 Physical findings

3   Laboratory: recovery of organisms from blood cultures must be obtained for a diagnosis of septicaemia neonatorum
   a Cultures to detect specific organism
      (1) Blood
      (2) Urine
      (3) Spinal fluid
      (4) Umbilical stump
      (5) Skin lesions
      (6) Nose, throat, rectal
      (7) External auditory canal
      (8) Gastric fluid
   b White blood cell count and differential — nonspecific test; may be difficult to interpret
   c Blood chemistries — sugar, calcium, pH, electrolytes
   d Acid-base studies
   e Bilirubin
   f Serum immunoglobulin estimation
4   Chest x-ray — may demonstrate pulmonary infection
5   When suspected that infection was acquired in utero, the placenta should be saved for histological examination and culture.

Complications

1   Meningitis — very common complication
2   Shock
3   Adrenal haemorrhage
4   Osteitis and septic arthritis
5   Metabolic derangements
6   Pneumonia
7   Urinary tract infection
8   High mortality rate

Treatment

Antibacterial Therapy (based on the identified organism)

1   Before the specific organism is identified, and after cultures have been obtained, the antibacterial therapy is based on the more common causative agents and their anticipated susceptibilities
   a Knowledge of particular nursery offenders and their antibiotic susceptibilities is needed for proper drug selection.
   b Therapy duration is generally 5-7 days after clinical improvement, but may be as long as 3-4 weeks with complicated infections.

Supportive Therapy

1   Observation
2   Isolation, if indicated
3   Fluid and caloric maintenance
4   Other as indicated.

Nursing Objectives
(See also Intensive Care Nursing, p. 73.)

To practise measures which will prevent the transmission of infection in the nursery.

1   Practise careful handwashing technique and serve as a model of good technique.
2   Personnel with infection should avoid contact with infants.
    a Seek medical care for infection. (Cultures should be done.)
    b Remain out of the nursery.
    c Wear a mask when it is necessary to enter the nursery.
3   Teach parents and other persons entering the nursery proper handwashing and gown technique.
4   Maintain sterile technique when procedures demanding this technique are performed.
5   Promote general cleanliness of the nursery environment.
    Infected equipment and stagnant water provide excellent conditions for bacterial growth.

To observe infants for the vague symptoms which appear early in the course of sepsis.

1   Observe the following:
    a Lethargy, decreased activity, and loss of muscle tone
    b Poor feeding or refusal to feed
    c Temperature alterations, especially hypothermia.
2   Be consistent in planning for the care of infants to provide a means whereby these early symptoms may be detected.
    a Accurate charting of the infant's previous behaviour
    b Whenever possible assign the same nurse to care for an infant on successive days.
3   Report to the paediatrician the symptoms observed.
4   When neonatal sepsis is caused by B group streptococci, the disease may take one or two courses:
    a Early onset — within 12-24 hours after birth
    (1) Acute septicaemia with fulminant clinical course; high mortality and severe neurological sequelae in survivors.
    (2) There is generally a history of obstetric complications and the serotype of streptococci from mother's birth canal and infant are the same.
    (3) Signs and symptoms include respiratory symptoms — in particular, acute respiratory distress, hypoxia, leading to shock.

b Delayed onset — occurs 10 days after birth to 6-12 weeks
(1) Illness is severe and associated with meningitis.
(2) Normal obstetric history; probably acquired infection from environment.
(3) Disease is characterized by meningeal symptoms, including bulging fontanelle and seizures.

To observe for episodes of apnoea and initiate measures to stimulate respiration.

1 Observe the infant closely for apnoea. It may be necessary to observe the infant for several days and to nurse the baby on a special apnoea alarm mattress or with an alarm capsule attached to the abdominal wall.
2 Stimulate infant when apnoea does occur.
   a Slap feet and provide more vigorous stimulation if necessary.
   b Apply artificial ventilation using mask and bag or mouth-to-mouth resuscitation when spontaneous respiration does not occur within 15-30 seconds.
3 Report frequent periods of apnoea to paediatrician.
4 Record length of apnoeic episode and response to stimulation.

To observe the infant for convulsions which may occur with sepsis.

1 Immediately report to the paediatrician any twitching or convulsive activity.
   a Remain with infant.
   b Suction mouth and nose if infant has secretions or vomitus in his mouth.
   c Turn head to side.
   d Protect infant from banging against side of incubator or falling from radiant warmer.
   e Provide oxygen if cyanosis or respiratory distress occurs.
   f Administer any medication prescribed to control the convulsions.
2 Record the length of and the type of convulsion, the parts of the body involved, the infant's general appearance before and following the convulsion, and response to any therapy given.

To ensure that evaluation and diagnostic tests be initiated promptly and correctly to avoid altered results from contamination.

Since the infective organism must be recovered in blood cultures, strict aseptic technique in obtaining cultures is vital.

1 Peripheral venipuncture is location of choice (umbilical vessels are already contaminated and femoral vein offers possible contamination from perineum).
2 Cleanse skin with aseptic solution (e.g. iodine solution). For maximal aseptic effect, allow solution to dry.

To provide for the nutritional needs of the infant in order to provide for his caloric needs.

1   During the acute phase of the illness the infant may not be able to take or tolerate oral feedings.

   a Monitor the administration of intravenous fluids.

   b Provide for the sucking needs of the infant by providing him with a dummy.

   c Nasogastric feedings may be given to the infant.

2   Initiate oral feedings of infant formula as soon as the infant's condition improves.

   a Begin by offering small feedings and observe following responses:

     (1) Vomiting

     (2) Abdominal distension

     (3) Infant's interest in feeding and ability to suck

     (4) Whether the infant tires with feeding.

   b Daily feedings may be supplemented with nasogastric feedings.

   c Gradually increase the amount of feeding.

   Do not force feedings — vomiting associated with diarrhoea may result, leading to dehydration.

   d Resume regular feeding schedule based on infant's ability to tolerate feeding.

3   Hold the infant for feedings as soon as his condition warrants it.

To provide measures to maintain the infant's temperature within normal range.

1   Take infant's temperature at hourly intervals.

2   Adjust the incubator temperature to maintain infant's temperature between 36 and 37°C.

3   When infant is placed in an open cot, maintain temperature and cover the infant appropriately.

4   Report hypothermia or hyperthermia to the paediatrician.

To administer the prescribed antibiotic therapy to control the infection.

1   Administer the prescribed medications.

   a Be aware of the action and side effects of the specific medications.

   b Be aware of the route of excretion.

   c Be aware of drug incompatibilities.

2   Observe the infant's apparent response to therapy.

   a Note child's activity, feeding behaviour and weight.

   b Observe for the development of new symptoms.

To be prepared to assist with blood transfusions

Adult whole blood also provides specific factors which enhance the phagocytic abilities of neonatal leukocytes.

To observe for the occurrence of septic shock and report immediately.

1 Monitor blood pressure.
2 Check peripheral resistance in pulses in all extremities: note colour and temperature.
3 Monitor urine output for evaluation of renal function.

To provide for the emotional needs of the infant.

1 Place bright, colourful objects in the cot or incubator.
2 Talk gently and quietly while caring for the infant.
3 Touch and gently stroke the infant.
4 Encourage the parents to visit and allow them to hold the infant as soon as possible.

To involve the parents in the infant's care in the hospital and prepare them for the infant's discharge.

1 Encourage parents to visit the infant.
   a Show them how to hold and feed the baby.
   b Answer questions they may have regarding the infant's progress and care.
   c Provide them with an opportunity to explain their concerns.
2 Discuss symptoms of complications which may occur and should be watched for following discharge.
3 Give specific instruction regarding medications to be given at home.
4 Ensure that family health visitor is notified of impending discharge.

INFANT OF A DRUG-ADDICTED MOTHER

An *infant of an addicted mother* is one who is born to a mother who is narcotic and/or methadone dependent and who takes the drug or drugs in varying dosages for varying periods during her pregnancy.

Aetiology
Maternal use of narcotics or methadone or both drugs during pregnancy.

1 The drugs cross the placental barrier and enter the fetal circulation.
2 The supply of the infant is abruptly terminated at delivery.
3 Other agents, i.e. phenobarbitone, are also capable of causing withdrawal symptoms.

Clinical Manifestations (of Neonatal Withdrawal)
1 The degree of withdrawal symptoms the infant manifests may be related to

the duration of the mother's habit, the type and dosage requirements of her addiction, and her drug level immediately prior to delivery.

a The closer to delivery the mother received her last dose, the longer her addiction and the higher her dose need, the longer the delay of withdrawal symptoms, and the more severe the symptoms in the infant.

b Although heroin and methadone produce similar withdrawal symptoms in the infant, those same symptoms are generally more severe with methadone withdrawal — probably because of the high level of the mother's dose, the pharmacological characteristics of the drug itself, and the use by the mother of other drugs simultaneously.

2   Onset of symptoms
   a Heroin — several hours after birth to 3-4 days of life
   b Methadone — 7-10 days after birth to several weeks of life.

3   Cardinal signs of neonatal narcotic withdrawal:
   a Coarse, flapping tremors
   b Irritability
   c Prolonged, persistent, high-pitched cry
   d Restlessness/sleepiness.

4   Other signs and symptoms of acute withdrawal:
   a Vigorous, ineffective sucking; poor feeding
   b Excessive tearing; excessive sweating
   c Increased salivation
   d Sneezing, nasal stuffiness
   e Vomiting and/or diarrhoea
   f Muscle rigidity
   g Yawning
   h Convulsions — with methadone withdrawal
   i Tachypnoea with associated respiratory alkalosis
   j Exaggerated reflexes
   k Hyperpyrexia.

5   Prematurity
   High incidence of infants born to addicted mothers are preterm and/or small for gestational age.

Diagnosis

1   Thorough maternal history, including drug habits.
2   Physical assessment. Kahn's * criteria of tremulousness and irritability:
   a Grade I — signs recognizable but mild
   b Grade II — signs marked but only when infant is disturbed
   c Grade III — signs marked and occurring at frequent intervals, even when infant is undisturbed.

*Kahn E J *et al.*, The course of heroin withdrawal syndrome in newborn infants treated with phenobarbital or chlorpromazine, *Journal of Pediatrics*, 1969, 75: 485.

3   Laboratory
    a Urine for toxicologic studies
    b Blood glucose
    c Serum calcium, pH, and total protein
    d Acid-base status studies, respiratory alkalosis
    e Serological studies for syphilis
    f Appropriate cultures if systemic bacterial infection is suspected.
4   Many of the clinical signs of neonatal narcotic withdrawal are nonspecific
    and may indicate other problems: hypoglycaemia, hypocalcaemia, central
    nervous system disorders or haemorrhage, infection, other non-narcotic
    drug withdrawal.

Treatment

1   Narcotic antagonist for narcotic-induced respiratory depression at birth
    (morphine addiction)
2   Drug therapy in sufficient daily amounts to alleviate signs of narcotic with-
    drawal. Duration of therapy using gradually decreasing dosages may be
    from 4 to 40 days
    a Paregoric (camphorated tincture of opium) orally
    b Phenobarbitone (orally)
    c Chlorpromazine (Largactil)
    d Diazepam (Valium) intramuscularly

3   Supportive therapy as appropriate.

Complications

1   Intrauterine growth retarded infant (IUGR); small for gestational age (light
    for dates) infant; preterm infant
2   Fetal anoxia with meconium aspiration
3   Infection-associated maternal venereal disease or hepatitis.

Prognosis

1   The long-term biological effects on the infant of a drug-addicted mother are
    not fully known. These children may have:
    a Abnormal psychomotor development associated with intrauterine
    growth retardation
    b Behavioural disturbances such as hyperactivity, brief attention spans,
    temper tantrums.
2   The unstable environment which the drug-addicted mother (or parents)
    may provide is a major threat to the child's health and development.

Nursing Objectives

To be familiar with withdrawal symptoms in order to facilitate early diagnosis, which in turn will decrease incidence of morbidity and mortality of high-risk infants.

1 Recognize cardinal as well as other symptoms.
2 Identify infants likely to have symptoms.
3 Report to paediatrician any suspicious behaviour.

To ensure that prophylactic measures have been administered against ophthalmia neonatorum. There is a high incidence of gonococcal infection in drug-addicted pregnant women.

To ensure that diagnostic measures are carried out. Collect urine for toxicological studies within 24 hours after birth, since narcotic metabolites disappear rapidly.

To administer nursing care appropriate for the symptoms of withdrawal the infant is experiencing.

1 Irritability and restlessness, high-pitched crying
   a Swaddle.
   b Minimize handling — holding usually aggravates irritability.
   c Decrease environmental stimuli.
   d Organize care to allow for periods of uninterrupted sleep.
2 Floppy tremors
   a Protect skin from irritation and abrasions
      (1) Use sheepskin.
      (2) Change position frequently.
      (3) Give good frequent skin care — keep infant clean and dry.
3 Frantic sucking
   a Give dummy between feeds.
   b Protect infant's hand from excoriation.
4 Poor feeding
   a Give small, frequent feeds.
   b Maintain energy and fluid intake requirement for infant's weight.
5 Vomiting/diarrhoea
   a Position infant to prevent aspiration.
   b Provide good skin care to areas exposed to vomitus or stool.
6 Muscle rigidity — hypertonicity
   a Change position frequently to minimize development of pressure areas.
   b Use sheepskin.
   c Skin care.
7 Increased salivation and/or nasal stuffiness
   a Aspirate nasopharynx; suction tracheal mucus.
   b Provide frequent nose and mouth care.
   c Note respiration rate and characteristics and infant's colour.

8   Tachypnoea
    a Note onset and severity of accompanying signs of respiratory distress.
    b Position infant for easier ventilation — semi-Fowler's position; hyperextend head slightly.
    c Minimize handling.
    d Have resuscitative equipment available.

To record accurately and in detail all symptoms, including the following:

1   Time of onset
2   Duration and frequency
3   Severity
4   Treatment initiated and infant's response
    Example: extent of irritability, changes in feeding behaviour, tolerance of handling, characteristics and frequency of stool
5   Vital signs.

To maintain caloric and fluid requirement and balance.

1   Keep accurate intake and output records to prevent dehydration.
2   Maintain intravenous fluid as appropriate when infant experiences vomiting or diarrhoea.
3   Infant may feed better on demand schedule.
4   Infant may need increased calories due to increased activity.

To support drug therapy when used to control symptoms of withdrawal.

1   If diazepam is used, be alert for the appearance of jaundice.
    (Sodium benzoate is used as a preservative in this preparation and interferes with the binding of albumin with unconjugated bilirubin.)
2   Methadone withdrawal symptoms are frequently more difficult to control than those of heroin withdrawal.
3   Note appearance of side effects of depression from oversedation:
    a Respiratory distress
    b Lethargy
    c Decreased sucking activity
    d Hypotonia.

To protect the infant from pathophysiological processes to which he is predisposed because of being preterm or small infant for gestational age.

1   Hypoglycaemia
2   Hypocalcaemia
3   Hypothermia
4   Anoxia
5   Sepsis

To encourage multidisciplinary conferences in an attempt to treat the whole family.

1   Initiate early referrals as needed to social services and health visitor to provide for continuity of care after discharge.
    a The unstable environment into which the infant may be discharged offers a threat to the child's future well-being and development.
    b Discharge to foster home may be considered.
2   Evaluate mother's attitude toward her infant.
    a She may be able to accept the responsibility of her child and to accept help offered to her.
    b She may become nonfunctioning as a result of the birth of her infant; she may feel inadequate, angry, guilty or see the infant as an added burden.

To encourage parental involvement in the care of this infant.

Frequently the infant may not be discharged with the mother. Promote early mother-infant attachment and foster their relationship.

1   Encourage frequent mother-infant contact.
2   Have mother feed infant.
3   Pace the growth of the relationship between infant and mother based on the infant's progress and the mother's positive reactions.
4   Keep in mind that methadone and heroin can be detected in breast milk and may lead to permanent addiction of the infant should the mother breast-feed.

Parental Guidance

1   Carefully planned follow-up care for the infant is essential.
    a Explain to the mother the need for consistent follow-up care for her infant.
    b Infants of drug-dependent mothers are at risk; they may show failure to thrive, experience battering, or succumb to sudden infant death syndrome.
    c Involve the health visitor in the planning early in hospitalization. This early involvement may offer mother some security.
    d It is often difficult to maintain contact for follow-up.
2   The mother may be accepting of rehabilitation during the postpartum period. Contact appropriate people or provide appropriate information for her.
3   Help the mother understand what she should expect in infant's behaviour upon discharge.
    a Many infants are irritable and restless for several months after birth.
    b Discuss with the mother the feelings she may have as a result of a strained mother-child relationship.

NEONATAL OR PROLONGED SLEEP APNOEA OF INFANCY

Nonfatal apnoea of infancy is the cessation of breathing for more than 20 seconds, or a shorter episode associated with bradycardia, cyanosis, or pallor.

Near-miss sudden infant death syndrome is the term sometimes used to identify a condition in an infant, usually between 2 weeks and 6 months of age, who is brought to medical attention because of an unexplained frightening respiratory or cardiac event, usually occurring while the infant is asleep.

Aetiology

1   Unknown — may result from many different pathological processes.
2   Apnoea related to organic disorders:
   a Seizure disorders
   b Gastro-oesophageal reflux
   c Significant anaemia
   d Sepsis, severe infection
   e Hypoglycaemia
   f Impaired regulation of breathing.
3   Current theories relating to the cause of sudden infant death syndrome:
   a Prolonged sleep apnoea
   b Chronic oxygen deficiency
   c Enzyme abnormalities.

Although many feel that some near-miss infants or those with prolonged sleep apnoea are at risk from sudden infant death syndrome, a definitive causal relation between the two has not been scientifically established.

4   Characteristics that may identify infants at risk from sudden infant death syndrome include:
   a Prematurity
   b Neonatal conditions with apnoea
   c History of aborted sudden infant death syndrome
   d History of sudden infant death syndrome in family.
5   Characteristics of sudden infant death syndrome pattern include:
   a Prematurity
   b Preceding cold or upper respiratory infection
   c Peak age 2-4 months
   d Occurs in males more often than females, in a ratio of 3 : 2
   e Bottle fed with infant milk formula.

Clinical Manifestations

1   Infant is usually found by parents or caretaker to be:
   a Limp
   b Cyanotic
   c Pale

    d No respiration

    e Cool to touch

    f Normal muscle tone.

2 Some form of resuscitation may be required — mouth-to-mouth respiration or cardiopulmonary assistance.

3 Infant usually exhibits symptoms when asleep, although the syndrome may occur during waking hours.

4 Types of sleep apnoea include:

    a Central or diaphragmatic — chest movement ceases.

    b Upper airway — chest and diaphragm move but there is no air-exchange.

    c Mixed — upper airway apnoea follows one of central apnoea. Bradycardia is associated with upper airway and mixed apnoea.

Diagnostic Evaluation

It must be established that a primary life-threatening failure in physiological homeostasis has occurred, ruling out other medical problems could result in respiratory failure as a secondary cause. To accomplish this the following procedures are generally included:

1 Detailed history of the event including information concerning what happened, appearance of infant, type of intervention, how infant responded, conditions prior to the event, special past medical history, special family history

2 Medical evaluation of infant (physical examination)

3 Laboratory data — generally minimal history or examination indicates a specific line of inquiry:

    a Complete blood count with differential

    b Serum glucose

    c Electrolytes

    d Calcium and phosphate

    e Magnesium

    f Blood gases, as indicated

4 Chest x-ray

5 Electrocardiogram

6 Electroencephalogram (may not be routine) and neurological examination

7 Respiratory studies — a pneumogram 12- to 24-hour tape recording of small changes in electrical resistance with each breath or respiratory pattern; multichannel sleep test with continuous print-out

8 Continuous cardiac and apnoea monitoring for recurrence of event, prolonged apnoea, or bradycardia

9 Barium swallow for gastro-oesophageal reflux.

Management

1 Cardiopulmonary monitoring — is critical
2 Specific treatment of any underlying cause
3 Theophylline — may be used to decrease apnoeic spells
4 Long-term follow-up for physiological and neurological behavioural functions, support and counselling from health visitor and primary health care team.

Prognosis

1 Infants who have experienced near-miss sudden infant death syndrome may be at risk to recurrent apnoea, hypoxia, and sudden death.
2 Because of hypoxaemia that may have occurred, child should be assessed for learning difficulties (hearing, eyesight), discrete neurological impairments, personality disorders, etc.

Nursing Objectives and Management

To be prepared for the infant's admission.

1 Have all equipment, including apnoea monitor, ready for use.
2 Select a room that is clearly visible from the nursing station; the room should be quiet in order to reduce sensory stimulation, which may reduce the likelihood of a recurring episode.
3 The family has just experienced the extreme stress of feeling that their infant has almost died. Professional efficiency and empathy at the time of admission is reassuring and builds parental confidence in nursing care.

To obtain a nursing history with special attention to:

1 Parents' description of the events that preceded hospitalization, and their understanding of prolonged apnoea.
   a This information may provide clues for factors to observe during hospitalization and provides data for the development of a teaching plan.
   b It also allows for the correction of misinformation and misconceptions.
2 Have parents describe sleep patterns, feeding habits, prior health problems, immunizations, and medications; this information may provide data regarding possible influencing factors or causes of the condition.
3 Have parents describe a typical day in the life of the infant and the family unit. This provides important data on how home-monitoring may affect family life, and contributes to the effective development of home management and family teaching plans; it also provides a basis for continuity of care for the infant.

To orientate the parents to the unit and the equipment used in the infant's care.

1 Explain the visiting policy and encourage parents to visit as much as possible.
2 Parents must be willing and available for comprehensive instruction in their infant's condition and necessary interventions so that they feel competent in the infant's care prior to discharge.
3 Assignment of consistent nursing is helpful so that families can develop a trusting relationship that will help them deal with the emotional aspects of the diagnosis and the complexities of the treatment plan.
4 Preparing the parents for all diagnostic tests that will be performed helps reduce the fear surrounding these procedures.

To monitor constantly, and document any apnoeic event the infant may experience.

1 Condition of infant
   a Awake/asleep
   b Respirations — none, normal, shallow; colour of infant
   c Monitor reading — apnoea, bradycardia and rate, read off
   d Position of infant — limp, vomited, etc.
2 Intervention
   a Nothing — infant OK or self-corrected
   b Gentle stimulation
   c Vigorously shaken
   d Resuscitation.

To serve as a role model for the family in the following areas of infant care.

1 Use of the infant monitor (i.e. electrode placement, operation of controls, care of lead wires to prevent damage, etc.). Discussion of home-monitoring should not take place until it has been determined that this procedure will be used.
2 Methods of responding to alarms. Respond to all alarms immediately according to established procedures (i.e. observation and assessment of infant, stimulation, resuscitation, etc.).
3 Recording procedure — complete documentation of any apnoeic episode; record each time alarm sounds.
4 Administration of theophylline, if prescribed.
   a Observe for signs of toxicity: apical rate above 200, vomiting, and agitation.
   b Although the mechanism by which theophylline reduces or prevents apnoea in some infants is not understood, research indicates it may act by:
      (1) Inducing rapid shallow breathing
      (2) Increasing metabolic rate with an increase in alveolar ventilation in proportion to increased CO_2 production.
5 Continue the infant's normal activities whenever possible (i.e. holding him for feedings, playing with him, disconnecting him from monitor for

bathing); allow for continuation of usual eating or sleeping patterns. Simulating the home environment as much as possible will encourage deep-sleep patterns, which may stimulate apnoea in some infants (valuable diagnostic information).

To effectively prepare parents for eventual discharge of infant.

Since the parents have experienced at least one apnoeic episode prior to hospitalization, the fear of their infant's sudden death has been heightened. When discharged, the parents have direct and full responsibility for appropriate action should infant's breathing cease.

1 Assess what parents know and understand about apnoea. Correct any misconceptions and provide accurate information.
2 Make sure parents know about feeding precautions — frequent burping, no bottle in bed, upright position after feeding, elevation of the head of the bed.
3 Instruct parents in the administration of any medications (i.e. theophylline).
4 Teach cardiopulmonary resuscitation to parents as well as to another responsible person, relative, or friend, to provide some relief for parents from infant care.

To teach and prepare parents for home-monitoring, if necessary.

1 Show parents how to operate and maintain the monitor. Reinforce teaching by equipment supplier. Be sure they know how to contact monitor technician.
2 Describe apnoea recording procedure to be used (see above).
3 Teach methods of responding to alarms — what to observe (i.e. colour, presence or absence of breathing) and how to respond (gentle and vigorous stimulation, cardiopulmonary resuscitation).
4 Discuss adjustments in daily living that will be necessary. Start by identifying a typical family day, then discuss anticipated changes.
   a Emphasize that this responsibility must be shared by both parents.
   b Discuss the possible impact on siblings.
   c Caution parents to eliminate noises that would interfere with their ability to hear the alarm (i.e. showering, vacuum cleaning) when only one parent is present. Someone must always be available to hear and respond to the alarm.
   d Avoid travelling long distances alone with infant.
   e Encourage parents to maintain their relationship with one another by using another person trained in cardiopulmonary resuscitation to assume infant care occasionally.
5 Use anticipatory guidance in preparing parents for complication of home monitoring:
   a Increased anxiety and tension
   b Constant worry about the alarm — even when it does not go off
   c Fatigue

d Loss of 'normal, healthy child' — parents then grieve when given the diagnosis.

6   Emphasize the healthy aspects of the infant. Encourage parents to continue as many usual routines as possible. Provide specific things parents can do to encourage normal development and a healthy parent-child relationship.

7   Encourage parents to provide total care for their infant prior to discharge.

To continue to observe family dynamics.

1   Assess for family conflicts or problems that can be alleviated.

2   Families who are overly stressed or demonstrate a maladaptive response may require social service or psychiatric consultation.

3   Modification of the management plan may be indicated.

To document patient/family progress in order to facilitate comprehensive care and discharge planning.
Daily notes should include:

1   Frequency and type of monitor alarms; intervention required

2   Teaching

3   Family dynamics
    a Who visited and for how long
    b Description of parent-child interaction
    c Description of parent interaction
    d Amount of care done by parents
    e Assessment of parental competence in providing care.

To ensure adequate follow-up support.
Most families are frightened by the responsibility of home-monitoring and will require support after discharge.

1   Inform family health visitor and primary health care team prior to discharge.

2   Instruct parents regarding when and how to obtain assistance for medical, technical, and social problems.

3   Ensure that all appointments for follow-up are given in writing at a convenient time for the parents to attend.

4   Facilitate contact with other parents of infants with prolonged apnoea.

To be aware that successful outcome for every baby with prolonged apnoea cannot be certain, despite continuous surveillance with or without monitors and appropriate intervention.

To participate in community education regarding prolonged apnoea and sudden infant death syndrome.

Available Resources
Foundation for the Study of Infant Deaths, 23 St Peters Square, London W6 9NW

FURTHER READING

Books and Pamphlets

Briblecombe F S W (ed.), *Separation and Special Care Baby Units*, Spastics International Medical Publications, 1978.
Cockburn F Drillen C M, *Neonatal Medicine*, Blackwell Scientific, 1974
Evans H E Glass L, *Perinatal Medicine*, Harper & Row, 1978
Harvey D Kelnar C J, *The Sick Newborn Baby*, Bailliere Tindall, 1981
Klaus M H Farnoff A A, *Care of the High Risk Neonate*, Saunders, 1973
Klaus M H Kennell J H, *Maternal Infant Bonding*, Mosby, 1976
Lubcheno L O, *The High Risk Infant*, Saunders, 1976
Marshall R E *et al.*, *Coping with Caring for Sick Newborns*, Saunders, 1982.
Moffet H L., *Pediatric Infectious Diseases*, Lippincott, 1981
O' Doherty N, *Atlas of the Newborn*, MTP, 1979
Redshaw M, *et al.*, *Born too Early: Special Care for your Preterm Baby*, Oxford University Press, 1984.
Schaffer A Avery M E, *Diseases of the Newborn*, Saunders, 1983
Scipien G M, Comprehensive Paediatric Nursing, McGraw-Hill, 1979

Articles

Abnormal infants of diabetic mothers, *Lancet*, March 1980: 663-634
Blake A *et al.*, Transport of newborn infants for intensive care, *British Medical Journal*, 1975: 13-17
Blake A *et al.*, Parents of babies of very low birthweight: long term follow-up, on *CIBA Foundation Symposium* No. 33: 271
Bliss V J, Nursing care for infants with neonatal nectrotizing enterocolitis, *Maternal Care Nursing*, January/February 1976, 2:37-40
Cater J, Changing pattern of care of the newborn infant, *Journal of Maternal and Child Health*, December 1978: 426-430
Christensen A A, Coping with the crisis of a premature birth in one couple's story *Maternal Care Nursing* January/February 1977, 2: 33-37
Duncan J A Webb L Z, Teaching families home apnoea monitoring, *Paediatric Nursing*, May/June 1983: 171-175
Feeding infants of low birth weight. *British Medical Journal*, 3 November 1979: 1092-1093
Fraser A, Pregnancy and drug addiction, *Midwife, Health Visitor and Community Nurse*, May 1978: 132-135
Hughes-Davies T H, Conservative care of the newborn baby, *Archives of Diseases in Childhood*, January 1979, 54: 59-61
Lynch M A Roberts J, Predicting child abuse: signs of bonding failure in the maternity hospital, *British Medical Journal*, March 1977: 466-470

McClure G, Delivery from care of the preterm infant, *Journal of Maternal and Child Health*, December 1979: 460-470

Priestly E, Born too early or too small, *Nursing Mirror*, March 1979: 38-40

Richards M P M *et al.*, Caretaking in the first year of life: the role of father and mothers in social isolation, *Child Care, Health and Development*, 3: 23-36

Speidel B D, Adverse effects of routine procedures on preterm infants. *Lancet*, 22 April 1978: 864-865

Stanway P A, Successful beast feeding, *Midwife, Health Visitor and Community Nurse*, September 1978: 304-306

Stevens D Schreiner R L, Infants of diabetic mothers. *Journal of the Indian State Medical Association*, 1978, 71: 409-410

Sullivan T *et al.*, Determining a newborn's gestational age. *Maternal Care Nursing*, 1979, 4: 38-45

Tufts F Johnson F, Neonatal jaundice and phototherapy. *Canadian Nurse*, December 1979, 75 (11): 45-47

Turner B S Merenstein G B, Hemodynamic monitoring of the critically ill neonate. *Canadian Care Quarterly*, September 1979, 2: 77-78

Vogel M, When a pregnant woman is diabetic: care of the newborn. *American Journal of Nursing*, March 1979, 79: 458-460

Whiteside D, Proper use of radiant warmers. *American Journal of Nursing*, October 1978, 78: 1694-1696

4

CONDITIONS OF THE RESPIRATORY TRACT

OVERVIEW OF CHILDHOOD RESPIRATORY DISORDERS

Common Types of Respiratory Disorders

Examples of common childhood respiratory disorders can be found in Table 4.1.
The following disorders are included:

1 Bacterial pneumonia
2 Viral pneumonia
3 Pneumocystic carinii pneumonia
4 Mycoplasma pneumonia
5 Bronchiolitis
6 Croup

Nursing Objectives

To determine the severity of the respiratory distress that the child is experiencing.
Make an initial nursing assessment.

1 Observe the respiratory rate and pattern.
  a Count the respiration for one full minute.
  b Observe child for retractions, and note severity and location.
2 Observe the child's colour, and note any presence of cyanosis.
3 Observe for nasal flaring.
4 Evaluate the child's degree of restlessness, apprehension, and motor tone.
5 Note any wheezing, stridor, or hoarseness.

To provide a humidified environment enriched with oxygen in order to combat anoxia and to liquefy secretions.

1 Place child in a Croupette with cool mist or use ultrasonic mist tent (see Oxygen Therapy, p. 186).

Nursing Alert: At no time should the mist be allowed to become so dense that it obscures clear visualization of the patient's respiratory pattern.

2   Observe the child's response to this environment.
3   Place child in comfortable position to promote easier respiration.
4   Frequent changing of clothing and bed linen will prevent chilling and will provide comfort.

To provide the child with adequate hydration

1   Maintain the administration of intravenous fluids at the prescribed rate.
2   When the child is in severe respiratory distress, he is given nothing by mouth because of the danger of aspiration.
3   Offer the child small sips of a clear fluid when the respiratory status improves.
    a Note any vomiting or abdominal distension after the oral fluid is given.
    b As the child begins to take more fluid by mouth, notify paediatrician so that intravenous fluid rate may be adjusted in order to prevent fluid overload.
    c Do not force child to take fluids orally that he does not want, as this may cause increased distress and possible vomiting. Anorexia often accompanies acute febrile infection. Generally do not awaken a sleeping child just to give frequent fluids.
4   Record child's intake and output.
    a Measure urinary output and record.
    b Check relative density of urine.

To provide the child with both physical and psychological rest.

1   Disturb the child as little as possible by organizing nursing care, and protect him from unnecessary interruptions from other personnel.
2   Be aware of the age of the child and be familiar with his level of growth and development as it applies to hospitalization.
3   The presence of the child's parents will alleviate some of his apprehension.
4   Provide opportunities for quiet play as the child's condition improves.
5   Explain procedures and hospital routine to child as appropriate for his age.
6   Reduce anxiety and apprehension to aid in decreasing psychological distress, thus helping the child to relax and ease respiratory effort.

To provide good skin care excoriation from secretions, accompanying diarrhoea, and breakdown from confinement to bed.

To provide measures to improve ventilation of affected portion of the lung.

1   Change position frequently.
2   Provide postural drainage if prescribed.
3   Relieve nasal obstruction that contributes to breathing difficulty.
    Instil saline solution or other nose drops and apply nasal suctioning.

4 Crying in a young child can be an effective method for ventilating the lungs.
5 Coughing is a normal tracheobronchial cleansing procedure. Constant coughing can be relieved temporarily by allowing the child to sip water; use extreme caution to prevent aspiration.
6 Abdominal distension frequently accompanies respiratory infection and can be painful and a hindrance to respiration.
   a Place in semi-Fowler's position; encourage movement to promote passage of flatus.
   b If this is unsuccessful, a small enema or suppository may bring relief if distension continues to be painful.

To assist in the control of fever.

1 Antipyretics
2 Increase evaporation from skin with the use of a fan and tepid sponging.

To provide for adequate nutrition to meet the growth and development needs of the child.

1 Determine the child's food preferences.
2 Offer the child small meals.

To administer appropriate antibiotic therapy.

1 Observe for drug sensitivity.
2 Observe child's response to therapy.

To be alert for the appearance of specific complications that may accompany respiratory infection and notify paediatrician immediately (see Table 4.1).

To include parents in the planning of care and in caring for the child.

Recognize parents' anxieties. The mother may be exhausted from caring for her sick child prior to his hospitalization.

Parent Teaching

*When Your Child Has a Croup Attack**

Direct parents according to the pointers outlined below:
   If your child develops hoarseness and a croupy cough with a cold, or if he wakes up in the middle of the night with a croup attack, here is the way to handle it:

1 Take your child into the bathroom and close the door. Turn on the hot water in the shower or tub, and let the room fill up with steam. Sit with your child in the steam-filled bathroom, with the water still running, for 10 minutes. If he is still making croupy noise as he breathes, call the doctor.
2 After breathing has improved, use a cold-air vaporizer. If your child sleeps in a cot, place a sheet or umbrella over the top of the cot and direct the stream of

*From *Patient Care*, 1 November, 1984. © 1974, Patient Care Publications, Inc., Darien, Connecticut, USA. All rights reserved.

(continued on p. 318)

Table 4.1   Respiratory disorders

Condition and causative agent	Age and incidence	Clinical manifestation
Bacterial pneumonia		
1 Streptococcal pneumonia *Streptococcus pneumoniae* (Gram positive) This type of bacterial pneumonia is most frequent in children.	Birth-4 years Winter and spring (especially in patients with sickle cell disease and patients without spleens)	Mild upper respiratory infection (URI) with sudden symptoms Infants: refusal to eat; vomiting; diarrhoea; hypo- or hyper-thermia May be: tachypnoea; grunting; retractions; nasal flaring meningism may be present Older child; prodromal upper respiratory infection; headache; anorexia; malaise; dry cough; fever; restlessness; pleuritic pain; grunting with shallow, rapid respirations; possibly abdominal pain
2 Streptoccal pneumonia Beta-haemolytic streptococcus, Group A (Gram positive)	3-5 years	Commonly superimposed on febrile respiratory infection in a child already ill with a viral exanthem Shows sudden increased fever, worsening cough, chills, pleuritic pain, respiratory distress
3 Staphylococcal pneumonia Coagulase-positive *Staphylococcus aureus* (Gram positive)	Birth-2 years	History of predisposing factors; gradual onset with respiratory symptoms or sudden onset with systemic involvement (very toxic child) Presence of coarse, bubbly crepitations

Diagnostic evaluation	Medical treatment and nursing management	Complications
X-ray — patchy area around bronchi Positive cultures: sputum; nasopharyngeal secretions; blood	Benzyl penicillin Symptomatic: Rest, with gradually increasing exercise Antipyretics O_2 mist Position change Encourage oral fluids to prevent dehydration Physiotherapy with percussion and breathing exercises should be started early	Rare with antibiotic prescription May see: otitis media, sinusitis; empyema; bacteraemia
X-ray — usually patchy, but may show disseminated infiltrate WBC increased — polymorphic leukocytosis Erythrocyte sedimentation rate (ESR) increased Positive culture from respiratory secretions; Empyema fluid	Appropriate antibiotic Symptomatic	Empyema Pneumatocele to pneumothorax Permanent pulmonary fibrosis and pleural thickening (fibrothorax)
X-ray — patchy consolidation of one or more lobes; pneumatocele abscesses Culture: sputum or gastric aspirate, pulmonary fluid or lung aspirate WBC — elevated in older child	Flucloxacillin or cephaloridine Rapid treatment is important Symptomatic: special attention to fluid balance; treatment of pleural complications; treatment of anaemia Be alert to signs of tension pneumothorax: abrupt onset of pain; cyanosis, dyspnoea, diminished chest movement on one side	Empyema Pneumothorax Lung abscess Osteomyelitis Staphylococcal pericarditis Bronchiectasis

(continued)

Table 4.1   Respiratory disorders *(continued)*

Condition and causative agent	Age and incidence	Clinical manifestations
4 *Haemophilus influenzae*	6 months-3 years	Similar to other lobar pneumonias and bronchopneumonia with spasmodic cough; 'toxic' appearance
Viral pneumonia Respiratory syncytial virus (RSV) (most common) Parainfluenza virus Adenoviruses	Birth-2 years; higher incidence in female than in male Winter and early spring	Gradual onset following an upper respiratory infection RSV turns into extension of bronchiolitis Parainfluenza virus causes coryza, pharyngitis, cough; may succeed pneumonia Adenovirus causes pharyngitis and cervical adenitis; may succeed pneumonia
Pneumocystis carnii pneumonia *Pneumocystis carinii* — parasite of uncertain systematic status	Predisposing factors: Preterm infant; immature debilitated infant; infectious disease, especially cytomegalic inclusion disease; serious compromising disease, e.g. cystic fibrosis Children receiving immunosuppressive medication for malignant disease immunodeficiency disease, especially in children under 1 year of age	Onset is generally slow, taking 3-6 weeks to peak, with increasing tachypnoea, extreme greyish cyanosis, and dyspnoea Presence of predisposing factors Pyrexia

Diagnostic evaluation	Medical treatment and nursing management	Complications
Culture: blood; nasal secretions; WBC shows an increase — lymphocytosis X-ray — lobar consolidation (may also have pleural effusion)	Ampicillin Symptomatic: cough suppression	Empyema Bronchiectasis (rare)
X-ray — infiltration of one or more lobes is more extensive than clinical picture would suggest Culture: nasopharyngeal Increase titre of specific antibody	Broad-spectrum antibiotic therapy (until confirmation of organism is established) Symptomatic and supportive	
X-ray shows bilateral diffuse alveolar densities, especially perihilar Observe cysts in special stained smear in material obtained from lung biopsy (not reliable) Lung aspiration by needle Endotracheal brush catheter technique	Pentamidine isethionate Trimethoprim and sulphamethazole (cotrimoxazole) Supportive: maintain oxygen and respirations; administer immunoglobins; possibly withhold immunosuppressive chemotherapy; maintain fluid, electrolyte, and acid-base balance; maintain nutrition Intubation and ventilation may also be necessary to improve oxygenation Be alert to early signs and predisposing factors that will aid in early diagnosis. Carefully observe for adverse effects of drug therapy: abscess formation and necrosis of injection site	Pneumothorax from diagnostic tests, concomitant bacterial pneumonia or sepsis Death

(continued)

Table 4.1   Respiratory disorders *(continued)*

Condition and causative agent	Age and incidence	Clinical manifestations
Mycoplasma pneumonia (pleuropneumonia-like organism) Microorganisms with properties between bacteria and viruses	5-15 years	Onset is insidious: malaise, headache, low-grade fever, sore throat, irritating cough, vomiting, possible crepitation
Bronchiolitis Respiratory syncytial virus (RSV) Adenovirus Parainfluenza virus Influenza virus	Most common in infants and children under 6 months; may occur in child up to 2 years of age Greater incidence in males than in females Winter-spring	Onset is often gradual and associated with exposure to respiratory infection Coryza of 1-3 days; tachypnoea Intercostal and suprasternal retraction Expiratory rhonchi Dry cough Fever Cyanosis Possible dehydration

Diagnostic evaluation	Medical treatment and nursing management	Complications
	Hypoglycaemia Nephrotoxicity Hypotension Tachycardia Hypocalcaemia Nausea and vomiting Skin rash Anaemia Hyperkalaemia Thrombocytopenia	
X-ray shows peribronchial infiltrate in lower lobes Increase in complement fixation test Positive sputum culture	Tetracyclines are the treatment of choice Supportive: antipyretic cough suppression	
X-ray demonstrates overinfiltration of lungs Virological or serological studies to isolate virus on throat swab P_aO_2 decreases P_aO_2 increases (late finding)	Antibiotic therapy given to severely ill child until confirmation is established Himidified O_2 relieve arterial hypoxaemia Monitoring blood gases and correction of acidosis Possible ventilatory assistance Maintain fluid-electrolyte-acid/base and nutritional balance Most infants need intragastric feeding or intravenous fluids for several days Keep nasal airway open and clear of mucus to decrease respiratory difficulty, because infant is an obligatory nose breather Position baby in infant seat inside Croupette; it may provide some respiratory assistance Be alert to signs of impending respiratory acidosis and dehydration	Exhaustion and anoxia Secondary bacterial infection Pneumothorax and pneumomediastinum (occasional) Apnoeic spells Circulatory collapse

(continued)

Table 4.1   Respiratory disorders *(continued)*

Condition and causative agent	Age and incidence	Clinical manifestations
Croup Acute laryngitis, laryngotracheobronchitis (LTB) Parinfluenza virus 1-2-3 (most common virus) Respiratory syncytial virus Influenza virus Enterovirus Adenovirus	6 months-2 years Winter	Generally onset is gradual and progresses slowly, following one to several days after an upper respiratory infection Coryza Croupy cough Inspiratory stridor Hoarseness Low-grade fever Increasing respiration and pulse rate Apprehension, restlessness, anxiety Has difficulty in feeding
Epiglottis Bacterial: *Haemophilus influenza* type B (most common) Pneumococci *Staphylococcus aureus* Beta-haemolytic streptococcus	2-7 years	Onset and progression are rapid — may follow short duration of coryza Severe inspiratory stridor with marked supraclavicular and intercostal retraction Sore throat — refusal to eat, dysphagia; High fever 39-40°C; Drooling; respirations may be shallow; hoarseness; paleness and exhausted appearance may insist on sitting up — condition worsens when lying down; cherry-red epiglottis; apprehension; restlessness; anxiety

Diagnostic evaluation	Medical treatment and nursing management	Complications
History and clinical evaluation — Laboratory findings: PCO_2 increased (late finding), PO_2 decreased Normal — mild leukocytosis X-ray of neck — subglottic oedema (below vocal cords). Normal supraglottic structures	Ampicillin Supportive: high humidification with oxygen, as necessary; hydration; nebulized racemic epinephrine with or without IPPB; antibiotic therapy Teach parents home management of croup (see p. 309)	Airway obstruction Anorexia
History and clinical evaluation Laboratory findings: PCO_2 increased (late findings) PO_2 decreased Leukocytosis X-ray of neck — epiglottic oedema (above vocal cords); normal trachea and larynx	A paediatric emergency Supportive: endotracheal intubation or tracheostomy; cool humidification with oxygen Antibiotic therapy — ampicillin or chloramphenicol Observe carefully for signs and symptoms of increasing respiratory distress; have in readiness equipment for intubation or tracheostomy (see p. 184) Maintain adequate hydration; intravenous fluids may be necessary	Airway obstruction Death

(continued from p. 309)

vapour under the sheet. If he sleeps in a bed, place a card table over his head, and drape a sheet over the card table. Keep one side of the cot or table open so he won't get too hot.

3 Give your child liquids that you know he likes every hour he's awake. Drinking plenty of fluids is very important in helping him get over croup.

4 Let him choose the position in which he is most comfortable. Don't make him lie down. An infant seat may be comfortable for a small baby.

5 If your child continues to make noise as he breathes, keep watch over him. Call the doctor immediately if any of the following things happen:

a His symptoms get worse fairly fast — more noise, higher fever.

b He becomes very restless — sitting up, lying down, jumping about trying to find a comfortable position.

c You notice sharp movement of the soft area around his collarbones or just below the ribs.

d His lips or fingernails become bluish in colour.

e He appears to be very sick regardless of the degree of breathing difficulty.

ASTHMA

Asthma is a recurrent and reversible condition of the lungs in which there is airway obstruction due to spasm of the bronchial smooth muscle, oedema of the mucosa, and increased mucus secretions in the bronchi and bronchioles that has been brought on by various stimuli. Asthma may occur at any age and sometimes appears to commence almost from birth.

Classification of Asthma

1 *Acute attack* — sporadic in nature, with varying intervals of freedom from difficulty and with precipitating factors often readily defined.

2 *Latent asthma* — no outward signs or symptoms of asthma, but there is some shortness of breath on occasion, transitory wheezing on strenuous exercise, and wheezy râles heard during deep inspiration.

3 *Intractable asthma* — persistent wheezing requiring regular, daily medication, for either the control of symptoms or the ability to function.

4 *Status asthmaticus* — severe attack in which the patient deteriorates in spite of adequate treatment with sympathomimetic drugs.

Aetiology

The stimuli responsible for triggering attacks of asthma are as follows:

1 Antigen-antibody reaction (allergy to pollen, animal dander, feather pillows, foods)

2   Infection
3   Physical factors
    a Cold
    b Meteorological factors (i.e. humidity, sudden changes in temperature and barometric pressure)
4   Irritants
    a Dust
    b Chemicals
    c Air pollutants (e.g. sulphur dioxide, carbon monoxide, particulate matter)
5   Psychological or emotional factors
6   Exercise
Note: In more than half the cases, there is a family history of asthma, hay fever, eczema or urticaria.

Clinical Manifestations

1   The onset of an asthmatic attack may be gradual with nasal congestion, sneezing and a watery nasal discharge present before the attack.
2   Attacks may occur suddenly, often at night, when the child awakens with the following symptoms.
    a Wheezing which occurs primarily with expiration
    b Anxiety and apprehension
    c Diaphoresis
    d Uncontrollable cough.
3   With treatment the attack may be controlled. The asthmatic attack may progress, however, and the child will develop the following symptoms:
    a Increasing dyspnoea
    b Thick, tenacious mucus
    c Coarse and fine musical râles
    d Flaring of the alae nasi
    e Use of accessory muscles for respiration
    f Cyanosis
    g Hypercapnia
    h Increased heart and respiratory rates
    i Abdominal pain from severe coughing
    j Vomiting
    k Extreme anxiety and apprehension.

Incidence

1   The incidence of asthma in infancy exists but increases in children 3 years and older.
2   Childhood asthma may cease at puberty.

Altered Physiology

1 The turbinates warm and moisten all air which passes into the lung.
2 Inspired air contains particulate matter which is removed by the blanket of mucus present in the tracheobronchial tree. This mucus is kept moistened by inspired moist air.
3 The blanket of mucus is moved constantly upward by the propelling action of the cilia, and if mucus becomes thickened or inspissated it cannot be moved.
4 An increased local deposition and concentration of allergens occurs.
5 This produces intrabronchial accumulation and stagnation of mucus which is the primary cause of the respiratory embarrassment.
6 Chemical mediators in asthma:
a Primarily involved are histamine and SRS-A (slow-reacting substance of anaphylaxis). SRS-A appears after histamine release, and persists for a longer period. It is not inhibited by the action of the antihistamines.
b These materials are primarily responsible for changes in the blood vessels and mucus membrane in the bronchi and bronchioles, as well as for the initiation of bronchospasm.

Diagnostic Evaluation

1 Eosinophilia in peripheral blood, nasal secretions, and sputum
2 Polymorphonuclear leukocytosis in the presence of infection
3 Pulmonary function studies — diminished maximal breathing capacity, tidal volume and timed vital capacity or forced expiratory volume per second (FEV_1)
4 Determination of blood gases and pH — respiratory acidosis and later metabolic acidosis
5 Gross and microscopic examination of sputum — bronchial casts and eosinophilia
6 Full blood count
7 Chest x-ray — to exclude presence of other diseases; child may show hyperventilation during asthma attack
8 Routine skin testing may help determine allergic causes.

Complications

1 Bronchiectasis
2 Emphysema
3 Cor pulmonale
4 Infants (up to 2 years) — serious respiratory failure due to the stage of development of their anatomical structures and physiological mechanisms which are not able to cope with the insult and compensatory demands of the disease.

Treatment

1 Removal of suspected stimulus: allergen, irritant, exercise, emotional factors.
2 Desensitization in order to build up child's resistance to his allergens.
3 Drug therapy to control symptoms.
4 Supportive:
   a Adequate hydration
   b Adequate oxygenation
   c Appropriate treatment of any existing infection
   d Correct acid-base balance
5 Physiotherapy.

Nursing Objectives

To become informed regarding the child's clinical condition, symptomatology nursing needs, and the medical plan of care.

1 Make a base-line nursing assessment of the child's condition in order to determine the severity of the attack and the degree of respiratory distress.
   a Observe the child's breathing pattern:
      (1) Determine whether the expiratory phase of respiration is increased.
      (2) Determine whether the child is wheezing. (In severe attacks wheezing is audible at a distance from the child.)
      (3) Determine whether the child is using accessory muscles for breathing.
   b Assess the child's level of anxiety and apprehension.
   c Observe the flaring of the alae nasi.
   d Observe the child for the development of cyanosis, utilizing adequate light.
2 Determine the heart and respiratory rates; record and report to the paediatrician any significant change.
3 Discuss with the paediatrician the plan of medical care.

To provide measures to relieve the respiratory distress the child is experiencing.

1 Position the child in high Fowler's position to allow maximum lung expansion.
   a Raise the head of the bed to achieve high Fowler's position.
   b Place an overbed table padded with a pillow in front of the child and have him extend his arms over the table — this provides a comfortable position and allows maximum utilization of accessory muscles for breathing.
2 Administer oxygen when signs of air hunger are present as prescribed by the paediatrician.
   a Do not wait for the appearance of cyanosis before administering oxygen.
   b Oxygen must be administered with caution since the child with severe respiratory distress may be dependent upon his low PO_2 to stimulate spontaneous respiration. In the face of a rising PCO_2 and a potential CO_2

narcosis, the administration of oxygen may remove the last stimulus to spontaneous respirations.

3 Explain to the child the purpose of the oxygen equipment before oxygen is administered and allow the child to feel and touch the equipment.

4 Use aerosol bronchodilators.

To relieve the anxiety and apprehension which results from the respiratory embarrassment.

1 Place the child in a quiet, clean room, where he can be closely observed.

2 Provide the child with maximum reassurance.

   a Provide facilities for parents to stay with their child.

   (1) Keep the parents informed as to the child's progress — what is being done and why — in order to relieve their apprehension. Parental anxiety is readily transmitted to the child. NB: In some circumstances when emotional factors are the main triggering mechanisms of the asthma attack, it would not be advisable for parents to be resident during their child's stay in hospital.

   (2) Talk calmly and quietly to the child.

   (3) Assure the child that you will not leave him alone.

   (4) Ensure that the child has his favourite security object or cuddly toy and that it does not get mislaid.

3 Organize care so as to avoid disturbing the child any more than necessary.

4 When the child falls asleep, allow him to continue to sleep and do not disturb him unless absolutely necessary.

5 Evaluate the need for sedation.

To provide adequate hydration in order to liquefy bronchial secretions and maintain electrolyte balance.

(Dehydration occurs secondary to decreased fluid intake, excessive perspiration, increased respiration, and infection.)

1 Observe for signs of dehydration:

   a Lack of skin turgor

   b Lack of tears

   c Dry parched lips

   d Depressed fontanelle

   e Decreased urinary output — high relative density; concentrated appearance.

2 Maintain parenteral fluid administration.

3 Encourage oral fluid intake:

   a Determine child's fluid preferences.

   b Offer small sips of fluid frequently.

   c Avoid iced fluids which may provoke bronchospasm.

   d Avoid carbonated beverages when wheezing.

4 Allow the child to return to a normal diet as soon as possible.

5 Observe for signs of overhydration and pulmonary oedema.

To be aware of the action and side effects of drugs used in the treatment of asthma.

1   *Adrenaline* — relaxes bronchial smooth muscle and constricts bronchial mucosal vessels, thereby reducing congestion and oedema; acts as a bronchodilator.
   a The smallest dose affording relief should be used.
   b Side effects — insomnia, headache, nervousness, palpitations, precordial pain, hypertension, hypoxaemia, tachycardia, nausea, sweating, urinary retention. (It may potentiate aminophylline toxicity.)

2   *Ephedrine* — relaxes bronchial smooth muscle and constricts bronchial mucosal vessels, thereby reducing congestion and oedema. Acts as a bronchodilator.
   a Has the advantage of prolonged action and oral administration.
   b Side effects — same as for adrenaline.

3   *Pseudoephedrine*
   a Has prolonged action and can be administered orally.
   b Side effects — relatively free.

4   *Aminophylline* — bronchodilator
   a Toxic reaction may occur, but it is more likely to happen with prolonged overdose or when given in conjunction with adrenaline or ephedrine without reducing aminophylline dosage.
   b Side effects — irritability, excitability, continued dehydration, vomiting, haematemesis, proteinuria, stupor, convulsions, coma, death. Hypotension occurs with intravenous use.
   c Occasionally cyanosis and syncope may appear after only a small amount of the prescribed dose. This is considered an idiosyncracy, and the drug should be discontinued.

5   *Expectorants* — given as an adjunct to hydration; thins secretions and helps the child to cough productively.

6   *Corticosteroids* — anti-inflammatory agents
   a Produce beneficial effects only after several hours.
   b Used when other drugs fail to bring beneficial relief from an asthmatic attack.
   c Side effects — use for mild attacks may lead to suppression of adrenal activity. Prolonged use may lead to growth retardation and steroid dependence.

7   *Disodium cromoglycate (INTA) prophylaxis* — adjunct to existing treatment especially for steroid dependent children. It inhibits the release of histamine and the slow reacting substance anaphylaxis (SRS-A). It has a prophylactic action, it should not be used in an acute attack. The 4-hourly use of a spinhaler will prevent many asthmatic attacks. NB: It is impractical to train a child under 4 years to use a spinhaler effectively. Beclomethasone dipropionate may be used alone or in conjunction with disodium cromoglycate by inhalation.

8   During the transition from intravenous to oral bronchodilators respirations should be monitored carefully and frequently.

To encourage the child and his parents to practise measures which will help to maintain optimal health, to prevent acute attacks, to ameliorate chronic symptoms, and to prevent onset of progression of respiratory disabilities.

1   General health measures
    a Provide a well-balanced diet and increased fluid intake.
    b Assure sleep, rest and reasonable exercise; avoid fatigue and chilling.
    c Avoid known irritants.
2   Psychological measures
    a Attempt to keep child emotionally calm and at ease.
    b Maintain optimistic attitude.
3   Regular medical follow-up
    a Assure strict adherence to medication regimen.
    b Give prompt attention when infection is present and new or progressive respiratory symptoms appear.

To teach the child and involve the parents in the teaching of proper breathing habits.

(The exercises strengthen the diaphragm so that breathing will become much better and the total lung capacity will be increased.)

1   Instruct the child to clear his nasal passages before beginning exercises.
2   Each exercise should start with a short gentle inspiration through the nose, followed by a prolonged expiration through the mouth.
3   During inspiration, the upper portion of the thorax should be kept immobilized.
4   During expiration, abdominal muscles should be pulled in.
5   On no account should the child take a deep inspiration during the exercise, but instead he should see how long he can continue the expiration.
    a *Exercise I — Abdominal breathing*
    (1) Lie on back with knees drawn up, body relaxed and hands resting on upper abdomen.
    (2) Exhale slowly, gently sink the chest and then upper abdomen until retracted at end of expiration (through mouth).
    (3) Relax upper abdomen (bulges forward) while taking brief inspiration through nose (chest is not raised).
    Repeat 8-16 times; rest 1 minute; repeat.
    b *Exercise II — Side expansion breathing*
    (1) Sit relaxed in a chair and place palms of hands on each side of lower ribs.
    (2) Exhale slowly through mouth, contracting upper part of thorax, then lower ribs, then compress palms against ribs. (This expels air from base of lungs.)
    (3) Inhale, expanding lower ribs against slight pressure from hands.
    Repeat 8-16 times; rest 1 minute; repeat.
    c *Exercise III — Forward bending*
    (1) Sit with feet apart, arms relaxed at sides.

(2) Exhale slowly, drop head forward and downward to knees, while retracting abdominal muscles.

(3) Raise trunk slowly while inhaling and expand upper abdomen.

(4) Exhale quickly, sinking chest and abdomen, but remain erect.

(5) Inhale, expanding upper abdomen.

d *Exercise IV — Elbow arching*

(This exercise is performed between breathing exercises.)

(1) Sit leaning slightly forward, back straight, fingers on shoulders.

(2) Move elbows in circles forward, upward, backward, and downward. Repeat four to eight times; rest; repeat.

e *General instructions*

Perform exercises:

(1) In the morning before breakfast when child is feeling fresh

(2) At night, before getting into bed to clear the lungs before sleep, *and*

(3) At the first sign of an impending attack to prevent asthma from developing.

Note: Many patients can abort their attacks entirely by doing simple exercises gently. Should child become short of breath or wheeze slightly, take single dose of whatever medication relieved him before beginning the exercises. Exercise may occasionally produce wheezing or coughing at the end of exercise. It may distress the child, but with perseverance the mucus in the bronchial tubes becomes loosened and the patient may be able to cough it up with consequent relief of attack.

To assist the parents to develop a realistic attitude toward the child's illness.

1 Try to treat the child as a completely normal child who needs only a few additional restrictions imposed because of his illness.

   a Accept him as a unique individual with unique contributions to make.

   b Let him know he is capable, loved, and respected.

2 Allow child the same duties and rights as other children in the family.

3 Try to explain why he must watch for certain things and why he is restricted in some ways.

   a Give explanations instead of orders and show him confidence and respect.

   b Be honest with him and express empathy.

4 Teach child the symptoms of an asthma attack and how to relax.

   a Give explanations instead of orders and show him confidence and respect.

   b Be honest with him and express empathy.

   c Help him to express his feelings rather than use his illness as an excuse for physically aggressive hostility or manipulative behaviour.

5 Avoid overprotection and unnecessary surveillance.

6 Teach child gradually to manage for himself rather than to be dependent on parents.

   a Allow him actively to explore his limitations and capabilities.

   b Teach him all the symptoms of asthma — will aid in early treatment.

   c Encourage him to keep a daily diary of symptoms, activity, environment, etc., noting any changes.

d Explain to him what medications he is taking and why and when they are taken.

e Show him the importance of a regular exercise programme.

f Teach him to recognize signs of respiratory infection and to seek medical attention when appropriate.

g Encourage him to become involved in hyposensitization (if used). Perhaps he can even administer his own medications.

h Teach him the importance of increasing fluid intake, especially during an asthma attack when fluid is needed to compensate for fluid loss resulting from dyspnoea and diaphoresis.

7   If child is too much engrossed with his illness, he can be diverted with kindly scolding, friendly minimizing of his ailments, or by encouraging other interests, so that he forgets his troubles as much as possible. Encourage him to build on his interests; help him to find activities that will not hurt him.

8   Do not talk about child's illness any more than necessary — do not allow secrecy or whispering. Recognize the child's feelings about his illness and allow him to talk about them with parents and family.

9   Inform friends and relatives of problems so that the necessary consideration is given him. Plan a team conference involving mother, paediatrician, health visitor, school nurse, and teacher.

10 Create an atmosphere at home that is not full of nervousness or unrest — but is still not artificially calm.

11 Prepare child for approaching events (if burst of emotions have an effect on his illness).

12 Teach child special skills.

a Let him develop special hobbies and interests that can be combined with his illness.

b Remember that accomplishments that develop respect and admiration in peers are particularly desirable and aid in building self-confidence and a feeling of security.

13 Both parents and child feel greater assurance if they are aware of how the child should be treated at certain stages of the disease.

Have special instructions and medications on hand.

14 If the child takes medications for his allergy or specific symptoms, administer them in a matter-of-fact manner without making any fuss.

15 Child needs security, self-confidence, and love. (Do not force these on the child.) Exaggeration is never beneficial.

16 Provide information and literature for the family. Parents can be given the address of Children's Chest Circle, Tavistock House, Tavistock Square, London WCl.

To teach the child and his parents protective measures which will encourage environmental control and help to avoid the offending allergen.

1   Keep child's bedroom as free from dust as possible.

a Keep in bedroom only the furniture which is absolutely necessary.

b Remove upholstered furniture, curtains, carpets, pictures, books, toys, and unnecessary dust-collecting objects.

c Use washable curtains and cotton or synthetic rugs.

d Use cotton or synthetic blankets and washable bedspreads (not chenille or tufted types).

e Do not use insect or other sprays in the bedroom.

f Do not store outer clothing or household articles in bedroom cupboards.

g Enclose mattresses, box-springs, and pillows in dustproof covers (unless they are synthetic).

h Blankets and clothing that have been stored should be thoroughly aired before use.

2   Vacuum clean bed mattresses and the house once a week, preferably with windows open and when child is at school.

3   Avoid irritating odours such as paint, tobacco smoke, insect powders, pine oils and jellies, and irritating cooking odours.

4   If possible, use an exhaust fan in the kitchen to remove cooking odours.

5   Remove all overstuffed furniture and rugs.

6   Avoid sitting and playing on overstuffed furniture and down pillows.

7   Avoid carbonated drinks, such as ginger ale and colas (especially when wheezing).

8   Avoid any physical exertion that causes wheezing or excessive shortness of breath.

9   Avoid using irritating ointments on chest or in nose.

10   Avoid dusty and musty places (basements, storerooms, etc.).

11   Avoid felt rug pads because of animal hair content.

12   Purchase foam furniture and foam rubber pads if possible when refurnishing the home.

13   If home is heated by a circulating hot-air system, shut it off in the bedroom (use electric heater if necessary).

14   Take only drugs prescribed by the paediatrician.

15   Routinely carry out prescribed physiotherapy exercises.

16   Report for treatment as directed by paediatrician.

RESPIRATORY DISTRESS SYNDROME (HYALINE MEMBRANE DISEASE)

Respiratory distress syndrome is a syndrome of immature infants that is characterized by a progressive and frequently fatal respiratory disorder resulting from atelectasis and immaturity of the lungs.

About three out of every 1000 infants born alive die from respiratory distress syndrome.

Aetiology

The exact aetiology of respiratory distress syndrome is not clearly defined.

1   Adequate pulmonary function at birth depends upon the following:

a Adequate amount of surfactant (a lipoprotein mixture) lining the alveolar cells, which allows for alveolar stability and prevents alveolar collapse at the end of expiration.

b Adequate surface area in air spaces to allow for gas exchange, i.e. sufficient pulmonary capillary bed in contact with this alveolar surface area.

2   Respiratory distress syndrome is the result of decreased pulmonary surfactant.

3   Contributing factors — any factor that decreases surfactant, such as

a Prematurity and immature alveolar lining cells

b Acidosis

c Hypothermia

d Hypoxia

e Hypovolaemia

f Unknown factor.

Clinical Manifestations

Symptoms are usually observed soon after birth and may include

Primary Signs and Symptoms

1   Expiratory grunting or whining (when infant is not crying)
2   Sternal, substernal, and intercostal retractions
3   Nasal flaring
4   Tachypnoea
5   Hypothermia
6   Cyanosis when child is in room air (infants with severe disease may be cyanotic even when given oxygen), increasing need for oxygen
7   Decreased breath sounds and dry 'sandpaper' breath sounds — on auscultation of chest
8   As the disease progresses:

a Seesaw retractions become marked with marked abdominal protrusion on expiration.

b Peripheral oedema increases.

c Muscle tone decreases.

d Cyanosis increases.

(1) Body temperature drops.

(2) Short periods of apnoea occur.

(3) Bradycardia may occur.

e Asphyxia becomes more severe.

(1) Apnoeic episodes develop.

(2) Changes in distribution of blood throughout body result in pale grey skin colour.

Secondary Signs and Symptoms

1 Hypotension
2 Oedema of hands and feet
3 Bowel sounds absent early in the illness
4 Urine output decreased.

Pathophysiology

1 Surfactant lowers surface tension at alveolar surface, giving alveoli stability; at end of expiration, some of the air remains in the lung (called the functional residual capacity), thus requiring less negative pressure and exertion to take next breath. When surfactant is deficient, surface tension is higher and alveoli are unstable and collapse at end of expiration. There is decreased functional residual capacity; thus, the next breath requires almost as much effort as the first breath after birth.
2 Changes that accompany respiratory distress syndrome include:
   a Hypoxaemia
   b Metabolic and respiratory acidosis
   c Hypercapnia
   d Reduced lung volume and compliance.
3 Symptoms peak in about 3-4 days, at which time surfactant synthesis begins to accelerate and pulmonary function and clinical appearance begin to improve.
   a Moderately ill infants or those who do not require assisted ventilation show the following:
   (1) Slow improvement by about 48 hours.
   (2) Rapid recovery over the next 3-4 days; few complications.
   b Severely ill and very immature infants who require some ventilatory assistance:
   (1) Demonstrate rapid deterioration (see Clinical Manifestations, above).
   (2) Ventilatory assistance may be required for several days; chronic lung disease is a frequent complication.

Incidence

Respiratory distress syndrome occurs most frequently in:
1 Preterm infants (primarily weighing between 1000 and 1500g) and between 28 and 37 weeks gestation.
2 Infants of diabetic mothers
3 Infants delivered by caesarean section — probably related to underlying indication for surgery
4 Infants of mothers who have experienced intrauterine vaginal bleeding.

Diagnostic Evaluation

1 Laboratory tests
   a PCO_2 — elevated
   b PO_2 — low
   c Blood pH — low due to metabolic acidosis
   d Potassium — elevated
   e Calcium — low.
2 Chest x-ray — demonstrates a diffuse, fine granularity; air bronchograms show 'ground glass' appearance.
3 Pulmonary function studies — demonstrate stiff lung with a reduced effective pulmonary blood flow.

Treatment

1 Early recognition is imperative so that treatment may be instituted immediately.
2 The infant should be transported to a unit providing specialized care.
3 The objectives of treatment include supportive measures:
   a Maintenance of oxygenation — P_aO_2 at 60-80 mmHg (8-10.7 kPa)
   b Maintenance of respiration with ventilatory support if necessary
   c Maintenance of thermoneutral state
   d Maintenance of fluid, electrolyte, and acid-base balance
   e Maintenance of nutrition
   f Prophylactic or specific antibacterial therapy
   g Constant observation for complications
   h Care appropriate for small preterm infant.

Complications

1 Complications related to respiratory therapy:
   a Air leak: pneumothorax — pneumomediastinum, pneumopericardium, and pneumoperitoneum
   b Pneumonia — especially Gram-negative organisms
   c Pulmonary interstitial emphysema
2 Patent ducts arteriosus — left-to-right shunt
3 Cerebral haemorrhage — especially in infant less than 1500 g
4 Disseminated intråvascular coagulation
5 Chronic problems associated with long-term use of oxygen:
   a Bronchopulmonary dysplasia
   b Chronic respiratory infections
6 Tracheal stenosis.

Nursing Objectives

To check the birth history for pertinent information to assist in determining the intensity of observation and care that the infant may require.

1   The Apgar score 1 minute after birth and 5 minutes after birth
2   The type of resuscitation required
3   Any treatment or medication administered
4   Any medication or anaesthesia the mother received during labour
5   Estimated gestational age.

To make a generalized nursing assessment of the infant's condition immediately upon admission.

Early diagnosis is critical to increasing survival rate.

1   Record and report any findings to paediatrician immediately.
2   Determine the degree of respiratory distress.
    a Observe the type of retraction present.
      (1) Determine the type of retraction present.
      (2) Determine the degree and severity of retractions.
    b Count the respiratory rate for one full minute.
      (1) Observe and determine if respirations are regular or irregular.
      (2) Observe to determine if the infant experiences any periods of apnoea.
        (a) Note the length of apnoea.
        (b) Note what type of stimulation initiates breathing.
      (3) Note the infant's activity at the time respirations are recorded (e.g. crying, sleeping).
    c Listen for expiratory grunting or whining sounds from the infant when he is not crying. This partial Valsalva manoeuvre is expiration against a partially closed glottis in an attempt to maintain a positive end-expiratory pressure and functional residual capacity to prevent alveoli from collapsing.
    d Observe for nasal flaring.
    e Observe for cyanosis.
      (1) Note location of cyanosis.
      (2) Note if cyanosis improves with oxygen administration.
3   Determine the infant's cardiac rate and rhythm.
    a Count the apical pulse for one full minute.
    b Note any irregularity in the heart rate.
4   Observe the infant's general activity.
    a Determine if the infant is lethargic or listless.
    b Determine if the infant is active and responds to stimuli.
    c Determine if the infant cries.
5   Observe the infant's skin colour.
    a Note cyanosis as to degree and location.
    b Note evidence of jaundice.
    c Note skin mottling.

d Note paleness or greyness.
6   Observe the general appearance of the infant's body.
   a Note oedema and location (face, hands, feet, etc.).
   b Note any other abnormal appearance of body.
7   Check infant's body temperature.
8   Note any stool passed. Observe and record type of stool.
9   Note any urinary output.
   a Apply urine collecting bag to obtain sample of urine (see p. 141).
   b Observe colour of urine.
   c Check specific gravity of urine.
   d Record amount of urine.

To provide measures to relieve respiratory distress.

1   Have emergency equipment readily available for use in the event of cardiac or respiratory arrest.
2   Provide measures for monitoring ECG and respiratory rate.
3   Place the infant in an oxygen-rich environment.
   a Incubator with oxygen at prescribed concentration.
   b Plastic hood with oxygen at prescribed concentration.
   c Plastic hood with oxygen at prescribed concentration when using radiant warmer.
   d Measure oxygen concentration every hour and record.
4   Observe the infant's response to oxygen.
   a Observe for improvement in colour, respiratory rate and pattern, and nasal flaring.
   b Note response by improvement in pH, PO_2, and PCO_2 (arterial).
5   Observe closely for apnoea.
   a Stimulate infant if apnoea occurs.
   b If unable to produce spontaneous respiration with stimulation within 15-30 seconds:
      (1) Call for help.
      (2) Clear airway.
      (3) Hyperextend head.
      (4) Apply hand resuscitator attached to an oxygen supply, or apply mouth-to-mouth resuscitation (see p. 200).
      (5) Intubation may be necessary:
         (a) Record heart rate during intubation by paediatrician.
         (b) Initiate cardiac massage if severe bradycardia or asystole occurs.
         (c) Listen to breath sounds once intubated; make sure that they are equal bilaterally.
         (d) When infant is attached to appropriate ventilator: secure endo-tracheal tube; suction tube to maintain patency.
         (e) Continue to monitor vital signs.
   c Record events.

To be familiar with the methods of providing assisted or controlled ventilation and the nursing implications for each.

1 Positive and expiratory pressure (PEEP) (see p. 193)
2 Continuous positive airway pressure (CPAP) (see p. 191).
3 Positive or negative pressure incubator (see p. 191).
4 Face mask and bag.

To provide adequate caloric intake (80-120 kcal/kg/24 hours) as indicated.

1 Nasojejunal
2 Nasogastric
3 Parenteral nutrition.

To maintain the method used for the administration of intravenous fluids necessary to meet the metabolic demands of the infant.

1 Monitor flow.
2 Observe site for infiltration or infection.
3 If umbilical artery catheter is in place, observe for bleeding.
4 Record the amount of blood drawn for laboratory analysis (small infants can become anaemic from having large amounts of blood removed for samples).
5 Prepare and administer prescribed medications.

To maintain the infant's abdominal skin temperature between 36.0 and 36.5°C, thus minimizing oxygen consumption rate.

1 Adjust incubator or radiant warmer accordingly.
2 Avoid frequent opening of incubator.

To observe constantly and carefully for any complications that may occur from ventilatory assistance, prematurity, or the disease itself.

Record and report observations to paediatrician immediately.

To assist the paediatrician in other supportive measures used to treat the infant.

1 Ventilatory assistance, oxygen therapy
2 Endotracheal tube, suctioning, physiotherapy
3 Monitoring blood values
4 Monitoring vital signs and general condition
5 Monitoring machines.

To provide an environment that allows infant rest and minimal disturbance balanced with necessary procedures and treatment based upon the infant's condition.

Infants undergoing multiple procedures lasting 45-60 minutes have shown a moderate decrease in PO_2 on continuous PO_2 measurement.

To provide for the psychological needs of the infant with respiratory distress syndrome.

Do not neglect his need for tactile, visual, and auditory stimulation.

To support the parents of this critically ill infant.

1   Help them work through their grief.
2   Assist them with psychological, emotional, and physical attachment to the infant as appropriate. Encourage their participation in care.

Note: The preterm infant with respiratory difficulty should continue to be observed very closely and his therapy should be adjusted as his condition changes. When his condition stabilizes, resume care as for a preterm infant. (see p. 240).

CYSTIC FIBROSIS

Cystic fibrosis is a generalized disorder affecting the exocrine glands so that the substances they secrete are abnormally viscous, affecting primarily pulmonary and gastrointestinal function.

Aetiology

1   Condition is inherited as a Mendelian recessive trait.
2   Underlying cause of the abnormal secretions is unknown.

Clinical Manifestations

1   Diagnosis is frequently made prior to 6 months of age — can be made at any age.
2   Meconium ileus may be found in the newborn.
3   Other presenting signs:
   a Salty taste when skin is kissed.
   b Cough, wheezing
   c Failure to gain weight or grow in the presence of a good appetite
   d Stools are frequent, bulky, and foul-smelling
   e Protuberant abdomen — pot belly
   f Wasted buttocks
   g Vomiting following coughing
   h Recurrent pulmonary infection
   i Clubbing of fingers — in older child
   j Increased anteroposterior chest diameter.

Pathophysiology

1   The secretions of the exocrine glands are thick and sticky rather than thin and slippery.
2   Pulmonary involvement
   a Thick mucus clogs bronchi and bronchioles.

(1) Lungs over inflate.

(2) Atelectasis results.

b Associated infection occurs in lungs.

c Fibrotic changes occur in lungs.

3　Gastrointestinal involvement

    a Thick mucus plugs pancreatic ducts

    (1) Prevents pancreatic digestive enzymes from reaching the small intestine; thus, there is abnormality of stools, loss of foodstuff in faeces [fat and nitrogen (protein)] — malabsorption syndrome.

    (2) Digestion is impaired, especially of fats; nutritional failure results.

    b Meconium ileus in infant — bowel obstructed by thick intestinal secretions.

    c Biliary cirrhosis — intrahepatic biliary tract obstructed by thick secretions.

4　Involvement of sweat glands

    Secretions contain excessive amount of sodium and chloride, leading to excessive loss of these substances — especially in hot weather, when child experiences fever or becomes overheated with activity.

Diagnostic Evaluation

1　Check for family history of cystic fibrosis, failure to thrive, and unexplained infant death; check child's history and physical condition. Carefully listen for subtle information that may be suggestive of cystic fibrosis.

2　Measurement of sodium and chloride level in sweat — chloride level of more than 70 mEq/litre is virtually diagnostic.

3　Measurement of trypsin concentration in duodenal secretions — absence of normal concentration is virtually diagnostic.

4　Analysis of digestive enzymes (trypsin) in stool

    Level is lower — used for initial screening for cystic fibrosis.

5　Chest x-ray

    a May be normal initially.

    b Later shows increased areas of infection, overinflation, atelectasis, and fibrosis.

6　Analysis of stool for steatorrhoea. Microscopy reveals numerous globules of neutral fat.

7　Simple screening test for newborn consists of Dipstix testing for increased protein content of meconium. A positive result indicates that sweat test should be performed.

Treatment

1　Establish and maintain good nutrition.

    a Pancreatic enzyme supplement with each feeding

b Increased kilojoule (calorie) and protein intake
c Decrease in fat intake
d Daily intake of water-soluble vitamins.
2 Prevent and control pulmonary infection.
  a Antimicrobial therapy as indicated for pulmonary infection
  b Bronchodilators and vasoconstrictors — for relief of bronchospasm
  c Mist tent (ultrasonic nebulizer), expectorants, and mucolytic agents — decrease viscosity of secretions.

Nursing Alert: Mist therapy may cause airway resistance to increase in some patients.

  d Physiotherapy — bronchial drainage
    (1) Postural drainage
    (2) Breathing exercises
  e Lobectomy — resection of symptomatic lobar bronchiectasis to retard progression of lesion to total pulmonary involvement.
3 Promote normal growth and development.
  a Treat child as a normal person.
  b Encourage normal relationships with peers and family.
  c Promote positive self-image.

Complications

1 Pulmonary or respiratory infections (emphysema, atelectasis, pneumothorax, bronchiectasis)
2 Pancreatic fibrosis
3 Cor pulmonale
4 Biliary cirrhosis — portal hypertension, oesophageal varices, splenomegaly
5 Chronic sinusitis
6 Nasal polyps
7 Heat prostration
8 Fibrosis of epididymis and vas deferens in male; aspermia
9 Diabetes
10 Haemoptysis.

Nursing Objectives

To assist in the diagnosis and assessment of the child being evaluated for cystic fibrosis by careful observation, recording, and reporting.

1 Characteristics of stool
2 Respiratory status
3 General behaviour and activity.

To establish and maintain adequate nutrition to allow for growth and development.

1   Diet composed of food that is high in kilojoules, high in protein, and low to moderate in fat is usually recommended. (Absorption of food is incomplete.)

2   Fat-soluble vitamins in water-miscible solution are given in quantities that are two to three times the normal dose. (Child shows difficulty in absorption.)

3   Absent pancreatic enzymes are replaced with extracts of animal pancreas.
     a Give with each meal.
     b Mix with small portion of food for infant or small child (e.g. mashed banana). Never mix in milk formula for bottle fed infants as this may discourage the infant from feeding, due to its taste. Also if the feed is not completed, some of the medication will not have been given.
     c Offer the older child capsules or tablets.

4   Salt intake will need to be increased during hot weather or during excessive exercise when sweating increases, to prevent salt depletion and heat prostration and cardiovascular collapse.

5   Use patience when feeding child.
     a Child may be irritable and fussy.
     b Breathing may be difficult; coughing and vomiting may be common.

6   Supplemental diet that is readily absorbed and requires a minimum of digestive enzymes may be prescribed.

To assist in preventing or treating lung infection and to support respirations by thinning secretions and clearing them from the respiratory tract.

1   Intermittent aerosol therapy
     a Usually done prior to postural drainage. (Treatment may also be done following drainage).
     b Provides small amount of medication in droplet form to penetrate respiratory tract.
     c Treatment is three to four times daily.

2   Mist tent
     a Frequently used only with patients that have already used mist; not started on newly diagnosed patients.
     b High humidity loosens secretions.
     c Used primarily at night or nap time.
     d Check temperature often and maintain below 26.6°C.

3   Postural drainage
     a Usually follows aerosol therapy three or four times per day.
     b Treatment ideally done before eating to prevent vomiting or discomfort.
     c Place child in position that gives greatest access to affected lobes of lung and facilitates gravity drainage of mucus from specific lung area. The following positions are useful:
        (1) Leaning over side of bed
        (2) Infant held in lap.

d Clapping with cupped hands and vibrating for 1-2 minutes in each area loosens plugs of mucus.

e A relaxed patient will cough more easily; coughing should be encouraged after postural drainage.

Suctioning of an infant or young child may be necessary when child will not cough.

4   Breathing exercises

Have child exhale slowly to increase the duration of exhalation.

To understand what medications are given in treatment and why they are given.

1   Antibiotics

a Frequently given when a child is not doing well generally.

b Broad-spectrum antibiotics to treat unknown organism or before sputum culture result is available, if child has bronchiole infection or cough.

c Specific antibiotics to treat specific organism causing infection.

2   Expectorants are used to thin bronchial mucous secretions.

3   Bronchodilators are used to increase width of bronchial tubes, allowing free passage of air into lungs.

To give meticulous attention and care in hygiene to the patient.

1   Provide good skin care and position changes to prevent skin breakdown of malnourished child.

2   See that nappy area is clean to reduce offensive odour from stool and to prevent nappy rash.

3   Because child may perspire freely, change clothing as often as necessary to keep him dry.

4   Mouth care is important, since mucus is present so frequently.

5   Shampooing and bathing will provide comfort by removing sticky residue from mist and aerosol therapy.

6   Restrict contact with person with respiratory infection.

To aim at supporting the child's emotional psychological, and intellectual needs and development.

1   Explain each procedure (new or routine), medications, etc., to child in a manner that is appropriate for his age.

2   Allow child to show his frustrations, fears, and feelings by talking, complaining, or crying.

a Support him during these times.

b Comfort him by talking to him and holding him.

3   Provide diversional activities appropriate for age, during or in between treatments.

4   Older child may begin to take responsibility for treatments with minimal supervision.

5   Frequently the child will manifest his anger, fear, and other emotions by

resistance to chest physiotherapy. Allowing child to engage in normal activities (e.g. swimming) within his physical tolerance can help to redirect these feelings as well as to improve respiratory function.

To make and record observations of the child and his condition and behaviour which will give information concerning his condition.

1 Characteristics of stools: colour, size, consistency, frequency
2 Eating habits
   a Foods taken or refused
   b Appetite — good or poor
3 Coughing and description of secretions produced
4 Daily weight to determine weight gain or loss
5 General behaviour
   a Irritability
   b Cooperativeness
6 Conservation of energy — periods of rest, nonstrenuous activity.

To encourage parental participation in learning to care for and handle the child and to foster acceptance of the child and his illness by his parents and family.

1 Provide opportunities for the parents to learn all aspects of care of their child.
2 Note that all the support and help given the parents during hospitalization will make home care easier.
3 Initiate a health visitor referral, which provides the following:
   a Facilitates preparing the home for child's entry, both emotionally and physically.
   b Can assist family in properly carrying out treatments.
4 Initiate social work referral. The social worker can help parents to better understand their family situation and their feelings about their child and cystic fibrosis; she can arrange for financial assistance if appropriate. The worker can be an emotional support to the mother who may be physically and emotionally exhausted from caring for the child with cystic fibrosis.
5 Assist with interpretation of the disease to family and patient. Help them to talk about their feelings and fears. Be honest with parents and child; help them understand there may be gradual lung involvement.
6 Refer family to Cystic Fibrosis Research Trust, 5 Blyth Road, Bromley, Kent BR1 3RS.
   a Multidiscipline team approach and cooperation is vital.
   b Incorporate teaching programme into nursing care plan. Be consistent with information and methods.

Parental Teaching

Education of parents is important in preparing them to continue the child's care at home.

1 Parents must have a thorough understanding of the dietary regimen. Help them to know what types of foods the child is allowed to have and which foods are restricted. Talk about ways to make each meal or certain foods attractive. Discuss need for salt replacement.

2 Help parents to become thoroughly familiar with the pulmonary therapy regimen. Do not rush your explanation; take time to demonstrate and explain procedures. Then allow parents to demonstrate all the treatments to be done at home.

3 Help the family to plan the most normal family pattern of living in relation to treatment of their child.

   a Consider the marriage needs of the parents and the needs of other members of the family.

   b Encourage family activities, holidays, etc., during child's remission of symptoms.

4 Help parents to understand and to provide emotional support of their child. Explain that he will experience the usual problems of growing up as well as the problems of cystic fibrosis and hospitalizations. The child needs love, understanding, and security — not overprotection. He needs growing independence, peer relationships, and personal achievements.

5 Help parents understand the rebellious and uncooperative behaviour of their adolescent. It is a normal part of this age; however, it may be directed towards the illness and treatment. Be firm with the child — optimistic, yet realistic, understanding, and loving.

6 Help the parents understand the value of genetic counselling and support the information given to them through counselling.

7 Impress upon the parents the importance of regular medical follow-up care:

   a Routine immunizations and vaccinations given early in infancy

   b Continuing evaluation and supervision in home management

   c New developments through research that may change therapy

   d Detection or prevention of complications.

8 Inform parents of the future of their child in society.

   a With the medical advances that have occurred, there is every reason to believe that, depending upon pulmonary involvement and complications, the child with cystic fibrosis will grow to adulthood. When the child grows up, he may be smaller and shorter than expected.

   b Play and school participation depends upon severity of illness.

   c Have parents discuss the child's problem with the school nurse, teacher, and other responsible adults who have close contact with the child.

   d Encourage parents to allow the child to participate in as well as take additional responsibility for his own care and treatment as he gets older.

FURTHER READING

Books

Avery G B, *Neonatology*, Lippincott, 1980.
Burton L, *Family Life of Sick Children*, Routledge and Kegan Paul, 1975.
Forfar J O Arneil P, *Textbook of Paediatrics*, Churchill Livingstone, 1984.
Marks M I, *Common Bacterial Infections in Infancy and Childhood*, MTP, 1979.
Scipien G M, *Comprehensive Nursing Care*, McGraw-Hill, 1979.
Strang L B, *Neonatal Respiration*, Blackwell Scientific, 1978.
Swann I L Hanson C A, *Sport and the Asthmatic Child*, Butterworth, 1982.

Articles

Alexander M M Scott M S, Physical examination: chest and lungs, Part 12, *Nursing*, January 1975, 5: 44-48.
Barnes N D Roberton N, Lower respiratory tract infections, *Update*, June 1979: 1393-1406.
Bergner M Hutelmeyer C, Teaching kids how to live with their allergies, *Nursing*, August 1976, 6: 11-12.
Beswick K, The asthmatic child and his family — a general practice approach. *Maternal and Child Health*, July 1982: 288-291.
Butler S, Cystic fibrosis: helping the family to cope, *Nursing Times*, 14 November 1984: 400-402.
Eichenwald H F, Pneumonia syndromes in children, *Hospital Practice*, May 1976, 11: 89-96.
Ellis H, Top priority — the child with stridor, *Modern Medicine*, June 1979: 14-17.
Garvey J, Infant respiratory distress syndrome, *American Journal of Nursing*, April 1975, 75: 614-617.
Grabinar J, When a child can't stop wheezing: illustrative chart for diagnosis and treatment, *Modern Medicine*, 1978: 94-95.
Green C, A simple straightforward approach to childhood asthma, *Practitioner*, November 1979: 960-965.
Huch R *et al.*, Transcutaneous PO_2 monitoring in routine management of infants and children with cardiorespiratory problems, *Pediatrics*, May 1975, 57: 681-690.
Ind P W, Drug therapy in asthma, Parts 1 and 2, *Maternal and Child Health*, 1984: 284-288 and 318-320.
Lewis G M Lewis R A, The place of nebulizers in childhood asthma, *Maternal and Child Health*, January 1984: 34-41.
Lewis G M *et al.*, Croup — a cause for anxiety, *Update*, December 1979: 1195-1202.
Milner A D, Childhood asthma: treatment and severity, *British Medical Journal*, 17 July 1982: 155-156.
Norman A P, Screening for cystic fibrosis, *Journal of Maternal and Child Health*, June 1978: 199-203.
Peckham C, Childhood allergies, *Health and Social Services Journal*, February 1978: 170.
Peterson E, Helping the asthmatic child build a healthy self-image, *American Lung Association Bulletin*, June 1976, 62: 10-13.
Russell G, Cystic fibrosis: Parts 1 and 2, *Nursing Times*, March 1978: 486-489 and 538-541.

Sawley L, Children with asthma, *Nursing Mirror*, 26 October 1983: 27-29.

Schwachman H, Changing concepts of cystic fibrosis, *Nursing Mirror*, January 1974, 9: 143-150.

Siddal T *et al.*, Breathless babies who can't complain, *Nursing Mirror*, January 1980: 20-22.

Taeusch H W, New directions in the management of RDS, *Hospital Practice*, March 1975, 10:53-61.

Talabere L R, The development and implementation of a cystic fibrosis teaching plan, *Journal of the Association for the Care of Children in Hospital*, Autumn 1976, 5: 18-24.

Turner J, A parent's perspective [of cystic fibrosis], *Nursing Mirror*, 14 November 1984: 23-25.

Valman H B, Breathing difficulties in the newborn, *British Medical Journal*, December 1979: 1483-1485.

5

BLOOD DISORDERS

ANAEMIA

Anaemia refers to a deficit of red blood cells or haemoglobin in the blood. It is the most frequent haematological disorder encountered in children.

Aetiology

1 Blood loss
2 Impairment of red blood cell production
    a Nutritional deficiency
        (1) Iron deficiency
        (2) Folic acid deficiency
        (3) Vitamin B_{12} deficiency
    b Decreased erythrocyte production
        (1) Pure red cell anaemia
        (2) Secondary haemolytic anaemias associated with infection, renal disease, chronic disorders
        (3) Aplastic anaemias
        (4) Invasion of bone marrow
          (a) Leukaemia
          (b) Tumours
3 Increased erythrocyte destruction
    a Drugs and chemicals
    b Infections
    c Antibody reactions
    d Burns
    e Poisons, including lead poisoning
    f Abnormalities of the red cell membrane
    g Enzymatic defects, notably G6PD (glucose 6-phosphate dehydrogenase) deficiency
    h Haemolytic disease of the new born

i Abnormal haemoglobin synthesis
   (1) Abnormal haemoglobins - sickle cell disease
   (2) Thalassaemic syndromes.

Clinical Manifestations

1   Condition may be acute or chronic
2   Early symptoms
   a Listlessness
   b Fatigableness
   c Anorexia
3   Late symptoms
   a Pallor
   b Weakness
   c Tachycardia
   d Palpitations
4   Eventual symptoms
   a Mental and physical sluggishness
   b Cardiac enlargement and symptoms of congestive heart failure
   c Inability to carry out the usual childhood activities
5   Prognosis
   a Varies with the type of anaemia
   b Death may result because of cardiac failure.

Altered Physiology

General Considerations

1   Red cells and haemoglobin are normally formed at the same rate at which they are destroyed.
2   Whenever formation of red cells or haemoglobin is decreased or their destruction is increased, anaemia results.
3   The ability of the red blood cell to carry haemoglobin is decreased.
4   The ability of haemoglobin to oxygenate the tissues and remove carbon dioxide for excretion by the lungs is also decreased.
5   Less haemoglobin is available to act as a buffer in regulating the pH of the blood.

Specific Anaemias

1   Iron deficiency anaemia (hypochromic anaemia)
   a Iron deficiency occurs most commonly between the ages of 6 months and 2 years, but it also occurs frequently during adolescence.
   b Initially the neonate's iron requirements are usually met by reserves acquired during fetal life, but after 3 - 4 months of age, additional iron must

be derived from the diet.

c A positive iron balance is necessary for optimal formation of red blood cells.

d Results of iron deficiency:
 (1) Decreased haemoglobin formation
 (2) Red cells with less colour and smaller in size (hypochromic and micro-cytic)
 (3) Low plasma iron
 (4) Low body stores
 (5) Low levels of transferrin, which binds and transports iron.

e Causes of iron deficiency
 (1) Insufficient supply
  (a) Dietary insufficiency (most common)
  (b) Inadequate stores at birth (in preterm infants, twins)
 (2) Excessive demands
  (a) Growth requirements
  (b) Chronic illness
 (3) Blood loss
  (a) Haemorrhage
  (b) Parasitic infection
 (3) Impaired absorption (rare)
  (a) Diarrhoea
  (b) Malabsorption syndrome.

2 Megaloblastic anaemias

a Folic acid and vitamin B_{12} are necessary for the synthesis of nucleo-proteins which are essential for the maturation of red blood cells.

b Deficiencies of folic acid or vitamin B_{12} or disturbances in their normal metabolism interfere with the synthesis of nucleoproteins.

c Red blood cells are immature and larger than normal at every stage of their development (megaloblastic and macrocytic).

d The number of circulating red blood cells is decreased.

e Each red blood cell may carry a normal amount of haemoglobin.

3 Hypoplastic anaemias
 The bone marrow is unable to manufacture new red blood cells and haemoglobin at a rate necessary to maintain a normal concentration of these substances in the circulating blood.

4 Aplastic anaemia

a Formation of red blood cells stops altogether.

b There is usually an associated defective synthesis of other elements in the blood such as platelets and white blood cells.

5 Anaemia of infection

a Life span of the red blood cell is moderately decreased.

b The ability of the bone marrow to produce red blood cells is significantly decreased. (This is the principal factor in determining the degree of anaemia.)

6   Haemolytic anaemias
   a The red blood cells are destroyed at abnormally high rates.
   b The activity of the bone marrow increases to compensate for the shortened survival time of the red blood cells.
   c Products of red cell breakdown increases with haemolysis.
   d Jaundice results when the liver is unable to clear the blood of the pigment resulting from the breakdown of haemoglobin from destroyed red cells.
   e Bone marrow hypertrophies and occupies a larger than normal share of the inner structure of bones.
7   Sickle cell disease (see p. 351).

Nursing Objectives

To make a baseline assessment of the child's condition.

1   Examine skin and mucous membranes for evidence of pallor.
2   Estimate the child's current functional level, including exercise tolerance and level of frustration.
3   Question parents regarding the child's normal level of activity, any symptoms that they have observed (pallor, decreased appetite, excessive fatigue, etc.), ways that their child indicates frustration, fatigue.
4   Obtain a history related to possible causative factors:
   a Dietary habits
   b Persistent infection, chronic disease
   c Access to drugs, poisons, etc.

To build up resistance to infection.

1   See that child maintains good general body hygiene.
2   Provide a diet high in vitamins, kilojoules (calories), and iron.
   a Be aware of the child's food preferences and plan his diet accordingly.
   b Offer small amounts of food at frequent intervals.
   c Reward the child for positive attempts to eat.
   d Allow the child to participate in selection of foods for each meal. This will encourage his motivation to eat, as well as being a basis for good dietary habits for the future.
   e Avoid tiring activities and unpleasant procedures at mealtimes.
   f Make mealtimes as pleasurable as possible. (Refer to section on Nutrition, p. 36.)
   g Provide food supplements and vitamins when necessary.
3   Ensure adequate rest.
   a Plan nursing care to allow for lengthy periods when the child is not disturbed by hospital routines, procedures, treatments, etc.
   b Observe for early signs of fatigue such as irritability, hyperactivity, etc.
   c Encourage sedentary rather than active projects.
4   Avoid exposure to other children with colds, infections, etc.

To administer blood and maintain the transfusion.

1   The procedure is similar to the administration of intravenous fluids. (See p. 155.)
2   Packed cells are frequently administered to enable the child to receive a high concentration of erythrocytes in a small quantity of fluid, and so avoid overloading the circulatory system.
3   Take special precautions.
    a The patient's name, hospital number, and blood type must correspond with the information on the blood container from the blood bank.
    b Identifying information such as donor type and number, patient's name on the blood label, kind of blood, and expiration date should always be checked by two people, one of whom must be a qualified nurse.
    c The blood should be checked for abnormal cloudiness or colour.
    d The child's temperature should be taken as a baseline measurement before the transfusion is begun.
    e If the intravenous infusion is continuous, the tubing should be flushed with normal saline before and after blood is administered and when medications must be given (a separate infusion line for intravenous medications is preferable).

Nursing Alert: Medications should not be given in the infusing blood itself. Blood should never be given with a dextrose and water solution, because haemolysis and clotting in the intravenous tubing can occur.

    f The rate of flow should be carefully regulated to prevent circulatory overload, especially in those children receiving multiple transfusions.
    g The same blood should not be left running over a long period of time (usually over 4 hours).
    h Recommendations of the blood bank for storage and administration of blood should be followed explicitly.
4   Observe the child for signs of transfusion reaction.
    a Reaction usually occurs within 15-20 minutes from the start of the transfusion.
    b Signs and symptoms:
        (1) Restlessness
        (2) Irritability
        (3) Chills
        (4) Elevation of temperature
        (5) Increased central venous pressure
        (6) Sudden changes in pulse and respiration
        (7) Rash or change in the colour of the skin
        (8) Changes in the appearance or quantity of urine output
        (9) Haemorrhagic phenomena
        (10) Headache, with pain in back or chest with sensation of tightness in the chest.

To minimize the child's anxieties and ensure his cooperation during hospitalization.

1   Allow the child to handle equipment used for tests and procedures (tourniquets, syringes, etc.).
2   Explain all procedures and the treatment plan to the child in a way that he can understand. Encourage mother or father to be present.
3   Allow the older child to look through a microscope at a blood smear.
4   Permit the child to cleanse the area for a venipuncture or finger prick.

Nursing Management of Specific Anaemias

Iron Deficiency Anaemia

1   Administer iron as ordered by the paediatrician.
  a Oral iron preparations
    (1) Administer between meals to minimize gastric distress.
    (2) Administer with a dropper or straw or dilute with water or fruit juice to prevent staining of the teeth. Dental stains can be removed by brushing the teeth with sodium bicarbonate or hydrogen peroxide and then rinsing with water.
    (3) Observe for side effects:
      (a) Gastric distress
      (b) Colic pain
      (c) Diarrhoea.
    (4) Caution the mother that iron medication causes the child's stools to be dark green or black.
    (5) Stress to parents the importance of continuing the iron therapy according to the paediatrician's directions even though the child may not appear ill.
    (6) Warn parents that medications containing iron are a leading cause of poisoning in children. The medication should always be stored well out of reach.
  b Intramuscular iron preparations. Rarely indicated in paediatric practice, but when prescribed the nurse should be aware of the following:
    (1) Dosage
      (a) Calculated by the paediatrician.
      (b) Depends on the child's weight and haemoglobin level.
    (2) Special precautions
      (a) Should be injected into a large muscle, preferably the buttock.
      (b) Injection sites should be recorded and rotated.
      (c) The injection site should not be massaged.
        Any pressure on the site may force the medication out of the muscle into the subcutaneous tissue.
        Walking will help absorption.
      (d) Parenteral iron should be administered with discretion and only to

those children whose anaemia is not amenable to oral iron therapy.
(e) Parenteral iron is contraindicated in children sensitive to the preparation or in anaemias other than iron deficiency anaemia.
(3) Technique of administration
(a) Use a separate needle to withdraw the medication from the ampoule and for injection.
(b) Use a needle which is 5 cm long.
Medication must be injected deeply into the muscle to avoid staining the tissue.
(c) Allow 0.5 ml of air in the syringe before injecting.
(d) Retract the skin over the muscle laterally before inserting the needle.
This will leave a curved needle track afterwards and help to prevent leakage from the muscle into the subcutaneous tissues.
(e) Insert the needle and withdraw the plunger to check against entry into a blood vessel.
(f) Inject the medication and the 0.5 ml of air following the injection-to clear the needle and prevent leakage of the medication along the injection track when the needle is withdrawn.
(g) Wait 10 seconds after injection before removing the needle.
(4) Observe for side effects
(a) Local
Pain at the injection site
Skin discoloration
Local inflammation with lymphadenopathy
(b) Systemic toxicity (occurs within 10 minutes of injection)
Muscle and joint pain
Nausea and vomiting
Sweating
Tachycardia
Bronchospasm with dyspnoea
Circulatory collapse, hypotension and dizziness.

Nursing Alert: Because of the possibility of anaphylaxis, a test dose should be given before initiating parenteral iron therapy.

2   Initiate and reinforce good dietary habits.
   a Determine from parents the type and amount of foods customarily eaten, the feeding methods, and the child's reaction to eating.
   b Introduce foods rich in iron such as meat, fortified cereals, vegetables, and fruits.
   c Do not allow the child to drink excessive quantities of milk at the exclusion of other foods that contain more iron. Limit milk intake to 1 litre per day.
   d Provide vitamin supplements if necessary. Vitamin C appears to enhance the absorption of iron.
   e Explain the reasons for diet change to parents in language they can understand. Visual aids and pictures may be helpful.

f Assist parents to select iron-rich foods that are acceptable to the child, within the family's food budget, and culturally acceptable.

g Make mealtime a pleasurable experience. (Refer to section on Nutrition, p. 36.)

3 Investigate social and economic problems which may contribute to the child's disease. Refer to the family's health visitor in order that the mother and the family can receive support.

Note: Parents should be warned of the need to store iron tablets in a locked cupboard out of reach of any small children.

Anaemia of Infection

1 Provide supportive care relative to the underlying disease.
2 Administer antibiotics as prescribed.

Megaloblastic Anaemias

Administer folic acid or vitamin B_{12} as prescribed.

The commonest cause of folic acid deficiency is inadequate intake. Deficiency may complicate malabsorption syndromes or arise as a complication of the therapeutic treatment with folic acid antagonists, e.g. methotrexate in leukaemia. Increased requirements for folic acid occur with prematurity and in chronic haemolytic anaemia.

1 Folic acid (pteroylmonoglutamic acid)
    a Dosage — must be determined by trial for each patient
    b Route
        (1) Oral route is preferred.
        (2) May be administered intramuscularly if malabsorption is suspected.
    c Toxic effects — none.
2 Vitamin B_{12} (hydroxocobalamin)
    This deficiency may arise as a result of inadequate diet, e.g. with vegans, as this vitamin is found only in animal tissues and milk. May also occur as a consequence of inadequate absorption due to small bowel disease or lack of the intrinsic factor.
    a Dosage — regulated by individual trial for each patient
    b Route
        (1) Intramuscular injection is preferred.
        (2) Oral administration is also possible. (This method is more expensive and less reliable.)
    c Side effects — none.
    d Points of emphasis
    Regular administration of the medication is essential. Parents may be tempted to miss injections because their child is not in distress before the injection or does not feel significantly better after it.

Family Education

1 Discuss general hygiene measures, including adequate rest, diet, sunshine, fresh air.
2 Encourage regular dental evaluations.
3 Explain that infection may be prevented by dressing the child according to the weather and keeping him away from persons with colds, sore throats, and other infections.
4 Teach parents how to administer medication.
5 Advise parents of need to keep outpatient appointments with paediatrician.

SICKLE CELL DISEASE (SICKLE CELL ANAEMIA)

Sickle cell disease occurs typically in the negro, but is also observed in people from the Mediterranean, Middle East, and India. It is a severe, chronic haemolytic anaemia occurring in persons homozygous for the sickle gene. The clinical course is characterized by episodes of pain due to the occlusion of small blood vessels by sickled red cells. Persons heterozygous for the sickling gene are said to possess sickle cell trait which is associated with a benign clinical course.

Aetiology

1 Genetically determined, inherited disease.
2 Each person inherits one gene from each parent which governs the synthesis of haemoglobin (see Tabel 5.1).

Table 5.1 Transmission of sickle cell disease

Genotype of parents	Probability of abnormal haemoglobin in offspring (%)		
	Normal	Trait	Disease
One parent with trait	50	50	0
Both parents with trait	25	50	25
One parent with trait, one parent with disease	0	50	50
Both parents with disease	0	0	100

Clinical Manifestations

Symptoms

1 Children are rarely symptomatic until late in the first year of life.
2 Clinical manifestations are sporadic.

    a Child may be asymptomatic for several months.

    b Periods of crisis occur at variable intervals.

    c Precipitating factors of crisis include:

      (1) Dehydration

      (2) Infection

      (3) Trauma

      (4) Strenuous physical exertion

      (5) Extreme fatigue

      (6) Cold exposure

      (7) Hypoxia.

3   Signs of crisis:

    a Loss of appetite

    b Paleness

    c Weakness

    d Fever

    e Pain in abdomen, back, joints, and/or extremities

    f Swelling of joints, hands, and/or feet

    g Jaundice.

Thrombocytic Crisis

1   Small blood vessels are occluded by the sickle-shaped cells, causing distal ischaemia amd infarction.

2   Extremities

    a Bony destruction

    b Periosteal reaction

    c Ulbers

3   Spleen

    Abdominal pain

4   Cerebral occlusion

    a Strokes

    b Hemiplegia

    c Blindness

5   Pulmonary infarction

6   Pulmonary thromboses

7   Cardiac decompensation

8   Impaired liver function

9   Convulsions, cerebral infarction

10 Retinal damage, blindness

11 Growth failure

12 Delayed puberty

13 Decreased life span.

Sequestration Crisis

1   Large amounts of blood become pooled in the liver and spleen

2   Spleen becomes massively enlarged
3   Signs of circulatory collapse develop rapidly
4   Frequent cause of death in infant with sickle cell disease.

Aplastic crisis

Bone marrow ceases production of red blood cells.

Chronic Symptoms

1   Jaundice
2   Gallstones
3   Progressive impairment of kidney function
4   Fibrotic spleen
5   High susceptibility to salmonella, osteomyelitis, and pneumococcal septicaemia.
6   Delayed puberty
7   Decreased life span.

Prognosis

1   Depends on severity of the disease
2   No known cure
3   Decreased life span
     Death occurs frequently before age 20.

Altered Physiology

1   Each haemoglobin molecule consists of four molecules of haem folded into one molecule of globin.
2   Each globin molecule consists of two alpha chains and two beta chains.
3   The amino acid sequence on the beta chain is altered in sickle cell haemoglobin.
     Valine is substituted for glutamic acid in the sixth position.
4   Sickle cell haemoglobin aggregates into elongated crystals under conditions of low oxygen concentration.
5   This distorts the membrane of the red blood cell causing it to assume a crescent or sickle shape.
6   Sickled red cells are fragile and are rapidly destroyed in the circulation.
7   Anaemia results when the rate of destruction of red cells is greater than the rate of production.

Diagnostic Evaluation

1   Stained blood smear
     a Done by finger prick.
     b Sickle cells are viewed under the microscope on a stained smear of blood.

   c Cells are seen only in persons with sickle cell anaemia (not sickle cell trait).
2   Sickling test
   a Finger prick to obtain blood.
   b Drop of anticoagulated blood placed under cover slip with paraffin wax. Allow cells to metabolize at room temperature.
   c As pH falls and oxygen is utilized, sickle cells may be observed.
   d Does not distinguish between person with sickle cell trait and disease.

Note: The finding of a positive sickling test should therefore lead to:

3   Electrophoresis
   a Requires venepuncture.
   b Haemoglobin is subjected to an electric current which separates the various types and determines the amounts present.
   c A person is diagnosed as having sickle cell trait if two types of haemoglobin are demonstrated in approximately equal amounts.
      A person is diagnosed as having sickle cell anaemia if the majority of his haemoglobin is sickle haemoglobin.

Preventive Measures
1   Every black child admitted to the hospital should be tested for sickle cell anaemia.
2   Parents at risk should be counselled regarding the genetic aspects of sickle cell anaemia.
3   All siblings of any child who is admitted to the hospital with sickle cell anaemia should be tested for the disease.

Nursing Objectives

To dilute the blood and reverse the agglutination of sickled cells within the small blood vessels.
1   Maintain intravenous therapy if indicated. (See procedure for the administration of intravenous fluids, p. 155.)
2   Increase the amount and frequency of liquid intake.
   a Offer fruit juice, water, milk, etc.
   b Offer child a choice in selection of fluids and method of drinking (straw, etc.).
3   Record the child's intake and output accurately. (Total his intake and output every 8-12 hours.)
4   Assist with a partial exchange transfusion if required.
      This technique is designed to remove some of the sickled cells and replace them with normal ones.

To reduce the child's fever which may aggravate déhydration.

1   Make frequent assessments of the child's temperature.
2   Administer antipyretic drugs as ordered by the paediatrician.
3   Refer to the section on fever, p. 105.

To alleviate the child's pain during a crisis.

1   Identify effective measures to alleviate pain by questioning parents and by personal trial and error. Consider any of the following measures:
    a Carefully position and support painful areas.
    b Hold or rock the infant.
    c Distract child by singing to him, reading him stories, providing play activities.
    d Provide familiar objects. Encourage parents to stay and share in care.
    e Bathe child in warm water, applying local heat or massage.
    f Give suitable medications.
    g Maintain bed rest.
2   Share effective methods of reducing pain with other nursing staff and family.

To treat associated or precipitating infections.

1   Treatment will depend on the specific nature of the infection.
2   Administer antibiotics as prescribed by the paediatrician.

To provide an optimal environment for the child during hospitalization.

Be certain that the child is kept warm and protected from infection.

To administer blood in cases of severe anaemia.

1   Refer to information on blood transfusion, p. 347.
2   Be especially alert for signs of transfusion reaction, which is a very serious problem.

To decrease surgical risk.

1   Administer preoperative blood transfusion(s) as prescribed.
    Preoperative blood is usually prescribed to suppress the formation of new sickle cells and to reduce the threat of anoxia.
2   Prepare the child emotionally for surgery.
3   Maintain adequate hydration before and after surgery.
4   Avoid sedatives and analgesics which depress the respiratory centre.
5   Observe the child closely for evidence of infection, especially of the respiratory tract.

To provide emotional support to the child and his parents.

1   Encourage parents to talk about their child, his disease, and how they feel

about it.

a Expect such feelings as guilt, shock, frustration, depression, and resentment.

b Accept negative feelings.

c Emphasize that the child's disease is no one's fault.

d Counsel parents concerning ways to recognize and alleviate their child's apprehension.

e Provide factual information so that parents are prepared to answer their child's questions.

   (1) The recessive nature of the inheritance should be explained.

   (2) Make certain that parents understand the difference between sickle cell trait and sickle cell anaemia.

2 Alleviate the child's anxieties concerning his illness.

a Role playing and play activities are useful in identifying his fears, according to his age.

b Explain what is happening to him in a way that he can understand.

3 Stress the positive aspects of his disease.

a Sickle cell disease does not affect intelligence.

b Between periods of crisis the child can usually participate in peer group activities with the exception of some strenuous sports.

4 Encourage quiet activities in which the child can excel — art, painting, leather work, metal and woodworking, chess, etc.

5 Plan for the child to continue his education.

   Encourage parents to discuss their child's school work with the hospital school teacher.

6 Refer to social worker and health visitor for ongoing support and counselling.

To make certain that the child receives coordinated and continuous care.

Send a nursing care summary to the health visitor or school nurse who will work with the child after he is discharged from the hospital.

Patient or Parental Health Teaching

1 Provide factual information about the disease and its cause. Encourage questions.

2 Discuss the genetic implications of sickle cell disease and offer genetic counselling to the family.

3 Instruct parents in ways that they can help their child to avoid sickling episodes.

a Do not allow the child to become chilled or to wear tight clothing that might impede circulation. Avoid severe competitive exercise.

b Instruct child and parents to avoid areas of low oxygen concentration such as high mountains and unpressurized aeroplanes.

c Do not utilize drugs that could cause acidosis or contract blood vessels.

d Be certain that the child receives regular medical supervision, including all the normal childhood immunizations.

e Provide prompt treatment of cuts, sores, mosquito bites, etc. Notify the paediatrician if the child is exposed to an infectious disease.

f Maintain good dental hygiene and be certain that the child receives frequent dental checkups.

g There is an increased need for folic acid to be given as chronic haemolysis can result in a deficiency of this vitamin.

4 Teach parents that the child has the same needs as a normal, healthy child for a balanced diet, good fluid intake, adequate rest, and daily exercise. The child will learn his own activity limitations and will rest when he becomes fatigued. He should not be pampered, but should receive the same love, discipline, privileges, and responsibilities of a normal child of his age.

5 Teach parents the signs of mild crisis:

   a Fever

   b Decreased appetite

   c Irritability

   d Pain or swelling in abdomen, extremities, back.

6 Instruct parents regarding home management of mild crisis.

   a Encourage adequate hydration. Teach techniques for increasing fluid intake.

   b Administer antipyretic medications.

   c Encourage rest.

   d Keep the child warm.

   e Seek medical advice if pain becomes severe or if intravenous therapy is required for the child.

7 Teach parents the signs of severe crises:

   a Pallor

   b Lethargy and listlessness

   c Difficulty in awakening

   d Irritability

   e Severe pain

   f High fever or a moderate fever that persists for 2 days.

8 Instruct parents to have emergency information available to those involved in the child's care (school nurse, teacher, babysitter, family members, etc.).

   a Name and phone number of family doctor.

   b Child's blood type, allergies, medications, and hospital registration number.

   c Name of informed neighbour or relative to be notified in an emergency.

   d Discuss the genetic implications of sickle cell disease with the child early, so that when he is old enough, he can avail himself of counselling concerning marriage and family planning.

Agencies

1   Sickle Cell Society, c/o Brent Community Health Council, 16 High Street, Harlesden, London NW10 4LX
2   Organization for Sickle Cell Anaemia Research (OSCAR), 200a High Road, Wood Green, London N22 4HH.

HAEMOPHILIA

Haemophilia is an inherited, congenital blood dyscrasia which is characterized by a disturbance of blood clotting factors. It appears in males but is transmitted by females.

Aetiology   (Table 5.2)
1   Hereditary
2   Sex-linked, recessive trait
   a Caused by a gene carried on the X chromosome, one of the sex chromosomes.
   b Transmitted by asymptomatic females who carry the haemophilic gene on one of their X chromosomes.
   c Appears in males who have the haemophilic gene on their only X chromosome.
   d Affected males may carry a latent form of the disease to female offspring.
   e Very rarely may appear in females if a female carrier mates with a male haemophiliac.
3   Spontaneous mutations may cause the condition when the family history is negative for the disease.

Table 5.2   Transmission of haemophilia

Genotype of parents	Probability of abnormality in offspring (%)				
	Female			Male	
	Normal	Carrier	Haemophiliac	Normal	Haemophiliac
Female carrier/ normal male	50	100	0	100	50
Noncarrier female/ haemophiliac male	0	100	0	100	0
Female carrier/ haemophiliac male	0	50	50	50	50

Clinical Manifestations

General Considerations

1 Seldom diagnosed in infancy unless excessive bleeding is observed from the umbilical cord or after circumcision.
2 Usually diagnosed after the child becomes active.
3 Varies in severity depending on the plasma level of the coagulation factor involved.
   a Children with factor levels of less than 1% of normal are considered severe haemophiliacs and often demonstrate severe clinical bleeding.
   b Children with factor levels of above 5% but less than 25% of normal are considered moderately afflicted. These children may be free of spontaneous bleeding, and may not manifest the potentially severe bleeding disorder until after trauma.
   c Children with factor levels of 25-50% of normal are considered mildly afflicted. They usually lead normal lives and bleed only with severe injury or surgery.
   d Degree of severity tends to be constant with a given family.

Clinical Signs and Symptoms

1 Easily bruised
2 Prolonged bleeding from the mucous membranes of the nose and mouth or from lacerations
3 Spontaneous soft-tissue haematomas
4 Haemorrhages into the joints — especially elbows, knees, and ankles (haemarthrosis)
   a Causes pain, swelling, limitation of movement
   b Repeated haemorrhages may produce degenerative changes with osteoporosis and muscle atrophy
5 Spontaneous haematuria
6 Gastrointestinal bleeding
7 Intracranial haemorrhage (rare).

Complications

1 Airway obstruction due to haemorrhage into the neck and pharynx.
2 Intestinal obstruction due to bleeding into intestinal walls or peritoneum.
3 Compression of nerves with paralysis due to haemorrhaging into deep tissues.
4 Intracranial bleeding.
5 Secondary complications associated with therapy — liver disease, immunological problems, thrombotic complications.

Prognosis

1 Uncertain.

2　Cycles may occur with periods of little bleeding followed by periods of severe bleeding.

3　Death may result from intracranial haemorrhage or from exsanguination following any serious haemorrhage.

Diagnostic Evaluation

1　Routine bleeding and clotting tests — often normal
2　Partial thromboplastin time (PTT) — prolonged
3　Prothrombin consumption — decreased
4　Thromboplastin generation — increased
5　Specific assays for clotting factors — abnormal.

Altered Physiology

1　Haemophilia results from the absence, deficiency, or malfunction of anti-haemophiliac globulin or factor VIII.

2　These blood clotting factors are necessary for the formation of prothrombin activator (thrombokinase or thromboplastin) which acts as a catalyst in the conversion of prothrombin to thrombin.

a The rate of formation of thrombin from prothrombin is almost directly proportional to the amount of prothrombin activator available.

b The rapidity of the clotting process is proportional to the amount of thrombin formed.

3　Other bleeding disorders closely resembling classical haemophilia:

Disorder	Clotting Factor
Haemophilia B (Christmas disease)	Factor IX (plasma thromoplastin component)
Haemophilia C	Factor XI (plasma thromboplastin antecedent)

Nursing Objectives

To provide emergency care for bleeding wounds.

1　Cleanse wound thoroughly.
2　Immobilize the affected part.
3　Apply local measures for control of bleeding.

a Apply pressure on the area.

b Place fibrin foam or absorbable gelatine foam in the wound.

4　Administer cryoprecipitate or plasma concentrate containing the necessary factor. NB: This should be given by rapid infusion (30 minutes) since anti-haemophiliac globulin has a short life in solution at room temperature. (See procedure for the administration of intravenous fluid, p. 155, and for blood transfusion, p. 347.)

Stop the transfusion if urticaria, headaches, tingling, chills, flushing, or fever occur.

5 Keep the child quiet during treatment.
   a Remain calm.
   b Sedate the child if necessary.
6 Take special precautions.
   a Suturing should be avoided if possible.
   b Cauterization is always contraindicated.

To provide supportive care for the child with haemarthroses.

1 Control bleeding:
   a Immobilize the joint in a position of slight flexion.
   b Elevate the affected part.
2 Alleviate pain:
   a Administer sedatives or narcotics as ordered by the paediatrician.
   b Avoid excessive manipulation of the child.
   c Use a bed cradle to keep the weight of the bedcovers off the affected part.
   d Apply ice packs.
   e Administer blood or plasma as directed by the paediatrician.

Nursing Alert: Aspirin is contraindicated since it decreases platelet adherence and may increase bleeding.

3 Prevent further bleeding.
   a Continue immobilization of the joint. (A bivalve plaster cast may be necessary.)
   b Maintain the child on bed rest. (Careful handling of the child is essential.)
4 Prevent permanent deformities and crippling:
   a Begin gentle passive exercise and massage of the joint after the bleeding has been controlled for at least 48 hours.
   b Refer the child for physiotherapy on an outpatient basis if this is indicated by:
      (1) Presence of persistent deformity
      (2) Need to use orthopaedic devices such as crutches, braces, splints, etc.
      (3) Need for specialized programmes such as electrical stimulation, increased physical exercises.
   c Reconstructive orthopaedic surgery may be required.
5 Assess the child for evidence of disease progress:
   a Increased pain
   b Further swelling of joints
   c Limitation of movement
   d Flexion contractures.

To prevent haemorrhage during nursing procedures.

1 Temperature taking
   Insert the thermometer very gently.

2 Administer medications orally whenever possible.
3 Injections should be avoided wherever possible, but if they prove necessary the following should be observed:
   a Choose intramuscular injection sites carefully and rotate them.
   b Inject the medication slowly.
   c Apply pressure to the area for 5 minutes.

To maintain a safe environment during hospitalization.

1 Pad cot rails.
2 Inspect toys for sharp or rough edges.
3 Supervise small children when they are ambulatory.
4 Utilize protective devices which the child brings from home. (Many children wear helmets, knee pads.)
5 Continually assess environment for potential hazards.

To provide emotional support to the child and his family.

1 Permit the child to participate in as many normal activities as possible within the realm of safety.
2 Allow the child to handle equipment used in his care.
   Use play to help the young child adjust to his illness by 'transfusing' his teddy bear, etc.
3 Encourage the child's continuing education despite long periods of hospitalization and absence from school.
   Have parents bring assigned books from the child's own school to the hospital school.
4 Encourage parental participation in the child's care.
   a Refer to section on family-centred care, p. 66.
   b Assess parent's attitudes and understanding about the disease. Clarify information if necessary.
   c Teach parents aspects of their child's care which must be continued after discharge. Have them practise appropriate techniques with nursing supervision until they achieve competence and are comfortable in the situation. (See Patient or Parent Health Teaching on p. 363.)
5 Counsel the parents concerning:
   a Feelings of guilt at having given birth to the child or resentment at having to care for him.
   b Refer the parents to a social worker if indicated.
6 Introduce the child and his family to other haemophiliac families.
   a Contact the Secretary, Haemophilia Society, 16 Trinity Street, London SE1, for further information about support groups.
   b Numerous specialized haemophilia centres have been established in the UK.
7 Convey confidence to the patient and his family; they often are fearful of the diagnosis and need support.

8 Initiate a primary health nursing referral, if appropriate, to health visitor and school nurse.

Patient or Parent Health Teaching

1 Protecting the child from trauma:
   a Select toys which are soft and without rough edges.
   b Pad the sides of cots, playpens, etc.
   c Guard against child's falling when he is learning how to stand and walk.
      (1) Remove potential sources of injury from furniture.
      (2) Pad child's knees and buttocks.
      (3) Use a helmet for the child's head.
   d Supervise play closely.
   e Inform the child's teacher, school nurse, other adults, and playmates of his condition so that his activities will be appropriately restricted.
   f Have the child wear a medic-alert bracelet. This should be worn at all times, so that in the event of trauma or emergency the attendant medical staff may be alerted.
   g Do not administer aspirin to the child.

2 Emergency treatment for haemorrhage
   a Immobilize the part. This may be done with splints or an elastic compression bandage. (These materials should be immediately available in the home.)
   b Apply ice packs. Parents should keep two or three plastic bags of ice immediately available in the ice compartment of the fridge.
   c Transport the child to his treatment centre.
3 Regular medical and dental supervision
   Preventive dental care is important and hospitalization is often necessary for extensive dental work and extractions.
4 Diet
   Diet is important to avoid excess weight which places additional strain on the child's weight-bearing joints and predisposes him to haemarthrosis.
5 Information concerning the disease itself
   The child should be helped to understand the exact nature of his illness as early as possible.
   Special attention should be given to the signs of haemorrhage, and the child should be told of the need to report even the slightest bleeding to an adult immediately.
6 Preventing emotional crippling by overprotection — this can be more disabling than the effects of the disease itself.
   a Promote the sense of independence and self-care within the patient's limitations.
   b Encourage healthful activity and reasonably aggressive pursuits — helps patient to cope with anxiety-driven behaviour.

Reinforce self-judgement of child or teenager in selection of safe physical activities.

c Help parents understand the importance of vocational guidance for their child — emphasis given to occupations using intellect or skills rather than physical effort.

d Refer to section on family stress in paediatric illness, p. 66.

7 Because of the use of blood components in the treatment of haemophilia, there is a risk of hepatitis. Watch for the early signs and symptoms 6 weeks after treatment: headache, pyrexia, anorexia, vomiting, abdominal pain and tenderness. Parents should seek medical advice immediately.

8 Genetic counselling and family planning services should be offered to the family.

9 Home care programme

a Home care programmes teach parents and children to administer plasma therapy at home when a haemorrhage episode begins.

b Advantages of home treatment:
(1) Earlier recovery of joint functions
(2) Greater self-sufficiency for patient and family
(3) Fewer absences from school or work
(4) Less anxiety related to travelling.

c Indications for home treatment:
(1) Frequent need for transfusions
(2) Poor access to emergency care
(3) Need for prophylactic therapy.

d General criteria for acceptance into programme:
(1) Willingness to learn venepuncture technique
(2) Demonstrated ability to follow directions
(3) Ability to manage transfusions
(4) Acceptance of the necessity for follow-up care
(5) Emotional stability sufficient to accept the responsibility.

e Teaching is usually done by the nurse in the speciality clinic in liaison with the primary health care team and includes instruction and practice in the following:
(1) Storage and preparation of replacement factors
(2) Venepuncture technique
(3) Transfusion management
(4) Record keeping.

f Hospital nursing responsibilities:
(1) Screen patients and families who may be eligible for home care programmes
(2) Facilitate appropriate self-management by children and families enrolled in home care programmes if hospitalization becomes necessary. Establish communication with the clinic nurse.

For additional information regarding home care programmes, including teaching guidelines, refer to further reading below.

Agencies
Haemophilia Society, 16 Trinity Street, London SE1.

FURTHER READING

Books

Biggs R (ed), *The Treatment of Haemophilia A and B and von Wilebrand's Disease*, Blackwell Scientific Publications, 1978.
Boone D C (ed), *Comprehensive Management of Hemophilia*, Davis, 1978.
Johnson S H, *High Risk Parenting*, Lippincott, 1979.
Tetrault S, *A Child with Sickle Cell Disease — His Hobbies and Activities*, Centre for Sickle Cell Disease, Howard University, 1977.
Whaley L Wong D, *Nursing Care of Infants and Children*, Mosby, 1979.
Willoughby M L N, *Paediatric Haematology*, Churchill Livingstone, 1977.

Articles

Chessells J M, The anaemic child, *Practitioner*, September 1978: 349-354.
Kenny M W, Sickle cell disease, *Nursing Times*, September 1980: 1582-1584.
McFarlane J, The child with sickle cell anaemia: what his parents need to know, *Nursing*, May 1975, 5: 29-33.
Oliver R A M, Investigating the child who bleeds or bruises easily, *Modern Medicine*, June 1980: 74-78.
Stableforth P, Aspects of haemophilia, *Journal of Maternal and Child Health*, October 1978: 334-336.
Stuart J *et al.*, Improving prospects for employment of the haemophiliac, *British Medical Journal*, May 1980: 1169-1172.

6

CARDIOVASCULAR DISORDERS

CONGENITAL HEART DISEASE

Congenital heart disease is a structural malformation of the heart or great vessels, present at birth.

Incidence

The congenital heart disease rate is 0.8% of live births in England and Wales.

Aetiology

1 Exact cause is unknown.
2 Results from abnormal embryonic development of the persistence of fetal structure beyond the time of normal involution.
3 Possible causes:
   a Fetal and maternal infection occurring during first trimester of pregnancy
   b Teratogenic effects of drugs and radiation
   c Maternal dietary deficiencies
   d Hereditary in some cases.
4 Frequently associated with other congenital defects.

Common Congenital Heart Malformations (Table 6.1)

Acyanotic

1 Obstructive lesions
   a Pulmonary stenosis
   b Aortic stenosis
   c Coarctation of the aorta
2 Left-to-right shunts

Table 6.1   Congenital heart abnormalities

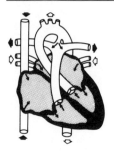

Patent Ductus Arteriosus

The patent ductus arteriosus is a vascular connection that, during fetal life, short circuits the pulmonary vascular bed and directs blood from the pulmonary artery to the aorta. Functional closure of the ductus normally occurs soon after birth. If the ductus remains patent after birth, the direction of blood flow in the ductus is reversed by the higher pressure in the aorta.

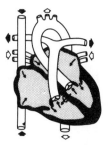

Ventricular Septal Defects

A ventricular septal defect is an abnormal opening between the right and left ventricle. Ventricular septal defects vary in size and may occur in either the membranous or muscular portion of the ventricular septum. Due to higher pressure in the left ventricle, a shunting of blood from the left to right ventricle occurs during systole. If pulmonary vascular resistance produces pulmonary hypertension, the shunt of blood is then reversed from the right to the left ventricle, with cyanosis resulting.

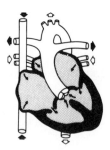

Truncus Arteriosus

Truncus arteriosus is a retention of the embryological bulbar trunk. It results from the failure of normal septation and division of this trunk into an aorta and pulmonary artery. This single arterial trunk overrides the ventricles and receives blood from them through a ventricular septal defect. The entire pulmonary and systemic circulation is supplied from this common arterial trunk.

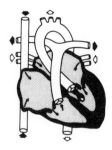

Subaortic Stenosis

In many instances, the stenosis is valvular with thickening and fusion of the cusps. Subaortic stenosis is caused by a fibrous ring below the aortic valve in the outflow tract of the ventricle. At times both valvular and subaortic stenosis exist in combination. The obstruction presents an increased work load for the normal output of the left ventricle blood and results in left ventricular enlargement.

(continued)

Table 6.1   *(continued)*

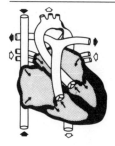

Coarctation of the Aorta

Coarctation of the aorta is characterized by a narrowed aortic lumen. It exists as a preductal or postductal obstruction, depending on the position of the obstruction in relation to the ductus arteriosus. Coarctations exist with great variation in anatomical features. The lesion produces an obstruction to the flow of blood through the aorta causing an increased left ventricular pressure and workload.

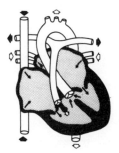

Tetralogy of Fallot

Tetralogy of Fallot is characterized by the combination of four defects: (1) pulmonary stenosis, (2) ventricular septal defect, (3) overriding aorta, (4) hypertrophy of right ventricle. It is the most common defect causing cyanosis in patients surviving beyond 2 years of age. The severity of symptoms depends on the degree of pulmonary stenosis, the size of the ventricular septal defect and the degree to which the aorta overrides the septal defect.

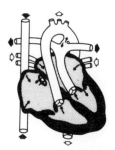

Complete Transposition of Great Vessels

This anomaly is an embryological defect caused by a straight division of the bulbar trunk without normal spiraling. As a result, the aorta originates from the right ventricle, and the pulmonary artery from the left ventricle. An abnormal communication between the two circulations must be present to sustain life.

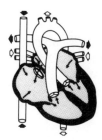

Atrial Septal Defects

An atrial septal defect is an abnormal opening between the right and left atria. Basically, three types of abnormalities result from incorrect development of the atrial septum. An incompetent foramen ovale is the most common defect. The high ostium secundum defect results from abnormal development of the septum secundum. Improper development of the septum primum produces a basal opening known as an ostium primum defect, frequently involving the atrioventricular valves. In general, left to right shunting of blood occurs in all atrial septal defects.

(continued)

Table 6.1   *(continued)*

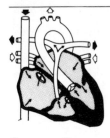

Tricuspid Atresia

Tricuspid valvular atresia is characterized by a small right ventricle, large left ventricle and usually a diminished pulmonary circulation. Blood from the right atrium passes through an atrial septal defect into the left atrium, mixes with oxgenated blood returning from the lungs, flows into the left ventricle and is propelled into the systemic circulation. The lungs may receive blood through one of three routes: (1) a small ventricular septal defect, (2) patent ductus arteriosus, (3) bronchial vessels.

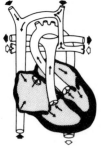

Anomalous Venous Return

Oxygenated blood returning from the lungs is carried abnormally to the right heart by one or more pulmonary veins emptying directly, or indirectly through venous channels, into the right atrium. Partial anomalous return of the pulmonary veins, to the right atrium functions the same as an atrial septal defect. In complete anomatous return of the pulmonary veins, an interatrial communication is necessary for survival.

   a Atrial septal defect
   b Ventricular septal effect
   c Patent duct arteriosus

Cyanotic

Right-to-left shunts
  1   Tetralogy of Fallot
  2   Tricuspid atresia
  3   Transposition of great arteries.

Aortic Valve Stenosis

Aortic valve stenosis occurs when there is obstruction to the left ventricular outflow at the level of the valve. This is the most common form of aortic stenosis, others being hypertrophic subaortic stenosis and supravalvular stenosis.

Physiology
  1   Blood flows from the left ventricle through the obstructed aortic valve into the aorta.
  2   Left ventricular pressure increases to overcome the resistance of the obstructed valve.

3 Myocardial ischaemia may occur as a result of an imbalance between the increased oxygen requirements of the hypertrophied left ventricle and the amount of oxygen that can be supplied to the myocardium.

Clinical Manifestations
1 Rarely symptomatic during infancy; infant may develop congestive heart failure.
2 Older children may experience chest pain, dyspnoea, and fatigue with exertion.
3 Narrow pulse pressure.
4 Weak peripheral pulses.

Diagnostic Evaluation
1 Auscultation:
   a Ejection click at fourth interspace to the left of the sternum
   b Harsh, low-pitched systolic ejection murmur
2 Chest x-ray — dilated ascending aorta and varying degrees of left ventricular enlargement
3 Electrocardiogram — left ventricular hypertrophy: strain pattern (T-wave inversion) is evidence of severe stenosis
4 Cardiac catheterization
5 Angiography.

Complications
1 Congestive heart failure
2 Myocardial infarction
3 Bacterial endocarditis
4 Sudden death.

Treatment
Aortic valvulotomy or prosthetic valve replacement (indicated for children who are symptomatic or have evidence of left ventricular strain on electrocardiogram) with a prosthesis in adult life.
Note: Bacterial endocarditis can convert asymptomatic aortic stenosis into gross aortic regurgitation with severe heart failure. Scrupulous dental hygiene is required and antibiotic cover given if dental extractions are needed.

Pulmonary Stenosis

Pulmonary stenosis refers to any lesion that obstructs the flow of blood from the right ventricle.

Pathophysiology

1 Blood flows from the right ventricle through the obstructed pulmonary valve into the pulmonary artery.
2 Right ventricle pressure increases to maintain normal cardiac output.
3 Right ventricle hypertrophy and occasionally left atrial enlargement occur.
4 Various degrees of tricuspid insufficiency occur in severe cases.

Clinical Manifestations

1 Generally asymptomatic; child may have decreased exercise tolerance.
2 With severe obstruction, child may have dyspnoea, generalized cyanosis.
3 May complain of pericordial pain.

Diagnostic Evaluation

1 Auscultation
  a Systolic ejection murmur over pulmonic area
  b Often will hear an ejection click and a widely split second sound
2 Chest x-ray right ventricular enlargement, main pulmonary artery enlargement, normal pulmonary vascularity, and normal left side; in severe stenosis, right atrial hypertrophy is also observed.
3 Electrocardiogram - right ventricular hypertrophy; severe cases may demonstrate a Q wave in the right pericordial leads and T-wave inversion (strain pattern).
4 Cardiac catheterization.
5 Angiocardiography.

Complications

1 Anoxic spells in infants with severe lesions
2 Bacterial endocarditis
3 Sudden death at any age.

Treatment

1 Surgery (valvulotomy) is generally indicated for all patients with severe stenosis and for symptomatic patients with moderate stenosis.
2 Asymptomatic children with moderate pulmonic stenosis should be evaluated at regular intervals for the progression of lesion.

Coarctation of the Aorta

Coarctation of the aorta is a narrowing or constriction of the vessel at any point. Most commonly, the constriction is located just distal to the origin of the left subclavian artery in the vicinity of the ductus arteriosus.

Altered Physiology

1 The narrowing of the aorta obstructs blood flow through the constricted segment of the aorta, thus increasing left ventricular pressure and workload.
2 Collateral vessels develop, arising chiefly from the branches of the subclavian and intercostal arteries, bypassing the coarcted segment of the aorta and supplying circulation to the lower extremities.

Clinical Manifestations

1 Usually asymptomatic in childhood — growth and development are normal
2 May demonstrate:
   a Occasional fatigue
   b Headache
   c Nose bleeds
   d Leg cramps.
3 Absent or greatly reduced femoral pulsations.
4 Hypertension in upper extremities and diminished blood pressure in lower extremities.
5 Symptoms secondary to hypertension (rare in children).
6 Severe anomalies cause symptoms in infants, including growth failure, tachypnoea, dyspnoea, peripheral oedema, and severe congestive heart failure.

Diagnostic Evaluation

1 Auscultation — nonspecific systolic murmur heard along the left sternal border
2 Chest x-ray — cardiomegaly (preductal), or enlarged left ventricle, dilated ascending aorta, and possibly enlarged left atrium (postductal); rib notching is a common finding in children over 8 years of age
3 Electrocardiogram — right ventricular hypertrophy (preductal) or varying degrees of left ventricular hypertrophy (postductal)
4 Cardiac catheterization
5 Angiography.

Complications

1 Cerebral haemorrhage
2 Rupture of the aorta
3 Infective endocarditis
4 Congestive heart failure.

Treatment

1 Infants — vigorous management of congestive heart failure and surgical correction is indicated for infants who present in the first 6 months of life with heart failure.
2 Asymptomatic older child — surgical resection is recommended for children between the ages of 3 and 6 years with significant coarctation.
3 Surgery — resection of the coarcted segment and end-to-end anastomosis or graft.

Patent Ductus Arteriosus

Patent ductus arteriosus is the persistence of a fetal connection (ductus arteriosus) between the pulmonary artery and the aorta.

Altered Physiology

1 During fetal life, the ductus arteriosus allows most of the right ventricular blood to bypass the nonfunctioning lungs by directing blood from the pulmonary artery to the aorta.
2 After birth, with the initiation of respiration, the ductus arteriosus is no longer necessary. It should functionally close within several hours after birth and anatomically close within several weeks after birth.
   a The smooth muscle in the wall of the ductus arteriosus contracts to obliterate the lumen.
   b Within several weeks after birth, degenerative changes occur in the ductus arteriosus and it becomes a cord of fibrous connective tissue (ligamentum ateriosum).
3 When the ductus arteriosus remains patent, oxygenated blood from the higher pressure systemic circuit (aorta) flows to the lower pressure pulmonary circuit (pulmonary artery) through the patent ductus arteriosus.
4 The volume of blood that the heart must pump in order to meet the demands of the peripheral tissues is increased. A greater volume burden is placed on the lungs and eventually on the left heart.

Clinical Manifestations

1 Small patent ductus arteriosus — usually asymptomatic.
2 Large patent ductus arteriosus — may develop symptoms in very early infancy.
   a Slow weight gain
   b Feeding difficulties
   c Frequent respiratory infections
   d Congestive heart failure.

Diagnostic Evaluation

1 Auscultation — continuous machinery-like murmur at the left intraclavicular area.
2 May have a wide pulse pressure and/or bounding posterior tibial and dorsalis pedis pulses.
3 Chest x-ray — may be normal; may demonstrate cardiomegaly, large aortic knob, increased pulmonary vascularity, and prominence of the left atrium and left ventricle.
4 Electrocardiogram — may be normal; may demonstrate left ventricular hypertrophy.
5 Cardiac catheterization.
6 Angiocardiography.

Complications

1 Congestive heart failure
2 Infective endocarditis.

Treatment

1 Surgical division of the patent ductus arteriosus:
   a In early infancy if congestive heart failure develops and cannot be controlled
   b Electively by 2-3 years of age
   Note: Indomethacin appears to trigger the natural closing of the ductus. It has been used successfully in some premature infants. If this success is sustained, this approach may replace surgery as the treatment of choice for some of these patients.

Atrial Septal Defect

Atrial septal defect is an abnormal opening in the septum between the left atrium and the right atrium.

1 *Ostium secundum type* — located in the centre of the atrial septum.
2 *Ostium primum type* — large gap at the base of the atrial septum frequently associated with deformities of the mitral and tricuspid valves and/or a small, high ventricular septal defect.

Altered Physiology

1 The pressure in the left atrium is greater than the pressure in the right atrium and promotes the flow of oxygenated blood from the left atrium to the right atrium.
2 The oxygenated blood that flows through the defect enters the right atrium

and mixes with the systemic venous blood returning to the lung. The blood flow through the shunt recirculates through the lung, thus increasing the total blood flow through the lung.

3   The major haemodynamic abnormality is volume overload of the right ventricle.

4   If the pulmonary resistance is great, this may increase right atrial pressure, thus causing a reversal of the shunt, with unoxygenated blood flowing from the right atrium to the left atrium. (This situation will produce cyanosis.)

Clinical Manifestations

1   Ostium secundum type — generally asymptomatic even when this defect is large

2   Ostium primum type — generally asymptomatic, although the following may occur:
   a   Slow weight gain
   b   Tiredness
   c   Dyspnoea with exertion
   d   Frequent respiratory infections
   e   Congestive heart failure.

Diagnostic Evaluation

1   Auscultation
   a   Systolic, medium-pitched ejection murmur heard best at the second left interspace.
   b   Fixed widely spaced second sound.
   c   May have mid-diastolic filling sound at the lower left sternal border.

2   Chest x-ray — prominent main pulmonary artery, right atrial and right ventricular enlargement, increase in vascular markings of the lungs.

3   Electrocardiogram — may demonstrate right ventricular hypertrophy and/or left axis deviation (ostium primum defect.)

4   Cardiac catheterization.

5   Angiocardiography.

Complications

Complications are rare in children

1   Infective endocarditis
2   Cardiac failure
3   Pulmonary hypertension
4   Coronary artery disease
5   Atrial fibrillation.

Treatment
Surgical closure with cardiopulmonary bypass by suture or patch.

Ventricular Septal Defect

Ventricular septal defect is an abnormal opening in the septum between the right and left ventricles.It may vary in size from very small defects (Roger's defect) to very large defects, and may occur in either the membranous or muscular portion of the ventricular septum

Altered Physiology

1   The pressure in the left ventricle is greater than the pressure in the right ventricle and promotes the flow of oxygenated blood from the left ventricle to the right ventricle.
2   The oxygenated blood that flows through the defect mixes with the blood returning from the right atrium. The blood flow through the shunt recirculates through the lung, thus increasing the total blood flow through the lung.
3   The major haemodynamic abnormalities are:
    a Increased right ventricular and pulmonary arterial pressure
    b Increased blood flow to the right ventricle, pulmonary arteries, left atrium, and left ventricle.
4   If the pulmonary resistance is great, this may increase right ventricular pressure, thus causing a reversal of the shunt with unoxygenated blood flowing from the right ventricle to the left ventricle (this situation, termed Eisenmenger's complex, will produce cyanosis).

Clinical Manifestations

1   Small ventricular septal defects — usually asymptomatic (many close spontaneously)
2   Large ventricular septal defects — may develop symptoms as early as 1-2 months af age:
    a Slow weight gain
    b Feeding difficulties
    c Pale, delicate-looking, scrawny appearance
    d Frequent respiratory infections
    e Tachypnoea
    f Excessive sweating
    g Congestive heart failure.

Diagnostic Evaluation

1   Auscultation — harsh holosystolic murmur, heard best at the fourth interspace to the left of the sternum
2   Chest x-ray — possible enlargement of the right ventricle, definite enlargement of the main pulmonary artery, increased pulmonary vascular mark-

ings, and enlargement of the left atrium and ventricle
3 Electrocardiagram — left ventricular hypertrophy, may have right ventricular hypertrophy
4 Cardiac catheterization
5 Angiocardiography.

Complications
1 Effective endocarditis
2 Congestive heart failure.

Treatment
1 Medical management of congestive heart failure if this occurs in infancy.
2 If congestive heart failure is intractable to medical management, surgical closure is indicated.
3 Patients with pulmonary arterial hypertension require early surgery (before 2 years of age) to avoid irreversible pulmonary bed changes.
4 Surgery is contraindicated in patients with Eisenmenger's complex.

Tetralogy of Fallot

Tetralogy of Fallot consists of four abnormalities: (1) right ventricular-outflow stenosis or atresia, (2) ventricular septal defect, (3) overriding of the aorta, and (4) right ventricular hypertrophy.

Altered Physiology
1 Obstruction of the blood flow from the right ventricle to the pulmonary circulation is caused by obstruction at the pulmonary valve level or the infundibular area of the right ventricle below the pulmonary valve.
2 Unoxygenated blood is shunted from the right ventricle through the ventricular septal defect directly into the aorta.
3 The right ventricle is hypertrophied because of high right ventricular pressure.

Clinical Manifestations
1 The clinical manifestations are variable and depend on the size of the ventricular septal defect and the degree of right ventricular outflow obstruction.
2 Cyanosis
   a Initially, the shunt through the ventricular septal defect is mainly from the left to right. Many infants with this defect are not cyanotic at birth, but they develop cyanosis as they grow and as the stenosis becomes relatively more severe

b Cyanosis may at first be observed only with exertion and crying, but during the first years of life, the child may become cyanotic at rest

c Infundibular stenosis may be minimal so that cyanosis never develops ('pink tetralogy')

3 Clubbing of the fingers and toes

4 Squatting (a posture assumed by children with this defect once they have reached the walking stage)

5 Slow weight gain

6 Dyspnoea on exertion

7 Hypoxic spells, transient cerebral ischaemia.

Diagnostic Evaluation

1 Auscultation
    a Single second sound
    b Systolic ejection murmur at the second and third interspaces to the left of the sternum

2 Inspection — prominent left chest with right ventricular heave

3 Chest x-ray
    a Heart size normal
    b Pulmonary segment small and concave ('boot-shaped heart')
    c Diminished pulmonary vascular markings

4 Electrocardiogram — right axis deviation; right ventricular hypertrophy

5 Cardiac catheterization

6 Angiocardiography

7 Laboratory data
    a Polycythaemia
    b Increased haematocrit.

Complications

1 Congestive heart failure — may occur in newborn but is uncommon beyond infancy

2 Infective endocarditis

3 Cerebral vascular accident (due to thrombosis or severe hypoxia)

4 Brain abscess

5 Iron deficiency anaemia.

Treatment

The objective of treatment is to improve oxygenation of arterial blood.

1 Palliative
    a *Waterston shunt* — anastomosis between the posterior lateral aspect of the ascending aorta and the right pulmonary artery
    b *Blalock-Taussig shunt* — anastomosis between the right or left subclavian

artery and the right pulmonary artery

2   Total correction
a Removal of shunt if previously performed.
b With cardiopulmonary bypass, ventricular septal defect is repaired and right ventricular-outflow obstruction is relieved.
c Total correction is increasingly being advocated for all infants in whom pulmonary arteries are of sufficient size.

Transposition of the Great Arteries

Transposition of the great arteries occurs when the pulmonary artery originates posteriorly from the left ventricle and the aorta originates anteriorly from the right ventricle.

Altered Physiology

1   This defect results in two separate circulations; the right heart manages the systemic circulation and the left heart manages the pulmonary circulation.
2   In order for life to be sustained, there must be an accompanying defect which provides for the mixing of oxygenated and unoxygenated blood between the two circulations.
3   The mixing of oxygenated and unoxygenated blood occurs through one or more of the following shunts:
a Atrial septal defect
b Ventricular septal defect
c Patent ductus arteriosus
d Patent foramen ovale.

Clinical Manifestations

1   Cyanosis, usually developing shortly after birth (degree dependent upon the type of associated malfunctions)
2   Shallow rapid respirations and tiredness
3   Slow weight gain
4   Clubbing of fingers and toes
5   Congestive heart failure may develop.

Diagnostic Evaluation

1   Auscultation — murmurs may be absent in infancy; may be murmur of an associated defect
2   Chest x-ray — cardiomegaly, narrow mediastinum, increased vascular markings (decreased vascular markings in children with associated pulmonary stenosis)

3   Electrocardiogram — right axis deviation, right atrial hypertrophy, right ventricular hypertrophy)
4   Laboratory tests:
    a Polycythaemia
    b Increased haemoglobin and haematocrit
5   Cardiac catheterization
6   Angiocardiography.

Complications

1   Congestive heart failure
2   Infective endocarditis
3   Brain abscess
4   Cerebral vascular accident (due to thrombosis or severe hypoxia)

Treatment

1   Vigorous medical management of congestive heart failure.
2   Palliative procedures
    a *Rashkind procedure* — the creation of an atrial septal defect with a balloon catheter during cardiac catheterization
    b *Blalock-Hanlon procedure* — surgical creation of an atrial septal defect
    c Pulmonary artery banding (indicated for infants with ventricular septal defects with large pulmonary blood flow)
3   Complete correction
    a *Mustard procedure* — with cardiopulmonary bypass, the atrial septum is removed and a baffle of Dacron velour and/or pericardium is sutured in place in such a way that the pulmonary venous blood is directed toward the right ventricle and the systemic venous blood is directed toward the left ventricle (usually done before 2 years of age, before pulmonary vascular disease develops).
    b *Rastelli procedure*
    (1) Surgery of choice for transposition with ventricular septal defect and left ventricular outflow-tract obstruction.
    (2) With cardiopulmonary bypass, the ventricular septal defect is closed in such a way that the left ventricle communicates with the aorta. The pulmonary artery is ligated, and the right ventricle is connected to the distal portion of the pulmonary artery by means of a valve bearing tubular graft.

c Recent procedures have been developed for anatomical correction of transposition of the great arteries by direct contraposition of the transposed vessels. This may become the preferred treatment in the future.

Tricuspid Atresia

Tricuspid atresia is a condition in which there is: (1) atresia of the tricuspid valve so that there is no communication between the right atrium and right ventricle, (2) interatrial septal defect, and (3) a hypoplastic right ventricle.

Pathophysiology

1   Blood from the systemic circulation is shunted from the right atrium through an interatrial communication to the left atrium and then to the left ventricle.
2   Pulmonary blood flow is established either through a patent ductus arteriosus, bronchial circulation, or a ventricular septal defect.

Clinical Manifestations

1   Severe cyanosis in the neonatal period
2   Respiratory distress
3   Clubbing
4   Hypoxic spells
5   Delayed weight gain
6   Right heart failure may occur.

Diagnostic Evaluation

1   Auscultation
    a Second sound usually single
    b Commonly no murmur or murmur of associated defect
2   Chest x-ray — diminished pulmonary vascular markings; may demonstrate enlarged right atrium, left atrium, left ventricle, and aorta
3   Electrocardiogram — right atrial, left atrial, left ventricular hypertrophy, left axis deviation
4   Echocardiogram — demonstrates diminuitive right ventricular chamber and no tricuspid valve
5   Cardiac catheterization
6   Angiocardiography.

Complications

1   Cerebrovascular accidents
2   Brain abscess
3   Bacterial endocarditis.

Treatment

1   Complete surgical correction — not possible at this time.
2   Palliative procedures to increase pulmonary blood flow:
    a *Waterston shunt* — anastomosis between the ascending aorta and right pulmonary artery
    b *Glenn procedure* — side-to-end anastomosis of the superior vena cava to the right pulmonary artery
3   Fontan's operation, performed on children aged 8-12 years, consists of a homograph valve placed at the juncture of the inferior vena cava and right atrium and another at the site of the anastomosis of right atrial appendage and pulmonary artery.

Treatment and Nursing Management of the Child with a Congenital Heart Defect

Nursing Objectives

To become informed concerning the child's symptomatology and the plan of medical care.

1   Obtain a thorough nursing history to become familiar with the child and his family in order to recognize normal and abnormal patterns (colour, respirations, murmur, feeding, exercise tolerance, etc.).
2   Discuss with the paediatrician his plan for medical care.
3   Make a baseline nursing assessment of the child's condition.
    a Observe and record information relevant to the child's growth and development (motor coordination, muscular development, emotional maturity).
        (1) Compare data with that for siblings, other family members.
        (2) Plot appropriate information on growth chart.
    b Observe and record the child's level of play:
        (1) Observe the child at play:
            (a) Is play interrupted to rest?
            (b) How does he play as compared with his peers?
            (c) Does he squat during play? (Squatting is a characteristic position a cyanotic child assumes when resting after exertion.)

(2) Observe infant while feeding.

Does the infant stop feeding to rest or does he fall asleep during feeding?

c Observe the child's skin and mucous membranes for colour changes.
(1) Skin
    (a) Colour changes vary from pink, dusky, mottled, to cyanotic.
    (b) Earlobes are good indicators of the degree of oxygen saturation.
    (c) Circumoral cyanosis occurs with oxygen deprivation.
    (d) Nailbeds are good indicators of colour change.
(2) Mucous membranes
    Lips and tongue indicate colour change because they are very vascular areas and contain superficial blood vessels: *mucous membranes are the best places to observe for cyanosis.*
(3) Record where cyanosis was observed (localized or generalized), where it was observed and the duration (continuous or intermittent, whether variable with exercise).

d Observe for clubbing. (Rounding of the fingers, especially the thumbnails, with thickening and shininess of the terminal phalanges — may occur in cyanotic children by 2-3 months of age.)

e Observe for chest deformities:
(1) Visible pulsations
(2) Left- or right-sided prominence.

f Observe respiratory pattern:
(1) Remove any clothing or covers which obscure visualization of the chest.
(2) Count respirations for at least 30 seconds.
(3) Count respirations while a child is at rest; if unable to soothe the child, note that he is crying, irritable, etc.
(4) Observe for increased respiratory rate, grunting, retractions, nasal flaring, irregularity of respirations.
(5) Record all signs of respiratory distress including change from usual pattern, when it occurred, duration, etc.

g Palpate the child's pulses.
(1) Radial or dorsalis pedis is difficult to feel in newborn.
(2) Femoral pulsations are easily felt in the inguinal region and can be compared with brachial pulsations.
(3) Record the strength of the pulse (full, bounding, weak, or faint).
(4) When a pulse is difficult to locate, mark its location with a pen to facilitate locating it next time.

h Record vital signs (apical pulse, blood pressure, respirations):
(1) Have child quiet for baseline vital signs.
(2) Record which extremity is used for blood pressure measurement.
(3) Refer to vital sign procedure (see p. 99).

To provide adequate nutritional and fluid intake to maintain the growth and developmental needs of the child.

1 Feed slowly in a semi-erect position; burp infants after each 30ml.
2 Utilize soft teats with large holes which make it easier for the infant to suck.
3 Provide small frequent feedings.
4 Feeding should generally be completed within 45 minutes or sooner if infant tires.
5 Provide foods which have high nutritional value.
6 Determine the child's likes and dislikes and plan meals with the dietician, taking into consideration the child's preferences.
7 Observe the child at mealtime; does a poor appetite represent a lack of interest in food or does the child become fatigued while eating?
8 Report vomiting and specify the amount, type, relationship to feeding or to medications.
9 Report diarrhoea and specify type and amount.
10 Maintain adequate hydration in the cyanotic child when he is vomiting, has diarrhoea or fever, or is exposed to high environmental temperatures since polycythaemia predisposes him to thrombosis.

To prevent infection.

1 Prevent exposure to communicable disease, including exposure to children with upper respiratory infections, diarrhoea, wound infections, etc.
2 Check with parents to be certain that the child's immunizations are up to date.
3 Practice careful handwashing technique and teach this to the child.
4 Report temperature elevation, diarrhoea, vomiting and upper respiratory symptoms promptly.
5 Be certain that the child receives prophylactic medication for subacute bacterial endocarditis before any invasive diagnostic or treatment procedures and dental work.

To prepare the child for diagnostic and treatment procedures.

1 Explain to the child what is going to be done in simple terms (refer to section on hospitalized child, p. 56).
2 Encourage the child to express his fears and fantasies verbally or through play.
3 Diagnostic procedures may include:
   a Electrocardiogram
   b Vectorcardiogram
   c Phonocardiogram
   d Echocardiogram

    e Chest x-ray
    f Barium swallow
    g Cardiac catheterization and angiocardiography
    h Complete blood count
    i Platelet count
    j Blood gases.

To explain to the child about his heart condition as early as the child can understand.

1   Discuss with the parents the importance of being truthful with the child about his heart condition.
2   The time to tell the child is generally when the child begins asking questions as to why he visits the doctor so frequently and why the doctors listens to his heart so closely.
3   The child's questions should be answered truthfully in a simple way.

To relieve the respiratory distress associated with increased pulmonary blood flow or oxygen deprivation.

1   Determine the degree of respiratory distress:
    a Infants — respirations greater than 60 per minute are indicative of respiratory difficulty.
    b Young children — respirations greater than 40 per minute are indicative of respiratory difficulty.
    c Observe the regularity of the respiratory pattern.
    d Observe for retractions (drawing in of the soft tissue in the rib interspaces or below the costal margin with each inspiration; may be barely visible, mild or severe).
    e Observe for nasal flaring, listen for grunting.

2   Include specific information in nursing record:
    a Number of respirations per minute
    b Regularity of respirations
    c Type and severity of retractions
    d Presence of nasal flaring, grunting
    e Response to oxygen therapy
    f Response to positioning
    g Colour changes
    h Irritability or anxiety observed.

3   Position the child at 45° angle to decrease pressure of viscera on the diaphragm and increase lung volume.
    a Infant — place in an infant seat.
    b Children — elevate head of the bed and support the arms with pillows.
4   Pin nappies loosely; provide loose fitting pyjamas or nightdress for older children. If own clothes are worn, ensure that they are loose around the neck,

arms and waist.

5 Feed slowly allowing frequent rest periods:

a Rapid respirations and frequent coughing predispose the child to aspiration.

b May require nasogastric feeding.

c Observe for abdominal distension which may increase respiratory difficulty.

6 Hyperextend the infant's or child's head.

7 Suction the nose and throat if the child is unable adequately to cough up secretions.

8 Provide oxygen therapy as indicated.

To relieve the hypoxic spells associated with cyanotic types of congenital heart disease (primarily tetralogy of Fallot).

1 Observe for hypoxic spells (attacks of acute oxygen deprivation), characterized by:

a Increased rate and depth of respiration

b Increasing cyanosis

c Murmur that becomes less intense, may disappear

d Bradycardia

e Progressive limpness and syncope

f May result in convulsions.

2 Be aware that these attacks frequently occur in the morning after awakening from sleep, during or after crying, during or after defaecation, or during or immediately following feeding.

3 Once an attack is recognized, call for assistance and immediately:

a Place child in knee-chest position.

b Administer oxygen via mask.

c Be prepared to administer medications as prescribed:

(1) Morphine sulphate

(2) $NaHCO_3$ (sodium bicarbonate) to correct acidosis

(3) Propranolol

d Assume a calm, reassuring attitude.

4 Observe child closely following recovery from an attack. Encourage fluid intake.

5 Record observations in the following areas:

a Condition and activity before the attack

b Response to positioning and medication

c Vital signs during and after attack.

To improve oxygenation so that body functions may be maintained.

1 Provide a safe, effective oxygen environment (refer to procedure on oxygen therapy, p. 186).

2 Explain to the child how oxygen will help him and orient him to equipment before it is used on him (e.g. tent, mask).

3   Observe the child's response to oxygen therapy:
   a Improvement of colour
   b Change in rate and character of respiration
   c Change in anxiety level.
4   Observe the child's response while he is being weaned from oxygen.
   Reduce litre flow gradually and observe response after each reduction.
5   Measures which are directed to relieve respiratory distress will aid in improving oxygenation.

To reduce the workload of the heart since decreased activity and expenditure of energy will decrease oxygen requirements.

1   Organize nursing care to provide periods of uninterrupted rest.
2   Avoid unnecessary activities such as frequent, complete baths, and clothing changes.
3   Prevent excessive crying:
   a Use dummy
   b Encourage mother to hold and cuddle baby. In her absence the nurse should do this
   c Feed when hungry
   d Keep baby comfortable.
4   Explain to the child the need for rest.
5   Provide diversional activities that require limited expenditure of energy.
6   Avoid discussing the child's condition or the condition of other children in the presence of the child.
7   Support the child during diagnostic and therapeutic procedures.

To observe the child for symptoms of congestive heart failure which occur frequently as a complication of congenital heart disease.
(For nursing management, refer to section on congestive heart failure, p. 390.)

1   Respiratory distress (tachypnoea, retractions, nasal flaring, grunting, voice changes)
2   Tachycardia, gallop heart rhythm
3   Fatigue (as evidenced by poor feeding in infants)
4   Oedema (periorbital oedema is observed in infants; older children develop swelling of hands and feet)
5   Weight gain
6   Irritability
7   Sweating
8   Liver enlargement
9   Splenomegaly
10 Orthopnoea
11 Neck vein distension (rarely seen in infants)
12 Murmurs (may appear, or the characteristics of previously heard murmur may change)
13 Cyanosis (may occur)

14   Pulmonary râles (may occur).

To observe for the development of symptoms of infective endocarditis which may occur as a complication of congenital heart disease.

1   Be aware of the symptoms of infective endocarditis:
   a Spiking fever
   b Petechiae
   c Anorexia
   d Pallor
   e Fatigue.
2   Be aware of the need for infective endocarditis prophylaxis for selected children undergoing surgery, dental work, and laceration repair.
3   For nursing management, refer to section on infective endocarditis, p. 403.

To observe for the development of thrombosis which may occur as a complication of cyanotic heart disease.

1   Be aware of the signs and symptoms of thrombosis:
   a Irritability and restlessness
   b Convulsions, coma, neurological signs
   c Paralysis
   d Rapid onset of oedema
   e Anuria, oliguria, haematuria.
2   Be aware that thrombosis is more likely to occur during phases of acute dehydration, fever, and vomiting.

To prepare the parents to care for the child following discharge.

1   Instruct family in necessary measures to maintain child's health.
   a Complete immunization
   b Adequate diet and rest
   c Prevention and control of infections
   d Regular medical and dental checkup
   Child should be protected against subacute bacterial endocarditis and given antibiotic to cover for dental treatment.
   e Regular cardiac checkups.
2   Teach family about the defect and its treatment:
   a Pathophysiology and natural history
   b Signs and symptoms of disease progress
   c Signs and symptoms of complications that might be anticipated
   d Signs of infection, dehydration
   e Medications and side effects
   f Special diets
   g Emergency precautions related to hypoxic attacks, pulmonary oedema, cardiac arrest (if appropriate).
3   Encourage the parents and other persons (teachers, peers, etc.) to treat the

child in as normal a manner as possible:

a Avoid overprotection and overindulgence.

b Avoid rejection.

c Facilitate performance of the usual developmental tasks within the limits of the child's physiological state.

   With most congenital cardiac defects it is not necessary to restrict the child's activity; the child will rest when he becomes tired and then resume his play.

d Prevent adults from projecting their fears and anxieties on to the child.

4   Refer to health visitor or school nurse as appropriate.

To refer the family to appropriate resources.

1   Social worker
2   Chaplain
3   Parents and organized parents groups
4   Chest, Heart and Stroke Association, Tavistock House North, Tavistock Square, London WC1.

CONGESTIVE HEART FAILURE

Congestive heart failure occurs when the cardiac output is inadequate to meet the metabolic needs of the body and results in accumulation of excessive blood volume in the pulmonary and/or systemic venous system.

Aetiology

1   Congenital heart disease (primary cause in the first 3 years of life).
2   Acquired heart disease — rheumatic heart disease, endocarditis, myocarditis.
3   Non cardiovascular causes — acidosis, pulmonary disease, central nervous system disease, anaemia, sepsis, hypoglycaemia

Clinical Manifestations

1   Dyspnoea and tachypnoea
2   Tachycardia
3   Orthopnoea
4   Peripheral oedema — often scrotal or periorbital

5 Feeding difficulties, anorexia
6 Restlessness
7 Tires easily
8 Pallor
9 Weight gain
10 Diaphoresis
11 Growth failure
12 Nonproductive, irritative cough
13 Neck vein distension
14 Hepatomegaly.

Pathophysiology

1 For any number of reasons, cardiac output is inadequate to meet the oxygenation and nutritional requirements of vital organs.
2 Various compensatory mechanisms occur:
  a Stroke volume increases and cardiomegaly develops.
  b Tachycardia occurs in an effort to maintain adequate stroke volume.
  c Catecholamines are released by the sympathetic venous system that increase systemic vascular resistance and venous tone and decrease cutaneous, splanchnic and renal blood flow.
  d Glomerular filtration decreases and tubular reabsorption increases, causing diminished urinary output and sodium retention.
  e Diaphoresis occurs.
3 Cardiac output decreases further as compensatory mechanisms fail.
4 The pulmonary vascular bed is not emptied efficiently, causing engorgement of the pulmonic system with subsequent pulmonary hypertension and oedema.
5 There is diminished blood return to the heart, with venous congestion and a rise in venous pressure.

Diagnostic Evaluation

1 Palpatation:
  a May have weak peripheral pulses.
  b Hepatomegaly (feature of right heart failure).
  c Abnormal precordial activity may occur.
2 Auscultation:
  a Gallop rhythm (frequent)
  b Cardiac murmurs may or may not be present
  c Râles (infrequent in infants).

3   Chest x-rays — cardiomegaly; may demonstrate pneumonia.
4   Laboratory data:
   a Dilutional hyponatraemia
   b Hypochloraemia
   c Hyperkalaemia.

Complications

1   Respiratory infections
2   Pulmonary oedema
3   Intractable congestive heart failure
4   Myocardial failure.

Nursing Objectives

To improve myocardial efficiency.

1   Administer digoxin as ordered by the paediatrician.
   a Digoxin is given to infants and children in very small amounts. Be aware of criteria for careful calculation of dose.
   b Count apical pulse for one full minute before administering.
     Be aware of the heart rate at which the paediatrician wants the medication withheld.
   c Report vomiting, which may occur following administration of digoxin, to determine if paediatrician desires dose to be repeated.
   d Observe for the development of premature ventricular contractions when digoxin is initially started; report this to paediatrician.
   e Be aware of signs of digitalis intoxication.
     (1) Altered emotional status, 'digitalis blues'
     (2) Decreased appetite
     (3) Bradycardia
     (4) Arrhythmias, especially coupled beats
     (5) Gastrointestinal symptoms, especially vomiting.

To reduce energy requirements.

1   Organize nursing care to provide periods of uninterrupted rest.
2   Avoid unnecessary activities such as frequent complete baths and clothing changes.
3   Prevent excessive crying.
   a Offer dummy to infant.
   b Hold baby, or encourage mother to cuddle her baby.
   c Eliminate sources of distress (e.g. hunger, wet nappies).

4   Explain to the child the need for rest.
5   Provide diversional activities that require limited expenditure of energy.

To remove accumulated sodium and fluid.

1   Administer diuretics as prescribed by the paediatrician.
    a Be aware of the side effects of the prescribed medication.
    b Weigh the child at least daily to observe response.
    c Maintain an accurate record of intake and output. Record urine relative density.
    d Encourage foods such as bananas and orange juice that have a high potassium content to prevent potassium depletion associated with many diuretics.
        (1) Hypokalaemia may cause weakened myocardial contractions and may precipitate digoxin toxicity.
        (2) Oral potassium supplements may be indicated when a child is on diuretics for an extended period of time.
2   Restrict sodium intake
    a The child is usually placed on a low sodium diet.
    b Be aware of the prescribed diet and the amount of sodium in foods and fluids offered to the child.
    c Question the child about his likes and dislikes so that the diet can be made as appealing as possible.
    d Interpret the diet and its purpose to the child and his parents.
    e Infants may require low sodium formulas.

To relieve the respiratory distress associated with pulmonary engorgement.
Refer to section on Congenital Heart Disease, p. 367.

To improve tissue oxygenation.

1   Administer oxygen therapy — refer to procedure, p. 186.
2   Maintain the infant in a neutral thermal environment.

To provide adequate nutrition to meet the caloric requirements of the child.

1   Provide foods which the child enjoys in small amounts, because he may have a poor appetite because of liver enlargement.
2   Infant feeding:
    a Feed frequently in small amounts.
    b Feed slowly in a sitting position, allowing frequent rest periods.
    c Supplement oral feeding with nasogastric feeding if the infant is unable to take adequate amount by mouth.
    d Record the amount of formula taken.
    e Place the child in an infant seat following feeding to prevent pressure of the viscera on the diaphragm.
    f Observe for distension and vomiting following feeding.

To decrease the danger of infection.

1   Practise careful handwashing technique.
2   Avoid exposure to other children with upper respiratory infections, diarrhoea, etc.
3   Report such changes as pyrexia, diarrhoea, vomiting, and upper respiratory symptoms promptly.

To observe for signs of disease progress or response to treatment.

1   Record and report in detail presence or disappearance of signs and symptoms.
2   Monitor vital signs frequently and report any significant changes.

To explain the condition and treatment to the child and family.

1   Utilize terminology that the child and/or parents can understand.
2   Correct misinterpretations — parents and children frequently interpret congestive heart failure to be synonomous with myocardial infarction, or they may fear that the heart is about to stop beating.

To prepare the parents for the care of the child at home.

1   Describe symptoms to be aware of and reported.
2   Teach them how to administer medications and about the side effects.
3   Explain dietary and/or activity restrictions.
4   Explain methods to prevent infection.
5   Refer to health visitor or school nurse as appropriate.

NURSING CARE OF THE CHILD UNDERGOING CARDIAC CATHETERIZATION

Cardiac catheterization involves introducing a radio-opaque catheter into a vein or artery in the groin or in the arm, either percutaneously or by means of a cutdown. The catheter is advanced into the cardiac chambers and vessels, where pressures are measured and samples for oxygen concentration are obtained. The procedure is usually done in conjunction with angiography, the injection of radio-opaque material into various chambers of the heart.

Purpose

1   To establish the diagnosis of cardiovascular defect.
2   To identify the severity of the defect.
3   To evaluate the effects of the defect on cardiovascular function.

Preoperative Nursing Management

1   Reinforce explanations of the procedure to the child and parents.
    a Provide specific information about:
        (1) Time of the test
        (2) Preparation for the procedure (nil by mouth, sedation, etc.)
        (3) Site of venepuncture (if known)
        (4) What the child will see (atmosphere of the catheterization room)
        (5) What will be expected of the child during the procedure
        (6) Routines after the procedure.
    b Detail, length, and timing of explanations should be appropriate to the child's age and level of cognitive development.
        (1) Photographs or a miniature replica of the cardiac unit and equipment may facilitate understanding of explanations. Utilize role play.
        (2) Older children and parents may benefit from an opportunity to see the room where the procedure will be done.
        (3) It is helpful for some children to handle the mask and other equipment that will be used.
    c Parents should be provided with an opportunity for private discussion of the anticipated procedure.
2   Maintain adequate hydration (especially important for children with cyanotic heart disease).
    Offer fluids just prior to nil by mouth period.
3   Cleanse proposed catheterization site thoroughly. Clean fingernails and/or toenails.
4   Obtain baseline set of vital signs — including blood pressure — just prior to the time of catheterization.
5   Administer sedation if ordered.
    a Secure side rails up after the child has been medicated. Encourage parents to stay.
    b Observe child closely for depressed respirations.
Note: Some units carry out cardiac catheterization under a general anaesthetic. For preparation, see p. 83.

Postoperative Nursing Management

1   Monitor vital signs frequently and report:
    a Sudden drop in blood pressure
    b Changes in pulse rate or rhythm
    c Increased or decreased respirations
    d Faintness, weakness
    e Elevated temperature.
2   Observe for complications resulting from damage to the vessels through which the catheter was passed.
    a Check the dressing or puncture site for bleeding.

b Observe site for redness, swelling, pain, or induration.

c Observe for numbness, pallor, decreased temperature, decreased motion, cyanosis, or mottling of affected extremity.

d Palpate pulses in affected extremity and compare with pulses in the opposite extremity.

3 Keep the child warm to avoid the risk of hypothermia.

This is especially important for small infants and children who may already be hypoxic because of their cardiac condition.

4 Maintain the child in a reclining position for several hours after catheterization to avoid:

a Possibility of sudden drop in blood pressure that may accompany an abrupt assumption of an upright position

b Bleeding at the site of the catheter entry.

5 Offer fluids as soon as the child is able to take them to avoid dehydration.

This is especially important for cyanotic children who are polycythaemic and prone to thrombus formation.

6 Reinforce discharge information. Parents should be informed about:

a Care of the incision, puncture site

b Dressing change (if any)

c Activity limitations (if any)

d Observation for and reporting of late complications (especially infection)

e Follow-up medical care

f Ensure that all instructions are written down for parents to refer to on return home.

7 If the child is a candidate for surgery, utilize appropriate opportunities to prepare him and his family for the experience.

a Encourage contact with children who are convalescing from surgery.

b Answer immediate questions of the parents.

CARDIAC SURGERY

Principles of Nursing Care

Preoperative

1 Prepare parents for the experience prior to the day of admission for surgery.

a Parents frequently ask questions about:

(1) What to tell the child

(2) When to begin preparation

(3) What to bring to the hospital

(4) Anticipated sequence of events

(5) Separation — rooming-in, whether or not to leave at night, etc.

b Utilize opportunities for teaching — visits to outpatients, contact with other parents and their children.

2 Prepare child for what he will experience during hospitalization.

a Consult with parents prior to beginning explanation. Their desires regarding how much information to give the child should be respected, and they should be active participants in preparation of the child.

b Most children need information in a language they can understand about:

(1) Preparation for surgery:

(a) Diagnostic tests

(b) Antibacterial skin preparation or baths

(c) Nil by mouth period

(d) Injections — antimicrobials and/or sedatives

(e) Time of the surgery

(f) Transportation to operating theatre

(2) Postoperative expectations:

(a) Incision (location)

(b) Chest tube

(c) Dressings

(d) Nasogastric tube

(e) Intravenous infusions

(f) Monitors

(g) Endotracheal tube, ventilator

(h) Suctioning

(i) Oxygen equipment

(j) Pain (ability to relieve)

(k) Bed scale (may fantasize that it is a stretcher to return child to the operating theatre)

(l) Appearance of intensive care unit; visiting regulations for parents.

c Have child practise coughing and deep breathing exercises (refer to procedure, p. 177).

d Detail, length, and time of explanations should be appropriate to the child's age and level of cognitive development.

(1) Photographs and a miniature replica of the intensive care unit may facilitate understanding of explanations.

(2) Older children and parents often benefit from an opportunity to see the intensive care unit.

(3) It is helpful for some children to have an opportunity to manipulate some of the equipment which will be used.

e Test the child's comprehension of teaching by asking him simple questions, having him place equipment on a doll, demonstrating coughing and deep breathing, and other similar activities.

f Allow opportunity for the child to express his concerns, either verbally or in play situations.

3 Provide opportunity for private discussions with the parents about the anticipated surgery.

a Parents need the same type of information as their child. They also need information about the following:

(1) Scheduled time of surgery

(2) Whether or not they can accompany their child to the operating theatre

(3) Waiting area

(4) Usual length of surgery

(5) Intensive care unit expectations and policies, facilities for staying overnight, availability of meals, etc.

b Provide emotional support to parents and answer their questions so that they are in the best position to support their child.

(1) Parents may need help dealing with guilt feelings that they had a role in causing the disease, that they did not seek medical advice soon enough, etc.

(2) Parents frequently have fears that the child will suffer excessive pain or die.

(3) Parents may ask technical questions relating to such matters as the heart-lung machine, and the type of material used for patching defects.

(4) Parents are sometimes hesitant about signing the consent form for cardiac surgery, especially if the child is asymptomatic.

4   Observe closely and report any signs of infection or inflammation (upper respiratory infection, hoarseness, pyrexia, vomiting, diarrhoea, skin lesions, etc.).

5   Perform appropriate nursing activities associated with congenital heart disease (refer to pp. 383-390).

Postoperative

1   Send the nursing history and care plan to the intensive care unit and discuss the child and family with appropriate personnel to ensure continuity of care.

2   Refer to Intensive Care, p. 73.

3   Be aware of specific complications which may occur following surgery for the following congenital heart lesions.

a Patent ductus arteriosus (rare)

(1) Recurrent laryngeal nerve injury

b Coarctation of the aorta

(1) Paradoxical hypertension

c Atrial septal defect

(1) Atrial arrhythmias

(2) Transient or permanent heart block

d Ventricular septal defect (VSD)

(1) Complete heart block

(2) Recurrent VSD

e Tetralogy of Fallot

(1) Low cardiac output

(2) Pulmonary insufficiency

(3) Complete heart block

(4) Recurrent VSD

(5) Residual pulmonary outflow tract obstruction

f Transposition of great arteries (Mustard procedure)

(1) Superior vena cava obstruction

(2) Pulmonary venous obstruction, pulmonary oedema

(3) Complete heart block

(4) Residual atrial shunts

(5) Arrhythmias

g Aortic stenosis

(1) Aortic insufficiency.

4 Support parents during the time that the child is in the intensive care unit.

a Accompany parents when they first visit their child following surgery. Since this may be traumatic, do not force them to maintain lengthy contact with the child.

b Address parental concerns and answer questions such as:

(1) How they should react to their child

(2) Amount of parental participation that is beneficial

(3) Fears and fantasies during the lengthy periods of waiting

(4) Concern for other children and families

(5) Technical questions

c Provide the parents with the phone number of the intensive care unit if they elect to leave.

d Make certain that parents have a comfortable place to sleep if they elect to stay at the hospital.

e Reassure parents that it is normal for children to regress following such extensive surgery. Explain what this might mean with an appropriate example.

Following Transfer

The following considerations apply to the child who has been transferred from the intensive care unit:

1 Observe for late complications.

a Respiratory

(1) Continue coughing and deep breathing exercises.

(2) Ambulate child as tolerated.

b Infection

(1) Monitor temperature at regular intervals.

(2) Observe incision(s) for redness, swelling, drainage.

c Congestive heart failure

Refer to Nursing Objectives, p. 392.

2 Provide emotional support to child and parents:

a Explain procedures, medications, special diet to child and parent.

b Encourage the child to attend to his personal needs as he is able.

c Allow the child to make some decisions in order to give him a feeling of control.

d Provide the child with appropriate diversion and play materials.

e Encourage parental participation in the child's care.

(1) Teach parents those aspects of the child's care which they can assume (e.g. coughing and breathing exercises).

(2) Discuss usual convalescent expectations of patient with parents (e.g. fatigue, itching at incision, emotional reactions).

3   Prepare the child and parents for discharge.

a Active, parental participation in the child's care facilitates discharge teaching.

b Provide the family with oral and written discharge recommendations including:

(1) Activity restrictions.

(2) Care of incision.

(3) Medications — exact amount and times of administration.

(4) Special diet (low sodium is often indicated) and how this can be achieved.

Dietician will advise and provide suitable literature and diet sheets.

(5) Emotional reactions — child may demonstrate:

(a) Regression in toilet habits, feeding and other learned skills

(b) Nightmares

(c) Increased dependency

(d) Decreased appetite

(e) Demanding behaviour — need to set limits.

(6) Observation for complications:

(a) Fever

(b) Increased heart rate

(c) Chest pain

(d) Shortness of breath

(e) Problems with the incision

(f) Vomiting or diarrhoea.

c Ensure that the family health visitor is informed prior to discharge.

MYOCARDITIS

Myocarditis is an inflammatory disease of the heart. In some instances, the inflammatory process is confined to the myocardium (isolated myocarditis), while in other conditions, such as acute rheumatic carditis, myocarditis is part of a pancarditis.

Aetiology

1 Often unknown
2 Coxsackie B virus (most common paediatric cause)
3 Rheumatic fever
4 Other infectious agents — viruses, bacteria, fungi, spirochetes, rickettsiae, and parasites
5 Toxic causes — diptheria endotoxin, chemotherapeutic agents
6 Various multisystem diseases.

Clinical Manifestations

1 Variable, depending on age of child, extent of inflammation, and capacity of myocardium to recover; varies from total absence of clinical manifestations to sudden, unexpected death.
2 Neonate — often presents with sudden onset of congestive heart failure. Signs include respiratory distress, tachycardia, pale skin which is cool and clammy, peripheral cyanosis, diaphoresis, oedema, and enlarged liver.
3 Older child.
   a Onset may be rapid with sudden temperature elevation, dyspnoea, and rapid pulse.
   b Onset may often be insidious, with complaints of fatigue, low-grade fever, respiratory illness, malaise, and gradual development of cardiac findings.

Pathophysiology

1 The inflammatory process interferes with the effectiveness of myocardial contractility.
2 Cardiac enlargement occurs, and congestive heart failure frequently results.
3 Residual myocardial fibrosis may occur, causing subsequent myocardial insufficiency and cardiac enlargement.
4 Prognosis is related to age at onset, extent of inflammation, response to therapy, and presence or absence of recurrences.

Diagnostic Evaluation

1 Auscultation
   a Heart sounds often indistinct, muffled, or dull.
   b Systolic murmurs frequently present.
   c Gallop rhythm possible.
   d Pulmonary râles may be heard.
2 Palpation
   a Peripheral pulses often rapid, weak, thready.
   b May demonstrate pulsus alternans — a pulse in which there is a regular alternation of weak and strong beats.

c May have hepatomegaly.

3   Chest x-ray — shows generalized cardiomegaly involving all four chambers of the heart. Pulmonary venous congestion is often visualized, and pneumonitis may be present.

4   Electrocardiogram is variable; it often demonstrates low voltage QRS complex throughout all frontal and precordial leads. It may reveal arrhythmias, conduction disturbances, and S-T segment and T wave changes.

5   Laboratory tests — cultures of blood, stool, nose, and throat; serial antibody testing.

Nursing Objectives

To control the underlying disease causing myocarditis.

1   Administer specific therapy for treatable conditions such as diptheria, rheumatic fever, toxoplasmosis, and trichinosis.

2   Administer steroid therapy as prescribed by the paediatrician.
      a Be aware that steroids are generally not recommended except for the treatment of rheumatic myocarditis with cardiac failure — to suppress the inflammatory process associated with connective tissue disorders, or in situations that are considered life-threatening.
      b Prepare the child and his family for any expected side effects of steroid therapy:
         (1) Body appearance may change — e.g. rounding of facial contours
         (2) Localized fat deposits
         (3) Appearance of acne or excessive hair
         (4) Weight gain with linear markings appearing in the stretched skin.
      c Be aware of serious side effects of steroid therapy and report promptly:
         (1) Gastrointestinal bleeding, ulcer
         (2) Hypertension and the tendency to accumulate water and sodium within tissues
            (a) Provide a low sodium diet.
            (b) Weigh child daily — report sudden weight gain.
         (3) Diminished resistance to infection; may mask symptoms of infection.

Nursing Alert: Do not place child with an infectious disease in the ward with children receiving steroid therapy. Restrict visitors and personnel with infectious diseases from contact with the child.

To treat congestive heart failure.

1   Refer to section on congestive heart failure, p. 390.

2   Be aware that children with myocarditis frequently show increased sensitivity to digitalis and may require a lower dose. Assess for the toxic symptoms.

To observe for the development of cardiac arrhythmias.
1   Be aware that children with myocarditis are prone to develop arrhythmias.
2   Initiate continuous cardiac monitoring if there is evidence of the development of an arrhythmia. If appropriate, transfer the child to the intensive care unit.
3   Have equipment for resuscitation, cardiac defibrillation, and cardiac pacing available in the event of life-threatening arrhythmia.

To provide supportive nursing care to the severely ill or dying child.
Refer to section on the dying child, p. 89.

To evaluate the child for evidence of response to treatment or progression of disease.
1   Observe for the development or disappearance of signs of congestive heart failure.
2   Monitor and record child's pulse, respirations, and blood pressure at frequent intervals.
    a   Count pulse for one full minute. Record rate and rhythm.
    b   Monitor the pulse when the child is asleep.

INFECTIVE ENDOCARDITIS
Infective endocarditis refers to infection of the endocardial surface of the heart or the intimal surface of certain arterial vessels. It is a rare condition which is usually associated with pre-existing cardiovascular disease (congenital or rheumatic) but may develop in a normal heart during a course of septicaemia.

Principles of Nursing Management
1   Although any child with heart disease is at risk for developing endocarditis, those most at risk are children with:
    a   Ventricular septal defect (especially a small VSD).
    b   Surgically created shunts such as Waterston or Blalock shunts.
    c   Patent ductus arteriosus.
    d   Semilunar valve stenoses.
    e   Coarctation of the aorta.
    f   Tetralogy of Fallot.
    g   Rheumatic heart disease.
2   Long-term (usually at least 4-6 weeks) intravenous administration of antibiotics is indicated in all cases.
    a   Careful management of intravenous therapy is essential.
    (1) Refer to Intravenous Therapy Procedure, p. 155.
    (2) Drugs must be administered according to schedule to maintain constant therapeutic levels.

(3) The paediatrician should be notified immediately if the intravenous infusion infiltrates into the tissues so that it can be restarted.

(4) Heparin locks may be utilized to allow the child freedom of movement between intervals of medication.

b Appropriate measures should be initiated to help the child maintain his level of development during the lengthy hospitalization.

(1) Refer to The Hospitalized Child, p. 56.

(2) Arrange for continuation of school work.

(3) Facilitate interaction with family, including siblings.

(4) Provide diversional activities that will help the child feel a sense of achievement and satisfaction.

(5) Facilitate contact with peers through written correspondence, telephone, or selected visiting.

3   Prevention is an important nursing responsibility.

a Procedures which increase the risk of bacteria gaining access to the bloodstream include:

(1) Tooth extraction, oral surgery, and periodontal procedures.

(2) Tonsillectomy and adenoidectomy.

(3) Bronchoscopy.

(4) Instrumentation of the genitourinary tract.

(5) Surgery or instrumentation of the lower gastrointestinal tract.

(6) Childbirth.

b Children with congenital or rheumatic heart disease should receive prophylactic antibiotics in conjunction with these procedures to reduce bacteraemia and prevent bacterial infection.

c The child and family should be instructed regarding the importance of good dental hygiene.

d Families of children with heart disease should be instructed about prevention of endocarditis, as well as about signs and symptoms of the disease.

FURTHER READING

Books

Forfar J O Arneil P (eds), *Textbook of Paediatrics,* Churchill Livingstone, 1984.

Hutchinson J, *Practical Paediatric Problems,* Lloyd Luke, 1980, Chapters 14 and 15.

Moss A J *et al., Heart Disease in Infants, Children and Adolescents,* Williams & Wilkins, 1977.

Petrillo M Sanger S, *Emotional Care of Hospitalized Children,* Lippincott, 1980, pp. 173-186.

Scipien G *et al., Comprehensive Paediatric Nursing,* McGraw-Hill, 1979.

Symposium on Pediatric Cardiology, *Pediatric Clinics of North America,* November 1978, 25 (4).

Articles

Botwin E, Should children be screened for hypertension? *Maternal Care Nursing Journal*, May/June 1976, 1: 152-159.

Chiswick M, Patent ductus arteriosus in premature babies, *British Medical Journal*, December 1981: 1490-1491.

Cogen R, Preventing complications during cardiac catheterization, *American Journal of Nursing*, March 1976, 76: 401-406.

Edwards M, Payton V, Cardiac catheterization: technique and teaching, *Nursing Clinics of North America*, June 1976, 11: 271-281.

Ferguson A W, Recognizing cardiac failure in infancy, *Update*, September 1979: 519-526.

Giboney G S, Ventricular septal defect, *Heart and Lung Journal*, May 1983: 292-299.

Hallidie-Smith K A, The significance of systolic murmurs in infancy and childhood, *Journal of Maternal and Child Health*, April 1979: 268-270.

Jordan S C, Heart disease in children, *Update*, October 1979: 933-944.

McCartney F, A better deal for newborns, with congenital heart disease, *Archives of Disease in Childhood*, April 1979: 268-270.

McKenzie S, Examination of children: cardiovascular system, *Journal of Maternal and Child Health*, June 1979: 232-234.

Posey R, Creative nursing care of babies with heart disease, *Nursing*, October 1974, 4: 40-45.

Ross A, Cardiac surgery in infants with congenital disorders, *Nursing*, December 1981, No. 32.

Scott O, The child with an innocent heart murmur, *Practitioner*, March 1978 : 403-405.

Sutherst J R, Fetal circulation, *Nursing Times*, March 1975: 413-415.

7

ALIMENTARY TRACT DISORDERS

DENTAL CARIES

Dental caries involves loss of tooth structure or the formation of a cavity as a result of bacterial attack — first on the enamel, which is the hard surface of the tooth, and then progressing inward towards the pulp.

Aetiology and Pathophysiology

Bacteria

1   Acidogenic organisms — decalcify the hard tissue by producing acids upon the tooth surface.
2   Proteolytic organisms — digest the product of tooth surface (decalcification thus produces odour and discoloration).
3   Leptotrichae organisms — form structures on the smooth tooth surface which houses acidogenic organisms.

Contributing Factors

1   Age — most susceptible age groups are children and adolescents.
2   Diet — large intake of simple sugars between meals.
3   Familial tendency to tooth decay.
4   Lack of proper oral hygiene.
5   Poor state of health (illness alters the normal bacteriostatic quality of saliva).

Clinical Manifestations

1   Decay is acute and rapidly penetrates the tooth in children.
2   Caries occurs where food debris collects:
    a Pits and fissures
    b Between teeth
    c At neck of tooth

3   Discoloration of teeth.
4   Decay odour.
5   Pain, abscess, or infection.

Treatment

1   Removal of decay and restoration of tooth surfaces involved.
2   Removal of diseased tooth or teeth that are decayed beyond restoration.

Complications

As a result of missing teeth or multiple caries, the child may experience many problems:
1   Poor nutrition
    a Refusal to eat foods that need chewing
    b Teeth drift and cause malocclusion
2   Faulty speech habits and articulation
    a Weak jaw muscles
    b Abnormal alveolar bone development
3   Psychological problems
       Embarrassment caused by appearance of teeth and oral odour
4   Oral foci of infection
       Subacute bacterial endocarditis may result in child with congenital heart disease.

Nursing Objectives and Health Teaching

Hospitalization of a child for treatment of dental caries is likely only when special behaviour difficulties are anticipated in treatment, when medical problems complicate dental treatment or when extensive repair is necessary.
(See Preventative Paediatrics, Dental Care, p. 46.)

To prevent dental caries in all patients.

To know that there is a direct relationship between incidence of dental caries in children and dental health education or knowledge of parents.

1   Assess parental knowledge and use opportunities to teach parents preventive care.
2   Encourage parental participation with the young child during teeth brushing exercise.

To know the principles of good oral hygiene and practise them when caring for each paediatric patient.

1   Encourage mouth rinsing or teeth brushing after eating.

Brush before bedtime to decrease bacteriogenic activity in the warm, undisturbed mouth during sleep.

2 Encourage proper brushing of teeth.

a Brush crosswise with a soft bristled brush.

b Electric tooth brush cleans teeth and stimulates the gingivae.

3 Supervise brushing in young children. (Dentrifice is not necessary.)

To know the value of good nutrition and its effect in preventing dental caries.

1 No in-between meal snacking of refined sugar foods. No gum chewing, except of sugar-less gum.

a Improves appetite at meals.

b Substitute fresh fruit for refined sugars. (No sweets between meals; give after meal before brushing.)

2 Discourage a bottle at bedtime or before sleep.

Residue is left on teeth during long periods of sleep and results in rampant decay.

To know the value of periodic dental examination and preventive measures used to decrease decay.

1 Encourage patient and parent to participate in regular dentist visits.

a Regular visits for cleaning and checking for decay; repair if necessary. First visit is to familiarize the young child with the dentist and equipment.

(1) Usually age 18-30 months — or when all primary teeth have erupted

(2) Should not be when child has toothache

b During childhood and adolescence visits are every 3-6 months. New decay appears suddenly in multiple area and advances rapidly.

2 If fluoridation is not supplied in community water, topical application is advisable.

a Most effective when applied on newly erupted teeth.

b Fluoride makes enamel more resistant to decay as it strengthens calcification of the developing dental tissue.

To keep the adolescent aware of his diet and its effect on dental decay.

1 Keep in mind diet fads and peer group pressure.

2 Have patient keep a dietary record for 1 week. Then evaluate it against an example of a good nutritious diet. Encourage patient to make his own evaluation.

Parental Teaching

1 After assessment of parental knowledge has been made, embark on teaching programme.

Main areas of concern:

    a Proper technique of dental hygiene
    b Value of good nutrition
    c Value of fluoridation
    d Importance of regular visits to the dentist every 3-6 months.
2 Further information can be obtained from:
    a British Dental Association, 64 Wimpole Street, London W1
    b General Dental Council, 37 Wimpole Street, London W1.

CLEFT LIP AND PALATE

Cleft lip and palate results when fusion involving the first brachial arch fails to take place during embryonic development. The incidence of cleft lip and palate in UK is approximately 1 per 1000 live births.

Aetiology

1 Failure of embryonic development — cause not known
2 Heredity factor: the siblings of a child with cleft lip have a 1 in 30 chance of being affected.

Altered Physiology

1 The lip and palate develop independently; thus, any combination of defects can occur.
    a Cleft lip
    (1) Varies from a notch in the lip to complete separation of the lip into the nose
    (2) May be unilateral or bilateral.
    b Isolated cleft palate
    (1) Cleft of uvula
    (2) Cleft of soft palate
    (3) Cleft of both soft and hard palate through roof of mouth
    (4) Unilateral or bilateral
    c Cleft lip and palate combined
    Any degree of involvement
    d Submucous cleft
    (1) Muscles of soft palate are not joined
    (2) Not recognized until child talks; cannot be seen at birth.
2 Associated problems
    a Eating
    (1) Suction cannot be created for effective sucking
    (2) Food returns through the nose
    b Nasal speech

c Lack of normal dental function and appearance

d Repeated bouts of otitis media with subsequent hearing loss.

Clinical Manifestations

1 Physical appearance of cleft lip or palate:
   a Incompletely formed lip
   b Opening in roof of mouth.

Nursing Objectives — Newborn

To show acceptance of the baby.

1 The nurse must maintain her composure and not show shock when handling the infant. The manner in which the nurse handles the baby can make a lasting impression on the parents.

   a The baby with a cleft lip can be unattractive and can cause shock when first seen.

   b When showing the baby to parents for the first time, support them by accepting both the baby and the parents' feelings. (Parents may be grieving about the perfect infant they did not have and may harbour ambivalent feelings about this baby.)

   c Be supportive of parents by reassuring them that reparative surgery can be done with much success. The surgeon and orthodontist cooperate closely, and treatment may not be complete until the child is fully grown.

   (1) The time when reparative surgery is done depends on the paediatric surgeon and the condition of the baby.

   (2) Lip surgery may be done several hours after birth or when the infant is 2-3 months of age or has gained 4.5 kg.

2 Surgery of the palate is done between 12 and 18 months of age. Prior to this a dental prosthesis may be fitted to align the parts of the maxilla which form the alveolar arch. Each time the baby sucks he presses on the prosthesis and through it on the maxillary bone, thus expanding the arch. After each feed, the prosthesis is removed and washed under a running tap. Oral toilet is carried out. The lips, gums, palate and nasal septum are inspected for any signs of pressure.

   At the age of 12-18 months, speech patterns have not been set, yet growth of involved structures allows for improved surgical repair.

To establish and maintain adequate nutrition for growth and development.

1 Encourage the mother to breast feed as soon as possible. Expressed breast milk may be given if infant is unable to latch-on and suck at the breast.

2 Babies with just a cleft lip may feed well if a regular teat with enlarged holes is used.

3   With certain types and combinations of cleft lips and palates, the baby is unable to create a vacuum and is thus unable to suck. However, when a prosthesis is fitted this problem is basically overcome. To make feeding easier, the following may be used:

    a Ordinary teat with enlarged holes.

    b Use of a double teat, i.e. one placed on top of the other.

4   Feed the baby in an upright sitting position to decrease possibility of fluid being aspirated or returned through the nose.

    a Burp frequently during feeding because these babies swallow a great deal of air.

    b Avoid repeated removal of teat from infant's mouth because of fear of choking, as this only frustrates the infant causing him to cry and increasing chances of aspiration.

5   Advance diet as appropriate for age and needs of the baby. Eating often improves when solids are introduced, since they are easier for baby to manipulate.

To prevent infection in the child so that surgery will not have to be delayed.

1   Avoid patient contact with anyone who has an infection.
2   Change the baby's position frequently.
3   Clean the cleft after each feeding with clear water and a cotton-tipped applicator.

To assist parents in preparing to take the newborn home from the nursery before lip and palate surgery has been done.

Health Teaching

1   Prepare mother for home feedings. She should have several days to practise feeding in order to become familiar with the baby's pattern.

    a Home equipment should be used in the hospital.

    b Mother should be aware of difficulties with feeding and how to handle them:

        (1) Infant feed returning through the nose

        (2) Respiratory distress

        (3) Longer time necessary for feeding.

    c Suggest that about a week or so prior to scheduled admission for surgery, mother begin using feeding technique preferred by the surgeon for postoperative feeding:

        (1) Side of spoon

        (2) Toddler cup.

2   Encourage parents to prepare siblings at home for the arrival of this baby if they have been unable to visit. (Pictures of the new baby might be suggested.)

3   Initiate a referral to the family's health visitor to continue emotional support and teaching programme at home.

4   Parents should know what plans have been started for surgical treatment.
5   Social work referral may be indicated.
   a To listen to mother express her concerns regarding management at home with a handicapped child.

To be aware of the complexity of long-range care and the importance of the many disciplines involved in the eventual outcome.

The nurse should know all the ramifications and potential problems for this child and his family.

1   The organization of trained professional people from the many disciplines that become involved include: paediatrician, plastic surgeon, general dentist, orthodontist, medical-social worker, nurse, speech therapist and psychologist.
2   Long-term follow-up and reparative surgery:
   a Chronic otitis media and hearing loss
   b Lip, palate, and orthodontic repair
   c Speech therapy
   d Psychological insult to the child.
3   Financial burden on the family, e.g. due to loss of overtime earnings because of frequent visiting, cost of rates, etc.
4   Psychological trauma to the family.

To emphasize the importance of the mother's role in caring for the child during outpatient treatment and the many hospitalizations required.

Mother can offer a great deal of security to the child when he is subjected to the trauma and frightening experiences of treatment.

Preoperative Care of the Child with a Cleft Lip

To prepare the infant for postoperative care so that it will be familiar to him, less frightening and easier for him to accept after surgery.

1   Practise the feeding method to be used as preferred by the surgeon:
   a Toddler cup
   b Side of spoon.
2   The use of elbow restraints for short periods of time:
   a Let the child play with them if he is old enough.
   b Allow mother to become involved in their use.
3   Help the infant get used to being on his back or propped on his side for long periods of time.

To prepare the mother (parents) as to what to expect when she sees the child postoperatively.

1   Explain the use of the Logan bow (a curved metal wire that prevents stress on the suture line) and restraints.

2 Encourage mother to be with the infant especially when he wakes up from anaesthesia to offer him security and comfort.

Postoperative Care of the Child with a Cleft Lip

To administer good postoperative care based on general principles and to observe for usual postoperative complications.

To prevent injury to the suture line of the lip.

1 Elbow restraints are the most effective way to prevent busy hands from reaching the lip, yet still allow some freedom of movement.
   a Pad restraint and place it from the axilla to inner aspect of the wrist.
   b Remove restraints occasionally, one at a time, to exercise the arms.
2 Logan bow, Elastoplast or Band-Aid placed cheek-to-cheek across top of lip prevents lateral tension.
   Prevent wetting tape, or it will loosen.
3 Prevent baby from crying, because crying also increases tension on the suture line.
   a Encourage mother to hold and cuddle infant.
   b Keep the infant dry, fed, and comfortable.
4 Position infant on his back or propped on his side to keep him from rubbing his lip on the sheets. An infant seat may be useful for variety in position, comfort, and entertainment. Provide for appropriate diversional activity, hanging toys, mobiles, etc.

To maintain adequate nutrition and fluid intake for weight gain, growth and prevention of dehydration.

1 Postoperatively feeding will have to be accomplished without tension on the suture line.
   a The first feed postoperatively should be dextrose.
   b Use side of spoon (never put spoon in mouth), toddler cup.
   As the baby should have been introduced to the feeding method of choice preoperatively, little difficulty should be met.
2 Advance slowly to bottle (breast) feeding as indicated by the surgeon's preference, usually after about 72 hours. Baby should be encouraged to suck more efficiently with the lip repaired.
3 Encourage mother to participate as much as possible in the care of the infant. It is good for both infant and mother to continue their relationship.

To keep the suture line clean, to decrease infection and remove crust formation which enlarges the resulting scar.

1 The sutures are removed 3-14 days after surgery. Clean suture line at least twice a day with normal saline.

2 Gently dry by patting. May be left open to the air.
3 Water should be given after feeding to clean the mouth. Excessive salivation may occur and saliva may dribble down the chin causing excoriation. Drying and applying a barrier cream will help to prevent this.

Preoperative Care of the Child with a Cleft Palate

Before admission to hospital for cleft palate repair, the nurse should ensure that the mother has taught her child to drink from a cup. In order to promote healing of the palate repair bottle feeds or a dummy should not be given.

To be familiar with growth and development as well as the emotional and psychological needs of the toddler, 12-18 months old. (This is the age most common for palate repair.)

1 Primary objectives for palate repair are to improve speech and dental function.
2 This toddler age is selected because the anatomical structures involved are still growing.
3 The toddler finds the hospital strange and frightening. (See p. 60.)
   a Encourage mother to stay with the child if possible.
   b Encourage play.

To prepare the child for postoperative care; if he is familiar with the procedures and routines he will be less frightened and more likely to cooperate.

1 Use elbow restraints frequently for short periods of time. Allow child to handle these.
2 Feed him in the manner in which he will be fed postoperatively.

To prevent infection by keeping the child away from anyone with infection.

To prepare the parents as to what to expect when they see the child postoperatively.

Include the parents in the preparation of the child. Then, with the parents alone discuss in more depth what to expect.

Postoperative Care of the Child with a Cleft Palate

To administer good postoperative care and to observe for possible postoperative complications.

1 Breathing with a closed palate is different from child's customary way of breathing.
2 Note respiratory effort.
3 Croup tent with mist may be used. This decreases occurrence of respiratory problems and provides moisture to mucous membranes which may become dry because of mouth breathing.

To prevent injury to the suture line in the mouth.

1   Use elbow restraints.
2   Do not put anything into the mouth. Do not allow the use of straws, eating utensils, fingers.
3   Prevent the child from crying. Blowing, sucking, talking, and laughing put strain on suture line.

To keep the suture line and mouth clean to prevent infection.

1   Keep mouth moist to promote healing and provide comfort.
2   Rinse mouth after each feeding.

To maintain adequate nutrition for growth and to promote healing.

1   Diet progresses from clear liquids to full liquids to soft foods
       Soft foods are usually continued for about 1 month after surgery at which time regular diet is started, excluding hard food.
2   Check weight periodically to see if adequate nutrition is being maintained.
3   Feed the child in the manner used preoperatively (cup, side of spoon). Never use straw, teat, plain syringe.

To administer antibiotics as prescribed.

The mouth and suture line are constantly contaminated.

To provide opportunities for social relationships and play as soon as possible.

1   While the child must be restrained, he especially needs to have some stimulation and diversional activity.
2   The continued presence of the mother and a satisfactory relationship with the nurse can minimize frustration and discomfort from surgery and restraints.

To continue support of parents who have already encountered many frustrations in caring for the child, and to foster continual parental acceptance of the child and his handicap.

1   Solicit assistance of social worker if appropriate; mother may talk about problems she is having raising a handicapped child.
2   Sincerely compliment the parents for the good work they have already done with this child.
3   Help parents understand that this child can live a normal life in the community.

To begin discharge planning and health teaching soon after admission so parents can learn how to care for the child at home.

1   Continued protection of the mouth.
       a May need to use elbow restraints, particularly at night time during sleep for a few weeks.

b Child this age will put everything into mouth — restrict this. Provide diversional activities.

c No sucking or blowing.

2 Diet of soft foods will need to be continued. Do not give lollipops.

3 Infection must be prevented.

Continue to clean mouth after eating.

Parental Teaching

1 There are three specific periods when parental teaching is vitally important for continual, effective management of the child:

a Management of the child with cleft lip and palate not yet repaired

b Preparing for lip or palate surgery

c Preparing for patient's discharge following surgery.

2 In each case specific instructions need to be given in the following areas:

a Good nutrition and feeding techniques

b Proper oral hygiene

c Prevention of injury to operative site

d Prevention of infection

e Plan for follow-up, especially after surgery

f Psychological and social development of child — including speech therapy.

3 Other members of the family must be considered.

a The child with a cleft lip or palate should not be thought of as sick, but as a child who has special needs to promote his individual growth and development. But he does not require attention all the time.

b The family should be included in his care, but they also must have a life of their own.

c The parents need time to themselves.

4 Help the parents realize that even though rehabilitation of the child is long drawn-out, the child can live a normal life.

Long-range planning should include detailed communication between the family and various disciplines.

(1) Collaborative effort between disciplines determines the effectiveness of each discipline.

(2) Parents may need help in understanding the value of each discipline for the future well-being of their child.

Speech therapy is often one area where the value is not completely understood.

OESOPHAGEAL ATRESIA WITH TRACHEO-OESOPHAGEAL FISTULA

Oesophageal atresia is failure of the oesophagus to form a continuous passage from the pharynx to the stomach during embryonic development. *Tracheo-oesophageal fistula* is the abnormal connection between the trachea and oesophagus.

Incidence

One in 3000 live births in the UK.

Aetiology

1   Failure of embryonic development
2   Cause unknown in most cases.

Clinical Manifestations

1   Pregnancy complicated by hydramnios
2   Low birth weight
3   Excessive amount of secretions
   a Constant drooling
   b Large amount of secretions from nose
4   Intermittent cyanosis
      Aspiration of accumulated saliva in blind pouch
5   Abdominal distension
      Inspired air from trachea passes through fistula into stomach.
6   If fed, the infant will respond violently after first or second swallow.
   a Infant coughs and chokes.
   b Fluid returns through nose and mouth.
   c Cyanosis occurs.
   d Infant struggles.
7   Inability to pass catheter through nose or mouth into stomach — tip of catheter will stop at blind pouch, or atresia.
Note: Be aware of coiling of catheter; coiling may make catheter *appear* to be descending into stomach.

Pathophysiology

Classification of Oesophageal Atresia

Type I   Proximal and distal segments of oesophagus are blind; there is no connection to trachea — 10-15% of cases.
Type II   Proximal segment of oesophagus opens into trachea by a fistula; distal segment is blind — very rare.

Type III   Proximal segment of oesophagus has blind end; distal segment of oesophagus connects into trachea by a fistula (most common; discussion is limited to this type — 80-90% of cases).

Type IV   Oesophageal atresia with fistula between both proximal and distal ends of trachea and oesophagus — very rare.

Type V   Both proximal and distal segments of oesophagus open into trachea by a fistula; no oesophageal atresia (H-type) — not usually diagnosed at birth.

Type III — Tracheo-oesophageal Fistula (TOF)

1   Child is unable to swallow effectively.
2   Saliva or formula accumulates in upper oesophageal pouch and is aspirated into airway from spillover.
3   Regurgitation of gastric acid through distal fistula.
   a Abdominal distension occurs as a result of air entering the lower oesophagus via the fistula and passing into the stomach, especially when child is crying.
   b Gastric distension may be severe enough to cause respiratory distress by elevation of the diaphragm.

Diagnostic Evaluation

1   Recognize infants at risk for TOF. Two major groups are at risk:
   a Infants with polyhydramnios
   b Low birth weight infants.
2   Observations of specific symptoms manifested by infant.
3   Inability to pass a stiff, radio-opaque 10-14 Fr. catheter into stomach through nose or mouth.
4   X-ray, flat plate of abdomen and chest — reveals presence of gas in stomach and tip of catheter in blind pouch.

Complications Associated with TOF

1   Pneumonitis — secondary to: (a) salivary aspiration, (b) gastric acid reflux
2   Concomitant lesions
   a Congenital heart disease
   b Gastrointestinal anomalies, particularly imperforate anus
   c Skeletal and muscular deformities
3   Low birth weight

Treatment

1   Immediate treatment:
   a Propping infant to prevent reflux
   b Suctioning of upper oesophageal pouch.

2   Appropriate treatment of any existing pathological processes — either acquired complications, such as pneumonitis, or complications from concomitant lesions, such as congestive heart failure.

3   Surgery

   a Prompt primary repair: division of fistula and oesophageal anastomosis of proximal and distal segments.

   b Short-term delay — subsequent primary repair: used to stabilize infant and to prevent deterioration when patient's condition contraindicates immediate surgery.

   c Staging: initial fistula division and gastrostomy with later secondary oesophageal anastomosis. Approach may be used with very small preterm infant, very sick neonate, or when severe congenital anomalies exist.

Nursing Objectives — Preoperative

To position baby with head and chest elevated 20-30° to prevent or decrease reflux of gastric juices into the tracheobronchial tree.

This position may also ease respiratory effort by dropping distended intestines away from the diaphragm.

Prone position will allow gastric juices to pool anteriorly away from oesophagus. Turn frequently to prevent atelectasis and pneumonia.

To assist in removing nasopharyngeal secretions from oesophageal blind pouch and to support infant's respiration.

1   Intermittent nasopharyngeal suctioning or indwelling Replogle tube (double lumen tube) or sump tube with constant suction is used.

   a Tip of tube is placed in the blind pouch.

   b Replogle or sump tube allows air to be drawn in via a second lumen and prevents tube obstruction by mucous membrane of pouch.

   c Maintain indwelling tube patency by irrigating with 1 ml normal saline frequently.

   d Change indwelling tube as needed and at least once every 12-24 hours; alternate nostrils. Take care to prevent necrosis of nostrils from pressure by catheter.

2   Place infant in incubator or radiant warmer with high humidity to aid in liquefying secretions and thick mucus. Give mouth care.

3   Administer oxygen as needed.

4   Be alert for indications of respiratory distress:

   a Retractions

   b Circumoral cyanosis

   c Restlessness

   d Nasal flaring

   e Increased respiration and heart rate.

To administer antibiotics and other medications prescribed.

Give to prevent or treat associated pneumonitis.

To monitor parenteral fluids as prescribed in order to prevent dehydration and electrolyte imbalance (see p. 149).

1   Supplies water, kilojoule (calories) and mineral requirements.
2   The infant does not receive oral feedings.

To observe infant carefully for any change in condition; report changes immediately.

1   Check vital signs, colour, amount of secretions, abdominal distension, and respiratory distress.
2   Also be alert for complications that can occur in any neonate or preterm infant.

To prevent infection by using the principles of isolation.

Incubator may be used for environmental isolation.

To be available and to recognize need for emergency care or resuscitation.

Accompany infant to x-ray or operating room in an incubator with portable oxygen and suction equipment.

To administer supportive nursing care that will prevent any deterioration of infant's condition and will assist in preparation for surgery.

1   Careful observations, recording and reporting of any signs or symptoms that may indicate additional congenital anomalies or complications.
2   Maintain infant temperature in thermoneutral zone.
3   Gastrostomy tube may be placed prior to definitive surgery to aid in gastric decompression and prevention of reflux.

Postoperative Care

There are two types of surgery considered for oesophageal atresia with tracheo-oesophageal fistula: (1) fistula division and oesophageal anastomosis (called *primary repair*) and (2) palliative surgery temporarily using a gastrostomy and cervical oesophagostomy until the infant gains weight so that a bowel transplant or anastomosis can be done. Generally the nursing care is essentially the same for either procedure.

To administer good postoperative care and to observe for signs of possible complications.

To maintain a patent airway to prevent oxygen starvation, apnoea, and aspiration of secretions.

1   Request that surgeon mark a suction catheter, indicating how far the catheter can be safely inserted without disturbing the anastomosis.

a Suction frequently — every 5-10 minutes may be necessary; at least every 1-2 hours.

b Observe for signs of obstructed airway.

2   Administer chest physiotherapy.

a Change infant's position by turning; stimulate him to cry so that he fully expands his lungs.

b Head and shoulders elevated 20-30°.

c Mechanical vibrator (to minimize trauma to anastomosis) may be used 2-3 days postoperatively followed by more vigorous physical therapy after third day. Care should be taken not to hyperextend the neck, thus causing stress to operative site.

3   Continue use of incubator or radiant warmer with humidity. Either device does the following:

a Provides an environment in which infant can maintain temperature in thermoneutral zone.

b Provides humidity to liquefy secretions.

c Allows for observation of and easy access to infant.

4   Be prepared to function in an emergency.

Have emergency equipment available:

(1) Suction machine, catheter

(2) Oxygen

(3) Laryngoscope, endotracheal tubes in varying sizes.

To be aware of type of chest drainage present, which may be determined by surgical approach, and provide appropriate care.

1   Retropleural — small tube in posterior mediastinum; may be left open for drainage.

2   Transthoracic — chest tube placed in pleural space and connected to suction.

a Keep tubing free from clots; keep it unkinked and without tension.

b If break occurs in the closed drainage system, clamp tubing close to infant immediately to prevent pneumothorax.

To assist in maintaining adequate nutrition to promote healing, growth, and development.

Feedings may be given by gastrostomy, or nasogastric tube into the stomach, depending upon the type of operation performed and the infant's condition.

1   Gastrostomy feeding

a Gastrostomy feeding can be started prior to oesophageal healing — adequate nutrition is an important factor in healing.

b Gastrostomy feedings may be continued until infant can tolerate full feedings orally.

c Care should be taken not to allow air to enter stomach, thereby causing gastric distension and possible reflux.

d Check with surgeon before allowing infant to suck on dummy during gastrostomy feeding.

2   Nasogastric feeding — see p. 130.
  a Tube should be aspirated hourly.
  b Left on free drainage for 24 hours after operation.
  c Displacement of tube is prevented by passing atraumatic silk through tube at nostril level then tape silk to cheeks.
3   Oral feedings may begin 6-14 days postoperatively following anastomosis.
  a Feed slowly to allow infant time to swallow.
  b Use upright sitting position.
  c Burp frequently.
  d Demand feeding may be more successful and pleasant for the infant than strictly scheduled feeding.
  e Do not allow infant to become overtired at feeding time. Note cardiac rate.
  f Try to make each feeding a pleasant experience for the infant.

To care appropriately for cervical oesophagostomy.

1   Keep the area clean of saliva.
  a Wash with clear water.
  b Place an absorbent pad over the area.
2   As soon as possible allow infant to suck a few millilitres of milk at the same time gastrostomy feeding is being done. Advance infant to solid foods as appropriate if oesophagostomy is maintained for a few months.
  a Encourage sucking and swallowing.
  b Familiarize infant with food, so that when he is able to eat orally, he will be used to it.
3   If neck skin becomes sore, a swab should be cultured to isolate causative organisms. Commonly due to *Candida*, therefore local nystatin treatment should be given.

To be aware of impending complications of oesophageal repair.

1   Leak at the anastomosis (development of mediastinitis, pneumothorax, and saliva in chest tube).
  a Hypothermia or hyperthermia
  b Pneumothorax
    (1) Severe respiratory distress
    (2) Cyanosis
    (3) Restlessness
    (4) Weak pulses
2   Stricture at the anastomosis
  a Difficulty in swallowing
  b Vomiting or spitting up of ingested fluid
  c Refusing to eat
  d Fever — secondary to aspiration and pneumonia
3   Recurrent fistula

    a Coughing, choking, and cyanosis associated with feeding
    b Excessive salivation
    c Difficulty in swallowing associated with abnormal distension
    d Repeated episodes of pneumonitis
    e General poor physical condition — no weight gain
4   Atelectasis or pneumonitis
    a Aspiration
    b Respiratory distress.

To provide for the infant's emotional and social needs.

To the extent of hospitalization and long-term care puts a strain on the normal opportunities in these areas (see Intensive Care Nursing, p. 81).
1   Hold and cuddle infant for feedings and/or after feedings.
2   Encourage mother (parents) to cuddle and love infant.
3   Provide for visual, auditory, and tactile stimulation as appropriate for infant's physical condition and age.

To encourage parental participation in learning to care for and handle the infant and to foster acceptance of the child by his parents and family.

1   Provide opportunities for the parents to learn all aspects of care of their baby.
2   Initiate a teaching programme for the parents early. Offer them available literature and help them become familiar with community resources.
3   Initiate a referral to health visitor or district nurse, for continuity of care in the home.
4   Encourage parents to talk about their feelings, fears, and concerns.
5   Help to develop a healthy parent-child relationship.
    a One parent should be resident.
    b Frequent visiting, if unable to be resident.
    c Phone calls to ward staff.
    d Physical contact of child and parents.
    e Encourage other members of the family to visit.

Parental Teaching

1   Teach carefully and thoroughly all procedures to be done at home. Show parents how; then watch return demonstration of the following procedures:
    a Gastrostomy feedings and care
    b Oesophagostomy care with feeding technique
    c Suctioning.
2   Help parents understand the psychological needs of the infant for sucking, warmth, comfort, stimulation, and love. Suggest that activity be appropriate for age.
3   Encourage parents to keep outpatient appointments and help them learn to recognize possible problems:

a Dilatation of oesophagus to treat stricture at the site of the anastomosis
b Raspy cough for 6-24 months
c Eating problems, especially when solids are introduced
d Repeated respiratory tract infection
e Occurrence of stricture at site of anastomosis weeks to months later — recognized by difficulty in swallowing; spitting of ingested fluid; fever.
4   Help parents understand the need for good nutrition.

HYPERTROPHIC PYLORIC STENOSIS

Hypertrophic pyloric stenosis is congenital, progressive hypertrophy of the muscle of the pylorus, causing partial obstruction of the stomach outlet.

Clinical Manifestations

Onset is within the first 2 months after birth. Far more common in males; the ratio is 6-7 males : 1 female. Usually manifests after first 2 weeks of life during which the infant appears to thrive.
1   Vomiting — onset may be gradual and intermittent or sudden and forceful. The following characteristics may be noted:
     a Occasional, nonprojectile vomiting at first, gradually increasing in frequency and intensity
     b Projectile vomiting, not bile-stained
2   Constipation — decreased quantity of stools
3   Loss of weight or failure to gain weight
4   Visible gastric peristaltic waves, left to right
5   Excessive hunger — willingness to eat immediately after vomiting
6   Dehydration — electrolyte disturbance with alkalosis
7   Decreased urinary output
8   Palpable pyloric tumour in upper right quadrant of abdomen.

Altered Physiology

1   Increase in size of the circular musculature of the pylorus with thickening (size and shape of an olive). The pylorus muscle becomes elongated and thickened and is enlarged — about twice the usual size.
2   Hypertrophy of the pylorus musculature occurs with narrowing of the pyloric lumen.
3   Constriction of the lumen of the pyloric canal (at the distal end of the stomach to become dilated).
4   Gastric emptying is delayed; vomiting after feeding and obstruction also occur.

Diagnostic Evaluation

1 Palpation of pyloric mass ('olive') in conjunction with persistent, projectile vomiting with associated alkalosis. Observation of peristaltic waves passing from left to right across the infant's upper abdomen whilst feeding.
2 Tests for metabolic alkalosis — due to loss of hydrochloric acid and potassium from vomiting
  a Serum sodium — increases
  b Serum chloride — decreases
  c Serum potassium — decreases
  d Serum pH — increases above 7
  e Serum CO^2 — increases.
3 Routine urinalysis — urine becomes alkaline and concentrated.
4 Blood haematocrit and haemoglobin — elevated due to haemo-concentration.
5 Flat film of abdomen — dilated, air-filled stomach, nondilated pyloric canal.
6 X-ray examination with barium
  a Narrowing of pyloric canal
  b Delayed gastric emptying time
  c Enlarged stomach
  d Increased peristaltic waves
  e Gas distal to stomach.

Treatment

Treatment may be medical or surgical. Whilst Rammstedt's operation is the treatment of choice, medical treatment can be successful with the use of atropine methonitrate before feeds. However, most centres reserve medical treatment for mild cases, those infants who do not develop symptoms until 6-8 weeks of life or for those who have other abnormalities, as it may be necessary to maintain treatment for several weeks leading to prolonged hospitalization.

Nursing Objectives — Preoperative Care

To assist in restoring hydration and electrolyte balance.

1 Intravenous therapy is usually initiated (see p. 155). Electrolytes are added to solution for replacement.
2 Careful observation of output, amount and characteristics.
  a Urine (check specific gravity)
  b Vomiting
  c Stools.
3 Accurate daily weight — serves as a guide for calculating need for parenteral fluid.

To prevent or decrease the likelihood of vomiting.

1   A gastric washout with normal saline immediately prior to surgery to remove gastric residue. Nasogastric tube is then left in position on free drainage.
2   Oral feedings may be continued, if surgery is delayed.
    a Feed small, frequent feedings, slowly.
    b Burp frequently.
3   Proper positioning.
        Prop patient in upright position.
        (1) Elevate head of bed, mattress, or infant seat at a 75-80° angle.
        (2) Place slightly on right side — to aid in gastric emptying.
        (3) Handle gently and minimally after feeding.

To make frequent, accurate observations of the infant's condition.

1   Dehydration
2   Vomiting
3   Stools and urine output
4   Vital signs.

Nursing Alert: Respiratory rate may be irregular with apnoea when patient is in severe alkalosis.

To provide comfort for the infant.

1   Mouth care — wet lips
        Let infant suck on dummy.
2   Physical contact or nearness of the mother or nurse.
3   Audio or visual stimulation may be soothing.
4   Minimal palpation of pyloric olive — will decrease risk of postoperative wound infection from bruising abdominal wall and excoriation of tissue in operative site.

To support parents who are usually very concerned and worried.

1   Mother may feel guilty, i.e. she may feel she has a poor feeding technique.
        Help her understand that she did not do anything to cause this deformity.
2   Prepare parents for surgery of their child.
    a Be honest with them.
    b Inform them of the expected postoperative appearance of the infant.
    c Show them where the operating room and recovery room are located and where to wait during surgery.
3   Encourage parents to maintain a good relationship with the infant. Allow them to hold infant.
4   Encourage them to get some rest.
        Mother may be tired and frustrated because of the extensive care she has had to give to the child.

Postoperative Care

To give good postoperative care and to observe for the usual postoperative complications (see p. 85).

To monitor parenteral fluids in order to maintain hydration.
Intravenous therapy may in some instances be continued until adequate oral intake is obtained.

To assist in resuming oral feedings.
1 Feeding is usually resumed 2-6 hours after operation.
   a Feedings usually start with small, frequent feedings of glucose water and slowly advance to full-strength milk feeds. The breast-fed infant is put to the breast 4 hours after operation, but allowed only half of normal time. Gradually, over the next 24 hours, the time is extended to normal.
   b Report any vomiting — the amount and characteristics.
   c Feed slowly and burp frequently.
   d Note how feeding is taken and if food is retained.
   e The amount of feeding is increased as the time interval between feedings is lengthened.
2 Continue to elevate infant's head and shoulders after feeding for 45-60 minutes for several feedings after surgery.
       Place on right side to aid gastric emptying.
3 Regurgitation may continue for a short period after surgery.

To encourage parents to resume care — especially feeding — of their infant.
1 This will help to restore their confidence in caring for their baby.
2 This activity provides an opportunity for the nurse to teach.
3 If the mother was breast feeding resume this as soon as possible.

Parental and Health Teaching

1 Help parents to understand that surgery has corrected the pyloric stenosis.
   a Discharge of baby will be from 2-5 days after operation when the baby is gaining weight.
   b Proper care of the operative site can be done by the mother. Sutures are removed (if nonabsorbable materials have been used) at home by the district nurse.
2 Since this may be a new mother, and the infant may be under 6 weeks of age, the mother may need help with routine infant care. Inform health visitor prior to discharge.

COELIAC DISEASE

Coeliac disease, also called gluten-induced enteropathy, 'is a permanent inability to tolerate dietary wheat and rye gluten.'*

Aetiology

1   Unknown. Although the relationship of gluten to mucosal abnormalities is established, the way in which these mucosal changes occur is not clear.
2   Genetics
   a Familial incidence
   b Mode of inheritance is not clear, probably autosomal recessive with incomplete penetrance.
3   Environmental inference likely — role of other 'allergens' unclear.
4   Current theories being investigated include the following:
   a Immunological (autoimmune vs. specific immune abnormality)
   b Search to identify deficient enzymes that digest gluten.

Clinical Manifestations

The age and mode of presenting signs and symptoms are extremely variable. Diagnosis is most commonly made by 6-24 months of age; however, it can be made in the adult.
1   3-9 months of age
   a Acutely ill
   b Severe diarrhoea and vomiting
   c Failure to thrive.
2   9-18 months of age (age when 'typical' coeliac appearance is seen)
   a Impaired growth
     (1) Normal growth during early months of life
     (2) Slackening of weight and weight loss follow
   b Abnormal stools
     (1) Pale
     (2) Soft
     (3) Bulky
     (4) Having offensive odour
     (5) Greasy — steatorrhoea
     (6) May increase in number
   c Abdominal distension
   d Anorexia
   e Muscle wasting — most obvious in buttocks and proximal parts of limbs
   f Hypotonia
   g Mood changes — ill humour, irritability, temper tantrums, shyness
   h Mild clubbing of fingers
   i Vomiting — often occurring in evening

* Anderson C M, Burke V, *Paediatric Gastroenterology*, Blackwell Scientific Publications, 1975, p. 175

3 Older child

    a Signs and symptoms often related to nutritional or secondary deficiencies resulting from disease.

    b May have abnormal stools and growth impairment.

    c May have colicky abdominal pain with constipation and large, pale stools.

4 Manifestations secondary to malabsorption

    a Anaemia

    b Hypoproteinaemia with oedema

    c Hypocalcaemia

    d Hypoprothrombinaemia — resulting from impaired vitamin K absorption

    e Disaccharide intolerance — with acid-sugar containing stools (secondary to the altered small bowel mucosa).

5 Coeliac crisis — most often seen in very young child and toddler (although rare)

    a Profound anorexia

    b Severe vomiting and diarrhoea

    c Weight loss

    d Marked dehydration and acidosis

    e Immobility

    f Grossly distended abdomen

        (1) Fluid rattle is present.

        (2) Abdomen flattens with passage of large liquid stool.

        (3) Patient appears shock-like.

    g Looks profoundly depressed.

Pathophysiology

1 Characteristics of coeliac disease include

    a Impaired intestinal absorption

    b Histological abnormalities of the small intestine

    c Clinical and histological improvement with wheat- and rye-free (possibly also barley- and oat-free) diet

    d Recurrence of clinical manifestations and histological changes after reintroduction of dietary gluten.

2 Histological changes in mucosa of small bowel, especially duodenum and jejunum resulting from dietary gluten include

    a Irregularity of epithelial cells

    b Loss of normal villous pattern

    c Obliteration of intervillous spaces which are infiltrated with plasma cells and eosinophils

    d Loss of epithelial cell brush border.

3 This mucosal damage results in

    a Disaccharidase deficiency

b Depression of peptidase activity.
4   Subsequent malabsorption probably results from
    a Decreased area of absorption in small bowel
    b Impaired enzyme activity.
5   The severity of symptoms of the disease depends upon the length of intestine with histological changes.
    a The extent of affected intestine is variable.
    b Generally, proximal small intestine mucosal damage is most severe and condition decreases in severity distally.

Diagnosis

1   Thorough evaluation of history and general status of child
2   Small bowel biopsy using a Crosby capsule — demonstrates abnormal mucosa
3   Determination of fat absorption
4   Measurement of haemoglobin levels — reduced
5   Prothrombin time — before intestinal biopsy
6   Radiological studies — skeletal x-rays commonly show
    a Demineralization
    b Retarded bone age.
7   Evaluation of clinical and histological response to withdrawal of and reintroduction of gluten. Reintroduction of gluten is indicated when:
    a Diagnosis was made on clinical manifestations only.
    b An infant with milk protein intolerance responded adversely to gluten (temporary gluten intolerance).

Treatment

1   *Life-long* gluten-free diet
    a Avoid *all* foods containing wheat or rye gluten. The exclusion of barley and oats is controversial; however, it is often wise to err on the safe side or to offer specific challenges and to test with biopsy.
    b The small intestine mucosa will always respond abnormally to dietary gluten, even though clinical signs may not be immediately evident.
    c Biopsy reverts to normal with appropriate diet.
2   Adequate kilojoule (calorie) intake.
3   Supplemental vitamins and minerals:
    a Folic acid for 1-2 months
    b Vitamin D
    c Iron for 1-2 months
4   Reduction of fat intake (rare).
5   Possible elimination of lactose from diet for 6-8 weeks — based upon reduced disaccharidase activity.

6   Treatment of coeliac crisis
   a Intravenous restoration of electrolyte balance and fluid for replacement of blood volume
   b Steroids
   c Parenteral hyperalimentation with amino acids, medium chain triglycerides, and glucose — for short periods of time may be necessary.
   d Initial oral feedings may need to be disaccharide or completely sugar free.

Complications

1   Recurrence of symptoms if diet is not followed
2   Possible predisposition to malignant lymphoma of small intestine at later age, if diet restrictions are terminated.

Nursing Objectives

To follow explicitly the dietary regimen which has been accurately calculated by the dietician to include enough kilojoules (calories) for weight gain yet to exclude wheat and rye glutens that produce enteropathy.

1   Initial diet is high in protein, relatively low in fat, and starch-free.
   a Milk protein or skim milk is sweetened with sucrose or banana powder.
   b Infants and young children may have a problem in intestinal fat absorption; therefore, fat intake may be reduced.
2   Proteins and sugars should be added gradually.
   a Individual foods are added one at a time at several-day intervals. Foods included and added are lean meat, cottage cheese, egg white, and raw ground apple.
   b Starchy foods are added to diet last.
   c Wheat and rye are never added to diet.
3   The child is given nothing by mouth during the initial treatment of coeliac crisis or during diagnostic testing.
4   If the child is ambulatory, take special precautions to ensure that he does not eat restricted foods.
5   Child may have anorexia; feeding him can be difficult.
   a Make mealtime pleasant.
   b Serve small, attractive portions.
   c Do not force him to eat.
6   Note carefully child's reaction to food. Close observation of child's responses to food may reveal other intolerances. Note and record:
   a Intake, foods refused
   b Appetite
   c Change in behaviour after eating
   d Characteristics and frequency of stools

e General disposition — behaviour improvement often seen within 2-3 days after diet control initiated.

7   New foods may be temporarily eliminated if symptoms increase.

To prevent infection in this child who is malnourished, anaemic and very susceptible to respiratory infection, which in turn will increase indigestion.

1   Avoid exposing the child to anyone with an infection of any kind.
2   Child usually perspires freely and has subnormal temperature with cold extremities.
  a Keep him dry.
  b Cover child lightly when ward is cool.
3   If child remains quiet in bed, change his position frequently because he is prone to upper respiratory infections.
4   Promote good hygiene.

To be aware of child's behaviour or change in behaviour and to care for him accordingly.

1   Diet and eating have a direct effect on behaviour. A hungry child may be irritable.
2   Behaviour is indicative of how the child is feeling.
3   The child is prone to mood swings — from having temper tantrums to being very timid, nervous, or unstable.
  a Allow child to express his feelings freely. Provide different types of media for child to express himself.
    (1) Older child talks or complains.
    (2) Baby cries and whines.
  b The nurse must exhibit patience.
  c Socialize routine procedures.
4   Record changes in behaviour, especially in relation to eating and diet.
5   Avoid conflicts or emotionally upsetting situations; these may precipitate diarrhoea, vomiting, and coeliac crisis.

To meet the child's emotional and psychological needs and to provide diversional activities appropriate for the age of patient and severity of disease.

1   This child may be withdrawn and indulge in self-play.
     Provide opportunity for play with other children, especially when child begins to feel better.
2   Frequently, play is more passive than active.
     Activity may be very exhausting. Provide appropriate material for constructive activities.
3   The toddler may cling to infantile habits for security.
     Allow this behaviour; it may disappear as his physical condition improves and he feels better.
4   The nurse must show the child she understands his mood swings and irritability by being patient with him. He needs a great deal of emotional satisfaction and support.

5   Offer the child other sensory stimulation to compensate for lack of eating pleasure.

To support the parents and to foster continuing parental acceptance of the child, his disease, and his behaviour.

Help parents maintain a healthy relationship with their child. The most important aspect in working with parents and child is to stress health and family counselling.

1   Encourage parents to visit and care for the child as much as possible. Comforting and holding the child can be very helpful. Child needs much love and understanding, especially from his parents.

2   Start teaching parents early about the disease and how they should care for the child at home.
   a Acquaint them with available literature, parent groups, and community resources.
   b Initiate health visitor referral to provide for continued support and teaching at home.

3   Listen to parental concerns and questions.
   a Give simple, honest answers.
   b Reinforce what the paediatrician has told them.

4   Allow parents to continue to maintain what other responsibilities they may have outside the hospital. Do not insist they stay at the hospital and attend only to this child.

5   Help parents to understand that after initial rapid weight gain further improvement may be slow.

To be aware of the signs and symptoms of coeliac crisis and to attend to the child's care according to medical plans.

1   Initial treatment.
   a Replace fluids and electrolytes by parenteral therapy.
   b Give nothing by mouth, especially if child is vomiting. Nasogastric tube may be required.
   c Observe the child carefully.

To be familiar with the medications used in treatment of coeliac disease and their implications.

1   Vitamins A and D — not absorbed well
2   Vitamin B complex and vitamin C — given if child is receiving antibiotics
3   Iron — given if child is anaemic
4   Vitamin K — for hypothrombinaemia and bleeding
5   Calcium lactate — given if milk is restricted from diet.

Parental Teaching

1   Help parents to understand what coeliac disease is and how it is controlled by diet.

a Provide a specific list of restricted foods as well as foods the child is allowed to eat.

b Teach mother (parents) how to read labels on foods to identify those containing wheat and rye glutens, thus avoiding them.

c Help mother become comfortable and proficient in situation problem-solving (e.g. What can be done when her child is invited to a birthday party where cake will be served? Bake gluten-free cupcakes and take to party).

d Provide opportunity for mother, dietician, and nurse to come together and talk about diet. At the same time foster a positive feeling toward dietary controls.

e Be certain parents understand the importance of the vitamin regimen.

f Help parents understand the importance of continued adherence to diet, even though the child is feeling well, eating well, and has normal stools. Advancing diet too rapidly may result in a setback.

2 Impress upon parents the importance of regular medical follow-up.

   Encourage the parents to seek prompt medical attention if the child has an upper respiratory tract infection which might trigger coeliac crisis if untreated.

3 Encourage parents to practise good hygiene to prevent infection.

   This child is especially prone to infection because of malnutrition and anaemia.

4 Help parents to understand that the emotional climate in the home and around the child is vitally important in maintaining the child's medical and physical stability.

   a Parents must exhibit patience with the child.

   b Have parents set defined limits of behaviour for the child; everyone in the family should know what they are.

   c Avoid conflicts or any emotional upsets in front of the child.

   d Social worker may need to become involved if there is domestic disharmony.

   e Other children and their needs must also be considered in the total family picture.

5 Help parents to understand that the child's physical condition and behaviour problems are related to the disease.

   a Parents may feel guilty or ambivalent towards the child.

   b Show them how they may avoid becoming overprotective of the child.

6 Help parents to understand that the disorder is life-long; however, changes in the mucosal lining of the intestine and in general the clinical condition of their child are reversible when dietary gluten is avoided.

7 Inform parents about the Coeliac Society of the United Kingdom, PO Box 181, London NW2 2QY. Help them to become familiar with the society.

DIARRHOEA

Diarrhoea is an excessive loss of water and electrolytes that occurs with passage of one or more unformed stools. It is a symptom of many conditions and may be caused by many diseases (see Table 7.1).

Aetiology

Often the cause is difficult to determine; occasionally it is unknown. The numerous causes of diarrhoea in infants and young children include:

1 Acute and infectious factors
   a Bacterial
       (1) Enteropathogenic *Escherichia coli*
       (2) *Salmonella*
       (3) *Shigella*
   b Viral
       (1) Enteroviruses — ECHO viruses
       (2) Adenoviruses
       (3) Human reovirus-like agent (HRVL)
   c Normal intestinal tract inhabitants act as pathogens in certain circumstances, i.e. after ingestion of antibiotics
   d Fungal — *Candida* enteritis
   e Parasitic
   f Protozoal
2 Noninfectious factors
   a Allergy to certain foods — milk, wheat protein
   b Metabolic disorders
       (1) Coeliac disease
       (2) Cystic fibrosis of pancreas
   c Disaccharidase deficiencies
   d Infant exposed to overfeeding; displaying emotional excitement and fatigue
   e Direct irritation of gastrointestinal tract by foods
   f Inappropriate use of laxatives and purgatives
3 Mechanical disorders
   a Malrotation
   b Incomplete small bowel obstruction
   c Intermittent volvulus
4 Congenital anomalies — Hirschsprung's disease.

Clinical Manifestations

Classification of Diarrhoea

1 Mild diarrhoea — hospitalization may not be indicated

2   Severe diarrhoea with gradual onset
3   Severe diarrhoea with sudden onset — incidence of death is high.

Symptoms

All classifications have similar symptoms, the severity of which is dependent upon intensity of diarrhoea and type of onset.

1   Fever — low grade to 41.1°C
2   Anorexia
3   Mild and intermittent to severe vomiting
4   Stools
    a Appearance of diarrhoea varies from a few hours to 3 days
    b Loose and fluid in consistency
    c Greenish or yellow-green colour
    d May contain mucus, pus, or blood
    e Frequency varies from 2 to 20 per day
    f Expelled with force; may be preceded by pain
5   Behaviour change
    a Irritability and restlessness
    b Weakness/pallor
    c Extreme prostration
    d Stupor and convulsions
    e Flaccidity
6   Respirations
    a Rapid
    b Hyperpnoeic
7   Dehydration
    a Little to extreme loss of subcutaneous fat
    b Up to 15% total body weight loss
    c Urinary output decreases or stops
    d Poor skin turgor and dry skin
    e Fontanelles and eyes sunken
    f Collapse imminent, low blood pressure, high pulse.

Pathophysiology

1   The particular aetiology of diarrhoea does not influence the potentially dangerous cycle of events as much as does the virulence of the organism and the general condition of the child.
2   The effects of diarrhoea present more of a threat to infants and young children than to the older child and adult.
    a Extracellular fluid volume is proportionately larger in the infant and young child.
    b Nutritional reserves are relatively smaller in the young child.

(continued on p. 440)

Table 7.1   Some malabsorption syndromes — based on types of stool

Disease	Diagnostic studies	Aetiology
Watery stools		
1 Disaccharide intolerance		
a Lactose (lactose → glucose, galactose) ↑ enzyme: lactase	1 Stool pH 2 Stool reducing substances 3 Lactose intolerance test 4 Enzyme assay	Primary congenital absence of enzyme lactase Secondary — any disease that damages epithelium of small intestine, e.g. gastroenteritis cow's milk sensitivity, coeliac sprue
b Sucrose (sucrose → glucose, fructose) ↑ enzyme: sucrase	1 Stool pH 2 Stool reducing substances 3 Sucrose tolerance 4 Enzyme assay	Primary — congenital absence of enzyme sucrase Secondary — any disease that damages epithelium of small intestine
2 Monosaccharide intolerance (glucose-galactose)	1 Stool pH 2 Stool reducing substances 3 Glucose — galactose tolerance tests 4 Trial carbohydrate elimination, using fructose	Primary — congenital defect in glucose transport Secondary — damage to and decrease of epithelium of intestine from acute gastro-enteritis or persistent diarrhoea; showing intolerance to fructose and glucose
3 Cow's milk protein sensitivity	1 Lactose tolerance test 2 Elimination of cow's milk from diet 3 Rechallenge with cow's milk will produce same symptoms.	Unknown Sensitivity to cow's milk
Parasites (Strongyloidiasis roundworm)	Examination of intestinal content for rhabtidiform larvae	*Strongyloides*
Giardia lamblia (protozoan)	Stool examination for *Giardia* cysts; duodenal aspirate for trophozites	Protozoan *Giardia lamblia*

Signs and symptoms	Treatment and nursing management*
Infant: watery, acidic diarrhoea; vomiting; failure to grow Older child (also): abdominal pain, cramps, abdominal bloating, nausea Fermentative diarrhoea when child exposed to lactose in diet	Elimination of all sources of lactose from diet. 1 to several weeks
Infant: watery, acidic diarrhoea, vomiting; failure to grow Older child (also): abdominal pain, cramps, abdominal bloating, nausea Fermentative diarrhoea when child exposed to lactose in diet	Elimination of sucrose from diet
	Primary — elimination of foods containing glucose from diet; feed foods containing fructose Secondary — elimination of diet containing fructose and glucose; administration of intravenous fluid and electrolytes until monosaccharide transport mechanisms are active
Gradual onset of watery or blood-tinged mucoid diarrhoea Steatorrhoea Vomiting Fever	Elimination of all sources of cow's milk protein If sensitivity appears by 6 months of age, tolerance of cow's milk resumes at 1-2 years of age
Skin red where larvae penetrate Cough, dyspnoea, patchy pneumonia for 2-3 weeks Abdominal pain, nausea, vomiting; watery stools Epigastric pain	Thiabendazole orally Topical thiabendazole to skin lesions
Persistent or intermittent watery diarrhoea Abdominal distension, poor weight gain, malabsorption syndrome Older child show coeliac picture	Metronidazole (Flagyl)

(continued)

Table 7.1 *(continued)*

Disease	Diagnostic studies	Aetiology
Fatty Stool		
Cystic fibrosis, coeliac sprue (see above discussion) Pancreatic insufficiency and bone marrow failure (Schwachman syndrome)	Pancreatic enzymes abnormal; sweat test normal; neutropenia	Familial pancreatic enzymes are probably reduced
Short-bowel syndrome		Inadequate absorptive surfaces Extensive bowel resection; increase in gastric acidity and production rate (hypersecretion), which in turn may inactivate pancreatic enzymes
Biliary tract obstruction		Biliary atresia Choledochal cyst Obstructive neonatal hepatitis
Normal stools		
Juvenile pernicious anaemia (vitamin B_{12} malabsorption)		Absence of intrinsic factor activity — cannot absorb vitamin B_{12}

3   Major alterations in physiology

    a Dehydration — extracellular fluid loss — results from the following:
      (1) Large loss of fluid and electrolytes in watery stools
      (2) Losses with repeated vomiting
      (3) Decreased fluid intake
      (4) Increased insensible fluid losses from skin and lungs resulting from fever and rapid respirations
      (5) Continued urine excretion
    b Electrolyte imbalance
      (1) Potassium — varies
      (2) Chloride; sodium; hypotonic, isotonic, or hypertonic dehydration may occur
    c Acid-base imbalance. Metabolic acidosis may result from
      (1) Large losses of potassium, sodium, and bicarbonate in stools
      (2) Impairment of renal function.

Diagnostic Evaluation

1   Thorough history of onset of diarrhoea and cause
2   Evaluation of general physical appearance and condition of child, including weight

Signs and symptoms	Treatment and nursing management[*]
Frequent infections Poor growth Stools — bulky, loose and frequent	Exogenous pancreatic enzyme therapy
Steatorrhoea Malnutrition	Intravenous alimentation Supplemental oral feedings of predigested formula, advancing slowly Supplemental vitamins A, D and E in water-miscible form Vitamin K, if prothrombin time indicates
Steatorrhoea Malabsorption of fat-soluble vitamins	Surgical correction if possible Medical treatment 1 Formula containing medium-chain triglycerides 2 Large doses of vitamins A, D and E in water-miscible form
Megaloblastic anaemia Failure to thrive Psychomotor retardation	Monthly vitamin B_{12} injection

[*] Nursing care plans can be adapted from discussions on diarrhoea, coeliac disease, and cystic fibrosis. (from Ament M E, *Journal of Pediatrics*, 1976, 81: 685, published by Mosby, with permission.)

3 Studies to establish nature of patient's condition
  a Electrolyte status and kidney function
    (1) Serum sodium
    (2) Serum chloride
    (3) Serum potassium
    (4) BUN (blood urea nitrogen)
  b Acid-base imbalance
    (1) Serum pH (acidosis)
    (2) Serum CO_2 content or combining power
  c Plasma volume by haematocrit and haemoglobin; also complete count, sedimentation rate, and culture
  d Urinalysis
  e Stool pH, reducing substances
4 Studies to determine cause of diarrhoea
  a Bacteriological cultures of stool
  b Bacteriological cultures of rectal swab
  c Serological studies for viral pathogens or direct visualization under electron microscope.

Treatment

1   Prevent spread of disease — suspect disease to be communicable until proven otherwise. Isolation; use barrier nursing precautions.
2   Supportive care — maintain hydration and electrolyte balance; record intravenous fluids, weights, fluid loss from diarrhoea and output.
3   Specific antimicrobial therapy
    Complications:
    (1) Dehydration
    (2) Protracted diarrhoeal state
    (3) Transient lactase deficiency — lactose intolerance.

Complications

1   Direct disturbances caused by diarrhoea itself:
   a Dehydration
   b Acidosis
   c Hypernatraemia
   d Alterations in potassium levels
2   Infection:
   a Local — i.e. site of cutdown, injection site
   b Respiratory tract
   c Middle ear (otitis media)
3   Nervous system, haemorrhage
4   Iatrogenic
   a Potassium depletion — 'washing out'
   b Hypernatraemia — sodium chloride overload
   c Oedema — excessive amount of parenteral fluids.

Nursing Objectives

To monitor intravenous fluid therapy (both amount and rate), which has been appropriately calculated by the paediatrician.

1   Fluid ordered as maintenance or replacement depending upon degree of patient's dehydration, must be checked by two nurses, one of whom must be qualified.
2   Fluid is calculated carefully so as not to overload circulatory system.
   a Check flow rate and amount absorbed hourly and totally.
   b Check intravenous site at regular intervals for infiltration or improper flow so site can be changed as necessary.
3   Use appropriate protective devices to prevent patient from moving and injuring himself or causing intravenous infusion to malfunction.
4   When preparing solution for therapy, use sterile solution and equipment.
5   Weigh patient daily to serve as a guide for specific fluid needs and current patient status.

6   When oral feedings are given in conjunction with intravenous fluid, careful adherence to prescribed volume is vital to prevent circulatory overload.

To provide physical comfort for the patient.

1   If protective devices are used, passive range of motion may help to keep patient's joints from stiffening.
2   While the patient is given nothing by mouth, special mouth care should be administered. An infant may find comfort in sucking a dummy. Burp him frequently to help expel air he has swallowed during sucking.
3   Change position and give good skin care to prevent lesions that may occur because of dehydration. Change soiled nappies quickly, because diarrhoeal stool will cause excoriation. Clean perineum thoroughly after each stool; application of ointment to skin may help protect it from contact with stool. Ointment must be completely removed after each stool. Leave buttocks exposed to air whenever possible. Avoid chilling.

To make frequent observations and be constantly alert to the patient's condition.

Record and report any changes immediately. Careful observations can give clues to improvement or deterioration in the patient's condition and can serve as a guide to medical care. Axillary temperature only should be recorded in the young infant with diarrhoea.

1   Note any changes in vital signs. Observe for any complications.
2   Note stool characteristics and number:
     a Abnormal constituents
     b Foul odour
     c Test stool for pH, reducing substances, and blood.
Note: Stool specimens and/or rectal swabs will be required for bacteriological and possible virological investigations.

3   Note activity and level of consciousness.
4   Note vomiting — frequency and characteristics.
5   Record urinary output — amount, frequency, and characteristics.
6   Check for presence of oedema.
7   Assess child's behaviour to determine how he feels.
     a Eating and restful sleep indicates he feels fairly good.
     b Crying or legs drawn up to abdomen usually indicates pain.

To prevent spread of infection by using good handwashing, gown and barrier techniques as indicated by hospital policy.

1   Many hospitals use isolation technique for children admitted with diarrhoea until the cause has been determined. (Infectious pathogens can spread rapidly and easily among infants and young children.)
2   Follow hospital policy as to care of nappies.

To meet the emotional and psychological needs of the patient.

1   Hospitalization is frightening — especially when it is sudden, as with diarrhoea.
2   Many treatments and procedures are painful — give reassurance to the child before, during, and after them.
   a Talk to the child.
   b Hold him and comfort him after the procedure.
   c Explain to him in language appropriate for his age what is to be done.
3   Provide some means of pleasant stimulation, entertainment, or diversion — especially while he must remain in bed.
   a Infant — mobile, musical toy.
   b Young child — read to him, something appropriate for age.
4   A hungry child is not easily comforted. Physical closeness may be helpful.
   a Petting, stroking.
   b Holding and rocking.

To provide and assist in resuming adequate energy and volume oral intake.

1   If diarrhoea is mild, oral electrolyte solution may be given. (Do not advance too quickly — base administration of solution on number of stools.)
2   Fluid is usually advanced slowly from clear liquids to half-strength formula or skim milk, to regular diet. Older child may advance more rapidly.
3   As diet is advanced, note any vomiting or increase in stools and report it immediately. Oral feedings should not be resumed too early or advanced too rapidly, because diarrhoea may recur.

To provide support for the family, especially the mother.

1   Reassure the mother that she is not the cause of her child's illness.
2   Explain procedures and need for treatment in easy-to-understand language. Be sure family understands the following:
   a Why infant's hair was shaved off a small area of scalp for an intravenous infusion
   b Reason for not giving the child anything to eat or drink
   c Need for protective devices.
3   Allow mother (parents) to care for and comfort the child as much as possible.
4   Allow her to leave the hospital and attend to other family members and matters. Invite parents to call the hospital when they cannot be there. Provide facilities for mother/father to be resident if they wish to do so.
5   Initiate a community nurse referral, especially if other children at home are ill or if home conditions have precipitated the diarrhoea.

Parental Teaching

1   After the cause of the diarrhoea is determined, it may be necessary to teach proper artificial feed and bottle or food preparation, handling, and storage.

It is especially important to be certain that the mother knows proper formula and bottle sterilization procedures.

2   Parents may need help in understanding the symptoms of a sick child.
3   Help parents understand the importance of medical care and general good hygiene.

HIRSCHSPRUNG'S DISEASE

Hirschsprung's disease (congenital aganglionic megacolon) is a congenital absence of the parasympathetic ganglion nerve cells from within the muscle wall of the intestinal tract, usually at the distal end of the colon.

Incidence

Occurring in about 1 in 5000 live births in England and Wales and is one of the most common causes of intestinal obstruction in the newborn.

Aetiology

1   An arrest in embryological development affecting the migration of parasympathetic nerves (innervation) of the intestine, occurring prior to the 12th week of gestation.
2   The cause is unknown — may be familial.

Clinical Manifestations

1   Appearing at birth or within first few weeks of life:
   a   No meconium passed
   b   Vomiting — bile-stained or faecal
   c   Abdominal distension
   d   Constipation
   e   Overflow-type diarrhoea
   f   Anorexia
   g   Temporary relief of symptoms with enema
2   Older child — symptoms not prominent at birth:
   a   History may reveal constipation at birth
   b   Distension of abdomen — progressive enlarging
   c   Thin abdominal wall — superficial veins are visible
   d   Peristaltic activity observable
   e   Constipation
     (1) Never has faecal soiling
     (2) Relieved temporarily with enema
   f   Stool appears ribbonlike, fluidlike or in pellet form

g Failure to grow
  (1) Loss of subcutaneous fat
  (2) Appears malnourished; perhaps has stunted growth.

Altered Physiology

1 Absence of or reduced number of ganglion cells in the intestinal tract muscle wall, usually the distal end of the colon.
2 No peristalsis occurs in the affected portion of intestine.
  a This section is usually narrow; therefore no faecal material passes through it.
  b The intestine above the affected section has an accumulation of faecal material.
3 Proximal to the narrow affected section, the colon is dilated.
  a Filled with faecal material and gas.
  b Hypertrophy of muscular coating.
  c In newborn may see ulceration of mucosa.
4 Abdominal distension and constipation result.

Diagnostic Evaluation

1 Rectal examination — exhibits absence of faecal material
2 Barium enema
  a Narrow segment of intestine proximal to anus
  b Dilated intestine proximal to narrow segment
3 Rectal biopsy — absence or reduced number of ganglion nerve cells.

Treatment

Definitive treatment is removal of the aganglionic, nonfunctioning, dilated segment of the bowel, followed by anastomosis.

1 Initially a colostomy is performed.
2 Definitive surgery may be delayed until age 9-12 months or until child is 6.8-9.0 kg.

Complications

1 Prior to primary surgery
  a Enterocolitis — a major cause of death; also occurs after surgery
  b Hydroureter or hydronephrosis
  c Caecal perforation
2 Postoperative
  a Enterocolitis
  b Leaking of anastomosis and pelvic abscess
  c Temporary sudden inability to evacuate colon.

Nursing Objectives — Preoperative Care

To assist in emptying the bowel and in preparing for surgery.

1 Rectal washouts daily; sometimes enemas may be required.
   a Procedure for enema in infant is similar to that in adult, except that less fluid and pressure are used.
   b Chemotherapeutic agents used to reduce the bacterial flora.
   c Normal saline solution should be used for rectal washouts.
   d Carefully note return from irrigation and degree of abdominal distension.
   e If enema is not expelled, siphoning may be indicated.
2 Note and record frequency and characteristics of stools.
3 Prevent injury to mucosa by taking axillary temperature.

Nursing Alert: Tap water enemas or rectal washouts should never be given as large quantities may be absorbed through the rental mucosa leading to water intoxication.

To observe for abdominal distension and its effect on patient's condition.

1 Note any change in degree of distension before and after irrigation. Record if location of distension changes, i.e. upper or lower abdomen.
2 Respiratory embarrassment may result from abdominal distension.
   Elevate head and chest of infant by tilting mattress.
3 Note degree of abdominal tenderness.
   a Legs of infant drawn up
   b Chest breathing.
4 Note colour of abdomen and presence of gastric waves.

To assist in establishing and maintaining hydration and adequate nutrition so that growth and weight gain may take place.

1 Monitor parenteral fluids appropriately.
2 Feeding may cause additional discomfort because of distension and nausea.
3 Offer small, frequent feedings. (Low-residue diet will aid in keeping stools soft.)
   a Appetite is poor.
   b Child must be fed slowly.
   c Provide as comfortable a position as possible for child during feedings.

To provide emotional and psychological support needed by the child.

1 Encourage mother to visit. Provide facilities for her to be resident if she wishes to do so.
2 Irritable child may be calmed by holding and rocking.
3 Provide suitable diversion appropriate for age.

To obtain a dietary history regarding food and eating habits.

1 This will contribute to planning dietary alterations.
2 Eating problems are common with Hirschsprung's disease.

To care properly for patient when nasogastric tube is used to aid in decreasing abdominal distention.

1 Note drainage from nasogastric tube and chart characteristics.
2 Check for patency.
  a Saline irrigations may be requested.
  b Carefully record input and output.
  c Note increasing distention; measure abdominal girth.
3 Give adequate mouth care.
4 Alternate nares when changing nasogastric tube every 24 hours. (Use minimal amount of tape to prevent skin irritation.)

Postoperative Care

One of two surgical procedures may be done in treatment of Hirschsprung's disease; (1) primary resection of aganglionic segment and anastomosis of the proximal ganglionic bowel to the rectal stump; or (2) temporary colostomy above the narrowed section; when condition of child is stabilized or weight of 8.17 - 13.62 kg is obtained, resection is done and colostomy closed (most common). Most commonly performed are Swenson's and Duhamel's operations.

To give good postoperative care and to observe for possible postoperative complications.

(See p. 85.)

To prevent infection.

1 At the site of surgical wound:
  a Dressing change, using sterile technique.
  b Prevent contamination from nappy.
    (1) Apply nappy below dressing.
    (2) Change frequently.
    (3) Prevent perianal and anal excoriation by frequent changing, thorough cleansing, and use of ointments.
  c Use careful handwashing technique.
  d Report any redness, swelling or drainage, evisceration, or dehiscence immediately.

2   Of the tracheobronchial tree and lungs:
    a Frequently suction secretions as indicated by the child's condition.
    b Encourage frequent coughing and deep breathing.
    Allow infant to cry for short periods.
    c Change position frequently to increase circulation and allow for aeration of all lung areas.

To properly care for colostomy and to understand its purpose.

1   Proper functioning of colostomy:
    a Note drainage from colostomy — characteristics, frequency, faecal material or liquid drainage.
    b Note abdominal distension.
    c Measure fluid loss from colostomy as the amount will affect fluid replacement.
2   Signs of obstruction from peritonitis, paralytic ileus, handling bowel, or swelling:
    a No output from colostomy
    b Increased tenderness
    c Irritability
    d Vomiting
    e Increased temperature.
3   Good skin care to prevent breakdown around colostomy:
    a Change soiled dressing or nappy frequently.
    b Wash skin with clear water.
    c Use karaya gum, aluminium paste, Maalox, Tinc Benz Co (Friar's balsam) or other means to protect skin from contact with secretions.
    d Keep area open to air occasionally.

To prevent abdominal distension.

1   Nasogastric tube may be used immediately postoperatively and left on free drainage.
    a Check patency (see above).
    b Watch for increasing abdominal distension.
    c Measure fluid loss as amount will affect fluid replacement.
2   Once oral feeding is begun, usually after about 24 hours when gastric aspirate has diminished, the nasogastric tube will be removed.
    a Avoid overfeeding.
    b Burp frequently during feeding.
    c Proper positioning after feeding.

To continue taking axillary temperatures.

1   Avoids injury.
2   Allows for more accurate reading.

To continue to provide emotional support to the patient. (See p. 436, diarrhoea.)

1   Recognize the effects of immobility, decreased handling and decreased activity; these would all be abnormal for a healthy infant.
2   Allow baby to derive some satisfaction from using a dummy. Hold him often during this time if condition permits.
3   Prepare parents for what they will see postoperatively (i.e. equipment, dressings, stoma).

To help parents understand and accept the child and the disease, as well as all that has happened.

1   Even a temporary colostomy can be a difficult procedure to accept and to learn to care for.
    a Support parents when teaching them to care for the colostomy.
    b Try to help them treat the baby or child as normally as possible.
2   Encourage parents to talk about their fears and anxieties.
        Anticipating future surgery for resection may be confusing and frightening.
3   Refer to health visitor prior to discharge to help parents care for child at home away from the comfortable situation of the hospital.

Parental Teaching

1   Begin early to teach thoroughly and carefully what the colostomy is for, how it works, and how to care for it and the child.
    a Parents may also need to know gastrostomy feeding techniques as well as procedures for care and dilation of anus.
    b Allow parents to try these procedures long before infant is to be discharged.
    c Emphasize the importance of treating the child as normally as possible to prevent behaviour problems later.
2   Encourage close medical follow-up and general good health hygiene:
    a Nutrition
    b General growth and development
    c Immunizations.

Stoma Care

Colostomy and ileostomy care in the infant and young child should take into account:

1   Colostomy irrigation is not part of management in small children. Irrigation is primarily for the purpose of regulating the colostomy to empty at regular intervals. Since children have bowel movements at more frequent intervals, this type of control is not feasible. Irrigation should only be done in preparation for tests or surgery and occasionally for the treatment of constipation.

2   Dehydration occurs quickly in the infant or small child; therefore, it is particularly important to observe drainage for amount and characteristics. It should be measured to provide for an accurate basis for computation of fluid replacement.

3   Prevention and treatment of skin excoration around the stoma is of primary concern and is a nursing challenge. With the advent of better skin shields and equipment that is designed especially for the paediatric patient, keeping an ostomy appliance in place is much less of a problem than it has been in the past. Through careful application and by trying different types of pouches until a proper fit is obtained, most children can be kept clean and dry for at least 24 hours between changes. This is a very significant factor in preventing skin breakdown and subsequent infections in the peristomal area. It is helpful to remember, however, that in the infant, dressings must be checked frequently:

   a Dressings and collection bags may not adhere well or stay in place.
   b Skin breakdown is more frequent.
   c Infant elimination is more frequent than in the older child.

GUIDELINES: CHANGING AN ILEOSTOMY APPLIANCE
(This procedure is uncommon in children.)

Purposes

1   To prevent leakage (bag is usually changed every 2-4 days).
2   To permit examination of skin around stoma.
3   To assist in controlling odour if this presents a problem.

Time

1   Early in morning before breakfast or 2-4 hours after a meal when the bowel is least active.
2   Immediately if patient is complaining of burning or itching underneath the disc or has pain around the stoma.

Equipment

1   Duplicate ileostomy appliance with belt/disposable bags
2   Soap, water, and washcloth
3   Karaya powder, karaya ring (self-adhering appliance); double-faced adhesive discs are best
4   Dressings
5   Receiver.

Procedure

Nursing Action	Rationale/Amplification
Preparatory Phase	
1 Have patient assume a relaxed position.	1 Encourage child and parental participation and understanding so that eventually he will be able to change appliance himself.
2 Explain details of this activity to child and parents if present.	
3 Expose ileostomy area; remove ileostomy belt.	
4 Position lamp; wash hands.	
Performance Phase	
1 Remove disc slowly from skin.	1 Solvent is not used, because it is damaging to skin.
2 Wash skin with warm water and soap using a soft washcloth. Observe stoma for its colour and condition.	2 Patient could take a shower or bath at this time. If stoma is discharging, cover with a dressing and seal with Micropore tape.
3 Moisten a karaya gum washer; wait until it is tacky and then apply over the stoma.	3 Karaya gum protects the skin while permitting healing underneath.
4 If Stomahesive or ReliaSeal are used , follow specific instructions in package insert. Be sure skin is thoroughly dry.	4 These are effective hypoallergic skin barriers.
5 Apply adhesive disc on the faceplate of the pouch against washer; press firmly for a few minutes until adherence is assured.	5 Seal-tight adherence results only when both parts are tacky before being pressed together.
6 Check the pouch bottom for closure; use rubber band or clip provided.	6 Proper closure controls leakage.
Follow-up Phase	
1 Dispose waste materials.	
2 If disposable bags are not used, clean ileostomy bag by washing in soap and water.	2 Preserve life of appliance and control odour.
3 Soak in deodorant solution; or rinse in solution of 60 ml distilled vinegar to 1 litre water.	3 Deodorizing agents should be effective but not destructive to rubber.

Note: Encourage child to participate according to his level of understanding.

Agencies

Parents can be given the address of The Ileostomy Association of Great Britain, 149 Harley Street, London W1, for advice and contact with other families in which a child has an ileostomy.

Colostomy

A *colostomy* is a temporary or permanent opening of the colon through the abdominal wall (an abdominal anus). Placement of the colostomy will influence the nature of the discharge. The *stoma* is that part of the colon that is brought above the abdominal wall in a colostomy.

Purposes

1 As a lifesaving measure in neonates with imperforate anus.
2 It can be a temporary measure to protect an anastomosis, e.g. in Hirschsprung's disease.

GUIDELINES: FOR COLOSTOMY CARE

Immediately following surgery until the wound is healed and sutures removed the colostomy may be cared for by using an aseptic technique with nonadherent dressings. Later, on surgeon's instructions, a suitable colostomy bag may be applied.

Procedure

Nursing Action	Rationale/Amplification
1 Explain procedure to parents and child, according to age and development.	1 Will encourage parental participation and acceptance.
2 Place child in comfortable position.	

Method

1 Remove bag slowly and carefully.	1 To prevent skin damage.
2 Wash and dry skin around stoma. A healthy stoma is bright red and protrudes approx. 1.5-2 cm ($\frac{1}{2}$-1 inch)	
3 Spray the stoma up to the margin of the colostomy with Tinc Benz Co (Friar's balsam).	3 To prevent skin contamination with faeces and avoid excoriation.
4 A karaya gum ring is applied to skin around colostomy. Can be trimmed to size for small babies. Should fit snugly around the colostomy. A bag is fitted and changed as necessary.	4 This will avoid leakage of faecal matter.

Note: Whenever possible encourage parental participation.

Follow Up Phase

1   Dress child appropriately and continue daily routine.
2   Clear away waste materials.

Note: A colostomy is usually of a temporary nature in young children. With good support and teaching, parents can learn to manage this at home until further surgery is indicated to correct the abnormality.

Parents can be referred to the Colostomy Welfare Group, 38 Eccleston Square, London SW1, for advice and contact with other families in which a child has a colostomy.

INTUSSUSCEPTION

Intussusception is the invagination or telescoping of a portion of the intestine into an adjacent, more distal section of the intestine.

Aetiology

1   Not usually known
        May be due to increased mobility of intestine and hyperperistalsis present in young children.
2   Possible contributing causes in older child:
    a Meckel's diverticulum
    b Polyps, cysts in the bowel
    c Malrotation of intestines
    d Acute enteritis
    e Abdominal injury
    f Abdominal surgery; intestinal intubation
    g Cystic fibrosis
    h Coeliac disease.

Clinical Manifestations

1   Incidence is rare in first month of life.
    a 4-10 months is most common age of onset (50-70%).
    b 1-2 years of age — frequency of occurrence is high.
2   Onset is sudden.
    a Paroxysmal abdominal pain
    b Currant jelly-like stools
        (1) Blood and mucus present in stool
        (2) One or more stools with this characteristic
        (3) Presence of bloody mucus on finger following rectal examination
    c Vomiting
    d Increasing absence of stools

e Increasing abdominal distension and tenderness
f Sausage-like mass palpable in abdomen
g Dehydration and fever
h Shock-like state
    (1) Rapid pulse
    (2) Pale skin
    (3) Marked sweating.

Altered Physiology

1 Mesentery is pulled into intestine when invagination occurs.
2 Progressive to obstruction
    a Intestine becomes curved, sausage-like — blood supply is cut off.
    b Bowel begins to swell — haemorrhage may occur.
    c Complete intestinal obstruction results — necrosis of involved segment.
3 Classification of location.
    a *Ileocecal* (most common) — ileum invaginates into ascending colon.
    b *Ileocolic* — ileum invaginates into colon.
    c *Colocolic* — colon invaginates into colon.
    d *Ileo-ileo* — (enteroenteric) small bowel invaginates into small bowel.

Diagnostic Evaluation

1 General condition and appearance of child; history
2 X-ray examination
    a Flat plate of abdomen — reveals staircase pattern (invagination appears like stair steps on x-ray)
    b Barium enema under fluoroscopy — coil-like appearance of bowel.

Treatment

1 Hydrostatic reduction of telescoped bowel with barium enema used during first 48 hours after onset.
2 Surgical reduction of intussusception; resection if bowel is gangrenous.

Nursing Principles — Preoperative Care

To assist in maintaining or restoring hydration and electrolyte imbalance.

Monitor parenteral fluids. (See p. 155, Intravenous Therapy.)

To prevent vomiting and aspiration.

1 Nurse in semirecumbent position.
2 Stomach may be deflated by insertion of nasogastric tube.
3 Maintain patency of nasogastric tube if one is inserted.
    a Irrigate at frequent intervals.
    b Note drainage and return from irrigation.

4 Patient is likely to be ordered nil by mouth.
   a Give mouth care.
   b Give infant dummy to suck.

To be aware of the patient's condition by frequent observations, thereby contributing to the total care of the patient.

1 Respirations are affected because of abdominal distension:
   a Grunting
   b Shallow and rapid if patient is in shock-like state.
2 Abdominal distension and unusual appearance of anus — intussusception may look like rectal prolapse.

Nursing Alert: When anus has an unusual appearance, take axillary temperatures to prevent injury.

3 Behaviour
   a Irritable — very sensitive to handling (Be gentle!)
   b Lethargic or unresponsive
   c Behaviour indicative of presence or absence of pain.

To prepare the child for surgery when he is shock-like or febrile.

1 Blood or plasma is given to restore circulating blood volume — observe for transfusion reactions.
2 Observe pulse rate carefully — safe range is below 140 per minute.
3 Reduce temperature — fever increases metabolism and makes oxygenation during anaesthesia more complicated.

To offer support to parents during this time of crisis and fear.

1 Encourage parents to verbalize their concerns.
2 Reinforce what the surgeon has told them. Help them to understand the reason for surgery.
3 Encourage them to be with child whenever possible.

Postoperative Care

To give good postoperative care and to observe for possible postoperative complications. (See p. 85.)

To be constantly alert for complications arising from surgery for intussusception.

1 Fever is usually present.
   a As a result of absorption of foreign protein
   b Absorption of bacteria through the damaged intestinal wall
2 Diarrhoea — from exposure to others who are infected
3 Shock
4 Dehydration

5   Toxicity
6   Peritonitis.

To assist in maintaining stomach decompression until first stool is passed.

1   See that indwelling nasogastric tube is functioning properly if present.
    a Tube may be connected to constant intermittent suction.
    b Note returns from drainage and irrigation.
2   Patient is usually given nothing by mouth for at least 12 hours postoperatively.
    Continue mouth care.
3   Note passing of flatus or stool and report — indicates peristalsis has returned to normal activity.
    Oral feedings may start.

To gradually resume full kilojoule (calorie) and volume oral intake appropriate for age and weight.

Progression will vary with surgeon and will depend upon whether bowel reduction or resection was surgical procedure.
1   Oral fluid is usually begun after the first stool is passed — about 2-3 days after surgery. When only a reduction was performed, oral fluid may be resumed when abdominal peristaltic activity is audible.
2   Give frequent, small feedings.
    a Start with glucose water or water.
    b Note and report any abdominal distension or vomiting.
    c Normal diet is gradually reintroduced.

To provide emotional support and meet the psychological needs of the child. (See p. 444, Diarrhoea.)

To support parents and to help them to maintain a good relationship with their child.

1   Encourage them to visit and call. Allow parents to become involved in caring for their child. Offer facilities for one or both parents to be resident.
2   Help parents to understand that recurrence is rare, but that certain short-term limits must be placed on the child's activity after discharge.

IMPERFORATE ANUS

The term *imperforate anus* is used to describe congenital 'abnormalities in the formation of the anorectal canal or in the location of the anus within the perineum'. *

Aetiology

1   An arrest in embryological development of the anus, lower rectum, and urogenital tract at the 8th week of embryonic life.

* Gryboski J, *Gastrointestinal Problems in the Infant,* Saunders, 1975, p. 506.

2   Cause unknown.

Types

1   Low imperforate anus — implies that the rectum has descended below the pubococcygeal line (puborectalis muscle) and is in normal anatomical relationship to levator sling and puborectus muscle.
   a Female
      (1) 90% of females with this condition present with low imperforate anus.
      (2) Fistula is present; rectum ends in fistula which presents in any location from low in vagina to normal position of anus.
   b Male
      (1) 50% of males with imperforate anus present with this type.
      (2) Perineal fistula is present and is located from anterior or normal position of anus to ventral surface of penis.
2   High imperforate anus — term implies that the rectal pouch is at or above the pubococcygeal line or the levator musculature.
   a Male
      (1) 50% of males with imperforate anus present with this type.
      (2) If fistula is present, it will usually communicate with the posterior urethra.
   b Female
      (1) 10% of females with imperforate anus present with this type.
      (2) Fistula will end high in vagina.

Clinical Manifestations

Condition is usually discovered immediately after birth or within several hours.
1   No anal opening.
2   Thermometer or small finger cannot be inserted into rectum.
3   Absence of meconium stool.
4   Green-tinged urine — if fistula is present (high, male)
5   Progressive abdominal distension.
6   Fistula is likely to be present.
   a Female — occurs between rectum and vagina or perineum.
   b Male — occurs between rectum and urinary tract, scrotum or perineum.
7   Other anomalies are likely, especially tracheo-oesophageal atresia. Other anomalies include those of the gastrointestinal tract, genitourinary system, cardiovascular system, and sacral vertebrae.

Diagnostic Evaluation

1   Visual examination

   a Presence of perineal fistula
   b Meconium coming from vagina or presence of meconium-stained urine.
2 General examination and/or presence of other associated manifestations
3 Urine examination for presence of meconium and epithelial debris —
   indicates presence of fistula
4 Micturating cystogram
5 Wangensteen-Rice x-ray (upside-down position)
   a Limited accuracy in locating rectal pouch
   b Useful only after infant is 24 hours of age.

Treatment

1 Low — female
   a Decompression of bowel with catheter irrigations
   b Dilatation of fistula for 8-12 months thereafter
   c Definitive repair
2 Low — male
   a Rectal cutback anoplasty or Y-V plasty
   b Local dilatation of fistula
3 High — male
   a Colostomy for decompression
   b Definitive pull-through surgery — deferred until about 1 year of age or
   when child attains 6.8-9 kg
4 High — female
   a Colostomy
   b Definitive repair usually done when infant is 1 year of age or 6.8-9 kg.

Complications

1 Rectal stenosis or prolapse, usually confined to mucosa
2 Separation of anastomosis
3 Urethral injury or stricture
4 Urinary retention and infection
5 Recurrent urinary fistulas
6 Faecal impaction or incontinence
7 Small bowel obstruction.

Nursing Objectives — Preoperative Care

To assist in maintaining stability in patient's general condition prior to emergency surgery.

1 Feedings are usually withheld.
2 Nasogastric tube may be passed to decompress the stomach, if indicated by
   child's condition.
3 Observe patient carefully for any signs of distress and report these to
   surgeon. Check vital signs frequently. Maintain temperature stability.

To observe the infant carefully for any other anomalies or changes in condition.

1 Use incubator or radiant warmer.
2 Observe for stool coming from a fistula.
3 Note that urine may be green-tinged.
4 Keep buttocks and perineal area clean.

Postoperative Care

Depending upon the location of the rectum (see types of imperforate anus), and sex of child, one of three surgical approaches may be used: (1) anoplasty, (2) temporary colostomy with definitive pull-through at a later time when child is older and larger, or (3) abdominal or sacroperineal pull-through.

To give good postoperative care and to observe for possible postoperative complications. (See p. 85.)

To provide appropriate care for perineal anoplasty.

1 Do not put anything in rectum.
2 Expose perineum to air.
3 Position baby for easy access to perineum for cleansing and minimal irritation to site, i.e. place baby on abdomen.

To provide good colostomy care and to prevent skin breakdown. (See p. 453, Hirschsprung's disease.)

To provide appropriate care for definitive pull-through surgery.

1 Carry out perineal care as stated above.
2 Provide proper care of gastrostomy or nasogastric tube used to decompress the gastrointestinal tract until peristalsis returns.
3 Provide proper care of bladder catheter, if used, and measure urinary output accurately.
4 Observe carefully for abdominal distension, bleeding from perineum, and respiratory embarrassment.

To maintain adequate nutrition as well as energy and fluid intake to prevent dehydration and electrolyte imbalance.

1 Oral feedings are usually started within 3-4 hours after an anoplasty.
2 Oral feedings are usually withheld until peristalsis returns. When primary repair is done, nasogastric suction may be maintained until feedings are started.
3 Monitor parenteral fluids (see p. 159).

To foster acceptance of the child and his diagnosis by his parents.

1 Assure parents that colostomy is temporary.
2 Encourage parents to become involved in care of the child and to give him the emotional security he needs.

3   Support teaching programme of surgeon for special care needed at home:
    a Colostomy care
    b Anal dilatation to prevent a stricture at site of anastomosis from scar tissue after instructions by paediatrician.
4   Initiate referral to health visitor.
5   Encourage parents to talk about their concerns.

Parental Teaching

1   Provide careful, thorough teaching of special care and procedures to be continued at home — colostomy care, anal dilatation. Develop a plan for return demonstration by mother. Liaise with health visitor about this, to ensure special care plan is appropriate to family and home environment.
2   Help parents to understand situations that may be encountered as a result of imperforate anus as the baby gets older:
    a Faecal impaction due to lack of sensation to defecate
    b Future surgery — if primary repair was not done
    c Toilet training
    d Inability to control faecal seepage from rectum.

ABDOMINAL HERNIA

A *hernia* is a protrusion of viscus through the wall of the cavity in which it is normally contained.

Umbilical Hernia

A common condition occurring in about 20% of newborn infants. Umbilical hernias sometimes appear within the early months of life, becoming more prominent during acts of crying and straining. They reduce easily and rarely strangulate.

Most umbilical hernias close spontaneously. Hernias that fail to do so may be repaired surgically in later childhood after the age of 3 years, and usually before commencing school.

Inguinal Hernia

The testis in the male descends from the abdominal cavity into the scrotum carrying with it peritoneum, thus forming a canal from abdomen to scrotum. Normally this tube closes completely. When this fails, descent of the intestine into it becomes possible, thus producing a hernia. A similar defect can occur in girls due to weakness of tissues about the round ligament.

Incidence

Occurs in a proportion of nine males to one female. Most often unilateral.

Clinical Manifestation

1   *Males:* Usually noticed as a scrotal swelling within a few hours of birth. Hernia more apparent when the infant cries.
2   *Females:* May appear any time, often associated with some discomfort.

Treatment

Elective surgical repair to prevent future complications, usually carried out in infancy depending upon the child's condition and family situation.

The hernial sac is ligated, excised and the inguinal ring repaired.

Irreducible Hernias

Occasionally the hernia becomes firm and tense due to a portion of the bowel becoming caught in the hernial sac with disruption of the blood supply resulting in oedema and discomfort.

Immediate conservative treatment is indicated. The head of the child should be placed lower than the buttocks, i.e. the foot of the cot is raised, and if necessary, sedation is given. Occasionally gallows-type extension to the legs may be applied. In the infant, a feed or use of a dummy may help to reduce crying, and abdominal tension. Applications of cool compresses may also be helpful in achieving reduction without surgical intervention. Force to the hernia should never be used to attempt reduction.

Strangulated Hernia

If the hernia is associated with pain and symptoms of obstruction (see p. 467), immediate surgical treatment is indicated, which may require the resection of gangrenous gut.

Preoperative Care

For elective surgery, normal preoperative preparation required, see p. 83.

If the hernia has become strangulated, intravenous therapy to correct dehydration will be required, see p. 155.

An indwelling nasogastric tube should be passed, and gastric aspiration maintained.

Antibiotics may be prescribed.

Postoperative Care

Simple Herniotomy

Feeds may be recommended 4 hours after surgery and the infant fit to go home later that day or on the following day.

Alert community nursing staff for removal of sutures, unless absorbable subcuticular sutures are used.

Herniotomy with Intestinal Resection

1 Continuation of intravenous therapy to maintain electrolyte balance.
2 Gastric aspiration maintained until bowel sounds return.
3 Gradual reintroduction of oral feeding, usually after about 24 hours, depending on bowel status and function.
4 Monitoring of vital signs at appropriately frequent intervals (see. p. 99).
5 Observation of wound and drainage.
6 Continue antibiotics as prescribed.
7 Provide suitable play activities according to interests and development. Encourage early mobilization (see p. 64).
8 Sutures removed 7-10 days according to wound healing.

Prognosis

Recurrence rate of inguinal hernia after herniotomy is less than 1%. However, an infant who presents with a hernia on one side may subsequently present with a hernia on the opposite side.

APPENDICITIS

Acute *appendicitis* is an inflammation of the appendix due to infection. It is almost always a surgical operation.

Incidence

May occur in any age group, although rare in first year of life.

Clinical Manifestations

1 Sudden, colicky pain in umbilical region, moving to right iliac where it becomes a dull ache.
2 Nausea and vomiting.
3 Commonly constipation, alternatively diarrhoea which may be quite severe.
4 The child looks ill with moderate pyrexia 40°C.

Note: If peritonitis develops, the child's condition shows considerable deterioration with high fever, tachycardia, dehydration, abdominal distension and ketosis.

Diagnostic Evaluation

1   Physical examination noting especially location and localization of pain, rebound tenderness, etc.
2   Blood studies with particular attention to white count; urinalysis.
     A white blood count reveals a moderate leucocytosis.
3   Careful history to rule out other possibilities.

Treatment and Nursing Management

Palliative Preoperative Care

1   Place child in comfortable position to relieve abdominal pain and tension — usually Fowler's position.
2   See that child takes nothing by mouth — to decrease peristalsis and allow stomach to empty preparatory to surgery. Note time and nature of last meal.
3   Frequently evaluate vital signs — to assess progression of infection.
4   Ensure that child understands preparations. Encourage parents to participate in care.

Parental Support

Explain need for surgery using words which they will understand. Offer facilities for them to be resident if they wish to do so.

Principles of Postoperative Care

Without Drainage

1   Following recovery from anaesthesia, modified Fowler's position is maintained (to suit age of child). Fluids and food given as tolerated. Analgesia given as needed.
2   Encourage early and gradual mobilization.
3   May be discharged home according to surgeon's instructions between 5th and 8th day postoperatively if good progress made.
4   Sutures removed 7th-10th day. Alert community nursing service for suture removal if child discharged home early.
5   Give guidance to parents about the need for their child to gradually increase physical activity. If of school age, may return to school 3-4 weeks after operation providing no complications.

With Drainage

1   Maintain the child in comfortable position, well supported by pillows.
2   Record accurately intake and output, including nasogastric aspirate.
3   Record vital signs. Be alert to any change in child's condition and its significance.

4   Observe and describe symptoms accurately: pain and tenderness have a tendency to shift and must be reported precisely. Give analgesia as indicated by child's condition.

5   Since nothing by mouth can be given until bowel sounds return, monitor intravenous infusion. Observe meticulous oral hygiene.

6   Administer antibiotics as prescribed.

7   Encourage deep breathing exercises (p. 178) and gradual mobilization.

8   Give wound and drain care according to child's condition and any specific instructions from the surgeon.

9   Be responsive to parents' anxiety, reassure them and their child in words which are meaningful to them.

10 Reduce parenteral fluids and give oral fluids and food when the following occur:

   a   Temperature and pulse rate come down.
   b   Bowel sounds return.
   c   Flatus is passed, or the child has bowel movement.

11 Prepare parents for discharge home when child is eating and drinking normally, reasonably active for age and development with the wound well healed.

Complications

Be alert for the possibility of complications. Report immediately any indication of infection, e.g. pyrexia, return of pain or acute tenderness.

MECKEL'S DIVERTICULUM

Meckel's diverticulum is a congenital abnormality of the ileum consisting of a blind pouch resembling the appendix.

Incidence

Present in about 2% of the population.

Significance

Meckel's diverticulum causes no symptoms unless some complication develops:

1   If the diverticulum is lined with gastric epthelium it may secrete acid gastric juice causing ulceration, with pain and anaemia.

2   The diverticulum may become attached to the abdominal wall or to other structures which may lead to volvulus, or intestinal obstruction.

3   The diverticulum may invaginate causing intussusception.

Treatment

Laparotomy with resection of diverticulum.

Nursing management and care similar to that for appendectomy (see p. 464).

INTESTINAL OBSTRUCTION

Intestinal obstruction is an interruption of the normal flow of intestinal contents along the intestinal tract. The block may occur in the small or large intestine, may be mechanical or paralytic, and may or may not compromise the vascular supply.

Types of Obstruction

1 Mechanical — a physical block to passage of intestinal contents without disturbing blood supply to bowel
   a Location
   b Extrinsic, e.g. hernia, intussusception
   c Intrinsic, e.g. haematoma, tumour
   d Intraluminal, e.g. foreign body, faecal or barium impaction, polyp
2 Paralytic (adynamic, neurogenic) ileus. Peristalsis is ineffective (diminished motor activity, perhaps because of toxic or traumatic disturbance of the autonomic nervous system); there is no physical obstruction and no interrupted blood supply.
3 Strangulation. Obstruction also compromises blood supply, leading to gangrene of the intestine.

Causes

1 Mechanical (extramural)
   a Adhesions — postoperative
   b Hernia
   c Malignancy
   d Volvulus (loop of intestine that has twisted)
2 Mechanical (intramural)
   a Haematoma
   b Intussusception (telescoping of intestine)
   c Stricture or stenosis (scarring)
3 Paralytic
   a Postoperatively after any abdominal surgery
   b Peritonitis, pneumonia
   c Wound dehiscence (breakdown)
   d Gastrointestinal tract surgery.

Altered Physiology

1 Disturbed physiological responses as a result of mechanical small intestine

obstruction results in increased peristalsis, distension by fluid and gas, and increased bacterial growth proximal to obstruction; the intestine empties distally.

2   Increased secretions into the intestine are associated with diminution in the bowel's absorptive capacity.

3   The accumulation of gases, secretions, and oral intake above the obstruction causes increasing intraluminal pressure.

4   Venous pressure in the affected area increases, and circulatory stasis and oedema result.

5   Bowel necrosis may occur because of anoxia and compression of the terminal branches of the mesenteric artery.

6   Bacteria and toxins pass across the intestinal membranes into the abdominal cavity, thereby leading to peritonitis.

7   'Closed loop' obstruction is a condition in which the intestinal segment is occluded at both ends, preventing either the downward passage or the regurgitation of intestinal contents.

Clinical Manifestations

Fever, peritoneal irritation, increased white blood cell count, pain and abdominal distension, toxicity and shock may develop with all types of intestinal obstruction.

Nursing Alert: Because of loss of water, sodium, and chlorides, signs of dehydration become evident: intense thirst, drowsiness, general malaise, aching; tongue becomes parched, face appears pinched, abdomen becomes distended. Shock may result (pulse increasingly rapid and weak, temperature and blood pressure lowered, skin pale, cold, clammy) ending in death.

Treatment and Nursing Management

The objective is to remove the obstruction, treat the fluid and electrolyte imbalance, relieve the distension, and prevent or detect early the complications of shock and peritonitis.

Initial Nursing Assessment and Care

1   Describe accurately the nature and location of the patient's pain, the presence of distension, the absence of flatus or defecation. The overview of symptoms is important in differentiating intestinal obstruction from other more benign conditions.

2   Monitor and record vital signs (including blood pressure).

3   Measure and record accurately all intake and output.

4   Save any stool that may be passed; this should be tested for occult blood.

5   Anticipate surgeon's request for urinalysis, haemoglobin determination, and blood cell counts.

6   Frequently determine the patient's level of consciousness; decreasing responsiveness may offer a clue to an increasing electrolyte imbalance.
7   Recognize the patient's concern and initiate measures to secure his cooperation and confidence in the staff: these include ascertaining his specific anxieties and providing him with therapeutic responses. Encourage parents to be present and participate in care.
8   Compare the child's state of orientation with his admission status; a lessening awareness of his environment may suggest his going into shock.
9   Minimize those factors that would enhance gastric secretions in order to prevent fluid loss (via nasogastric suction); avoid conversation about enticing meals and eliminate meals being served within his range of seeing or smelling.
10 Undertake measures to prepare the child for surgery, since most problems of mechanical obstruction require surgical correction.

Medical, Surgical and Nursing Management

1   Correct fluid imbalance by preparing for and maintaining intravenous therapy.
2   Administer antibiotics (neomycin and kanamycin) and possibly a broad spectrum agent to lessen the possibility of infection, particularly peritonitis.
3   Prevent infarction by carefully assessing status of child and vital signs. If pain increases in intensity, localizes or becomes continuous, it may herald strangulation.
4   Detect early signs of peritonitis, such as rigidity and tenderness, in an effort to minimize this complication.
5   Relieve obstruction by releasing, removing or repairing the cause of the obstruction; this is done surgically in most instances.
    a Resection of obstructing lesion and end-to-end anastomosis is done when no evidence of peritonitis and only minimal oedema exist; this requires a proximal colostomy to decompress new anastomosis.
    b Resection of all necrotic intestine is necessary.
    c A loop colostomy is done when relief is sought by drawing a proximal loop or segment of colon up to the skin surface and opening it as a colostomy; the distal portion of colon is treated later (see p. 453).

Specific Postoperative Nursing Care

1   To meet fluid, electrolyte and nutritional needs, administer prescribed amounts of fluids; keep accurate intake and output records. Gastric suction until bowel sounds return.
2   Frequently monitor vital signs; assess degree of pain. Administer analgesics as prescribed.
3   Introduce early mobilization, and the gradual introduction of feeding according to bowel status.
4   Wound and drainage care.
5   Administer antibiotics if prescribed.

6   Provide for normal activities according to age, development and general condition, e.g. play opportunities.

Further details of postoperative care, see p. 85.

HEPATITIS

Hepatitis is an inflammation of the liver caused by viruses.

Significance

1   From a community health point of view one is concerned with ease of disease transmission and morbidity.
2   From an educational point of view one is concerned with prolonged loss of time from school.

Preventive Measures

1   Stress importance of proper public and home hygiene.
2   Recognize merits of conscientious surveillance in the proper and safe preparation and dispensation of food.
3   Promote effective health supervision in schools.
4   Initiate and support health education programmes.

Types of Hepatitis

1   Type A hepatitis (infectious hepatitis, IH virus)
     Also called epidemic hepatitis, catarrhal jaundice, short-incubation hepatitis.
2   Type B hepatitis (serum hepatitis, SH virus)
     Also called homologous serum jaundice.

Diagnostic Evaluation

1   By radioimmunoassay test, the presence of hepatitis B antigen (HB_sAg) is detected in individuals who have infectious or serum hepatitis.
2   By the (HB_sAg) test, detection of hepatitis is possible before the patient becomes clinically ill.
3   Levels of SGPT (serum glutamic pyruvic transaminase) also rise 1-2 weeks before clinical jaundice occurs.

Type A Hepatitis

Epidemiology

1   Causative agent — filtrable virus
2   Mode of transmission
    a Faecal-oral route; respiratory possible
    b Blood transfusion, blood serum or blood plasma from a carrier or infected person
    c Contaminated equipment: syringe and needles
    d Contaminated food, milk, or shellfish, polluted water
3   Incubation — 3-7 weeks; average 4 weeks
4   Occurrence
    a Worldwide — sporadic or epidemic
    b Autumn and winter months
    c Usually in children over the age of 6 years and young adults.

Clinical Manifestations

1   Pre-icteric (prior to period of jaundice) phase
    a Headache, fever, anorexia, nausea, vomiting, abdominal tenderness, pain over liver, backache, myalgias
    b Respiratory manifestations often thought at first to be influenza
2   Icteric phase
    a Urine — dark; stool often light for several days
    b Liver — enlarged, often tender
    c Nausea, vague epigastric distress, heartburn, flatulence, anorexia.

Type B Hepatitis

Epidemiology

1   Causative agent
    a Filtrable virus
    b Hepatitis B antigen (HB_sAg)
2   Mode of transmission
    a Parenteral route
        (1) Blood/blood components transfusion from an infected person
        (2) Contaminated needles, syringes
    b Skin puncture — medical instruments
    c Mucosal transmission; dental instruments
3   Incubation — 6 weeks-6 months (average $2\frac{1}{2}$-3 months)
4   Occurrence
    a Worldwide
    b Recipients of blood and blood products
    c Intravenous drug abusers.

Diagnostic Evaluation

1 Viral studies
2 Liver function tests.

Treatment and Nursing Management

1 Isolate patient to minimize contacts; allow activity as tolerated.
2 Wear gloves; wash hands thoroughly.
3 Assist with venepunctures for laboratory diagnostic studies such as of transaminase and serum bilirubin levels.
4 Provide tissues and paper bags for nasal and throat secretions; incinerate.
5 Handle bedpan carefully; clean thoroughly and restrict its use to the same patient. Continue this pattern for at least 3 weeks.
6 Use disposable syringes and needles; label clearly all laboratory specimens as coming from a patient with hepatitis.
7 Provide diet that is nutritious and appealing to patient; small, frequent snacks may be in order.
   a Offer a large breakfast as anorexia worsens later in the day.
   b Offer frequent fluids with added glucose.
8 Administer alkalis to counteract gastric acidity.
9 Avoid sedatives; they are poorly handled by an inflamed liver.
10 Impress on the parents the importance of careful follow-up visits including laboratory and physical examinations until laboratory results have returned to normal levels.
11 Recognize that recovery is slow and prolonged; increase activities as tolerated.
12 Type A only: give gammaglobulin to close contacts of the patient, particularly members of the family.
13 Notify health visitor prior to discharge; alert school nursing service.

Health Teaching and Preventive Measures

Type A Hepatitis	Type B Hepatitis
Instruct parents to practise good personal hygiene.	Transfuse a patient only when justified
Employ proper safeguards to prevent use of blood and its components from infected donors.	Use blood substitutes when feasible. Use disposable needles and syringes; dispose of these carefully, using agreed unit procedure.
Screen food handlers carefully.	Use hyperimmune globulin.
Practise safe preparation and service of food.	
Use disposable needles and syringes; dispose of these carefully, using agreed unit procedure.	

Nursing Alert: Although type A hepatitis is usually spread by faecal and oral routes and type B hepatitis is usually spread by the parenteral route, BOTH TYPES MAY BE SPREAD BY ALL ROUTES!

JAUNDICE

Haemolytic Jaundice

Haemolytic jaundice is attributable to abnormally high concentration of bilirubin in blood exceeding the capacity of normal liver cells to excrete it.

1   Encountered in children (acholuric jaundice) with haemolytic transfusion reactions, congenital spherocytosis, autoimmune haemolytic anaemia, erythroblastosis fetalis, and other haemolytic disorders.
2   Bilirubin in the blood is unconjugated (indirect-reacting).
3   In faeces and urine, urobilinogen is increased; urine is free of bilirubin.

Extremely severe jaundice (unconjugated bilirubin elevated: 20-25 mg/100 ml) causes brain-stem damage in neonates.

Hepatocellular Jaundice

Hepatocellular jaundice is due to an inability of diseased liver cells to clear the normal amount of bilirubin from the blood.

Causes

1   Infection — epidemic infectious hepatitis, homologous serum hepatitis.
2   Drug or chemical toxicity.

Clinical Manifestations

1   Mildly or severely ill patient.
2   Lack of appetite, nausea, loss of vigour and strength, weight loss, moderate pyrexia.
3   Elevated SGOT (serum glutamic oxaloacetic transaminase) and SGPT (serum glutamic pyruvic transaminase) — two enzymes that are liberated with cellular necrosis and rise in bloodstream.
4   Rise in bilirubin. Alkaline phosphatase mildly elevated.
5   Abnormal serum proteins in prolonged illness; prothrombin time increased.
6   Headache and chills possible in infectious condition.
7   Cholesterol decreased in serum.

Obstructive Hepatic Jaundice

Obstructive hepatic jaundice is due to blockage of bile ducts. The condition is seen in the newborn due to congenital obliteration of the bile ducts; otherwise unusual in childhood.

Clinical Manifestations

Due to damming back of bile, which is reabsorbed by the blood
1   Skin jaundiced, sclerae yellow
2   Urine — deep orange colour
3   White or clay coloured stools
4   Pruritus.

Laboratory Evidence

1   Conjugated bilirubin and alkaline phosphatase levels are greatly raised.
2   Elevated SGOT (serum glutamic oxaloacetic transaminase) and SPGT (serum glutamic pyruvic transaminase).

Objectives of Nursing Management

To control pruritis and make child comfortable.
1   Apply soothing lotions and give cool baths.
2   Clothing should be light, cotton and loose.
3   Assist child in reducing need to scratch skin by providing activities which distract his attention; keep nails trimmed and clean; keep child in cool environment (utilize a fan in hot weather); ensure child has dummy comforter if appropriate to allay anxiety and restlessness; encourage parents to participate in care.

Diet

Glucose fluids only in the presence of nausea. Gradual introduction of light diet with increased intake of protein and low fat intake, until liver function improves.

Drugs

1   Administer antibiotics and supplementary water-miscible vitamins as prescribed.
2   Other chemotherapy, e.g. antihistamines, may be ordered.

Activity

Activity should be dictated by the condition of the child. In the early stages, bed rest is often needed. Later increasing activity may be provided, but recognizing that the child may tire easily, needing frequent rest periods.

Surgical Treatment

Prepare child for surgical investigation or operation (see p. 83).

Support for Parents and Family

Encourage parents to talk about their anxieties for their child, in what may be a protracted illness. Recognize that parents may feel depressed regarding long-term outcome and prognosis for future care.

THREADWORM (ENTEROBIASIS, OXYURIASIS)

The threadworm *(Enterobus vermicularis)* causes the most common form of intestinal worm infestation in the UK, and is most prevalent in children.

Clinical Problems

1 One threadworm may produce 5,000-15,000 eggs.
2 The ingested eggs hatch in the small intestine; embryos reach adulthood in the caecum.
3 The gravid female worm navigates down the large intestine and deposits eggs on the skin of the perianal area.
4 The eggs that survive are ingested and reach maturity in 2-6 weeks in the gastrointestinal tract.
5 Scratching leads to contamination of the hands and nails; hand to mouth contact results in reinfection.
6 Infective eggs may contaminate food and drink, bed linen, dust, etc.

Clinical Manifestations

(An infected person may be asymptomatic)
1 Intense itching (nocturnal) above the anus — from nocturnal migration of gravid females from anus and deposition of eggs in perianal folds of skin.
2 Restlessness, nervousness.
3 Vaginitis — from threadworm migration into the vagina.

Diagnostic Evaluation

1 Anal impressions on Sellotape slide taken in morning before going to toilet or bathing, so that ova deposited during the night will not be removed.
   a A parent may be taught the method so that the test may be carried out first thing in the morning.
   b Wash hands thoroughly.
2 Detection (inspection) of characteristic eggs about the anus.

Treatment

Treatment of the whole family with piperazine, pyrantel embonate or pyrvinium embonate (this turns stools blood red colour; parents should be warned about this).

Prevention of Reinfection; Health Teaching

1 All members of the family should be treated, or reinfection is apt to occur. Treat on the same day to eliminate cross-infection.

2   To prevent reinfection:
a Cut fingernails short — eggs may be obtained from beneath the nails of infected person.
(1) Avoid nail biting.
(2) Wash hands frequently during treatment period.
(3) Scrub nails with a brush, especially before going to bed.
b Wash hands with soap and water after using toilet and before meals.
c Wash around anal area upon arising (after diagnostic test).
d Infected child should wear snug-fitting cotton pants — to discourage contact of hands with perianal region and contamination of bed linen.
e See that infected person sleeps alone.
f Handle bedding and nightwear carefully — there are large numbers of infective eggs in a contaminated house that cause reinfection.
g Change bed linen and nightwear frequently.
h Reassure mother and family members that threadworms are not a sign of poor hygiene.

FURTHER READING

Books

Anderson C M Burke J, *Paediatric Gastroenterology*, Blackwell Scientific, 1975.
Avery G B, *Neonatology*, 1981.
Brimblecombe F Barltrop D, *Children in Health and Disease*, Baillière Tindall, 1978.
Harries J T, *Essentials of Paediatric Gastroenterology*, Churchill Livingstone, 1977.

Articles

Aggett P J A, The metabolic effects of massive intestinal resection in infancy and childhood, *Journal of Maternal and Child Health*, February 1979: 44-48.
Barnes N D Roberton N R C, Common gut problems in children, *Update*, April 1979: 885-892.
Cutting W, Oral treatment of diarrhoea in children, *Journal of Maternal and Child Health*, 1979: 276-281.
Duberly J King H, The nurse teacher and carer for mother and child, *Nursing Mirror*, August, 1978: 15-18.
Ellis H, Children with acute appendicitis, *Journal of Maternal and Child Health*, January 1978: 2-5.
Garrett G, The coeliac child, *Nursing Times*, November 1977: 1708-1710.
Glendinner B G, Congenital pyloric stenosis, *Journal of Maternal and Child Health*, June 1978: 220-224.
Huddart A G, The care and management of the newborn cleft palate infant, *Nursing Mirror*, January 1975: 61-65.

Irwin E C McWilliams B J, Play therapy for children with cleft palates, *Child Today*, May, June 1974, 3: 18-22.

Jolleys A, Meconium ileus, *Nursing Times*, May 1978: 833-834.

Jones P F, The acute abdomen in infancy and childhood, *Practitioner*, April 1979: 473-478.

Marnel P D, Vomiting in infancy, *Journal of Maternal and Child Health*, March 1979: 90-94.

Tripp J *et al.*, Gastroenteritis, a continuing problem, *Lancet*, July 1979: 276-281.

Walker-Smith J A, Chronic diarrhoea in childhood, *Archives of Disease in Childhood*, May 1980: 329-330.

Walker-Smith J A, Food allergy and bowel disease in childhood, *Midwife, Health Visitor and Community Nurse*, September 1984: 308-316.

Walker-Smith J A, Gastrointestinal disease in childhood, *Maternal and Child Health*, January 1985: 10-14.

Webster P, Stomas in childhood, *Journal of Community Nursing*, November 1981: 4-6.

8

KIDNEYS, URINARY TRACT, AND REPRODUCTIVE SYSTEM CONDITIONS

ACUTE GLOMERULONEPHRITIS

Glomerulonephritis refers to inflammation of the kidneys caused by an antigen-antibody reaction following an infection in some part of the body. Acute glomerulonephritis is predominantly a disease of childhood and is the most common type of nephritis in children.

Aetiology

1 Presumed cause — antigen-antibody reaction secondary to an infection elsewhere in the body
2 Initial infection
   a Usually either an upper respiratory infection or a skin infection
   b Most frequent causative agent — nephritogenic strains of Lancefield Group A beta-haemolytic streptococcus.
   c Infrequent causative agents:
      (1) Other bacteria
      (2) Viruses.

Altered Physiology

1 The organisms responsible for nephritis contain antigens similar to those of the basement membrane of the renal glomeruli.
2 Antibodies produced to fight the invading organism also react against the glomerular tissue.
3 The antigen-antibody combination results in an inflammatory reaction in the kidney.
   a There are proliferation and swelling of the endothelial cells of the glomerular capillary wall.
   b All of the glomeruli are involved, but the extent of proliferation varies among them.

4   Changes in the glomerular capillaries reduce the amount of the glomerular filtrate, allow passage of blood cells and protein into the filtrate, and reduce the amount of sodium and water that is passed to the tubules for reabsorption.

5   General vascular disturbances, including loss of capillary integrity and spasm of arterioles, are secondary to kidney changes and are responsible for much of the symptomatology of the disease.

Incidence

1   Unknown — milder cases are not recognized
2   More common in males than females
3   Most common in preschool and early school age groups
4   Rare in children under 1 year of age
5   Varies with the prevalence of nephritogenic strains of streptococci and the likelihood of cross-infection.

Clinical Manifestations

Onset

1   Usually 1-3 weeks after the onset of the initiating infection
2   May be abrupt and severe or mild and detected only by laboratory measures.

Signs and Symptoms

1   Urinary symptoms
    a Decreased urine output
    b Bloody or brown-coloured urine
2   Oedema
    a Present in most patients
    b Usually mild
    c Often manifested by periorbital oedema in the morning
    d May appear only as rapid weight gain
    e May be generalized and influenced by posture
3   Hypertension
    a Present in over 50% of patients
    b Usually mild, but occasionally more severe
    c Rise in blood pressure may be sudden
    d Usually appears during the first 4-5 days of the illness
4   Variable fever
    a May be high initially
    b Usually fluctuates at about 37.8°C for several days
5   Malaise
6   Mild headache
7   Gastrointestinal disturbances, especially anorexia and vomiting, often with abdominal and loin pain.

Diagnostic Evaluation

1   Urinalysis
   a Decreased output — may approach anuria
   b Microscopic or gross haematuria
   c High specific gravity
   d Protein
     (1) Variable
     (2) Usually below 3 g per day
   e White cells — moderate
   f Granular and cellular casts — especially red cell casts
2   Serum complement level — usually reduced
3   Blood urea nitrogen and creatinine — often mildly to moderately elevated
4   ASO or antistreptolysin O titre — elevated
5   Sedimentation rate — elevated
6   Chest x-ray — may show pulmonary congestion, and cardiac enlargement.
7   Renal function studies — normal in 50% of the patients.

Prognosis

1   Prognosis is generally good, but variable, and is not correlated with the severity of the disease.
2   Younger children generally have the best prognosis for complete recovery.
3   At least 95% of affected children recover completely.
   a Acute symptoms usually disappear in 1-3 weeks.
   b Blood chemistry is usually normal by the end of the second week.
   c Urine sediment may be abnormal for months or even years following the acute episode.
   d Sedimentation rate may remain elevated for several months.
   e Exacerbations may occur with acute infections during the recovery phase but usually do not alter the outcome.
4   Death during the acute phase is very uncommon, but may occur due to the effects of hypertensive encephalopathy or heart failure.
5   A small percentage of children develop chronic nephritis.

Complications

Occur infrequently.

Hypertensive Encephalopathy

1   Manifestations
   a Restlessness
   b Stupor
   c Convulsions
   d Vomiting

e Severe headache

f Visual disturbances

g Cranial nerve palsies

2 Cause — probably ischaemia secondary to vasospasm

3 No correlation with the degree of renal impairment or fluid retention

4 Duration

    a Usually 1-2 days

    b Ends spontaneously with decreased blood pressure.

Congestive Heart Failure

1 Cardiac failure may occur due to persistent hypertension, hypervolaemia, and peripheral vasoconstriction

2 Manifestations

    a Dyspnoea

    b Tachycardia

    c Gallop rhythm

    d Liver engorgement

    e Increased venous pressure

    f Changes in the electrocardiogram

    g Cardiac enlargement

    h Pulmonary oedema

3 Duration

    a Variable

    b Usually subsides rapidly with the onset of diuresis and the fall in blood pressure.

Uraemia

1 Manifestations

    a Evidence of acidosis

    b Drowsiness

    c Coma

    d Stupor

    e Muscular twitching

    f Convulsions.

Anaemia

Usually caused by hypervolaemia rather than a loss of red blood cells in the urine.

Nursing Objectives

To promote healing and prevent disease complications

1 No specific measures have been demonstrated to modify the inflammatory process.

2 General measures

a Maintain bed rest during the acute phase of the illness, at least until gross haematuria has disappeared and child is no longer hypertensive.

(1) Organize nursing activities to allow child to have periods of uninterrupted rest.

(2) Explain to the child why it is necessary for him to stay in bed. (Bed rest is often interpreted by the child as punishment.)

(3) Administer sedation if required to keep the child quiet and at rest.

(4) Provide diversion appropriate for the child's age.

(5) Place the child's bed in a position where he can watch the activities of the unit and other children.

(6) Provide alternative means of rest for children who are too young to understand the necessity of remaining in bed. These children may be more comfortable and rested sitting in a chair.

(7) Observe the child closely for fatigue once ambulation is begun.

b Protect the child from infection.

(1) Avoid placing the child in a room with patients who have fevers, upper respiratory infections, or any other contagious disease.

(2) Administer therapeutic doses of antibiotics as ordered by the paediatrician to eradicate existing infection.

(a) A 10-day course of intramuscular penicillin is often prescribed. May be followed by oral penicillin for a further 3 weeks.

(b) Points of emphasis.

Inject the medication into a large muscle.

Rotate the site of injection.

Observe the child closely for adverse reactions such as skin rash, urticaria, serum sickness, and anaphylaxis.

(3) Protect the child from chilling or overheating.

(4) Provide scrupulous daily hygiene, including mouth care. Keep the skin clean and dry.

c Provide a diet in conformity with the child's age and the recommendation of his paediatrician.

(1) A regular diet without added salt is usually prescribed during the acute phase in noncomplicated cases.

(2) A diet restricted in protein and potassium is necessary for children who demonstrate some degree of renal failure; those with raised blood urea levels.

(3) Fluids must be restricted in children with hypertension, raised blood urea levels, congestive failure, or renal failure.

(4) Explain all dietary restrictions to the child and his parents.

(5) Obtain a careful history of dietary preferences and patterns so that the child's meals can be as acceptable as possible.

(6) Place a sign indicating dietary restrictions on the child's bed so that anyone approaching him will be aware of his special needs.

(7) If the child is to be given a restricted amount of fluids, offer small

amounts of fluids spaced at regular intervals throughout the day and evening.

Use a cup of appropriate size for the amount of fluid being offered.

(8) Refer to section on nutrition, p. 36.

To observe and record disease progress.

1 Maintain a complete record of the child's intake and output.

a Measure fluids accurately in graduated containers. Do not estimate fluid intake or output.

b Place a sign on the child's bed to ensure that no urine is accidentally discarded and that all intake is recorded.

c Total the intake and output every 8 or 24 hours according to nursing care plan.

(1) Notify the paediatrician if output does not appear adequate.

(2) In children who are not toilet trained, a fairly accurate record of intake and output can be obtained by weighing nappies before and after micturition.

d Record other causes of fluid loss such as the number of stools per day, perspiration, etc.

2 Weigh the child daily.

a An increase in weight may indicate fluid retention.

b Weigh the child on the same scale and at the same time each day.

(1) It is usually advantageous to weigh the child before breakfast.

(2) The child should be weighed in a consistent manner, with minimal clothing.

3 Record the blood pressure at frequent intervals.

a Refer to the method for determining blood pressure, p. 102.

b A diastolic pressure of 13 kPa (100 mmHg) is an indication of concern and should be reported to the paediatrician immediately.

Place the child in bed and observe him closely for cerebral changes.

4 Observe for signs of complications:

a Increased blood pressure

b Fluid retention or oedema

c Changes in vital signs, especially more rapid pulse or respirations

d Changes in activity status, especially lethargy, restlessness, stupor, or coma

e Vomiting

f Visual disturbances

g Severe headache

h Convulsions.

5 Record appearance of urine.

Note the persistence of haematuria or whether the urine appears to be clearing.

To reduce hypertension

1 Limit the fluid intake according to the paediatrician's recommendation.
2 Maintain bed rest.
3 Administer antihypertensive drugs as ordered by the paediatrician.
   a Reserpine is the drug most frequently employed.
      (1) Route of administration
         (a) Oral, intramuscular, or intravenous
         (b) Initial control is usually achieved by intramuscular administration; the child is later maintained with oral medication.
      (2) Side effects
         Nasal stuffiness, dryness of mouth, diarrhoea.

Note: Phenobarbitone may be combined with reserpine.

To provide appropriate nursing care to the child with disease complications.

1 Encephalopathy
   Refer to the section on care of the child with seizures, p. 651.
2 Congestive heart failure. (Refer to the section on congestive heart failure, p. 390.)
3 Anaemia
   Refer to the section on anaemia, p. 343.
4 Renal failure
   a Maintain strict record of intake and output.
   b Weigh the child at frequent intervals.
      It may be necessary to weigh the child as often as every 8-12 hours.
   c Perform all nursing activities as for the child with uncomplicated glomerulonephritis.
   d Administer fluids as prescribed by the paediatrician.
      (1) Fluid intake is usually restricted to an amount equal to urinary output-plus insensible water loss (usually 300-400 ml per square meter of body surface area per day).
      (2) Fluid requirements must be recalculated frequently.
         These vary with such factors as the child's activity, sweating, vomiting, body temperature, metabolic rate, etc.
      (3) Some form of carbohydrate is usually ordered to prevent excessive breakdown of body proteins and to decrease the formation of ketones.
         (a) Fluids, such as ginger ale or syrups, should be offered to the child who can tolerate oral fluids.
         (b) Glucose solutions may be administered intravenously. (Refer to the procedure for the administration of intravenous fluids, p. 155).
   e Have appropriate electrolytes available for administration.
      (1) Electrolytes are usually not added to the diet unless indicated by low serum levels or known loss.
         Plasma concentrations of sodium, potassium, chloride, and bicarbonate and urea must be monitored at frequent intervals.

(2) Replacement of electrolytes is rarely indicated during the oliguric phase.

(3) Potassium intoxication may occur and is usually counteracted by the administration of sodium bicarbonate of a cation exchange resin (e.g. Resonium A) which exchanges sodium for potassium.

(4) Hypocalcaemia requires the administration of calcium.

f Assist with peritoneal or renal dialysis if this is required. (Refer to Guideline, p. 210.)

To provide emotional support to the child and his family during hospitalization.

1 Explain all aspects of the diagnostic tests and treatment in terms that the family can understand.
2 Formulate a nursing care plan which facilitates a consistent approach to the child's care.
3 Allow the child to make some decisions and to participate in his care. He may decide when he wants his bath and should be allowed to make some dietary choices, etc.
4 Maintain discipline. Establish and enforce appropriate limits for the child's behaviour.
5 Provide diversion appropriate for the child's age.
6 Arrange for the continued education of the school-age child.

To prepare the child and his parents for discharge.

1 Encourage as much family participation as possible during the child's hospitalization. (Refer to section on family-centred care, p. 66.
2 Help the family plan for adaptation of the child's nursing care to the home environment.
   a Review the medication schedule.
   b Arrange for family to meet dietician to suggest means of implementing sodium restricted diet.
      (1) Provide the family with a list of commercial foods and fluids which are normally high in sodium content, so that they can avoid these.
      (2) Help the parents to plan sample menus.
      (3) Provide suggestions for low-sodium cooking and baking.
   c Discuss activity and fluid restrictions if appropriate.
3 Make certain that the family has an appointment for continued medical supervision.
4 Initiate appropriate referrals.
   a Community health nursing team
   b School/education authority for continued education

Patient or Parental Teaching

1 Medical explanation of the disease process should be reinforced.

a The need for medical evaluation and culture of all sore throats should be emphasized.

b The family should be made aware of signs and symptoms of disease recurrence.

2 Tonsillectomy or other oral surgery should not be done for several months after the acute phase of glomerulonephritis.

If this type of surgery is necessary later, penicillin should be administered before and after the procedure to prevent bacterial spread.

NEPHROTIC SYNDROME

Nephrotic syndrome refers to a symptom complex characterized by oedema, marked proteinuria, hypercholesterolaemia and hypoalbuminaemia. Although there are many types of the disease, lipid nephrosis or so-called minimal disease is the most common in children.

Aetiology

1 The symptom complex results from large losses of protein in the urine, too great for the body to replenish by albumin synthesis.

2 The exact cause of the protein loss is unknown, but may result from a variety of disease states and nephrotoxic agents.

Altered Physiology

1 For unknown reasons the glomerular membrane, usually impermeable to large proteins, becomes permeable.

2 Protein, especially albumin, leaks through the membrane and is lost in the urine.

3 Plasma proteins decrease as proteinuria increases.

4 The colloidal osmotic pressure which holds water in the vascular compartments is reduced owing to decrease in amount of serum albumin. This allows fluid to flow from the capillaries into the extracellular space, producing oedema.

5 Accumulation of fluid in the interstitial spaces and peritoneal cavity is also increased by an overproduction of aldosterone, which causes retention of sodium.

6 There is increased susceptibility to infection because of decreased gamma-globulin.

7 Generalized oedema is responsible for most of the physical characteristics of the disease, including respiratory distress, gastrointestinal symptoms, umbilical and inguinal hernias, rectal prolapse, decreased ambulation, loss of body tissue, and malnutrition.

Incidence

1   Incidence about 1 in 50,000 children.
2   More common in males than in females.
3   The disease most commonly occurs in children aged between 1 and 7 years.

Clinical Manifestations

Onset

1   Insidious
2   Oedema is often the presenting symptom.
  a Initially, usually slight and inconstant
  b Usually first apparent around the eyes

Signs and symptoms

1   Irritability and depression
2   Gastrointestinal disurbances, including vomiting and diarrhoea
3   Anorexia — malnutrition may become severe
4   Severe, recurrent infections
5   Marked, recurrent oedema
  a Ascites may be severe.
  b Intense scrotal oedema is common.
  c Peripheral oedema is dependent and shifts with the child's position.
  d Striae may appear on the skin from overstretching.
6   Profound weight gain; the child may actually double his normal weight.
7   Decreased urine output during the oedematous phase.
8   Minimal haematuria and hypertension may be present.
9   Pallor — caused by the stretching of skin over the subcutaneous fluid, usually not proportional to the amount of anaemia.
10   Wasting of skeletal muscles may occur because of the continuous drain of plasma protein nitrogen into the urine.
11   Nephrotic crisis
  a Abdominal pain
  b Fever
  c Erysipeloid skin eruption possible
  d Symptoms subside within a few days
  e Often followed by spontaneous diuresis.

Diagnostic Evaluation

1   Urinalysis
  a Proteinuria — marked
  b Casts — numerous
  c Haematuria — absent or transient

2 Renal function tests — variable, often normal
3 Blood
  a Total serum protein — reduced
  b Serum albumin — reduced
  c Total serum globulin — normal or increased
  d Amino acid level — decreased
  e Anaemia — absent or slight
  f Sedimentation rate — elevated
  g Cholesterol and lipoproteins — increased
     (1) Alpha and beta fractions — increased
     (2) Gamma fraction — reduced.

Clinical Course and Prognosis

1 The severity and duration of the clinical course is variable.
2 Partial or complete remissions occur secondary to spontaneous or induced diuresis.
3 Most children experience a number of remissions and exacerbations over a period of 1-10 years.
4 The majority of affected children eventually have a complete recovery. Some children may have compromised renal function for life.
5 Death may occur from profound sepsis, progressive renal insufficiency, or congestive heart failure.

Nursing Objectives

To relieve oedema and other manifestations of the nephrotic state.

1 Administer steroids as prescribed by the paediatrician.
  a Steroid therapy is the preferred approach to treatment because steroids appear to affect the basic disease process in addition to controlling oedema.
  b Prednisone is usually the drug of choice because it is less apt to induce salt retention and potassium loss.
    There is no standard programme of therapy, but most children receive 2-4 mg/kg until complete remission occurs; this is followed by low-dose maintenance therapy or an intermittent schedule for 8-12 months.
  c Children with nephrotic syndrome may respond to steroid therapy in several ways:
    (1) Steroid sensitive — children respond to a single short course of steroids without evidence of relapse after cessation of therapy.
    (2) Steroid dependent — children respond incompletely or tend to relapse on lowered dosages of steroids and require additional supportive treatment.
    (3) Steroid resistant — children become resistant to steroid therapy or cannot be maintained in remission without developing serious side effects of treatment.

d Observe for evidence of side effects and complications of therapy.

   (1) Cushing's syndrome

   (a) Manifestations include increased body hair (hirsutism), rounding of the face (moon face), abdominal distention, striae, increased appetite with weight gain, and aggravation of adolescent acne.

   (b) The child should have access to a mirror so that he can observe gradual physical changes in his body.

   (c) The child and his parents should be provided with opportunities to discuss their feelings about the child's altered body image. Play therapy may be helpful for the young child.

   (d) It should be stressed that these physical changes are not harmful nor permanent, and will disappear after the steroid treatment is stopped.

   (2) Serious side effects and uncommon complications

   (a) Masking of infections
   The child should be observed very closely for signs of inflammation or infection.

   (b) Peptic ulceration
   Give medication with milk or an antacid.
   Test all stools with haematest.

   (c) Growth suppression

   (d) Precipitation of diabetes mellitus

   (e) Increased intracranial pressure manifested by headache, anorexia, vomiting, diplopia, and seizures

   (f) Osteoporosis

   (g) Cataracts

   (h) Thromboembolism

   (i) Adrenal suppression and insufficiency

Nursing Alert: No vaccinations or immunizations should be given during active episodes of nephrosis or while the child is receiving immunosuppressive therapy.

2   Administer immunosuppressive drugs as ordered by the paediatrician.

   a Cyclophosphamide is the drug of choice because its efficacy has been most thoroughly documented.

   b This therapy is generally reserved for children with steroid-dependent or steroid-resistant nephrosis because of severe side effects.

   c Observe for complications of therapy.

   (1) Decreased white blood count renders the child very susceptible to infection.

   (2) *Hair loss* — The child should be prepared for this complication and should be helped to deal with the change in body image. Head scarves or wigs may minimize the child's distress.

   (3) *Cystitis* — The drug should be given in the morning and large volumes

of fluid given orally to prevent concentration of the drug in the urine.
(4) Sterility may result in both sexes from long-term use.

3   Administer diuretics as recommended by the paediatrician.

   a Diuretics are occasionally effective in relieving massive oedema.

   b Be aware of those diuretics which may cause potassium depletion.

   (1) Offer foods high in potassium, such as orange juice or bananas.

   (2) Supplemental potassium chloride may be administered orally if the urine output is adequate.

Nursing Alert: Mercurial diuretics should not be administered intravenously to patients with nephrosis because fatalities have been reported.

4   Maintain the child on bed rest during periods of severe oedema.
    Refer to the section on acute glomerulonephritis, p. 481.

5   Administer a diet low in sodium and high in potassium.

   a Moderate sodium restriction is usually indicated. Excessively salty foods are excluded and extra salt is eliminated.

   b Potassium may be provided in juices, fruits (especially oranges, grapes, and bananas), and milk.

6   Restrict fluids as requested by the paediatrician.

   a Fluid restriction is usually imposed only during the extreme oedematous phases.

   b Restriction is carefully calculated at frequent intervals, based on the urine output of the previous day plus estimated insensible losses.

   c Offer small amounts of fluids spaced at regular intervals throughout the day and evening.
    Use a cup of appropriate size for the amount of fluid being offered.

   d Measure fluids accurately in graduated containers. Do not estimate fluid intake or output.

   e Place a sign on the child's bed to ensure that no urine is accidently discarded and that all intake is recorded.

   f Determine total intake and output every 8 or 24 hours according to nursing care plan.
    In children who are not toilet trained, a fairly accurate record of output can be obtained by weighing nappies before and after micturition.

   g Record other causes of fluid loss such as the number of stools per day, perspiration, etc.

7   Assist with abdominal paracentesis when this is required because of marked ascites. (See Guidelines, p. 492.)

To protect the child from infection.

1   Apply measures stated in the section on acute glomerulonephritis, p. 481.

2   Closely observe the child who is on steroids for signs of infection since this medication masks such symptoms.

3   Provide meticulous skin care to the oedematous areas of the body.
   a Bathe the child frequently and apply powder.
      (1) Areas of special concern are the moist parts of the body and oedematous male genitalia.
      (2) Support the scrotum with a cotton pad held in place by a T-binder if necessary for the child's comfort.
   b Position the child so that oedematous skin surfaces are not in contact.
   Place a pillow between the child's legs when he is lying on his side, etc.
   c Swab eyelids and cleanse the surrounding area several times daily to remove exudate.
   Elevate the child's head to reduce oedema.
4   If possible, avoid femoral venepunctures and intramuscular injections in the buttocks.
   In addition to the risk of infection the child may be predisposed to thromboembolism because of hypovolaemia, stasis, and increased plasma concentration of clotting factors.

To restore lost plasma and tissue proteins.

1   Offer a high protein, high kilojoule (calorie) diet.
   a Salt restriction is generally not necessary, except during periods of oedema and hypertension.
   b Fluid restriction is of little value in controlling oedema in nephrotic syndrome.
2   Obtain a complete history of dietary preferences and patterns so that the child's meals can be as acceptable as possible.
3   Place a sign on the child's bed indicating any dietary restrictions, so that anyone approaching him will be aware of his special needs.
4   Offer small amounts of high protein foods at frequent intervals.
   Permit additional amounts of food at the child's discretion.
5   Refer to section on nutrition, p. 36.

To observe for disease progress.

1   Apply nursing measures 'To observe and record disease progress', in the section on acute glomerulonephritis, p. 482.
2   Observe the child's entire body at frequent intervals for oedema.
   Record areas of transient oedema.
3   Record the amount and appearance of urine. Especially note:
   a Decreased urine output
   b Increased amount of protein
   c Cloudiness
   d Haematuria.
4   Observe for side effects of all medications.
5   Observe for indications of thrombosis and report these to the paediatrician immediately.

To provide emotional support to the child and his family.

1　Encourage frequent visiting.
　a Allow as much parental participation in the child's care as possible.
　b Refer to section on family-centred care, p. 66.
2　Allow the child as much activity as he can tolerate.
　a Bed rest should be enforced during periods of hypertension.
　b Balance periods of rest, recreation, and quiet activities during the convalescent phase.
　c Allow the child to eat his meals with other children.
3　Encourage the child to verbalize his fears.
　a Young children frequently fear abandonment by their parents or loss of body integrity. (The boy who is unable to see his penis because of extensive oedema may think that he has been castrated and needs reassurance that his body is intact.)
　b Refer to section on the hospitalized child, p. 56 .
4　Assist parents to verbalize their fears, frustrations, and questions.
　a Parents often express frustration regarding the uncertainties associated with the cause of the disease, the clinical course, and prognosis.
　b Parents may question the difference between nephritis and nephrotic syndrome.

To prepare for the child's discharge.

1　Begin discharge planning early.
　a Have the dietician discuss special diets with the parents. Encourage them to plan sample menus.
　b Encourage the parents to administer the child's medication prior to discharge.
　c Instruct parents about urine testing.
　d Provide suggestions regarding activity restriction at home.
2　Provide written discharge instructions concerning:
　a Diet
　b Prevention of infection
　c Skin care
　d Administration of medications
　e Activity restrictions
　f Urine testing
　g Appointment for continued medical supervision.
3　Initiate a community health nursing referral for continued support and counselling.

Parental Teaching

1　Reinforce medical interpretation of the child's disease. Stress the importance of attention to the details of the child's care and continued medical supervision.

2 Discuss the problem of discipline with the parents. Encourage them to set consistent limits on and expectations of their child's behaviour.
3 Emphasize the necessity of taking medication according to the prescribed schedule and for an extended period of time. Discuss complications encountered with steroid therapy.

GUIDELINES: ASSISTING WITH ABDOMINAL PARACENTESIS

Purpose

To withdraw fluid from the peritoneal cavity in order to relieve pressure symptoms and respiratory distress.

Equipment

1 Sterile equipment
   Hypodermic syringe
   Hypodermic and aspiration needles
   Novocain or lignocaine 1%
   Scalpel
   Trocar and cannula or Southey's tube with shield, stilletto and tubing
   Needle holder
   Suture needles and sutures
   Forceps
   Gloves
   Towels
   Graduated receptacle
   Cotton wool balls
   Gauze squares
   Abdominal dressing
2 Non-sterile equipment
   Preparation tray
   Test tubes
   Pail for the collection of fluid
   Waterproof protection for bed
   Abdominal binder
   Safety pins
   Adhesive tape

Procedure

Nursing Action	Rationale/Amplification
Preparatory Phase	
1 Explain procedure to parents, seek their cooperation. Mother or father may wish to be present during procedure. Show parent where best to sit to be able to talk to and comfort their child. Explain the procedure to the child in terms he can understand. Stress that he will feel better after the procedure.	1 To allay his fears and assure his cooperation.
2 Have the child empty his bladder just prior to the procedure.	2 To avoid puncturing the bladder during the procedure.
3 Secure the help of a second nurse if necessary.	3 To observe the child and assist the paediatrician during the procedure.
4 Position the child correctly:	
a Make him comfortable, sitting upright in bed well supported by pillows.	**a** Will help ascitic fluid to drain. Will ease dyspnoea.
b Hold his hands.	
Method	
1 Maintain the child's position.	1 To avoid injury.
2 Talk to the child frequently and hold his hands. Praise him for his cooperation.	2 To offer emotional support.
3 Observe the child's colour and respirations.	3 Symptoms of shock develop if too much fluid is removed.
Follow-up Phase	
1 Apply abdominal binder snugly.	
2 Record the amount and character of the drainage and the child's condition.	
3 Observe frequently for signs of shock and note the drainage on the bandages.	

URINARY TRACT INFECTION

Urinary tract infection refers to an infection within the urinary system. The lower urinary tract (urethra, bladder, or the lower portion of the ureters) or the upper urinary tract (upper portion of the ureters or kidney) or both may be involved.

Aetiology

1   Causative organisms
   a Gastrointestinal flora account for 75-85% of all cases.
     (1) *Escherichia coli* — most common causative agent
     (2) *Proteus*
     (3) *Aerobacter*
     (4) *Enterobacter*
     (5) *Klebsiella*
     (6) *Pseudomonas.*
   b Streptococci and staphylococci cause most other cases.
2   Route of entry
   a Ascent from the exterior (most common)
   b Circulating blood
3   Contributing causes
   a Obstruction, usually congenital
   b Infections elsewhere in the body
     (1) Upper respiratory
     (2) Diarrhoea
   c Poor perineal hygiene
   d Short female urethra
   e Catheterization and instrumentation
   f Entrance of an irritant into the bladder
   g Inherent defect in the ability of the bladder mucosa to protect it from microbial invasion.

Altered Physiology

1   Inflammatory changes occur in the affected portions of the urinary tract.
2   Clumps of bacteria may be present.
3   Inflammation results in urinary retention and stasis of urine in the bladder. There may be backflow of urine into the kidneys through the ureters.
4   There are inflammatory changes in the renal pelvis and throughout the kidney when this organ is involved.
5   The kidney may become large and swollen.
6   Scarring of the kidney parenchyma occurs in chronic infection and interferes with kidney function, particularly with the ability to concentrate urine.

7   Eventually, the kidney becomes small, tissue is destroyed and renal function fails.

Incidence

1   Most common renal disease in children.
2   More common in females than in males, ratio 6:1, except in the neonatal period, when both sexes are equally affected.

Clinical Manifestations

Onset

1   May be abrupt or gradual
2   May be asymptomatic

Signs and Symptoms

1   Fever
    a May be moderate or severe
    b May fluctuate rapidly
    c May be accompanied by chills or convulsions
2   Anorexia and general malaise
3   Urinary frequency, urgency, dysuria
4   Daytime or nocturnal enuresis
5   Dull or sharp pain in the kidney area
6   Irritability
7   Vomiting
8   Failure to thrive in infancy.

Diagnostic Evaluation

1   Urinalysis
    a Pus is present in abnormal amounts.
    b Casts, especially white cell casts, may be present and are indicative of intrarenal infection.
    c Haematuria — occurs occasionally.
2   Urine culture
    a Documentation of pathogenic organisms in the urine is the only means of definitive diagnosis.
    b A urine culture demonstrating more than 100,000 bacteria per millilitre indicates significant bacteriuria.
3   Renal concentrating ability — decreased
4   Urological and radiological studies
    A voiding cystourethrogram should be carried out and the intravenous pressure should be taken after the initial infection subsides to identify

abnormalities, which might contribute to the development of infection, and to identify existing kidney changes due to recurrent infection.

Prognosis

1   Generally good in uncomplicated cases.
2   Persistent infection may occur in patients with obstruction or urinary retention and may lead ultimately to renal failure.
3   There is a tendency for recurrence of both treated and untreated infections.

Nursing Objectives

To obtain a clean urine specimen for examination or culture.

1   A freshly micturated early morning specimen is most accurate. (This urine is usually acid and concentrated, which tends to preserve the formed elements).
2   Refer to the procedure for the collection of urine specimens, p. 126.
3   Catheterization may be necessary to obtain a sterile specimen in older girls.
     Defer this procedure whenever possible in order to avoid emotional trauma and the accidental introduction of additional bacteria.
4   Obtain a midstream specimen whenever possible.
5   The urine should be sent to the laboratory immediately or refrigerated to avoid a falsely high bacterial count.

To eradicate infective organisms.

1   Administer antibiotics as prescribed by the paediatrician.
2   Antibiotic therapy is generally determined by the results of urine cultures and sensitivities, and by the child's response to therapy.
3   Most frequently used antibiotics:
     a Sulphafurazole (Gantrisin)
       (1) Side effects and toxic effects
          (a) Nausea and vomiting
          (b) Dizziness, headache, drug fever, dermatitis
          (c) Blood dyscrasias
          (d) Oliguria, crystalluria, and anuria — result from precipitation of the drug in the renal tubules.
       (2) Contraindications
          (a) Drug sensitivity
          (b) Infants under the age of 2-3 months.

Nursing Alert: Keep the child well hydrated to avoid crystallization of the drug in the renal tubules.

b Ampicillin
  (1) Side effects
    (a) Diarrhoea
    (b) Nausea
    (c) Vomiting
    (d) Epigastric distress
    (e) Mild flatulence
    (f) Pruritis
    (g) Hypersensitivity reactions, including rash, urticaria, angioneurotic oedema, and anaphylactic reactions
  (2) Contraindications
    (a) Known hypersensitivity to other penicillins
    (b) Infections caused by penicillinase-producing staphylococci or other penicillinase-producing organisms
  (3) Points of emphasis
    (a) Package circular should be consulted for directions regarding reconstitution, administration, and storage of intramuscular and intravenous preparations.
    (b) Oral preparations should be administered at least 1-2 hours after meals to assure maximum absorption.

c Nitrofurantoin (Furadantin)
  (1) Side effects and toxic effects
    (a) Nausea and vomiting
    (b) Peripheral neuritis
    (c) Haemolytic anaemia
    (d) Sensitization
  (2) Contraindications
    (a) Anuria
    (b) Oliguria
    (c) Infants under 1 month of age
  (3) Points of emphasis
    (a) The drug may cause the urine to be amber or brown in colour.
    (b) Drug should be administered after meals or with a small amount of food to minimize nausea or vomiting.
    (c) Administration of the drug should be continued for at least 3 days after the urine becomes sterile.
    (d) Prolonged therapy should be closely monitored by clinical and laboratory means and the dosage regulated accordingly.
    (e) Recurrences of infections following the discontinuance of nitrofurantoin may occur more quickly than recurrences following sulphafurazole (Gantrisin) therapy.

Note: Other drugs which may be used according to the sensitivity of the causative organism include: cotrimoxazole, cephaloridine, naladixic acid, colistin, gentamycin and kanamycin.

To provide for symptomatic relief of the child's discomfort during the febrile period.

1   Maintain bed rest.
2   Administer analgesic and antipyretic drugs as prescribed by the physician.
3   Encourage fluids to reduce the fever and dilute the concentration of the urine.
    a Obtain a complete nursing history regarding the child's fluid preferences and method of taking them.
    b Administer intravenous fluids if necessary. Refer to Guidelines, p. 155.
4   Refer to section on care of the child with fever, p. 105.

To observe for progress of disease

1   Nursing notes should include:
    a Frequent recording of the child's temperature
    b Accurate measurement of intake and output
    c Description of the colour and odour of the urine, especially if it is abnormal
    d Presence of any of following symptoms:
       (1) Frequency of urination
       (2) Burning or pain with micturition
       (3) Enuresis
       (4) Urinary retention
    e General behaviour and activity status of the child
    f Signs of untoward or toxic effects of drugs
    g Pain, especially in the kidney area.

To provide emotional support to the child and his parents.

1   Reinforce medical explanations of the disease and its therapy.
2   Explain all diagnostic tests and procedures to the child before they are carried out.
3   Encourage the verbal child to talk about his experience and how he feels about it. Correct any misconceptions he may have.
4   Provide an environment that is as close to normal as possible during hospitalization. Include opportunities for the child to play.

To prepare the child and his family for discharge.

1   Discuss any treatment that will be required at home. Provide written discharge instructions regarding:
    a Rest

b Fluid intake
c Administration of medications
d Appointment for continued medical supervision.
2   Communicate or have the parents communicate with the school nurse if it is necessary for the child to receive medications at school.

Parental Teaching

1   Long-term therapy is often prescribed to prevent recurrence of urinary tract infections.
   a Schedules for prolonged therapy vary from several months to a year.
   b The infection should not be considered as eradicated until at least two negative cultures are obtained 4-6 weeks after cessation of therapy.
2   The child should be kept under continued medical surveillance because of the possibility of disease recurrence.
      Emphasis should be placed on the fact that even though this disease may have few symptoms, it can lead to very serious, permanent disability.
3   Spread of bacteria from the anal and vaginal areas to the urethra can be minimized in female children by cleansing the perianal area from the urethra back towards the anus.
4   Bubble baths should not be used because of the bladder-irritant effect of these soaps.
5   Encourage adequate fluid intake, especially water.
6   Encourage child to void frequently and to empty the bladder completely with each voiding.

ABNORMALITIES OF THE GENITOURINARY TRACT WHICH REQUIRE SURGERY

Exstrophy of the Bladder (Ectopia Vesicae, Ectopic Bladder)

In *exstrophy of the bladder* the posterior and lateral surfaces of the bladder and urethral outlets are exposed because of failure of the two sides of the lower abdomen to unite. The condition allows direct passage of urine to the outside. A rare congenital abnormality affecting predominantly males; the incidence is 1 in 50,000 live births.

Clinical Manifestations

1   Constant dribbling of urine excoriates the skin.
2   Ulceration of the bladder mucosa may occur.
3   There are usually associated defects, including separation of the pubic rami, defects of the bowel, epispadias, undescended testes or inguinal hernia in the male and cleft clitoris, separated labia or absent vagina in the female.
4   Affected children walk with a waddling or unsteady gait.

Treatment

1   Urinary diversion is indicated in many cases.
2   Complete correction by means of plastic surgery. The child can then micturate normally.
3   Plastic repair of the bladder, abdominal wall, and genitalia.
4   Surgery or braces to correct deformity of the pelvic girdle. Surgery is usually performed between 6 and 12 months of age, when construction of a bladder can be attempted.

Nursing Management

Preoperative Care

1   Protect the bladder area from trauma and irritation.
    a Position the infant on his back or side.
    b Cleanse the area frequently with mild soap and water.
    c Cover the defect with sterile gauze to which a bland ointment such as Vaseline has been applied.
    d Change the gauze covering and the infant's nappies frequently.
2   Observe the infant closely for signs of infection.
3   Teach the mother how to cleanse the area and protect the bladder.
        Ensure that a referral is made to the family health visitor for reinforcement of teaching and maternal support.
4   Collect urine specimens by holding the infant over a sterile bowl in a position which allows urine to drip into the container.
        A medicine dropper may also be used to collect urine from the opening in the bladder.

Postoperative Care
1   Maintain intravenous fluids until oral fluids can be given.
2   Maintain continuous catheter drainage into a closed system of drainage. Usually removed after 10 days.
3   Teach the child anal sphincter control to prevent seepage of urine.
    a Expect some soiling of his clothes.
    b Avoid causing him embarrassment when such accidents occur.
4   Observe for complications:
    a Urinary or incisional infections.
    b Fistulae in the suprapubic or penile incisions.
5   Long-term support will be necessary for many children and families to help them deal with such fears as appearance of genitalia, potential inability to procreate, and rejection by peers. Ongoing discussion groups for parents and children may be helpful.

Prognosis

Few children become fully continent. Many require further surgery and urinary diversion may become necessary in later life.

Patent Urachus

Patent urachus is persistence of the embryonic connection between the umbilicus and the bladder. In many patients only a cyst persists, located at the upper end of the tract, under the umbilicus.

Clinical Manifestations
1   Urine dribbles from the umbilicus when entire urachus is present.
2   Midline swelling is present in cases of a cyst.
3   Infection of urachal cysts is common.

Treatment
1   Eradication of infection
2   Removal of cysts
3   Surgical obliteration of the patent urachus.

Obstructive Lesions of the Lower Urinary Tract

Types of Obstruction

1 Urethral valves
    a Filamentous valves that obstruct urine flow
    b Most commonly found in males
2 Congenital narrowing of the urethra
3 Bladder neck obstruction
        Most common site of lower urinary tract obstruction
4 Meatal stricture
5 Severe phimosis (rare)
6 Neuromuscular dysfunction. (Refer to the section on spina bifida, p. 634.

Clinical Manifestations

1 Abnormal urination
    a Dysuria
    b Frequency
    c Enuresis
    d Dribbling
    e Reduced force of urine stream
    f Difficulty starting urine stream
    g Straining during urination
    h Abrupt cessation during urination.

Altered Physiology

1 Urinary tract becomes distended proximal to the point of obstruction.
2 The bladder dilates and hypertrophies.
3 Stasis of urine occurs.
4 The ureters become elongated, dilated, and tortuous.
5 Hydronephrosis and destruction of kidney tissue inevitably result.

Treatment

1 Eradication and prevention of infection. (See section on urinary tract infection, p. 494.)
2 Dilation of urethral stenosis or stricture.
3 Surgical relief of the obstruction.

Obstructive Lesions of the Upper Urinary Tract

Types of Obstruction
1 Stricture of a ureter.
2 Congenital absence of one ureter.
3 Duplication of the ureter of one kidney.
4 Compression of a ureter by an aberrant blood vessel.

Clinical Manifestations
1 Often asymptomatic. (There is seldom any problem with micturating.)
2 Vague symptoms such as failure to thrive may be present.
3 Urinary tract infections may be frequent.
4 Hypertension may occur.

Treatment
Same as for obstructions of lower urinary tract.

Hypospadias

Hypospadias is malposition of the urethral opening.

Altered Physiology

Males
1 The urethra opens on the lower surface of the penis, proximal to its usual site.
2 In severe cases, the urethra may open on the shaft of the penis, at its base, or on the perineum.
3 Frequently associated with congenital chordee in males — cord-like defect which extends from the scrotum up the penis and deflects the penis downward.

Females
The urethra opens into the vagina (rare).

Clinical Manifestations
1 Inability to pass urine with the penis in the normal elevated position.
2 Severe forms interfere with the ability to procreate.

Treatment

Plastic surgery.

Epispadias

Epispadias is another form of malposition of the urethral opening.

Altered Physiology

Males

The urethra opens on to the dorsum of the penis.

Females

The urethra opens into the vagina. Perineal examination shows a double clitoris (rare).

Note: Should be suspected in the presence of dribbling incontinence in the female child.

Clinical Manifestations

1   Inability to pass urine with the penis in the normal elevated position.
2   Severe forms interfere with penile erection and the ability to procreate.

Treatment

Corrective plastic surgery usually delayed until the infant is 1 year old.

1   The first stage of surgery is delayed until the infant is at least 12 months old when the chordee (fibrous tissue on the ventral surface of the penis).
2   Plastic reconstruction (the second stage) is delayed until the infant is 3-4 years.

Perineal Urethrostomy

In order to facilitate healing after surgery for hypospadias a perineal urethrostomy may be made. This is a temporary opening through the perineum into the urethra, into which a catheter is passed, allowing the drainage of urine but bypassing the operative site until healing is complete. The catheter is attached to sterile disposable tubing and bag. This should be changed daily using an aseptic technique.

Circumcision

Circumcision is the excision of the foreskin (prepuce) of the glans penis.

Clinical Indications
1   Usually done in infancy for hygienic purposes
2   Phimosis (inability to retract foreskin over the glans)
3   Paraphimosis (condition in which the foreskin cannot be reduced from a retracted position)
4   Recurrent infections of glans (balanitis) and foreskin
5   Personal desire of parents.

Pre- and Post-operative Care
See p. 83.

Postoperative Nursing Management
1   Watch for bleeding.
2   Change Vaseline gauze dressings frequently. Frequent nappy changes.
3   Watch for meatal ulceration, which causes pain, often retention of urine, occasional bleeding and may lead to meatal stenosis.
4   Clear written guidance should be given to the parents when the child is ready for discharge. This should include recognition of any complications and hygiene of the area. Follow-up appointments at outpatients should be given.

Hydrocele

Hydrocele is an abnormal accumulation of fluid within the scrotum around the testicle and within the two layers of the tunica vaginalis.

Causes
(Caused by defective or inadequate reabsorption of normally produced hydrocele fluid.)
1   Secondary to local injury, including hernia operation
2   Secondary to infection
3   Following epididymitis or orchitis; torsion
4   Idiopathic.

Clinical Manifestations
1   Enlargement of the scrotum
2   Usually painless until fluid accumulation is large enough to cause pressure.

Treatment

1　No treatment is required unless complications are present. Spontaneous cure often occurs in early infancy.
　a Circulatory complications involving testicle.
　b Painful large hydrocele which is uncomfortable and cosmetically unacceptable to the parents.
2　Surgical intervention: open operation for eversion of hydrocele sac or removal of hydrocele sac.

Complications

1　Haemorrhage into scrotal tissues
2　Infection.

Cryptorchidism (Undescended Testis)

Cryptorchidism is the absence of one or both testes from the scrotum. The testes may be located in the abdominal cavity or inguinal canal.

Aetiology

Caused by delayed descent, prevention of descent by some mechanical lesion, or endocrine disorders (rare).

Clinical Manifestations and Altered Physiology

1　Normal development of secondary sex characteristics.
2　Degeneration of the sperm-forming cells occurs after puberty because of the higher temperature of the abdomen compared with the normal location in the scrotum. Sterility results.
3　Emotional disturbances often occur when the child discovers that he is different from his peers.
4　Associated hernias are found in about 70-80% of the patients.

Treatment

1　Orchiopexy (placement of the testes in the scrotum)
2　Plastic surgery in patients with an absent testis
3　Administration of chorionic gonadotropin — has produced descent of the testes in some children. (Testes would probably have descended spontaneously in these cases.)

Nursing Management

Preoperative Care

1   Encourage the child and his parents to express their feelings about the condition.

Expect anxieties regarding sterility and homosexuality and perceptions of the child as defective or inadequate.

2   Discuss the condition and surgery frankly, in terms the child can understand.

  a Maintain a matter-of-fact attitude.

  b Clarify any misconceptions the child may have.

3   Provide privacy for medical examinations.

Postoperative Care

1   Maintain traction, if necessary.

  a Sometimes a suture is placed in the lower portion of the scrotum and is attached to a rubber band which is fastened to the upper aspect of the inner thigh by a piece of adhesive.

  b This traction anchors the testis to the scrotum and is removed in approximately 5-7 days. Alternatively the testis may be tethered to the inside of the scrotum.

2   Prevent contamination of the suture line.

3   Administer antibiotics as ordered to prevent infection.

Ambiguous Genitalia

Female Pseudohermaphroditism

1   Most common problem of sexual differentiation.

2   A deficiency of hydrocortisone results in adrenocortical hyperplasia and an overproduction of androgens.

3   *Manifestations* — masculinization of the external genitalia in the female infant.

4   *Treatment*

  a Administration of hydrocortisone in children with adrenal hyperplasia.

  b Corrective plastic surgery

This should be undertaken as early in life as possible, before social adjustment becomes a severe problem.

Male Pseudohermaphroditism

Type	Treatment
1 Normal female genitalia with testes internally (testicular feminization syndrome)	1 **a** Surgical removal of testes **b** Administration of oestrogens at puberty **c** Child reared as a girl
2 Predominantly male genitalia with testes internally	2 **a** Surgical removal of all nonmale structures **b** Child reared as a boy
3 Ambiguous genitalia due to damaged testes in fetal life	3 **a** Plastic reconstruction **b** Child reared as a boy.

True Hermaphroditism

1 May be either genetic males or females
2 Have both ovarian and testicular tissue
3 Genitalia are usually ambiguous
4 Gender choice is based on the infant's anatomy.
   Infant is usually reared as female.

Diagnostic Evaluation

1 Buccal smear to determine the presence or absence of sex chromatin
2 Endoscopy and x-ray studies to reveal presence, absence, and nature of internal genital structures
3 Chromosomal analysis to identify genetic sex
4 Biochemical tests of urinary steroid excretion patterns
5 Laparotomy or gonad biopsy.

Nursing Management

1 Recognize the situation as a social emergency.
   Support the parents while they wait for gender assignment of the infant. This should be done as soon as possible, but may require several days or weeks for results of studies.
2 Reinforce medical explanations of the anatomical problems and treatment. Approach the situation matter-of-factly.
3 Initiate appropriate referrals for family support and counselling. These may include:
   a Social work
   b Psychiatry
   c Community health nursing
   d Child guidance clinic
   e Genetic counselling.

Care of the Child Requiring Urological Surgery

Preoperative Care

1 Determine the child's fantasies regarding his illness and hospitalization. Correct any misconceptions that he reveals.

2 Provide an explanation of the anatomy and physiology of the urinary system in terms that the child can understand.

  a Use a body outline appropriate for the age of the child.

  b Explain how the child differs from the normal. Relate his defect to his symptoms whenever possible.

3 Explain all diagnostic tests prior to their occurrence. These may include: urinalysis, 24-hour urine collections, intravenous and retrograde pyelography, angiography, and cystoscopy.

  a Descriptions should include such information as:

  (1) Preparation required — fasting, enemas, etc.

  (2) Location of the test — operating theatre, x-ray department, etc.

  (3) Appearance and attire of personnel

  (4) Positioning

  (5) Anaesthesia

  (6) Pain or discomfort

  (7) Expectations following the procedure — diet, rest, urine collections, etc.

  b Determine the child's understanding of the procedure.

  (1) Ask him simple, direct questions.

  (2) Allow him to perform the procedure on a doll or demonstrate it on a diagram.

4 Explain the surgical procedure.

  a Explanations should include:

  (1) Preparation required — fasting, enemas, etc.

  (2) Description of the operating room including the appearance of the personnel

  (3) Anaesthesia. Allow child to handle masks, tubing, etc.

  (4) Postoperative appearance

    (a) Urinary drainage tubing and collection devices

    (b) Appearance of urine

    (c) Sutures

    (d) Bandages

    (e) Intravenous infusion.

  b Determine the child's understanding of his surgery and reinforce teaching when necessary.

5 Points of emphasis during the preparation:

  a The child is in no way to blame for his illness.

  b No other part of the body will be operated on.

Postoperative Care

1   Care for all catheters and urinary tubes according to hospital procedure. Maintain appropriate position of tubes.
2   Observe and record:
    a Amount and appearance of urinary drainage
    b Occurrence of bladder spasms
    c Symptoms of urinary or incisional infection.

Care of the Child who has an Ileal Conduit (Ileoloop)

Definition of the Procedure

One or both ureters are anastomosed to a segment of ileum, which then serves to carry urine to the external body surface of the abdomen.

Preoperative Care

1   Refer to the preceding section on the emotional preparation of the child and his family for urological surgery.
2   Allow the child to try on the ileal conduit apparatus in order to become familiar with it.
    Observe for discomfort and skin reactions to the adhesive or cement.
3   Administer antibiotics as prescribed by the surgeon.
    Be aware of the action, side effects, and contraindications of the prescribed therapy.
4   Provide the child and his parents with opportunities to express their fears and ask questions about the procedure.
    Expect worries related to sterility, location and appearance of the stoma, activity restrictions, clothing, and management.
5   Reassure the child and his parents that they will be taught to manage the conduit before leaving the hospital.
6   If appropriate, introduce the family to parents with a child who has had the same surgery.

Postoperative Care

1   Maintain the urinary collection apparatus. In the immediate postoperative period, urine is usually drained away by wide-bore catheter for several days in order to reduce the risk of leakage from the anastomoses, avoid ascending infection, and improve emptying of the ureters. Once the wound has healed satisfactorily, a urostomy collecting bag can be fitted.
    a Cleanse the area around the stoma with mild soap and water and dry it well.

b Keep the skin around the stoma completely dry during application of the appliance to ensure that it will remain attached.

c Place the adhesive plate of the appliance securely around the stoma.

The opening in the adhesive plate should be of a size that fits snugly over the stoma but does not compromise circulation.

d Empty the appliance every 2-4 hours or whenever it contains approximately 100 ml of fluid. (During the night the appliance may be attached via tubing to a collection bottle or a night bag.)

e Nursing observations related to the appliance:

(1) Leaking around the appliance

(2) Skin irritation

(3) Improper fit of the appliance.

f Points of emphasis:

(1) A properly applied apparatus should remain in place 3-5 days. It needs to be changed only when it begins to leak or becomes uncomfortable.

(2) It is normal for the urine to contain some mucus; it may be blood tinged.

2 Offer generous amounts of fluids to maintain hydration and keep the urine dilute and clear.

3 Carefully monitor intake and output.

Decreased urine output may indicate dehydration, obstruction of ureters, urine drainage into the peritoneal cavity, or compromised kidney function.

4 Observe for complications:

a Wound infection

b Leaking at the site of anastomosis

c Peritonitis

d Paralytic ileus

e Intestinal obstruction

f Stenosis of the stoma

g Fluid and electrolyte disturbances.

5 Assist the child and his family with problems related to altered body image.

a Assume a calm, understanding, and matter-of-fact attitude.

b Avoid outward expression of distaste.

c Keep equipment used in the management of the conduit out of sight to avoid embarrassment when visitors appear.

d Encourage the child to wear his own clothes so he is reassured that the appliance is invisible under clothing. Provide guidance on best styles to wear, e.g. pinafore-type dresses, dungarees. Avoid tight waist bands.

e Take precautions to prevent or eliminate odours, e.g. immediate cleansing of used collection bags, etc.

f Help the child and family to achieve control by teaching them to manage the care as soon as possible.

g Encourage early resumption of as many normal activities as possible.

Patient or Parental Teaching

1   Involve the child and his family in his self-care as soon as possible.
    Teaching should include how to assemble, apply, empty, change, and cleanse the appliance.
2   Explain that appliances can be adapted to meet individual patient's needs.
    Some experimentation will probably be necessary before the most suitable equipment can be identified.
3   Adequate daily fluid intake (approximately 125 ml/kg) is essential for maintaining good urine flow.
4   If disposable bags are not used, at least two appliances should be available, one in use and the other as a spare.
5   The appliance should be cleaned and aired regularly to avoid odour or crusting, with urinary crystals.
    a A mild soap and warm water should be used to clean the appliance.
    b Crusting can be removed by a solution of white vinegar and water (approximately 150 ml of white vinegar to a litre of water).
6   New appliances should be provided approximately every 6 months or whenever old ones begin to feel thin or worn, or disposable urostomy bags may be used.
7   Activity limitations are usually not necessary unless the child has associated physical problems.
8   Clothing may have to be altered slightly to fit over the pouch of the appliance.

Preparation for Discharge

1   Provide written information regarding the equipment that the child is using and where to obtain it.
2   Provide at least a 2-week supply of equipment for the family to take home.
    Advise the parents to obtain a prescription for new supplies before the old ones are depleted.
3   Initiate appropriate referrals:
    a Health visitor
    b School nurse.

FURTHER READING

Books

Brimblecombe F Barltrop D, *Children in Health and Disease*, Ballière Tindall, 1978.
Hellerstein S, *Urinary Tract Infection in Children*, Yearbook Medical, 1982.
James J A, *Renal Disease in Childhood*, Mosby, 1976.
Lieberman E, *Clinical Pediatric Nephrology*, Lippincott, 1976.

Morgan R, *Childhood Incontinence*, Heinemann, 1981.
Petrillo M Sanger S, *Emotional Care of Hospitalized Children*, Lippincott, 1980.
Scipien G *et al.*, *Comprehensive Pediatric Nursing*, 1979.

Articles

Barnes N D Roberton M, Urinary tract problems in childhood, *Update*, March 1979: 615-631.

Chambers T, When a child's kidneys fail, *Nursing Mirror*, December 1979: 38-39.

Chambers T, Urological emergencies: childhood problems, *Nursing Mirror* (Clinical Forum), 22 January 1981: XV-XVI.

Cross P, Urethral reimplantation: nursing care of the child, *American Journal of Nursing*, November 1976, 76: 1800.

Davidson-Lamb N Jones P F, Urinary tract infection in children, *British Medical Journal*, 4 August 1984: 299-303.

Dische S, Childhood enuresis-a family problem, *Developmental Medicine and Child Neurology*, October 1976: 323-330.

Esser J Peckham C, Nocturnal enuresis in childhood, *Developmental Medicine and Child Neurology*, October 1976: 577-589.

Fay J, Reflux and urinary obstruction, *Nursing Mirror*, October 1978: 41-44.

Horton C Devine C, Hypaspadias and epispadias, *Clinical Symposia*, 1977, 24 (3).

Kincaid-Smith P Dowling J P, Glomerulonephritis and the nephrotic syndrome, *Medicine*, November 1982 (23): 1070-1078.

McAloon J *et al.*, Management of childhood urinary tract infection in family practice, *British Medical Journal*, 9 June 1984: 1729-1730.

Nicholson R, Chronic renal failure, in a child, *Nursing Times*, June 1979: 99-999.

Saunders E L Chambers T L, The nephrotic syndrome in children, *Maternal and Child Health*, January 1983: 4-9.

Scott J, Paediatric urology, *Midwife, Health Visitor and Community Nurse*, October 1982: 411-422.

Stann J, Urinary tract infections in children, *Paediatric Nursing*, July August 1979: 46-49.

Valman H B, Urinary tract infection, *British Medical Journal*, 1 August 1981: 363-365.

Williams D I Morgan R C, Wide bladder syndrome in children, *Journal of the Royal Society of Medicine*, July 1978: 520-522.

9

SKIN PROBLEMS

BURNS

Burns are a frequent form of childhood injury. A second degree burn of 10% or more of the body surface in a child younger than 1 year, or a second degree burn of 15% or more of the body surface in a child over 1 year is considered a very serious injury. The effects of burns are not limited to the burn area.

Incidence and Aetiology

1 Burns outnumber all other causes of death during infancy, childhood, and adolescence, with the highest incidence of burns occurring in children under 5 years of age.
2 Causes of burns in children
  a Burns from hot water
    (1) Child (left unsupervised in bath) turns on the hot water tap
    (2) Child placed in bath of hot water that has not been tested
    (3) Spilling of hot coffee, tea on child; spilling occurs especially when pot handles stick out on top of stove
  b Burns from open flames
    (1) House fires
    (2) Child climbing up to stove — clothing catches fire
    (3) Child playing with matches
  c Electrical burns
    (1) Child playing with electrical outlets or appliances
    (2) Child playing with extension cords
    (3) Child playing on railway lines or in sidings
  d Caustic acid or alkali burns of mouth and oesophagus
    Child ingesting strong household cleaning products
  e Chemical burns of the skin
    Child playing with inflammable liquids, e.g. petrol, clothes cleaner, that come into contact with skin (often the liquid/substance then ignites)

f Burns inflicted upon the child as a result of child abuse
g Smoke inhalation and inhalation from plastic combustion.

Clinical Manifestations

1   The characteristics of burn wounds are classified as follows:
a First degree burns (partial thickness — superficial) involve superficial epidermis; the skin is pink or red in appearance and is painful to touch.
b Second degree burns (partial thickness — medium or deep) involve the entire epidermis; the skin is red, blistered, moist with exudate, and painful to pinprick or touch.
c Third degree burns (full thickness — subdermal) involve the dermis or underlying fat, muscle, or bone; the skin appears white, dry, or charred and is painless to touch.
Often it is difficult to tell the degree of burn, especially in the young child.
2   Symptoms of shock appear soon after the burn:
a Rapid pulse
b Subnormal temperature
c Pallor
d Prostration
e Low blood pressure.
3   Symptoms of toxaemia may develop within 1-2 days after the initial burn:
a Prostration
b Fever
c Rapid pulse
d Cyanosis
e Vomiting
f Oedema.

Note: These symptoms may progress to coma or death.

4   Burns of the respiratory tract result in symptoms of upper airway obstruction resulting from acute oedema and inflammation of the glottis, vocal cords, and upper trachea:
a Rapid breathing
b Dyspnoea
c Stridor
d Nasal flaring
e Restlessness.
5   Smoke inhalation may cause no initial symptoms other than mild bronchial obstruction during the initial phase following the burn. Within 6-48 hours the child may develop sudden onset of the following conditions:
a Bronchiolitis
b Pulmonary oedema
c Severe airway obstruction

d Damage from smoke inhalation — can present up to 7 days after the burn injury.

Treatment

The objectives of treatment are: to replace fluid loss from burn surface; to maintain circulation; to prevent renal failure; to prevent or treat infection; to aim toward early repair of the burn wound; to restore the child to the best possible state of physical and psychological functioning.

1 Calculation of the burn area
    a Evans' 'rule of nine' (used in assessment of extent of burns in adults) has proved quite inexact when applied to young children.
        (1) During infancy and early childhood the relative surface area of different parts of the body varies with age.
        (2) The younger the child, the greater the proportion of the surface area constituted by the head and the lesser the proportion of the surface area constituted by the legs.
    b Calculation of percentage of burn surface area is based on Lund and Browder's design (Figure 9.1).
2 Categorization of seriousness of burn is based on
    a Total area injured
    b Depth of injury
    c Location
    d Age of child
    e Condition of patient, i.e. level of consciousness
    f Previous medical history, i.e. chronic disease.

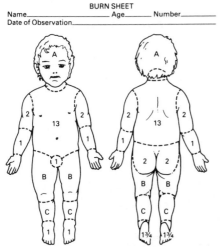

Relative Percentages of Areas Affected by Growth			
Area	Age 0	1	5
A = ½ of head	9½	8½	6½
B = ½ of one thigh	2¾	3¼	4
C = ½ of one leg	2½	2½	2¾

Figure 9.1 Calculation of burn surface areas. (From Pascoe D J Grossner M, *Quick Reference to Pediatric Emergencies*, Lippincott, 1978, with permission.)

Complications

Acute

1 Infection
   a Burn wound sepsis
   b Pneumonia
   c Urinary tract infection
   d Phlebitis
2 Curling's ulcer, gastrointestinal haemorrhage
3 Acute gastric dilation
4 Renal failure
5 Respiratory failure
6 Post-burn seizures
7 Hypertension
8 CNS dysfunction
9 Vascular ischaemia
10 Anaemia and malnutrition
11 Faecal impaction.

Long-term

1 Malnutrition
2 Scarring
3 Contractures
4 Psychological trauma.

Nursing Objectives

To recognize the symptoms of shock and to know support measures which are initiated to restore and maintain circulation.

1 Be alert to the symptoms of shock which occur very shortly after a severe burn.
   a Tachycardia
   b Hypothermia
   c Hypotension
   d Pallor
   e Prostration
   f Shallow respirations.
2 Monitor the administration of intravenous fluid, since major burns are followed by a reduction in blood volume due to outflow of plasma into the tissues.
   a Maintain the administration of plasma and intravenous fluid — usually lactated Ringer's solution is used during first 24 hours after injury.

b Obtain weight — this measurement is critical for accurate intravenous fluid volumes to be determined:

Infants and small children: 4 ml/kg per percentage burn

Older child: 2-3 ml/kg per percentage burn.

c Fluid loss from transcapillary leakage is greatest during the first 12 hours post-injury and diminishes to almost zero 12-24 hours post-injury. Fluid loss after 48 hours is due to vaporization of water from wound.

d Maintain the administration of other intravenous fluids, including albumin, once the plasma volume is restored.

3 Maintain an accurate record of intake and output.

   a Record time and amount of all fluids given.

   b Measure accurate urinary output every 30 minutes to 1 hour.

      (1) With severe burn injuries, an indwelling catheter may be used for the first 3 days.

      (2) Urine flow is a most helpful clinical guide to fluid replacement and kidney function.

      (3) Estimate urine output 1 ml/kg each hour or

      10-20 ml/hour under 2 years of age

      20-30 ml/hour 3-5 years of age

      30-50 ml/ hour over 5 years of age.

      (4) Check relative density.

      (5) Report diminishing urinary output.

4 Provide a rich oxygen environment in order to combat hypoxia, as necessary.

5 Provide sedation to relieve pain.

   a Sedatives must be given in very small amounts to children in order to prevent their depressant effect.

   b In severe burn injury, sedation should be given intravenously because of lack of absorption of intramuscular medication during emergency phase.

6 Provide a source of heat over the child's bed, since additional heat may be necessary to maintain body temperature.

7 Request laboratory results and record on special flow sheet.

   a Haematocrit or red blood cell count serves as a rough guide to the adequacy of initial treatment, since the loss of plasma results in concentration of red blood cells.

   b Electrolytes serve as a guide to fluid replacement.

8 Maintain close observation of vital signs in order to evaluate continuously the state of peripheral circulation.

   Report immediately any significant changes.

9 Observe for additional complaints or circumstances that might suggest associated

   a Gastrointestinal haemorrhage

   b Acute gastric dilatation may occur, especially if child has greater than 20% injury, associated injury, or tachypnoea. Nasogastric tube may be inserted to prevent vomiting, aspiration, and paralytic ileus.

    c Paralytic ileus — associated with circulatory problems in small children; may be alleviated with insertion of nasogastric tube.

10   Determine need for tetanus inoculation.

To observe for symptoms of respiratory distress and to initiate measures to alleviate distress.

1   Be alert for symptoms of respiratory distress:
    a Dyspnoea
    b Stridor
    c Rapid respirations
    d Restlessness
    e Cyanosis.

2   Provide an oxygen source in order to combat anoxia.

3   Report these symptoms.

4   Monitor blood gases.

5   Intubation or tracheostomy may be performed.

To provide scrupulous skin care in order to prevent infection and promote healing.

1   Burn treatment for full thickness wounds:
    a Exposure — maintains a dry surface, produces early formation of a protective eschar, and predisposes patient to less infection.
    b Occlusive dressing — burns are kept covered with dressings that have been soaked in a solution or topical medication is applied followed by dressing. First dressings may be left 2-3 days. Second dressings 7-10 days depending on child's clinical condition and surgeon's technique.
    c Primary excision of burn — necrotic eschar is immediately removed, allowing site to be grafted. Grafting may be postponed 24-48 hours.
    d Surgeons have their own preferences as to which method is used. The goals remain the same — to prevent infection, to remove dead tissue, and to provide for early closure of wound.

2   Maintain sterility in working with the burn area regardless of whether the open or closed method is used.

3   The Bradford frame or a turning bed frame may be used to facilitate skin care.
    a Provides a method for the collection of urine and faeces and maintains cleanliness of the burn areas and dressings.
    b Contractures may be prevented by maintaining functional position of extremities and good body alignment.
    c Two Bradford frames may be used to change position of the child from back to stomach and vice versa without having to handle the severely burned child.

4   Position the child and turn him frequently.

5   Apply protective devices to prevent the child from scratching the burn area.

6   Administer antibiotics as prescribed.
   a Prophylactic penicillin may be used against beta-haemolytic streptococci in the first 5-7 days.
   b Specific antibiotic therapy may be necessary for complicating infection.
7   Ensure that serial wound biopsy and quantitative cultures are done if prescribed.
8   Topical antibacterial therapy may be prescribed.
9   Heterograft or homografts are used to:
   a Restore water vapour barrier and decrease protein loss
   b Decrease pain
   c Decrease bacterial count at the wound as graft adheres to the site.

To monitor parenteral fluids to prevent electrolyte imbalance and dehydration.

1   Injury-induced fluid loss is greatest up to 48 hours post-burn, at which time reabsorption of these fluids results in diuresis if renal function is intact; accurate urinary output measurement is critical during this time.
2   Decreasing water loss by evaporation can be accomplished by keeping ambient air warm and moist, thus reducing high energy requirements and the chance of metabolic derangements. This, however, sets up an excellent environment for growth of *Pseudomonas.*
3   When parenteral hyperalimentation is used, there is increased risk of infection in the burned patient. Be alert to early signs and symptoms of infection.

To provide a high protein, high kilojoule (calorie) diet in order to provide nutrition necessary for healing and for the growth and developmental needs of the child.

1   Hypernutrition is important, because of the extreme hypermetabolism related to large burn injuries.
   a High kilojoule (calorie) — to support hypermetabolic state; protein synthesis
   b High protein — to replace protein lost by exudation; support synthesis of immunoglobulins and structural protein; prevent negative nitrogen balance
   c Vitamin and mineral supplement.
2   Anorexia is common in the burned child.
   a Tell child why eating is important if old enough to understand. Also explain to parents why increased intake of food and fluids is important.
   b Offer small amounts of food, perhaps four or five feedings rather than three per day.
   c Give him a choice of foods; determine his favourite foods.
   d Offer high protein, high kilojoule (calorie) dietary supplements.
   e Make meals a pleasant time, unassociated with treatments or unpleasant interruptions.
   f Nasogastric tube feedings may be necessary to supply high nutritive needs.

To ensure, with the physiotherapist, that a planned programme of physiotherapy is carried out to achieve the best possible rehabilitation.

1   Carry out physiotherapy procedures to minimize joint and skin complications:
   a Position — position joint in opposite direction of expected contracture.
   b Splints — aid joint positioning and decrease skin contractures and hypertrophy.
   c Exercise — gain and maintain optimal range of motion.
   d Pressure garment — aid circulation, protect newly healed skin, prevent and treat hypertrophic scar formation. It may be necessary to wear pressure garments for 12-18 months after injury, at which time healed skin has matured and become supple.
2   Plan the time each day for physiotherapy to be carried out.
3   Utilize play opportunities to help the child accept the programme (e.g. tricycle riding may be used as form of exercise).
4   Allow the child to be ambulatory as soon as he is able.

To prepare the child for the many painful surgical and other procedures that he must undergo.

1   Explain to the child and his parents what is going to happen before each procedure.
2   Explain to the child what will happen before he goes to the operating theatre, where he will wake up, and who will be there when he does wake up.
3   Explain and demonstrate what equipment will be used following surgery or other procedures.

To provide emotional support for the child who has been very frightened and traumatized by this painful experience.

1   The child may be suffering from all-encompassing physical pain for which he has no previous experience to prepare him; he becomes confused and frightened and he may regress. Coupled with physical pain is psychological pain resulting from isolation, separation from parents, reliving the experience of being burned, fear of rejection.
2   Encourage the child to talk about the way he feels.
   a The child may feel guilty and think that the burn is punishment for some wrong deed.
   b Allow the child opportunities at play where he may be able to begin to work out his feelings.
3   The child will be concerned about his appearance.
   a Continually inform the child that you love him even though he has a bad burn.
   b Encourage early contact with other children.
   c Adjustment to disfigurement can be long and painful.

4 Psychiatric consultation is very frequently necessary in order to assist the child to work out his feelings. Signs may include:
 a Persistent refusal to eat.
 b Resisting all nursing procedures.
5 Contact with the child's parents, siblings, and nurse will help him with his feelings of fear, isolation, and rejection.
6 Arrange for services of a schoolteacher for the school-age child as soon as his condition permits.

To support the parents during this very difficult time. They are under extreme stress, because a burned child creates a family crisis.

1 Use knowledge about the family's psychosocial status in planning care.
 a A medical social worker may offer beneficial psychosocial support to the family.
 b Be aware of siblings at home and that they may have needs that are being neglected as a result of this crisis.
2 Encourage parents to visit the child often; attempt to have them become actively involved in the child's care. Offer facilities for one or both parents to 'live in' if they are able to do so.
3 Give the parents the opportunity to discuss their feelings.
 Parents frequently feel very guilty because they did not give the child the appropriate supervision he should have had when the accident occurred.
4 Keep parents informed as to the child's progress. Notify family health visitor prior to discharge.

To be aware that rehabilitation is long-term.

1 Future scar revisions may be necessary.
2 Special skin care is necessary following burn injury.
 a Avoid exposure to sunlight.
 b Treatment for hypertrophic scar and keloid formation.
 c Use of lotions and creams to prevent drying, cracking, and itching.
3 Psychological support of the trauma resulting from the burn injury, the actual event and hospitalization.
4 A planned programme of physiotherapy will be needed.

ATOPIC ECZEMA (INFANTILE AND CHILDHOOD ECZEMA)

Atopic eczema is a term that describes any inflammatory dermatosis that is characterized by erythema, papulovesiculation, oozing, crusting, and scaling in various phases of resolution.

Aetiology and Incidence

1   Infantile eczema usually manifests itself between the second and sixth months of age, up to 2 years.
2   This type of dermatitis is the commonest, earliest manifestation of allergy.
3   Atopic eczema is not a disease but, rather, a reaction state of the skin.
4   The exact aetiology is not known. Many infants with eczema have a positive family history of allergy and later develop asthma or hay fever.
5   The following may be triggering factors affecting the day-to-day appearance of the lesions:
  a Bacterial, viral, or fungal infections
  b Particulate matter and contactant irritants
  c Environmental factors
    (1) Temperature and humidity
    (2) Inhalants
  d Foods
  e Emotional or physical stress — mother-child relationship
  f Drugs.

Clinical Manifestations

1   Infants — lesions
  a Erythematous, papular, and weeping lesions develop.
  b Oozing and crusting of the lesions occur.
  c Cheeks, forehead, neck, behind ears and the crawling surfaces of arms and legs are the areas most frequently involved.
  d Lesions are more concentrated on the head and body than on the extremities; however, they may progress to cover body.
2   Older children — lesions
  a Erythematous, papular, and weeping lesions develop.
  b Oozing and crusting of the lesions occur.
  c The flexor surfaces of the upper and lower extremities, antecubital and popliteal fossae, in addition to the face and neck and areas frequently involved.
  d As the disease becomes chronic, lichenification (leatheriness and hardening of skin) and hyperpigmentation develop.
3   Pruritus — may be mild or severe.
4   Excessive scratching may cause restlessness, sleeplessness, and irritability.
5   Excessive scratching may result in an inflammatory reaction and excoriation, bleeding, and subsequent infection.
6   The colour of lesions is red (possibly intense red).

Altered Physiology

1   The dermatitis involves the epidermis and the vascular layer of the cutis.

2   The dermatitis goes through a cycle involving areas of erythema, papules, vesicles, wheal reactions, and ultimately, scaling eruption.
3   With superimposed infection, there is exudation, pustulation, and crust formation.
4   Various stages of the disease can be present on different parts of the child's body.
5   The disease is subject to remissions and exacerbations.
6   Secondary infections may occur from scratching.

Diagnosis

1   Family history of allergies
2   Positive dermal reaction
3   Presence of circulation Prausnitz-Küstner antibodies
4   Tendency to develop blood eosinophilia
5   Clearing of skin with removal of specific allergen and reappearance of dermal reaction upon re-exposure.

Treatment

1   Symptomatic and supportive
    a Trial period of hypoallergenic diet to eliminate any responsible food
    b Avoidance by patient of any other known allergen
    c Control of any complicating skin infection
    d Relief of itching and irritability; sedation may be necessary
    e Measures to improve condition of involved skin:
       (1) Prevent scratching
       (2) Cleansing
2   Preventive — teach mother how to keep condition under control.

Complications

1   Acute infection — pyogenic infection may develop.
2   Long-term — eczema may progress to allergic rhinitis or asthma.

Nursing Objectives

To institute measures which prevent the child from scratching himself when he experiences severe itching in order to prevent further irritation and possible infection of the skin.

1   Clothes should be cool and loose. Avoid the use of wool and synthetic fibres wherever possible.
2   Keep child cool.
3   Trim finger and toe nails short, keep clean.

4   Provide safe toys that will not be used by the child to scratch himself. (Use soft playthings made of nonallergenic materials.)
5   Cotton hand mittens and socks may be worn, especially at night, to stop child scratching himself.
6   Anger and frustration are frequently displayed in violent scratching; therefore
   a Keep child comfortable, and occupied. Try to anticipate his needs.
   b Provide as much personal contact and supervision as possible when mother or father is not present.
   c Allow play activities that afford the child an opportunity to express his anger and frustration.
   d Provide infants with activity toys, mobiles, etc. A dummy to suck will provide soothing comfort.
7   Administer prescribed medications:
   a Sedatives
   b Antihistamines
   c Antipruritic agents.

Note: The use of local anaesthetics to relieve itching is contraindicated because of their potential for skin sensitization.

8   Very rarely, wrist, ankle or jacket restraints may be used but only when *absolutely essential* to prevent damage due to violent scratching. If used, they should be removed frequently and never left on during sleep.

To provide measures which will improve the condition of the involved skin.

1   Bathe the child by the prescribed method.
        Water and soap are often irritating. Ung. emulsificans aquosum should be used in daily bathing and washing. The child enjoys the pleasure and relief provided by bathing. Provide water toys for child to play with in bath.
2   Local skin care is aimed at removing the debris, and allaying the inflammatory reaction and pruritis.
   a Hydrocortisone lotion 1% with or without tyrothricin 1 in 1000. Local application to exudative lesions daily. Any dressing, if used, should be light and kept to the minimum. These are now usually unnecessary.
   b Hydrocortisone ointment 1% for dry eczema, applied twice daily.
3   Prevent skin irritation from bed clothing and bed linen.
4   Change nappies frequently to prevent skin excoriation.
5   Avoid extreme ambient temperatures.

To promote measures which will prevent contact with dietary and environmental allergens.

1   Review the child's chart and question the parents regarding known allergies.
   a Note the known allergens on the nursing records and place a tag on the head of the bed to indicate that the child has an allergy.
   b Inform the dietician as to the child's food allergies.

2 Avoid substances which have a high potential for sensitization.

a Foods such as milk, eggs, chocolate, wheat cereal, and orange juice are to be avoided.

b Wool and dust are to be avoided.

3 Observe the child's reactions when an elimination diet is prescribed.

a A minimal diet is ordered. Trial diet may be composed of:

(1) Milk substitute

(2) Rice cereal

(3) Two fruits

(4) Two vegetables

(5) Beef

(6) Aqueous multivitamins

(7) No egg products.

b A new food is added to the diet every 3-5 days, during which time the response to that food is observed.

c An allergic response occurring during this 3- to 5-day period indicates sensitivity to that food; that particular food is then eliminated from the diet.

d If no response is apparent, that food is added to the child's diet.

e Another food substance is then added, and the child is observed for the following 3- to 5-day period. This method is followed until the food allergen is determined.

4 Provide a substitute for cow's milk when the child is allergic to it.

a Goat's milk may be used.

b Commercial formulas made from meat or vegetable protein substances are available.

To protect the child from sources of infection.

Protect the child from exposure to sources of infection known to cause exacerbations and severe infections.

Contact with other children, visitors, and personnel who have the herpes simplex virus is to be avoided.

To provide the emotional support needed by any child his age who is hospitalized; provide love and attention and give the child freedom to express his feelings.

To assist the parents in providing for the child's care following hospitalization.

1 Explain to parents the usual causes of the problem. Help them to understand that eczema is chronic — that there is no cure — but that a therapeutic regimen can be followed that will control it.

2 Demonstrate the application of topical medications and the application of dressings, if any. Explain timing of bathing, application of skin lotions or ointments and the giving of any medications. Make bath time a 'fun time'.

3 Give specific information regarding diet. Emphasize the foods which are allowed rather than the foods to be avoided.

4   Additional information in home management may include the following:
   a Adequate rinsing of all clothes, bed linen, and nappies used by the child.
   b Control environment.
   c Avoid exposure to extreme heat or cold or to rapid changes in ambient temperature; avoid strenuous activity (can swim), soap, perfume, detergents, and stress.
   d Keep child's fingernails cut short and keep them clean.
5   Encourage the parents to hold and cuddle the child as much as possible to encourage the body contact that is frequently avoided because of protective devices and ointments.
6   Encourage the parents to discuss their feelings and concerns about the child's illness.
   a The appearance of the child may be very disturbing to them.
   b They need to be made to feel adequate in caring for the child at home.
7   A referral should be made to the health visitor to provide support to the family, especially during initial phases of adjustment.
8   The parents can be given the address of: The National Eczema Society, Mary Ward House, 5-7 Tavistock Place, London WCl.

IMPETIGO

Impetigo is an infectious disease affecting the superficial layers of the skin and is characterized by the formation of vesicles, crusts, or bullae.

Aetiology and Incidence

1   Bullous impetigo in neonate and infant — lesions are large, flaccid bullae containing pus and supernatant clear serum that rupture and leave raw edges. Lesions are more prominent in axillae and groin.
2   Impetigo contagiosa in older child — lesions appear with thick, yellow crusts.
3   Impetigo is usually caused by staphylococci or rarely by streptococci.
4   Occurs most frequently where personal hygiene is poor.
5   Occurs most frequently in children under 10 years of age.
6   Spread by contact — easily conveyed from person to person (using same handkerchief, towels, napkins, pencils, toys, etc.); plastic paddling pools in summer — when spilled water is replaced and no antiseptic or disinfectant is used.
7   Any abrasion of skin may serve as portal of entry.

Clinical Manifestations (of Impetigo Contagiosa)

1   Incubation period of 1-5 days.

2 Lesion first appears as pink-red macules that quickly change to vesicles which, in turn, enlarge, become pustular, develop crusts, and leave temporary superficial erythematous areas.

3 Face, scalp, and hands are commonly involved, but other areas may be affected.

4 Regional lymphadenopathy — common with secondary infection of insect bites, eczema, poison ivy, scabies.

5 Pruritus may occur.

Diagnosis

1 Aspiration and culture of bullae.

2 Culture after removal of crust.

Treatment

1 Treatment is based on the following:

a Aetiology and type of infection.

b Gentle removal of all crusts with saline or 1 in 1000 aqueous Hibitane solution to ensure penetration of topical antibiotics.

c The following may be used: fucidin, framycetin, neomycin (may be combined with bacitracin).

d The treatment should be repeated three times a day until clear.

e Systemic antibiotics — when severe or recurrent.

2 Prevention — avoid contact with sibling(s) of affected child.

Note: All members of the family in which a staphylococcal infection has occurred should be treated if they have a lesion (no matter how trivial) if the organism is to be eradicated from the patient's environment.

Nursing Objectives

To be aware of the appearance of the characteristic lesion of impetigo.

1 Observe the condition of the child's skin upon admission to the hospital.

2 Report any suspicious-appearing lesions.

3 Record the appearance and location of the lesion.

4 Initiate appropriate measures to prevent the spread of the infection.

a Place the child in a single room.

b Maintain barrier nursing technique.

5 Watch for the development of new lesions.

To provide measures to prevent secondary infections.

1 Provide mittens or protective devices to prevent the child from scratching the lesions.

2   Trim the child's fingernails and toenails.
3   Maintain cleanliness of fingernails and toenails.

To provide measures to assure the child's comfort until healing has occurred and the child is free from infection.

1   Hold child frequently.
2   Provide diversional therapy.
3   Administer medication and treatment to relieve itching.
4   Provide the child with a diet adequate to meet his growth and development needs.

To practise measures of general health and provide teaching for the child and his parents which will be helpful in preventing spread and further infection.

1   General measures to improve personal cleanliness should be encouraged.
2   Minor wounds should be adequately cleaned and treated.
3   The child should be isolated if at home.
4   The child should be kept out of school until the lesions have healed.

RINGWORM OF THE SCALP (TINEA CAPITIS)

Ringworm of the scalp is a fungal infection of the scalp and hair follicles.

Aetiology

1   Ringworm of the scalp is caused by different species of the *Microsporum canis* and *Tricophyton tonsurans*.
2   Ringworm of the scalp is seen primarily in children before puberty.

Clinical Manifestations

1   The lesions usually develop in the occipital, temporal, and parietal areas of the scalp.
2   Pruritus usually occurs in the area.
3   The involved areas of the scalp appear as patches, rounded or oval in outline, covered by scales and lustreless, irregularly broken hairs.
4   Single patches of multiple patches may occur.
5   Systematic manifestations are absent.
6   Evaluation
    a Wood's light — a filtered ultraviolet radiation causes microsporon infections to fluoresce with a brilliant, greenish light.
    b Microscopic evaluation of infected hair follicles — to identify *Trichophyton* which fluoresces poorly under Wood's light — spores visibly coat hair.

Altered Physiology

1   The fungal infection produces an inflammation of the scalp which causes alopecia and broken hairs.
2   The lesions of the scalp may have papulovesicular erythematous borders or may appear only as scaling with a few broken hairs.
3   Kerion, an acute inflammation which produces oedema, pustules, and granulomatous swelling, may occur.
4   The infection may be spread through child-to-child contact, as well as through the common use of towels, combs, brushes, hats. Infected cats, dogs, ponies, mice and hamsters kept as pets may be the source of the infection.

Treatment

1   Griseofulvin — an antifungal antibiotic which is administered orally.
2   Tolnaftate is a locally applied fungicide but should always be given in conjunction with systemic treatment.
3   Treatment is usually continued for 2-3 weeks. The child's lesions should then be examined daily under a Wood's light. After five successive negative examinations the child may return to school.
4   Duration of treatment is generally guided by periodic use of Wood's light or cultures.

Nursing Objectives

To recognize the characteristic lesions of ringworm of the scalp.

1   Observe the condition of the hair and scalp as a part of the routine assessment of the child on admission to the hospital.
2   Report suspicious-appearing lesions.
3   Record the appearance and location of the lesions.
4   Initiate the appropriate isolation techniques (as per hospital policy).

To be aware of the side effects of the medications used in the treatment of ringworm of the scalp.

1   Griseofulvin may produce headache, heartburn, nausea, epigastric discomfort, diarrhoea, and urticaria.
2   Record and report to the paediatrician any side effects observed.
3   A diet high in fat may be prescribed to enhance intestinal absorption.

To be aware of the case-finding measures to prevent additional cases and to identify the earliest evidence of infection.

1   All family contacts should be screened.
2   The school should be notified so that appropriate case-finding techniques may be initiated.

To be aware of the psychological trauma associated with loss of hair, especially in a girl, and to provide support as appropriate.

Use of wigs or scarves may provide some relief of anxiety.

To teach the child and his family methods to prevent further episodes.

1   Teach general hygiene measures — regular shampooing and bathing.
2   Advise them to avoid the sharing of hats, combs, brushes, etc.
3   Trace animal contacts; if appropriate arrange veterinary treatment.

PEDICULOSIS

Pediculosis is the infestation of human beings by lice.

Aetiology

1   Three types of lice affect human beings:
    a *Pediculosis capitis* — head louse
    b *Pediculosis corporis* — body louse (very rarely in children)
    c *Phthirus pubis* — pubic louse/crab louse (seldom found in children) can attach only to curly hair — pubes, axillae, eyebrows.
2   Each type of louse generally remains in the area designated by its name, but it may occasionally be seen in other areas of the body.
3   The infestation occurs in areas of filth and poverty, where personal cleanliness is neglected, baths are infrequently taken, and clothing is kept on the body for long periods of time.
4   Lice are transmitted by personal contact with people harbouring them or through contact with articles which temporarily harbour them.

Clinical Manifestations

1   Severe itching in the area affected is the primary symptom of pediculosis; scratch marks will be evident in these areas.
2   In children, pubic lice are found most frequently in the eyelashes and eyebrows.
3   Infested scalp areas may become secondarily infected from scratching.
4   Crusts, pediculi, nits and dirt may combine to cause a foul odour and matted hair.
5   Body lice may produce minute red lesions.

Altered Physiology

1 The eggs of lice (nits) are attached to the hair or clothing by a sticky substance which hardens. The eggs hatch within 1 week — the lice reach maturity within 1 month and are then capable of reproducing.
2 The lice on the skin produce itching; the longer the infestation persists, the more severe the skin reaction becomes and the more severe the lesions appear.
3 The lice live on clothing and go to the body for feeding; thus, they produce visible scratch marks and points of puncture.

Treatment

To eliminate and remove nits and pediculi (lice) and to treat the irritated skin.

Pediculosis capitis may be treated with Malathion or carbaryl according to manufacturer's instructions. Twelve hours after use of either preparation the hair is shampooed and the hair combed with a fine comb whilst still wet. It is advisable to treat all members of the household, particularly children, at the same time.

Note: It is not necessary after treatment to comb out the nits or eggs which can be uncomfortable for the child. These eggs die and any egg found more than a centimetre or so away from the scalp is harmless.

Nursing Objectives

To perform the treatments prescribed to destroy and eliminate the parasite.

1 Observe and record the response to treatment.
   a Note the change in the degree of discomfort caused by itching.
   b Observe infected areas for changes in the characteristics of the lesions.
   c Observe for systemic manifestations of infection.

To provide measures to prevent the child from scratching himself.

1 Provide mittens or protective devices to prevent the child from scratching.
2 Trim fingernails and toenails and keep them clean.
3 Provide the child with play activities or suitable occupation to distract him from itching.

To provide appropriate teaching for the family to prevent recurrent attacks.

To screen the family for parasitic infection.

SCABIES

Scabies is a disease of the skin produced by the burrowing action of a parasite mite resulting in irritation and the formation of vesicles or pustules.

Aetiology

1   Scabies is caused by the itch mite, *Sarcoptes scabiei*.
2   Scabies occurs most frequently in individuals living in areas of poverty, where cleanliness is lacking.
3   Scabies occurs as a result of direct contact with infected persons or by indirect contact through soiled bed linen, clothing, etc.

Clinical Manifestations

1   Itching, particularly at night, is the primary symptom. The itching is usually very severe.
2   Scratching frequently produces secondary skin infection.
3   Systemic manifestations are absent, unless they result from the secondary infection (i.e. fever, leucocytosis).

Altered Physiology

1   Both the male and female parasite live upon the skin
2   The female parasite burrows into the superficial skin to deposit her eggs.
3   The burrow is seen most commonly between the fingers but may occur in any natural fold of the skin or in pressure areas, e.g. heel of palm, axillary and buttock folds, male genitalia, female breasts.
4   The burrows may occur in any part of the body in infants and small children and are easily identifiable.
5   Pruritus occurs, and the scratching of the skin may produce secondary infection. Scattered follicular eruptions contain immature mites.
6   Inflammation may produce pustules and crusts.

Diagnosis

Presence on skin of female mite, ova, and faeces.

Treatment

The objective is to destroy the parasite, to relieve itching and to reduce skin irritation.

1   Benzyl benzoate
2   Gamma benzene hexachloride

In order successfully to treat scabies it is most important to:

1 Bath the child and dry afterwards.
2 Apply prescribed treatment over whole of body from neck down, taking particular care to work in between toes, fingers and other flexures.
3 After 24 hours repeat whole procedure.

Note: Clothing, underwear and bed linen should be changed and laundered. It is not necessary to send blankets or other garments for disinfection.

All members of the household should be treated at the same time. It is important to tell the parents that the papular lesions on the genitalia and around the axillae may persist for several months despite successful treatment. Irritation too may continue for a few weeks. (See p. 525 guidelines for managing irritation and scratching.)

Nursing Objectives

Same as for pediculosis, p. 533.

ORAL CANDIDIASIS (THRUSH) AND CANDIDAL NAPPY DERMATITIS

Oral thrush is a mycotic stomatitis characterized by the appearance of white plaques on the oral mucous membrane, the gums, and the tongue.

Candidal nappy dermatitis is a rash characterized by red, scaly, sharply circumscribed but moist patches with pustular satellite lesions.

Aetiology

1 Caused by *Candida albicans.*
2 Most frequently seen in newborns, but may be seen in older infants, usually as a complication of antibiotic therapy.
3 Maternal vulvovaginal candidiasis is the primary source of neonatal thrush.
4 The growth of the organisms is favoured by:
   a Lack of cleanliness
   b Malnutrition
   c Diabetes
   d Antibiotic treatment (destroys normal flora)
   e Neoplasms
   f Hyperparathyroidism
   g Lowered immunity, e.g. a child receiving immunosuppressive therapy.
5 The infection may be acquired from:
   a Contaminated hands
   b Contaminated feeding equipment
   c Contaminated bedding

    d Another patient.

6   Thrush frequently occurs in children with cleft lip and palate.

Clinical Manifestations

Thrush

1   The infant develops small plaques on the oral mucous membrane, tongue, or gums; these plaques appear like curds of milk but cannot be wiped out of the mouth.
2   Thrush often appears to cause the infant no pain or discomfort.
3   The mouth may be dry.
4   Occasionally, the infant may appear to have some difficulty in swallowing.

Candidal Nappy Dermatitis

1   Buttock rash consisting of erythematous maculopapular eruption with perianal distribution.
2   Generally causes discomfort, especially with wetting and cleansing.

Altered Physiology

Thrush

1   Spores lodge between epithelial cells and gradually separate the layers.
2   The infection then spreads to the surface of the mucous membrane.
3   Growth usually begins in several discrete areas of the oral mucous membrane with gradual spreading to the point where a continuous membrane may be formed.

Treatment

Thrush

1   1-2% aqueous solution of gentian violet swabbed in the mouth may be used.
2   Oral administration of nystatin in suspension three or four times daily, or miconazole gel.

Candidal Nappy Dermatitis

1   Keep dry and clean.
2   Expose buttocks to fresh air and sunlight whenever possible.
3   Topical application of nystatin or miconazole nitrate cream or ointment, or painting the nappy area with 1-2% aqueous solution of gentian violet.
4   Tyrothricin lotion 1 in 1000 to buttock lesions.

Nursing Objectives

To recognize the appearance of thrush and to be aware of the infant who is particularly susceptible to the development of the condition.

1   Newborns and infants who have particular susceptibility include:
   a Sick, debilitated infants
   b Infants who are on antibiotic therapy
   c Infants with cleft lip and palate, parathyroidism, and neoplasms.
2   Inspect mouth before every feeding for presence of thrush.
3   Report the appearance of thrush to the paediatrician and record this information on the nursing record.

To practise measures which prevent the development and spread of thrush.

1   Practise careful handwashing techniques.
2   Practise techniques which ensure that teats, bottles, or any other object which comes into direct or indirect contact with the infant's mouth is clean.

To recognize the appearance of candidal nappy dermatitis and report to paediatrician immediately.

To teach mothers (parents) the general principles of preventing nappy dermatitis.

1   Change nappy as soon as possible after wetting or soiling. Check nappy every hour in newborn.
2   Wash entire nappy area thoroughly and dry area before applying clean nappy.
3   Allow infant to go without a nappy for short periods. Expose buttocks to sunlight and fresh air whenever possible.
4   Use clean nappies that are soft to the touch and absorbent.
5   Use terminal aseptic rinse when washing nappies to neutralize ammonia produced when infant urinates.
6   Avoid powder and oil which tend to clog pores and cake on skin, retaining bacteria.
7   Use ointments as appropriate for condition of nappy area.
   a Protective
   b Soothing and protective. Metanium ointment or other commercially produced products for the purpose may be obtained from the chemist by the parents.
8   Avoid occlusive plastic coverings, tightly pinned or double nappies, all of which tend to increase production and retention of body heat and moisture.

FURTHER READING

Books

Black J A, *Paediatric Emergencies*, Butterworth, 1979, Chapters 4 & 5.
Jolly H, *Diseases of Children*, Blackwell Scientific, 1981.
Scipien G M *et al.*, *Comprehensive Pediatric Nursing*, McGraw-Hill, 1979.
Symposium on Pediatric Dermatology, *Pediatric Clinics of North America*, May 1978, 25 (2).

Articles

Campbell L, Special behavioural problems of the burned child, *American Journal of Nursing*, January 1976, 76: 220-224.
Gange R W, Bacterial skin infections, *Nursing Times*, January 1977, Supplement.
Hay R J Wells R S, Fungal infections of the skin, *Journal of Maternal and Child Health*, July/August 1978.
Launer J, Self-help society for eczema sufferers and their families, *British Medical Journal*, December 1976: 1494-1495.
Livesey R P, Principles of good diapering for parent education, *JOGN Nursing*, January/February 1976, 5: 25-27.
Morely W N, Napkin eruptions in infancy, *Journal of Maternal and Child Health*, April 1977: 144-148.
O'Neill J A, Evaluation and treatment of the burned child, *Pediatric Clinics of North America*, May 1975, 22: 407-414.
Rycroft R J, Eczema, *Nursing Times*, March 1977, Supplement.
Savedra M, Coping with pain: strategies of severely burned children, *Maternal and Child Nursing*, 1976, 5: 187-203.
Starkler L, Impetigo contagiosa, *Journal of Maternal and Child Health*, June 1977: 226-231.
Talabre L Graves P, A tool for assessing families of burned children, *American Journal of Nursing*, January 1976, 76: 225-227.
Trunkey D Parks S, Burns in children, *Current Problems in Paediatrics*, January 1976, 6: 3-51.

10

METABOLIC DISORDERS

JUVENILE DIABETES MELLITUS

Diabetes mellitus is a disorder of carbohydrate metabolism resulting in high serum levels of glucose and the spilling of glucose in the urine. The disease is also associated with abnormal metabolism of fat and protein.

Aetiology

1 Heredity appears to be a predisposing factor.
  a The exact mode of inheritance is complicated.
  b It appears that the genetic abnormality must be present in both parents for clinical manifestations of diabetes mellitus to develop.
2 Factors in addition to genetic ones are also involved in provoking the clinical manifestations of the disease.
3 Viral aetiology for juvenile diabetes has also been suggested.

Altered Physiology

1 The pancreas produces an insufficient amount of insulin.
2 The body is unable to oxidize glucose properly.
3 Protein and fat are oxidized at abnormal rates.
4 Hyperglycaemia results from the deficient oxidation of glucose and the inability of tissues to use glucose as fuel.
5 Glycosuria results when the serum level of glucose exceeds the renal threshold.
6 Diuresis is initiated and may progress to dehydration and impaired renal function.
7 Ketones accumulate in the blood when fat is oxidized at abnormal rates.
8 Ketones are excreted in the urine.
9 Acidosis occurs when ketosis is severe enough to lower the CO_2 combining power of the blood. Diabetic coma may result.

Clinical Manifestations

1 Rapid onset (usually over a period of a few weeks)
2 Major symptoms
   a Increased thirst
   b Increased appetite
   c Increased urination and often nocturia
   d Wasting
   e Tires easily
3 Minor symptoms
   a Skin and urinary tract infections
   b Dry skin
4 Diabetic acidosis
   a Precomatose state
      (1) Drowsiness
      (2) Dryness of skin
      (3) Cherry red lips
      (4) Increased respirations
      (5) Nausea
      (6) Vomiting
      (7) Abdominal pain
   b Comatose state
      (1) Extreme hyperpnoea (Kussmaul breathing)
      (2) Soft, sunken eyeballs
      (3) Rigid abdomen
      (4) Rapid, weak pulse
      (5) Decreased temperature
      (6) Decreased blood pressure
   c Circulatory collapse and renal failure may follow, resulting from the combination of lowered pH, electrolyte deficiency, and dehydration
5 Side effects
   a Stunting of growth
   b Failure to develop secondary sex characteristics.

Complications

1 Retinopathy and cataracts
2 Neuropathy
3 Renal disease
4 Increased incidence of gangrene, myocardial infarction, and stroke.

Nursing Objectives

To recognize signs of diabetic acidosis (see clinical manifestations) and to provide supportive care to the child should this develop.

1 Be aware of common causes of diabetic acidosis:
   a Untreated diabetes
   b Inadequate insulin coverage
   c Failure to adhere to the prescribed diet
   d Chronic or repeated infections.
2 Apply the principles of nursing care of the comatose child.
3 Maintain intravenous therapy. (See intravenous procedure, p. 155.)
   a Be prepared to administer intravenous sodium bicarbonate and potassium supplements.
   b Have intravenous glucose available should the child suddenly become hypoglycaemic.
   Care is taken to avoid reducing the blood glucose to hypoglycaemic levels.
4 Prepare soluble insulin for intravenous administration.
   a This may be 0.1 unit per kilogram body weight per hour.
   b Subsequent dosage depends on the degree of ketosis and repeated blood glucose levels.
5 Insert a nasogastric tube to relieve abdominal distension and prevent vomiting.
6 Monitor urine output exactly.
   Test urinary sugar and acetone of each specimen.
7 Provide emotional support to the child and his family.
   a Respond immediately to the child's needs for physical comfort.
   b Discuss the child's treatment plan and expected response with his parents to alleviate their anxiety.
8 Reinstitute oral feedings when the child is sufficiently responsive and the acidosis has disappeared as evidenced by absence of acetone in the urine.
   a This is usually after 12-16 hours of parenteral therapy.
   b Begin with a low fat, liquid diet.
   c Offer quantities of tea, fruit juice, or milk to replace the large amount of potassium lost during the acute phase of acidosis.
   d Observe closely for signs of hypoglycaemia or recurrent acidosis once oral feedings are reinstituted.
9 Begin a teaching programme with the child as soon as possible to allay his worries concerning his physical status, prognosis, and treatment.

To provide a diet adequate for the child's normal growth and development and sufficient to satisfy his appetite.

1 The prescribed diet is determined by the child's symptomatology, family and cultural characteristics, and paediatrician preference.
   a Diets range from relatively 'free' diets in which an exact intake is not prescribed to more rigid, strictly controlled diets.

b Most diets are restricted in carbohydrates. May be based on the exchange method.

c All diets must supply sufficient energy intake for activity and growth, sufficient protein for growth, and the required vitamins and minerals.

d Foods are distributed throughout the day to accommodate varying peak action of insulin.

Distribution may be adjusted for increased or decreased amounts of exercise.

2   Determine the child's usual dietary habits so that adherence to his controlled diet will be easier.

3   Include the child and his parents in his meal planning as soon as possible.

4   Allow the child normal activity while hospitalized so that the observed result of his dietary control will be valid.

5   Allow the child to eat with other children.

6   Make certain that the child adheres to his prescribed diet.

7   Make appropriate substitutions if necessary because of food preferences.

To administer insulin in an amount adequate to maintain the child's approximate glycaemic equilibrium.

1   The dose and kind of insulin are determined from the results of fractional testing of the urine for sugar and acetone.

2   Insulin should be given 30 minutes before the morning meal.

3   Be aware of the major types of insulin and their effect (Table 10.1).

4   Develop a systematic plan for injections which emphasizes rotation of sites. In this way, it will be several weeks before it is necessary to return to the same site.

a The upper arms and thighs are the most acceptable sites for injection in children, but the outer areas of the abdomen or hips may also be used.

b A diagram showing injection sites should be used to maintain the rotation (refer to Figure 10.1).

The sites can be checked off each day until the routine is familiar.

c Injections are begun at an upper corner of the area to be used.

d Subsequent injections are given about 2.5 cm apart, working in rows.

e When one row is completed, injections are begun in the next arm, leg, hip, or the abdomen,

f When the pattern is completed, injections are returned to the beginning area and a new row is started about 2.5 cm below the original row.

g Guidelines for site location are as follows:

(1) *Arms:* Begin below the deltoid muscle and end one hand breadth above the elbow. Begin at the midline and progress outward laterally using the external surface only.

(2) *Legs:* Begin one hand breadth below the hip and end one hand breadth above the knee. Begin at the midline and progress outward laterally using only the outer, anterior surface.

(3) *Abdomen:* Avoid the beltline and 2.5 cm around the umbilicus.

(4) *Hips:* Use the upper outer quadrant of the buttocks.

5   Be certain that the measuring scale of the syringe matches the unitage of the bottle of insulin.

     a Insulin is available in strengths of 20, 40, 80, and 100 units per millilitre.

     b The new U-100 insulin is preferred, since it is a purer form of insulin which is less likely to cause local allergic reactions or fat atrophy.

6   Use insulin that is at room temperature.

     a The bottle in use may be kept at room temperature without losing appreciable strength.

     b Extra bottles should be stored in the refrigerator.

7   Mix the solution by rotating the vial between the hands. Do not shake vigorously.

8   Administer insulin subcutaneously and not too near the skin to prevent local skin reactions and to promote absorption.

9   Following injection, exert firm pressure with a Mediswab or other medicated swab to prevent bleeding and massage the area to aid absorption of the medication.

Table 10.1   Types of insulin and their effects

Type of insulin	Onset (hours)	Maximal activity (hours)	Duration (hours)
Soluble insulin	$\frac{1}{2}$-1	2-3	4-6
Semi-Lente insulin	$\frac{1}{2}$-1	4-8	12-18
Isophane (NPH) insulin	1-1$\frac{1}{2}$	8-10	20-24
Lente insulin	1-2	14-16	24-26

10   Observe the skin closely for signs of irritation. Avoid the injection site for several weeks if signs of local irritation are observed.

11   Observe the skin for a rash indicating an allergic reaction to the insulin.

12   Be aware of factors which vary the need for the utilization of insulin, particularly exercise and infection.

     a Exercise

       (1) Tends to lower the blood sugar level.

       (2) Encourage normal activity, regulated in amount and time.

     b Infection

       (1) Increases the child's insulin requirement.

       (2) Be alert for signs of infection.

13   Encourage the child to express his feelings about the injections.

     The child may be helped to master his fear of injections by gaining control of the situation through play and active participation in the procedure.

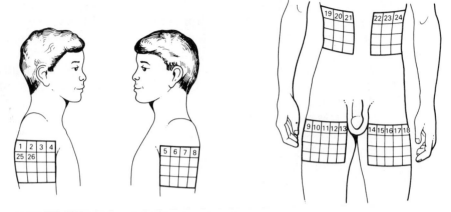

Figure 10.1   Rotating injection sites for insulin.

To be aware of the symptoms and treatments of hypoglycaemia.

1   Common causes
   a Overdose of insulin
   b Reduction in diet or increased exercise without a reduction in insulin
2   Symptoms
   a Sudden hunger
   b Weakness
   c Restlessness
   d Pallor
   e Sweating
   f Tremors
   g Dizziness
   h Visual disturbances
   i Odd behaviour
   j Dilated pupils
   k Unconsciousness
3   Treatment
   a Be prepared to give orange juice or other food containing readily available simple sugars.
   b Have 50% dextrose available for intravenous injection or glucagon available for intramuscular injection.

To test the child's urine regularly for sugar and acetone in order to determine the effectiveness of treatment.

1   Collect urine specimens four times daily, before each meal and before bed.
   a Because analysis is more accurate if the second micturated specimen is used, have the child micturate between 30 minutes and 1 hour before each of the specimens to be tested is obtained.

b Discard the first specimen and test the second.

c Since obtaining specimens from young children may be difficult, it may be preferable to test the urine with each micturition.

2 Record the results of urine testing accurately.

 a Use a form so that the information will be clear and readily available.

 b Help the child to understand how his disease is controlled by teaching him to test his own urine, record results, and report information to medical personnel or parents.

3 Be certain that the urine test is done according to the specific instructions for the method being used:

 a Correct time interval for reading results

 b Correct colour chart for brand of reagent

 c Correct storage, handling, and use of reagent

 d Do not use expired reagent; check expiration date.

To prevent infection.

1 Bathe daily.

2 Maintain meticulous skin care through such activities as frequent ambulation of the child and application of body lotion.

3 Keep fingernails and toenails clean and well trimmed.

4 Provide prompt treatment for any violations of the skin (bruises, abrasions, lacerations, etc.).

To foster acceptance on the part of the child that he is a normal, healthy person and able to compete with his peers.

1 Include the child and his parents in the treatment plan in its earliest stages.

2 Emphasize that daily management of his disease can become as routine as matters of personal hygiene.

3 Permit and encourage the development of the child's natural talents. Do not allow him to use his disease as a crutch.

4 Allow the child independence in his care as soon as possible, but provide the necessary direction.

5 Initiate a teaching programme for the child and his parents early. Offer them available literature.

6 If appropriate, group diabetic children together on the unit. Initiate group discussions for diabetic adolescents.

7 Invite parents to join a group of parents of diabetic children if such a group is available in the area.

8 Notify family health visitor or paediatric liaison health visitor prior to discharge, giving full details of the stage of acceptance by the child and his family of the condition.

Patient or Parental Teaching

Patient or parental teaching is one of the most important aspects in the nursing care of the diabetic child. Thorough instruction is essential in the following areas:

1   Influence of exercise, emotional stress, and other illnesses on both insulin and diet needs
2   Recognition of the symptoms of hypoglycaemia and diabetic acidosis and knowledge of related emergency management
3   Prevention of infection
    a Give frequent baths.
    b Attend to regular body hygiene with special attention to foot care.
    c Report any breaks in the skin. Treat them promptly.
    d Report infections promptly to the paediatrician.
    e Use only properly fitted shoes and socks; do not wear vinyl or plastic, which do not permit ventilation. Avoid calluses and blisters.
    f Dress the child appropriately for the weather.
    g Keep the child away from people with upper respiratory or other types of infection.
    h See that child receives regular dental check-ups and maintenance.
    i Follow routine immunizations according to the recommended schedule.
4   Urine testing
    a Demonstrate the procedure.
    b Have the child and his parent demonstrate to the nurse.
    c Allow the child to do the procedure under supervision until his accuracy is certain.
    d Encourage the child to assume responsibility for his own urine testing.
    e Help the child to develop an easy method of recording urine results, e.g. using coloured paints.
    f Be certain parents understand what results are desirable for the child and the appropriate action to take when test results are other than those desired.
    g Warn the parents of the caustic nature of Clinitest tablets if ingested. The agent should be kept away from young children.
5   Administration of insulin
    a Both the child and his parents should be taught how to do this procedure and what effects the various forms of insulin have.
    b Give parents an opportunity to express their feelings about the injection.
    c Explain the procedure simply and demonstrate it.
    d Discuss the procedure for rotation of sites and the rationale for this method.
    e Have the parent and the child practise insulin administration using an orange or similar object.
    f Allow the parent to practise by injecting himself with sterile water under supervision.
    g Have the parent inject his child under supervision.

h Have the child inject himself.

(1) Most children over the age of 8 can be taught to give insulin to themselves.

(2) Generally, the earlier this responsibility is given to the child, the easier it is for him.

i Carefully check the dosage measured by the child and his parent until you are certain of their accuracy.

6　Maintenance and sterilization of insulin equipment

a The use of disposable equipment should be encouraged, because it is easier and safer.

b Nondisposable syringes and needles must be sterilized in the following manner:

(1) Remove the plunger from the barrel of the syringe.

(2) Place them both into a strainer along with the needle.

(3) Place the strainer in a saucepan of water and boil for 5 minutes.

If the family does not have a strainer, the syringe parts and needle should be wrapped in gauze before being placed in water.

(4) Reassemble the syringe, being careful to touch only the outside of the syringe and the knob of the plunger.

(5) Slip the needle on to the syringe with a twisting motion, being careful to touch only the hub of the needle, never its point.

(6) Work the plunger back and forth several times to force out any water that remains in it.

7　Diet

a Review the prescribed diet with the family.

b Discuss acceptable modifications of exchanges.

c Allow the child to manage his own diet as early as possible.

d Emphasize that the diet is based on normal household foods. The purchase of special, expensive diabetic foods is usually not necessary.

e Stress that food labels must be scrutinized. A label of 'diabetic' or 'low-calorie' does not necessarily mean that the food is acceptable for the child.

f Give details to parents of the book published by the British Diabetic Association of the carbohydrate values of branded and proprietary foods.

8　Precautionary measures

a Have the child carry with him an identifying card which states that he has diabetes and includes his name, address, telephone number, and his family doctor's name and telephone number.

b See that the child has two lumps of sugar available in case of hypogly-caemia or insulin reaction.

c Have the family discuss the child's disease with the school nurse and with other responsible adults who are in close contact with the child (teachers, scout leaders, etc.).

d Advise the parents that vials of insulin and syringe kit should be kept on one's person when travelling, because baggage may be subjected to extreme temperatures and pressures incompatible with the stability of insulin, or may be lost or mislaid.

9   Agencies: British Diabetic Association, 10 Queen Anne Street, London WlM 0BD.

DIABETES INSIPIDUS

Diabetes insipidus is a disorder of water metabolism caused by a deficiency of vaso-pressin, the antidiuretic hormone (ADH) secreted by the posterior pituitary.

Aetiology

1   Deficient secretion of vasopressin (antidiuretic hormone).
    a Brain tumours, especially craniopharyngiomas
    b Central nervous system malformation or degenerative disease
    c Head trauma
    d Infection — including encephalitis, meningitis, many communicable diseases, and vaccination
    e Unknown cause
2   Failure of the renal tubules to respond to vasopressin (nephrogenic diabetes insipidus)
    a Hereditary (dominant) disease
    b More common in males.

Altered Physiology

1   Vasopressin normally acts on the distal tubules and collecting ducts of the kidney to facilitate reabsorption of water.
2   Pathology of the pituitary or hypothalamus results in a deficiency of vaso-pressin.
3   The kidney is unable to produce a concentrated urine without sufficient vasopressin.
4   Nephrogenic diabetes insipidus
    a Vasopressin secretion is normal.
    b The renal tubules do not respond to vasopressin.
    c The kidney is unable to produce a concentrated urine.

Clinical Manifestations

1 Onset — usually sudden
2 Symptoms
   a Depend on the age of the child and his primary lesion
   b Universal symptoms
      (1) Polydipsia (excessive thirst)
      (2) Polyuria (excessive urine output)
      (3) Inability to concentrate urine
   c Symptoms in infants
      (1) Excessive crying (quietened with water rather than additional milk)
      (2) Hyperthermia
      (3) Vomiting
      (4) Constipation
      (5) Rapid weight loss
      (6) Dehydration
      (7) Growth failure
   d Symptoms in older children
      (1) Excessive thirst which may interfere with play and sleep
      (2) Enuresis
      (3) Anorexia
      (4) Pale and dry skin
      (5) Reduced sweating
      (6) Viscid saliva.

Diagnostic Evaluation

Water Deprivation Test

1 The child fasts overnight and then is offered water until adequate hydration, stable weight, and free water diuresis are established.
2 All oral intake is then withheld for 6 hours.
3 Urine and serum osmolalities are determined prior to the beginning of hydration, at the start and termination of fluid deprivation. Serum sodium concentration and urine specific gravities may be substituted if osmometry is not available.
4 Positive results
   a Persistent excretion of dilute urine (osmolality less than 150 milliosmoles per kilogram; relative density less than 1.005).
   b A weight loss of 5% or more.
   c Increase in serum tonicity (osmolality greater than 290 milliosmoles per kilogram; sodium greater than 150 mEq/l = 150 mmol/l).

Vasopressin Sensitivity Test

A reduction of urine flow and an increase in urine concentration is observed following the administration of antidiuretic hormone.

Nursing Objectives

To prevent dehydration and restore electrolyte balance.

1 Nursing actions when the disorder is caused by a deficiency of vasopressin.
   a The most effective preparations available for treatment are synthetic analogues of vasopressin, these are given once or twice daily by nasal spray or dropper.
   b Pitressin tannate in oil may be used for replacement therapy.
   (1) Dosage — regulated by trial for each child.
   (2) Route of administration
      (a) Intramuscular
      (b) Never intravenous
   (3) Special precautions
      (a) Careful attention must be given to adequate suspension of the pitressin tannate in oil.
      (b) Hold the ampoule under hot water tap to reduce the viscosity of the suspending medium. (Immersion of the ampoule in boiling water destroys the hormone.)
      (c) Shake the ampoule vigorously until the active ingredient is smoothly dispersed.
      (d) Inject the medication with a 2.5cm No. 20-22 gauge needle.
      (e) Inject the medication deeply into the muscle.
      (f) Following injection, massage the area vigorously to aid absorption of the medication.
      (g) Establish a pattern of systematic rotation of injection sites.
      (h) Used with caution in patients with vascular disease or epilepsy.

Note: Pitressin may also be administered as a nasal spray, but the duration of its action is so brief that administration is required at 2-hour intervals.

2 Nursing actions when the disorder is caused by failure of the kidney to respond to vasopressin.
   a Administration of pitressin is ineffective.
   These children already produce a sufficient quantity of vasopressin.
   b Administer a low sodium, low solute residue diet to reduce the osmolar load on the kidney.
   c Administer chlorothiazide therapy as prescribed by the paediatrician.
   (1) May cause sodium diuresis which acts to promote proximal tubular sodium reabsorption.
   (2) If all sodium is reabsorbed proximally, none reaches the distal regions to permit formation of hypotonic urine and a degree of water economy results, but may lead to sodium depletion if reabsorption is ineffective.

To observe and record the child's response to therapy.

1　Intake and output
　　a Total the intake and output record every 8 hours.
　　b Record the relative density of urine at each micturition.
2　Temperature — be alert for the development of fever.
3　Skin turgor — decreased skin turgor is sign of dehydration.
4　Colour.
5　Appetite — record the child's intake accurately with each meal.

To participate in the diagnostic evaluation of diabetes insipidus.

1　Explain the purpose of appropriate laboratory tests and the protocol that the child and family will be asked to follow.
2　Supervise the child closely to avoid surreptitious fluid intake during fasting periods.
3　Observe the child closely for evidence of fluid and electrolyte disturbances while the test is in progress.
　　a Dehydration and shock may occur in severely affected children during the water deprivation test.
　　b Hypertonic dehydration may occur during the hypertonic saline test.
　　c Overhydration may occur in patients with primary psychogenic polydipsia during the vasopressin sensitivity test.
4　Collect urine specimens as requested by the paediatrician.
　　a Attempt to collect the urine on schedule.
　　b Record carefully:
　　　　(1) Time of collection
　　　　(2) Fluid intake (including intravenous fluids), if any
　　　　(3) Volume of urine
　　　　(4) Specific gravity of urine
　　　　(5) Weight of patient.

To provide emotional support to the family.

Prognosis depends on the underlying condition.

1　Hereditary and idiopathic types — favourable with adequate treatment.
2　Trauma — spontaneous recovery often occurs.
3　Tumour
　　a Varies with the site of the lesion and type of tumour.
　　b Needs of the family accentuated by many problems including surgery and facing the death of the child.

Patient or Parental Education

1　Explain the condition with specific clarification that diabetes insipidus and diabetes mellitus are very different disorders.

2   Teach parents the correct procedure for preparation and administration of injectable vasopressin.
3   Encourage the child to assume full responsibility for his care when he is old enough.
4   The child should wear a medic-alert tag, which identifies his condition.
5   The older child should carry nasal spray for temporary relief of symptoms if necessary.
6   The school nurse and other significant adults should be informed of the child's problem.

HYPOTHYROIDISM

Hypothyroidism is a metabolic disease resulting from deficient production of thyroid hormone. It may be either congenital (cretinism) or acquired (juvenile hypothyroidism).

Aetiology

Congenital

1   Embryonic defect with partial or complete absence of the thyroid gland
2   Defect in the synthesis of thyroid hormone
3   Destruction of fetal thyroid as a result of antigen-antibody reaction.
4   Iodide deficiency (endemic cretinism)
5   Toxic substances encountered during pregnancy causing maldevelopment or atrophy of the fetal thyroid gland. These may rarely include some medications administered during pregnancy.

Acquired

1   Hypoplasia of the thyroid gland
2   Partial defect in synthesis of thyroid hormone.
3   Autoimmune disease
4   Thyroidectomy
5   Medications
    a   Iodides
    b   Cobalt
    c   Thiouracil group of drugs
6   Iodine deficiency.

Clinical Manifestations

1   Approximately twice as common in females as in males.
2   Severity of clinical findings depends on the age at onset, extent of thyroid deficiency, and the particular individual.

3   Early signs and symptoms (several days or weeks after birth):
  a Prolonged physiological jaundice
  b Nasal obstruction and stuffiness
  c Feeding difficulties
  d Hoarse cry
  e Decreased intestinal activity — constipation
  f Poor muscle tone — umbilical hernia
  g Physical and mental sluggishness
  h Subnormal temperature
  i Possible heart enlargement
4   General appearance
  a Skin — dry, thick, scaly, coarse, cool, and pale
  b Facial characteristics
    (1) Bridge of nose — flat, broad, and undeveloped
    (2) Eyes — widely spaced with swollen eyelids
    (3) Anterior fontanelle widely open
    (4) Tongue — thick and protruding
  c Hair — frequently dry, coarse, brittle, slow-growing
  d Skeletal
    (1) Short, thick neck
    (2) Broad hands
    (3) Short fingers
    (4) Decrease in linear growth rate
5   Later signs and symptoms
  a Poor muscle tone
    (1) Protuberant abdomen
    (2) Lumbar lordosis
  b Delayed dentition
  Teeth decay easily
  c Delayed skeletal development
    (1) Short stature
    (2) Retarded bone age
    (3) Infantile skeletal proportions
      (a) Large head
      (b) Short extremities
  d Slow motor and mental development
    (1) Late sitting, standing, walking, talking
    (2) Late attaining normal milestones
    (3) Slow cerebral activity. (If severe hypothyroidism occurs before the age of 2 years, intelligence is often impaired.)
  e Retarded sexual development
  f Anaemia
  g Hypersensitivity to cold
  h Fatigue.

6 Clinical manifestations may be delayed in breast-fed infants until the child is weaned because of the thyroid hormone contained in breast milk.

Diagnostic Evaluation

1 X-ray shows retarded bone age.
2 Thyroid function tests are abnormal.
3 Neonatal screening is now possible with a highly sensitive radioimmunoassay for thyroxine or thyroid-stimulating factor.

Prognosis

1 Depends on the child's age at onset and the effectiveness of his therapy.
2 If untreated — becomes mentally handicapped and short.
3 When treated:
  a Normal physical growth and development occur.
  b Mental development is unpredictable.
    (1) The best results are obtained by giving continuous, full therapy as early as possible (within the first 3-4 months of life).
    (2) The best outlook is for children who have active thyroid tissue during the fetal life, have adequate treatment, and show a high family intelligence quotient.

Nursing Objectives

To administer L-thyroxine as the therapy of choice for the deficient hormone.

1 Dosage
  a Initally very low
  b Gradually increased to the maximum amount which the child can tolerate without producing signs of toxicity.
2 Route of administration
  Always administer by the oral route.
3 Special precautions
  a The total daily requirement is given as a single dose.
  b Administer the medication at the same time each day.
4 Observe for toxic effects:
  a Excitability
  b Tachycardia
  c Cramps
  d Diarrhoea
  e Fever
  f Vomiting.

To provide a complete, well-balanced diet.

1 Special problems related to nutrition
   a Anaemia
      (1) Increases the child's need for iron.
      (2) Include high quantities of meat, fish, poultry, eggs, enriched breads and cereals in the child's diet.
   b Increased skeletal development
      (1) Increases the need for additional vitamin D.
      (2) Encourage the older child to drink three to four glasses of milk daily.
   c Constipation
   Provide foods which are high in roughage such as raw fruits and vegetables; include bran.
2 Determine the child's dietary preferences and use this information to plan his menus.
   a Include the child in menu planning when this is possible.
   b Refer to section on nutrition, p. 36.

To prevent tooth decay.

1 Provide mouth care after each meal.
2 Discourage the intake of sweets, chewing gum, and fizzy drinks.

To provide emotional support to the child and his family.

1 Do not hurry the child.
2 Assess the child's capabilities and establish realistic expectations and limits.
3 Assist parents to adjust to alterations in their child's behaviour as he responds to treatment.
   The child may develop new enthusiasm for the naturally disturbing antics of childhood!

To provide support to the parents of a mentally handicapped child.

(Refer to section on mental handicap, p. 683.)

Patient or Parental Teaching

Medication

1 Give the medication conscientiously at the same time each day.
2 Adjust the dosage (by the paediatrician) to the needs of each individual child.
   a Regular medical follow-up and frequent re-evaluation are essential.
   b Dose may have to be increased during puberty and the reproductive period.
3 The medication must be continued throughout life.

4   Allow the parents to administer the medication during the child's hospitalization so that they will gain confidence in their ability to carry out the procedure.
5   Encourage parents to help the child accept increasing responsibility for his medications as he grows older.

Diet

1   Discuss the importance of a well-balanced diet.
2   Suggest sample menus. These should be economical and based on the family's normal dietary patterns.
3   Assist the mother of an infant with techniques of feeding.

Dental Care

1   Teach the child correct techniques for brushing his teeth.
    Stress that he should follow this procedure after each meal.
2   Encourage regular evaluations by a dentist (every 6 months).
    Refer the family to a dental clinic if necessary.

HYPERTHYROIDISM (THYROTOXICOSIS)

Hyperthyroidism is an endocrine disease resulting from an excessive secretion of thyroid hormone. It is frequently characterized by an enlarged thyroid gland (goitre) and prominent eyeballs (exophthalmos).

Aetiology

1   Unknown
2   Possible precipitating factors
    a   Autoimmune response
    b   Heredity
    c   Infection
    d   Psychological trauma.

Clinical Manifestations

1   Rare and less severe in children as compared to adults.
2   More common in females than males.
3   Onset is usually between 10 and 15 years of age (usually gradual onset).
4   Signs and symptoms
    a   Enlarged thyroid gland (goitre)
    b   Exophthalmos
    c   Nervousness and motor hyperactivity
        (1) Inability to sit still

  (2) Decreased attention span
  (3) Mood shifts
   (a) Irritable
   (b) Excitable
   (c) Cries easily
  (4) Sleep disturbances
d Increased appetite and food intake
e Weight loss or no weight gain
f Increased urinary excretion
g Skin
 (1) Warm
 (2) Moist
 (3) Flushed
h Muscular weakness and fatigue
i Tachycardia, palpitation and dyspnoea
j Increased systolic blood pressure; increased pulse pressure
k Accelerated growth rate
l Delayed sexual maturation
m Possible amenorrhoea in females
n Thyroid 'crisis' or 'storm' (very rare in children).

Diagnostic Evaluation

1 High serum levels of T_4 and T_3
2 T_3 uptake test — elevated
3 Radioactive iodine uptake — rapid
4 Basal metabolic rate increased
5 Thyroid stimulating hormone (TSH) values usually low.

Prognosis

1 Favourable in children who have passed through the therapeutic phase of hyperthyroidism with good immediate results.
2 Recurrence later in life.
 Recurrence risk cannot be accurately predicted; it depends on various factors in the therapeutic regimen.

Nursing Objectives

To avoid excitement

1 Provide a quiet environment.
 a Avoid assigning the child to a large ward or room with several other patients.

b Limit the number of playmates that the child has at any one time.
c Maintain a fairly constant schedule of daily activities.
d Sedate if necessary.
  (1) Barbiturates or tranquillizers are the drugs of choice.
  (2) Sedation may be especially beneficial at bedtime.
2 Encourage quiet rather than strenuous activities.
  Interest the child in diversionary activities which do not require lengthy mental concentration.
3 Maintain constant but gentle discipline.

To provide a diet high in protein, kilojoules (calories) and vitamins.

1 Offer between-meal snacks such as milk shakes.
2 Vitamin supplements may be necessary.
3 Offer foods which can be easily swallowed if the child is experiencing dysphagia.

To administer carbimazole, methylthiouracil.

1 These drugs block the production of T_4 and T_3 by the thyroid, thus controlling the symptoms.
2 Dose
  a Dosage must be individually regulated for each child.
  b It is essential to space the dose at regular intervals (every 6-8 hours) throughout a 24 hour period.
  Each dose is fully effective for only a few hours.
3 Observe for clinical response.
  a It is usually apparent in 2-3 weeks.
  b Exophthalmos may not reverse, but it should not advance.
  c Record disappearance of symptoms, including enlargement of the thyroid gland.
4 Observe for toxic effects. Report the following:
  a Fever
  b Mild, sometimes purpuric, papular rash
  c Headache
  d Nausea, abdominal cramps, diarrhoea
  e Pain and stiffness in joints, especially hands and wrists
  f Sore throat
5 Observe for relapse when the drug is discontinued.
  a Usually discontinued slowly after 1-2 years of administration.
  b Relapse usually occurs within 6 months of discontinuing the drug.
  c Treatment usually continued throughout early adolescence in pubertal children.

To demonstrate understanding of the child's physical and emotional problems.

1 The disease frequently has its onset during adolescence when the child is very concerned with his body image.
2 Encourage the child to talk about his disease and how he feels about it. Correct misinformation and misinterpretations as necessary.
3 Assist the adolescent girl to apply make-up which can significantly reduce the obviousness of her exophthalmos.
4 Discuss the child's disease and treatment with his parents, school nurse and teachers so that their demands and expectations will be realistic.

Patient or Parental Teaching

Medication

1 Allow the parent to administer the child's medication under supervision during his hospitalization to ensure accuracy after discharge.
2 Points of emphasis
   a The medication must be administered in the exact amount that was ordered.
   b Daily administration of the drug at regular intervals is essential.
   c The child must be observed for signs and symptoms of drug toxicity.

Medical Supervision

Close medical follow-up is necessary in order to evaluate the child's progress and regulate drug dosage.

FURTHER READING

Books

Bacon G *et al.*, *Paediatric Endocrinology*, Yearbook Publishers, 1982.
Craig O, *Childhood Diabetes and its Management*, Butterworth, 1982.
Craig O, *Childhood Diabetes: the Facts*, Oxford University Press, 1982.
Farquhar J W, *Diabetes in Your Teens*, Churchill, 1982.
Fletcher R F, *Lecture Notes on Endocrinology*, Blackwell Scientific, 1982.
Ramsay I, *Endocrinology and Metabolism*, John Wright, 1980.

Articles

Engle V, Diabetic teaching: how to win your patient's cooperation in his care, *Nursing*, December 1975, 5: 17.
Guthrie D, Exercise, diets and insulin for children with diabetes, *Nursing*, February 1977, 7: 48.

Guthrie D Guthrie R, Diabetes in adolescence, *American Journal of Nursing*, October 1975, 75: 1740.

Kaufman S, In diabetic diets, realism gets results, *Nursing*, November 1976, 6: 75.

McConnell E, Meeting the special needs of diabetics facing surgery, *Nursing*, June 1976, 6: 30.

McDonagh M, Adolescent diabetes mellitus, *Nursing Mirror*, November 1979: 38-40.

Robinson W, Home treatment is best for diabetic children, *Nursing Mirror*, October 1975: 36.

Rose V, Fun for the future; a diabetic children's camp holiday, *Nursing Times*, August 1977, 1304-1305.

Roskell V, Families with diabetic children, *Nursing Times*, December 1977, 1948-1951.

Schuman D, Assessing the diabetic, *Nursing*, March 1976, 6: 62.

Tattersall R, Why children develop diabetes, *Nursing Mirror*, August 1977: 28-30.

11

EYE, EAR, NOSE AND THROAT CONDITIONS

THE BLIND CHILD

Impaired vision (blindness) refers to insufficient or inadequate vision in varying degrees, which prevents a person from being able to perform the ordinary activities of daily living.

Aetiology

1. Familial factors
    Genetic determination
2. Antenatal or intrauterine factors
    a Rubella
    b Toxoplasmosis
    c Syphilis

3. Perinatal factors
    a Prematurity
    b Oxygen poisoning — retrolental fibroplasia
    c Infections

4. Postnatal factors
    a Injury or trauma
    b Infections
    c Inflammatory disease

Altered Physiology

1. Defective visual fields
2. Impaired colour vision
3. Decreased visual acuity
4. No vision — or a small percentage of vision (may have light perception).

Clinical Manifestations

Infant

1   No eye-to-eye contact, especially with mother
2   Abnormal eye movements
3   Does not follow objects at 2 months of age
4   Failure to locate distance objects at 6-12 months of age
5   Mother senses 'something is wrong'.

Older Child

1   Squinting, frequent blinking
2   Bumping into things
3   Frequent rubbing of eyes.

Diagnostic Evaluation

1   Legal definition — visual acuity 6/60 or less with correction
2   Tunnel vision — peripheral field of vision has an angular distance not greater than 20°.

Treatment

1   Surgical repair of defect
2   Glasses
3   Special training
    a Language development and acquisition
    b Mobility-perceptual motor training
    c Early stimulation therapy.

Nursing Objectives

The nurse may become involved with the blind child in the hospital in three critical situations: (1) before diagnosis has been made when she may detect a visual loss, usually in an infant; (2) at time of diagnosis; and (3) after diagnosis has been made and she is giving nursing care to the hospitalized blind child.

Detection: Early Care of the Blind Child after Diagnosis

To be familiar with the normal pattern of visual development and to be able to recognize deviations as well as manifestations of visual impairment

1   Knowing the stages of growth and development can be helpful in recognizing or suspecting visual impairment in the individual child.

2   The neonate has limited focal length of vision but will turn to light sources. At 3 months, he watches the human face and will scan surroundings. In other ways the infant's visual system is similar to an adult's, but seems to prefer the colours red and blue.
3   Be alert to and assess the child's response to visual stimulation.
   a Does the infant follow the human face or bright object with his eyes according to stage of development?
   b Does the infant reach for objects?
   c Does the 9- to 12-month-old child move around?

To be familiar with the causes of visual impairment and blindness in order to recognize from the history whether or not the child is in a high-risk stage.
1   Neonatal and perinatal factors
   a Prematurity
   b Oxygen therapy
   c Infections
2   Past infections — inflammatory diseases.

To record observations and report any suspicious behaviour by the infant or child indicating visual impairment.
1   Early diagnosis is the key to successful habilitation and optimal development of the child's capabilities.
2   The complication of complete withdrawal of the child can be avoided by early diagnosis and proper stimulation and emotional support.

To help the family of a newly diagnosed visually impaired child.
1   Parents must be allowed time to understand and accept what has happened.
2   Their lifestyle will have to change; they will need to find new ways to adjust socially and personally.

To work with the paediatrician and parents in helping the child master certain developmental tasks, thus aiding the child in achieving his fullest potential.
Parents need help in recognizing the clues the child presents indicating his need and readiness for new learning experiences. The child must also learn in his own natural way.

1   Continued communication must be fostered between parents, mother, and child.
   a Mother must learn techniques of touching, handling, and talking to her child.
   b Mother should make a special effort to help her baby associate her voice and body with receiving pleasure.
   c Encourage touching by both mother and baby during feeding times.

2　The child and parents must be helped to develop a discriminating relationship; specific consistent clues of handling the child can be built into behaviour.
a Each parent shares some special, individualized activity with the child.
b Voice and touch bring parents and child together.

3　The child must be allowed and encouraged to use his hands for exploring his world. Child must also learn appropriate use of hands.
a Give child objects of different shapes, sizes, and textures. Use toys that make noise and that are within reach and stay there.
b Give finger food to child during meals — when child is about 8 months of age or when he sits up.
c Extra tactile opportunities provided for child will compensate to some extent for loss of visual input.

4　The child needs to learn to become mobile.
a Mother's voice can encourage child to move towards her.
b A favourite toy placed in front of child can encourage him to move towards it.

5　The child needs much help in learning to talk.
a Expose the child to sounds that have a specific function — cleaning equipment, dishes.
b Mother should talk a great deal to the child. The child cannot benefit from gestures and facial expression used in language.

6　The child needs social exposure to his peers.
Nursery school can be very helpful.

To foster continuous acceptance of the child by his parents and to provide support for them.

1　Evaluate the parents' emotional status and offer them reassurance and explanations.
a Parental acceptance and a healthy home atmosphere are vitally important in helping the visually impaired or blind child to accept and adjust to his limitations.
b The child can sense his parents' approval or disapproval and the degree to which they love and accept him.

2　Help parents to understand and accept their responsibilities in the care of their child. Parents who have received appropriate information and guidance in handling their child can enrich the time spent with the child and prevent further handicapping and management problems. Indicate that they should do the following:
a Provide proper stimulation for the child to learn that which is ordinarily learned through vision. Frustration often occurs when child gives little feedback. Efforts may decrease as a consequence.
b The voice is often used to protect the child.

3   Help parents understand how they can develop the child's skills in interpreting information through the senses of hearing, touch, smell, and taste. They can learn to understand their blind child.
   a Hearing
      (1) Help child to determine distance by ringing a bell.
      (2) Familiarize him with appliances, birds, voices.
   b Touch
      Allow child to handle different textured materials.
   c Smell
      Acquaint child with flowers, perfume, kitchen odours.
   d Taste
      Help child distinguish different kitchen substances.
   e Memory
      Have child practise retelling stories, his telephone number, address, etc.
4   Initiate referral to the health visitor who can make their home visits to reinforce and interpret what mother has heard from the paediatrician and to encourage mother in her efforts.
5   Encourage parents to discuss their feelings about caring for a handicapped child at home.
      Initiate a social worker referral. (The social worker can help parents deal with their feelings.)
6   Help parents understand the problems the child faces and will face as he gets older.
   a Child will probably be delayed in development. There can be a delay of up to 5 months in creeping and 7 months in walking, even though posture and balance for such activities are similar to those of sighted child.
   b Child is likely to develop 'blindisms' — habits or mannerisms of blind children; these are a manifestation of inadequate impulse control.

To be familiar with the community resources and the professional team to be involved in habilitation of the visually impaired child.

Several types of educational programmes are available to the child, depending upon his confidence and coping abilities.

1   Residential schools.
   a Used when nothing is available in the local community.
   b Preferred when the home care of the child would be determined to his progress.
2   Day schools for the blind. (Child attends school during the day but lives at home.)
3   Ordinary school where blind child is integrated with sighted child. (Child receives special training in braille.)
4   Vocational programmes for the older child (training for some occupation).

To evaluate how well the child who was once able to see accepts visual impairment — in terms of his physical abilities and psychological dependence.

(Vision helps to maintain contact with reality.)

1   A serious impairment in relationships with people can result when the child is unable to express his innermost sentiments.
2   Allow the child to express his feelings, especially those of fear and anger. Talk, play, and certain activities help the child express these feelings.

Hospital Care of the Visually Impaired or Blind Child

Many of the important areas discussed above must be considered when caring for the child in the hospital situation. In addition, emphasis must be placed on the following objectives:

To interview the parents at the time of admission to learn as much as possible about the child and his care and activities at home.

1   Be aware of the child's schedule and activities during the day. Know what activities he can or cannot do, and what he likes to do.
2   Become familiar with how he is oriented to his new surroundings.
   a How much does he get about?
   b What precautions are necessary?
3   Be aware of how parents comfort and discipline the child.
      How does he comfort himself or seek security?
4   What special care or treatment must be continued while the child is hospitalized?
5   Share this information with nursing staff in a nursing care plan so continuity of care from home to hospital can minimize fear and frustration in the child.

To attend to the child's needs according to the medical problem that required his hospitalization.

To plan and provide for the appropriate type of play, activities programme and stimulation for the child.

1   Assess the child's level of growth and development and use the information obtained from the parents.
2   Allow the child as much independence as possible in his care, but provide guidance as necessary.
      Orient the ambulatory child thoroughly to his room and surroundings.
3   Encourage the development of the child's abilities. Avoid overprotecting him.
4   Provide activities that will increase his learning and give him pleasure (e.g. talking records).
5   Provide emotional preparation for procedures and surgery, as appropriate.

To meet the psychological and emotional needs of the visually impaired or blind child for protection and security against harm.

1   The nurse should always speak to the child prior to touching him so as not to frighten or startle him.
2   Always use a warm and gentle touch.
3   Explain strange sounds that may be frightening.
4   Plan frequent nurse-patient interactions to increase the child's sense of security.
5   Place items he needs and uses within his reach.
    a Familiar items that give the child security should also be close to him.
    b Tell him if they are moved.
6   During any procedure, talk to the child the entire time. Explain what is going on around him.

To avoid overemphasizing the child's handicap and to be unobtrusive about meeting his needs.
Allow the child to explore and learn about his new environment and the hospital.

To provide continual parental support

1   Encourage parents to become involved in the care of their child to help maintain or develop a healthy parent-child relationship.
2   Encourage parents to talk about their fears and feelings concerning this child. Help them relax.
    Parents can be invaluable in increasing the security and decreasing the fear the child may have as a result of being in a strange place.
3   Discuss realistically long-term and short-term planning for the child, i.e. educational opportunities.
    a Encourage parents to tell teachers, school nurses and adults responsible for his care about his special needs.
    b Avoid overemphasis on educational achievements.
4   Help parents understand that discipline, order and consistency are necessary in the child's environment to give him security.
5   Emphasize that the parents' role is to give this child love and physical care as well as to stimulate and influence him so he may have a satisfactory mental, social and emotional growth.
6   Help parents see that other members of the family must also be considered.
    a Their handicapped child does need special attention, but he does not need all the attention all the time.
    b Other members of the family should be included in his care, but they also have a life of their own and need as much attention from parents as they would have if the handicapped child were not present in the family.
    c Parents need time to themselves. They should be encouraged to go out alone together and to give time to their marriage.

7   Help parents realize that even though the development and progress of their blind child is long and drawn out, the child may be able to live a normal life in the community.
     a Are parents aware of and do they accept the short- and long-term goals?
     b Many blind people are successful as technicians and professionals in our society.

EYE DEFECTS REQUIRING SURGERY

Eye defects requiring surgery are (1) structural manifestations of the eye present at birth or (2) acquired conditions of the eye. They can be extraocular or intraocular conditions.

Aetiology

1   Congenital
     a Hereditary tendencies
     b Birth injury
     c Innervational factors
     d Intrauterine influences
2   Disease
     a Metabolic
     b Infection
3   Trauma to the eye.

Strabismus

Strabismus is the inability to balance the extraocular muscles; thus the eyes cannot function together at the same time.

Altered Physiology

1   The visual axis of only one eye goes to the object being observed. The person appears to be looking in two directions at once.
2   Specific deviations
     a Paralytic strabismus — muscles of one eye are underactive.
     b Concomitant strabismus — both eyes move, but the deviation between the eyes is always the same.
     c Convergent — manifested as 'cross-eye'.
     d Divergent — manifested as 'wall-eye'.
     e Vertical — vertical separation of visual axes.
     f Esotropia — one eye deviates towards the other eye.
     g Exotropia — one eye deviates away from the other eye.

Clinical Manifestations

1   Deviations of the eye (constant or intermittent)
2   Squinting
3   Closing one eye to see
4   Tilting head
5   Stumbling or clumsy behaviour
6   Inaccuracy in picking up objects
7   Double vision.

Complications

1   Amblyopia — poor vision in eye not used
2   Emotional problems resulting from cosmetic aspect of deformity.

Treatment

1   Corrective glasses
2   Patching nondiverging eye
3   Surgery
    Lengthening or shortening of extraocular structures

Nursing Management

See p. 571.

Cataract
Cataract is an opacification or milk-white appearance of the eye lens.

Altered Physiology

Inability of light to pass through the clouded lens in adequate amounts — loss of vision as lens becomes more opaque; loss of transparency.

Clinical Manifestations

1   Gradual diminution of visual acuity
2   Strabismus
3   Nystagmus
4   Grey opacities of lens.

Diagnostic Evaluation

Ophthalmoscopic examination reveals opacification of the lens.

Treatment

1 Medication — dilation of pupil with mydriatic eye drops
2 Surgery
   a Optical iridectomy
   b Lens fragmentation, irrigation, and aspiration.

Complications

Untreated Cataract

1 Bilateral cataract
   a Nystagmus
   b Stimulus-deprivation amblyopia
2 Unilateral cataract
   a Strabismus
   b Stimulus-deprivation amblyopia.

Following Surgery for Congenital Cataract

1 Retinal detachment several years later
2 Average vision only 20/70
3 Need for glasses or contact lenses to replace refracting power of lens.

Nursing Management
See p. 571.

Trauma
Trauma is injury to the globe, adnexa, and surrounding tissue of the eye as a result of blunt objects (cricket ball, rock) striking the eye area, or sharp items (scissors, knife) penetrating the eye area.

Altered Physiology

Blunt Injury

1 Subconjunctival haemorrhage and suffusion of blood into eyelid
2 Secondary haemorrhage days after injury
   a Accumulation of blood in anterior chamber and blocking of overflow channels
   b Rapid rise of intraocular pressure (glaucoma)
3 Retinal oedema, haemorrhages, and detachment.

Penetrating Injury

1 Loss of aqueous fluid, development of cataract

2   Bleeding into anterior chamber and vitreous
3   Retinal detachment.

Complications

Sympathetic ophthalmia — inflammation of the uninjured eye probably due to an allergic reaction to pigment released from injured eye. This condition can lead to significant visual loss.

Nursing Management of the Child Undergoing Eye Surgery

Nursing Objectives: Preoperative Care

To help the child and his parents to know and understand what the surgery entails.

(Explanations should be appropriate for the age of the child.)
1   Take a trip to the operating and recovery rooms if the child is not on bed rest due to trauma.
2   Practice applying eye patches for short frequent periods.
    a Allow the child to handle the equipment to be used, using a doll or teddy as 'patient'.
    b Explain that the patches will only be temporary.
3   Help the child become familiar with the protection devices if they are to be used postoperatively.
4   Discuss and practise postoperative exercises if feasible.
5   Relieve child's fears about pain by telling him that there will be only a little pain — as if something is in the eye.

To assess the child and his needs according to age and specifically to his eye problem.

1   Does the child have the ability to read or watch television?
2   Does the child wear glasses? When?
    Help him to learn to protect his glasses when not in use.

To provide as much comfort and reassurance to the child as possible to diminish his fears especially concerning hospitalization and impending surgery.

1   Room assignment can be significant.
    a A quiet room with subdued lighting can be more comfortable for trauma patients.
    b Placement in a room with other children (without infection) may be comforting for elective surgery patients.

2   Allow the child to have familiar tactile and auditory stimulating objects around him.
3   Provide facilities for mother or father to live in if they are able to do so.

Postoperative Care

To administer effective postoperative care and to observe for possible postoperative complications.
(See p. 85.) Be alert to care and consideration for specific eye defect.

1   Strabismus
    a Frequently child is discharged on the day following surgery, following recovery from anaesthesia.
    b Surgery is extraocular; no postoperative ocular rupture hazards exist.
    c Activity is not restricted.
    d Eye bandages may or may not be used.
    e Eyes will probably be blood-tinged and will drain. Eyes may feel uncomfortable. Black eye is normal, as a postoperative swelling.
    f Eyes may be difficult to open the morning after surgery. Gently separate lids from above and below. Do not force lids open. Tears will soften secretions.
    g Child may have photosensitivity.
2   Cataract or intraocular surgery
    a Child is generally positioned on his back; thus, prevention of aspiration is a concern.
    b Avoid sudden head movement, crying, and vomiting, because these increase intraocular pressure; they cause strain on sutures and subsequent bleeding.
    c Avoid surprising patient and making him jump. Avoid noises. Speak gently before touching child.

To prevent the child from pulling off the dressing and causing injury or contamination

1   Sedation may be warranted until the child becomes accustomed to having his eye continually bandaged.
2   Protective devices may be used only if necessary.
        Rest during the immediate postoperative period is necessary and a child struggling because of restraints can defeat their intended purpose.
3   Diet should be increased slowly to prevent vomiting; this could cause possible injury to the eye due to increased pressure.

To provide emotional and psychological reassurance and support to the child who is anxious because his eyes are bandaged, preventing him from seeing.

1   Encourage parents to be with child, especially when he is waking up from anaesthesia. If parents are not able to do this, someone should.
    a Sit with child, stroke him, and speak gently and softly to him.

b Let him hold a familiar object.

c Hold him if there are no contraindications to his being lifted and held.

2 Always speak to child before touching him so as not to startle him.
   Explain what is going to be done to him before doing it.

3 Tell the child what foods are on his tray.
   Allow him to finger feed himself.

4 Explain sounds. (Sounds in the world without sight can be very frightening.)

5 Reassure child that patches will be removed soon and he will be able to see again (if he is going to see).

6 Provide appropriate diversional activities for the child.

   a Read him stories.

   b Provide radio, record or cassette player.

   c Talk with him.

To administer appropriate eye medications and change dressing as prescribed.

1 First dressing may be done by the surgeon.

   a Strabismus — dressing removed day after surgery.

   b Cataract — dressing may be used for 2-6 days after surgery.

2 Be familiar with types of eye medications used.

   a Mydriatic — used to dilate pupil.

   b Miotic — constricts pupil and decreases increased intraocular pressure in early glaucoma.

   c Anti-inflammatory drugs.

   d Antibiotics.

3 Be familiar with the principles of instilling eye medications (drops, ointments, and irrigations).

   a Have room darkened — light may be uncomfortable.

   b Try to gain the confidence and cooperation of the child and reassure him by talking to him during the procedure.

   c Assistance may be necessary to stabilize child's head and prevent injury. Have child close eye; drop medication on to inner canthus; open eye and drop will roll in.

   d Irrigate from inner canthus outward.

   e To instil drops, pull lower lid down and drop medication on to conjunctiva from dropper parallel to lid. If drops are instilled on conjunctiva and not on cornea, patient tolerates medication better.

   f Do not force lid open.

   g Blot away excess fluid with tissue or cotton ball; do not rub eye.

   h Avoid contaminating dressing.

   i Always wash hands before and after contact with the eye for any procedure.

To involve parents and child in preparation for discharge.

1 Teach parents how to instill eye medications. (See above.)

2   Postoperative patches or glasses may be necessary.

Help parents and child understand the value and importance of the patching or glasses.

3   Encourage parents to contact the school nurse and other adults responsible for child's care to explain special exercises or specific care for the child.

4   Encourage follow-up as advised by the surgeon.

Parental Teaching

1   Help parents understand what was wrong with the child, what was done to help correct the problem and what the parental responsibilities are in continuing any recommended therapy with the child.

2   Be certain parents understand what special care is to be given and how it is to be accomplished.

TONSILLECTOMY AND ADENOIDECTOMY

Tonsillectomy and adenoidectomy is the surgical removal of adenoidal and tonsillar structures, part of the lymphoid tissue that encircles the pharynx. (The function of the tonsils and adenoids is to serve as a first line of defence against respiratory infection.)

Aetiology

1   Acute or chronic infection of tonsils and adenoids

2   Hypertrophy produces obstruction to:

   a Breathing

   b Swallowing

   c Eustachian tube.

Clinical Manifestations

1   Indications for tonsillectomy

   a Recurrent or persistent tonsillitis

   b Enlargement of cervical nodes

   c Peritonsillar abscess or retrotonsillar abscess

   d Suppurative cervical adenitis with tonsillar focus.

2   Indications for adenoidectomy

   a Chronic otitis media, impaired hearing

   b Recurrent acute otitis media

c Persistent rhinitis
d Grossly hypertrophied adenoids with persistent mouth breathing.

Note: It is not uncommon for more than one of these indications to be present in the same child.

Diagnostic Evaluation

Since bleeding is a likely complication of surgery to this highly vascular area, the following preoperative blood studies must be completed according to surgeons instructions:

1   Clotting time
2   Smear for platelets
3   Prothrombin time
4   Partial prothrombin time
5   Blood grouping
6   Haemoglobin estimation.

Nursing Objectives — Preoperative Care

To assess upon admission the psychological preparation of the child for hospitalization and surgery.

1   The child should know why he has been admitted to the hospital and what will happen to him.
2   When parents have not told the child about hospitalization, it may be because they cannot.
    a They do not know what will happen.
    b They do not know how to tell the child because of their own anxieties.
    c They do not understand the importance of telling the child the truth in order to perpetuate the child's trust in the parents.
3   Help parents in preparing the child by talking at first in general terms about hospitalization.
4   Child may have preconceived ideas from parents and peers about what to expect. (These may pose a threat to the child.)
    a Expose child to other children on the unit, especially those who have had and are recovering from surgery.
    b Correct any misunderstandings the child may have.
5   The preschool child is very vulnerable to psychological trauma as a result of this experience.
    a Tell the child the truth.
    b Include parents when helping the child.

To take nursing history from parents at the time of admission to obtain any pertinent information that would contraindicate surgery.

1   Infection
   a When was last recent infection?
   b Has child been exposed to any contagious diseases?
2   Safety
   a Does the child have any loose teeth?
   b Are there any bleeding tendencies in child or family?

To maintain adequate hydration prior to surgery, since blood loss may be extensive during surgery.

1   Encourage the child to drink fluids the night before surgery.
2   Usually nil by mouth is ordered at least 4 hours prior to surgery.

To prepare the child specifically (appropriate for age) for what to expect postoperatively.

1   Where he will wake up
2   Sore throat, emesis of blood, position
3   Medications/mouth wash
4   Fluid regimen.

To encourage mother to stay with her young child day and night of surgery or at least before surgery and when the child returns to his room and is waking up.

1   Prepare the mother as to what to expect when she sees the child postoperatively:
   a Vomiting
   b Colour
   c Crying, angry or frightened.

To know if the child has a history of chronic infection or rheumatic fever so antibiotics may be given pre- and postoperatively.

Postoperative Care

To administer good postoperative care based on general principles and to observe for usual postoperative complications
(See p. 85).

To assist the child in maintaining a patent airway, by draining secretions and preventing aspiration of vomitus.

1   Place child prone or semiprone before he becomes alert with head turned to side.
2   Allow the child to assume position of comfort when he is alert. (Mother may hold child).
3   Child may vomit old blood initially.

To observe the child constantly until he is awake, and then frequently thereafter; monitor vital signs and be alert to signs of haemorrhage.

1   Indications of haemorrhage (the most frequent complication)
    a Increasing rapid pulse
    b Frequent swallowing
    c Pallor
    d Restlessness
    e Clearing of throat and vomiting of blood
    f Continuous slight oozing of blood over a number of hours postoperatively.
2   Have emergency equipment readily available.
    a Suction equipment
    b Packing material.

To offer measures of comfort to the child

1   Cool liquids offer some relief from sore throat, as well as prevent dehydration and temperature elevation.
    a Give ice chips 1-2 hours after awakening.
    b Advance clear liquids cautiously until vomiting has ceased.
    c Offer cool, synthetic fruit juices and milk at first as they are best tolerated.
2   Give analgesic, especially to older child, half an hour before meals to aid swallowing.
3   Rinse mouth with cool water or alkaline solution mouth wash.

To provide opportunity for child to have as much rest as possible.

1   Encourage mother to be with the child when he awakens as he is usually frightened. (Mother's presence can be very comforting.)
2   When mother must leave, reassure the child she will return.
3   Keep child in bed in a quiet room or quiet area of the ward.

Parental Teaching

1   Explain and write instructions as to the care of the child at home after discharge.
    a Diet should still consist of large amounts of fluids as well as soft, cool nonirritating foods. (Supply list of suggestions.) Normal foods should be introduced 24-48 hours after surgery.
    b Bed rest should be maintained for a couple of days, then daily rest periods for about a week.
    c If signs and symptoms of impending trouble occur, the family doctor should be called immediately.
        (1) Earache accompanied by fever
        (2) Any bleeding, often indicated only by frequent swallowing
    d How to give any medications the surgeon may order.

e The child should be kept away from anyone with a cough, cold, or infection.
Crowded places, such as buses and cinemas, are best avoided.
2   Discuss with the mother (parents) what results they can expect from the surgery.
  a Decreased number of sore throats
  b Improvement in obstructive symptoms
  c Decreased incidence of cervical lymphadenitis
  d Improvement in nutritional status
3   Guide parents in helping the child make the hospital experience a positive one once he has returned home.
  a Talk about what happened.
  b Let child play out his feelings.
4   An outpatient appointment to see the surgeon should be given or sent to the parents on discharge.

OTITIS MEDIA

Otitis media is an infection of the middle ear.

Aetiology
1   Bacteriological
  a Pneumococci
  b Beta-haemolytic streptococci
  c *Haemophilus influenzae*
2   Secondary
  a Cold
  b Measles
  c Scarlet fever
3   Eustachian tube dysfunction
  a Obstruction
  b Abnormal patency.

Altered Physiology
1   Obstruction of the Eustachian tube by swelling of mucous membranes:
  a Air exchange does not take place between the pharynx and middle ear.
  b Obstruction impedes drainage of secretions to the nasopharynx.
2   Secretions and bacteria become trapped in the middle ear.
    Bacteria multiply rapidly in that environment.

3 Fluid and exudate replace air in the middle ear.
   a Eardrum bulges.
   b Tympanic membrane may rupture.

Clinical Manifestations

1 History of cold for several days
2 Fever
3 Older child
   a Pain in affected ear
   b Blurred hearing
   c Headache
   d Vomiting
4 Infant
   a May rub ear
   b Anorexia
   c Turns head from side to side
   d Diarrhoea.

Diagnostic Evaluation

1 Examination will reveal bulging of eardrum and lack of normal lustre; ruptured drum may be obscured by secretions.
2 Culture and sensitivity determination of drainage from ruptured drum in order to select appropriate antibiotic therapy.
3 Tympanometry — the use of an electroacoustic impedance bridge with which a tympanogram can be obtained. The tympanograms produced show the dynamics of the tympanic membrane, middle ear, Eustachian tube system.

Treatment

Medical

1 Antibiotics — appropriate for organism
2 Paracetamol or acetylsalicylic acid (antipyretic) for fever
3 Analgesic
4 Ear drops for relief of pain
5 Antihistamines and decongestant — to clear nasal pharyngitis and inflammation of Eustachian tube.

Surgical

1 Myringotomy — surgical incision of the tympanic membrane to allow drainage and relieve pressure

2 Grommet-tympanostomy tubes — small Teflon tubes are inserted into the middle ear through a myringotomy incision.
   a The tube projects through the drum into the external auditory canal.
   b This tube is a substitute for the Eustachian tube, allowing the following to occur:
   (1) Continuous ventilation of the middle ear
   (2) Drainage of fluid into the external auditory canal
   (3) Promotion of healing of lining membranes
   (4) Prevention of premature closing of incision.
   c The tubes may be left in place several weeks to several months. The perforation closes in about a week after the tubes are removed.
   d Hearing will improve in children with middle ear fluid.
   e Most common age for treatment is between 2 and 7 years.
   f Complications of grommet tubes include:
   (1) Recurring otitis media or suppurative otitis media
   (2) Plugging of tubes with blood, cerumen, or exudate
   (3) Early spontaneous extrusion of tube
   (4) Permanent perforations.
   g Specific postoperative considerations
   Do not allow water to get into ears (during swimming or bathing) because of the infection potential.

Complications
From untreated or ineffective treatment of acute otitis media

1 Chronic otitis media
2 Mastoiditis
3 Septicaemia
4 Meningitis and brain damage
5 Chronic otitis media with perforated eardrum may lead to impaired hearing or deafness.

Nursing Objectives

To administer medications and treatments as prescribed.

1 Give appropriate antibiotics according to sensitivity of organisms.
   Usual course of treatment is 10 days.
2 Instil nose drops and decongestant.
   May help to shrink mucous membranes and allow drainage from obstructed Eustachian tube.
3 Give ear irrigations and instil glycerine or oil for relief of pain, if ordered.
   a Child may need to be held, or 'mummy' restraint used.
   b For child under 3 years old — pull auricle down and back.
   c For child over 3 years old — pull auricle up and back.

d Position child so the affected ear is up — allows fluid to run on to the eardrum.

To prevent mixed infection and reduce the chances of complications arising from present infection.

1 Always wash hands prior to any treatment or contact with the ear.
2 Change position of the child as appropriate.
   a Position affected ear up to instil medications or to irrigate ear.
   b Position affected ear down to facilitate drainage when child is resting.
3 Clean any exudate present from myringotomy or perforated drum.
   Prevents excoriation from drainage.

To provide physical comfort for the child while continuing therapy.

1 Local heat
   a Use of a covered hot water bottle containing water not over 38.9°C will often help to soothe an older child's pain and discomfort.
   b Place child on side, with affected ear on top of bottle to facilitate drainage.
2 A mild analgesic may be necessary if child is restless and indicates pain.
3 Myringotomy may be done in cases where there is severe pain.
   Small incision of the tympanic membrane to relieve pressure and prevent a jagged opening from a spontaneous rupture.
4 Encourage fluid intake to help maintain hydration since the child may have a fever.

To observe for signs of complications and report them .

1 Mastoiditis
   a Pain behind affected ear
   b Increasing irritability
   c Onset or increase fever
   d Tenderness, redness, and swelling over mastoid area
2 Meningitis
   a Sudden onset of high fever
   b Stiffness of neck
   c Irritability
   d Headache
   e Lethargy
3 Chronic otitis media with perforation of tympanic membrane
   Usually not observed until follow-up care by surgeon

To provide emotional and psychological support appropriate for child's age and degree of illness.

1 Encourage child to participate in diversional activities.
2 Reassure child
   a Talk to him gently.

b Allow child to express his feelings, fears and frustrations by talking, playing, and drawing.

c Hold and rock the younger child.

3 Encourage parental visits and involvement in the child's care. Provide facilities for parents to be resident if they are able to do so.

To help the parents understand that prevention of recurring otitis media is vitally important for the future well-being of the child.

1 Explain the value of preventing and treating the common cold.
2 Removal of hypertrophied and infected adenoid tissue may be necessary at a later date at the recommendation of the surgeon.
3 Explain that the child may have decreased hearing for several weeks following this episode of illness.
4 Help parents learn what signs indicate recurrent otitis media and the need for immediate medical intervention. Prompt treatment can prevent permanent hearing loss.

To help parents and child understand treatment and expectations related to ventilating tubes.

1 Following surgery, antibiotic ear drops may be prescribed to aid in keeping tubes patent.
2 Hearing may not improve for 1-3 weeks postoperatively.
3 Tubes will remain in place from 2-10 months, and are designed to extrude into the external ear canal.
4 When tubes extrude, slight pain and a small amount of bloody drainage may occur.
5 Water should be prevented from entering the external ear canal — use properly fitting ear plugs, cottonballs coated with petroleum jelly, etc.
6 Stress the importance of regular medical follow-up to evaluate proper functioning of tubes.

THE CHILD WITH IMPAIRED HEARING

Impaired hearing occurs when there is a hearing loss in speech frequencies of over 20 decibels, and the child does not learn to talk in the normal way.

Aetiology

1 Unknown
2 Familial factors — genetically transmitted
3 Antenatal or intrauterine factors
   a Rubella
   b Pre-eclampsia or eclampsia
   c Drugs
   d Congenital syphilis

4 Perinatal factors
   a Prematurity
   b Anoxia at birth
   c Hyperbilirubinaemia
   d Erythroblastosis fetalis
5 Postnatal factors
   a Ototoxic drugs
   b Acquired disorders of the central nervous system
   c Acute infections
   d Injury
6 Chromosomal anomalies
   a Trisomy 13-14-15
   b Trisomy 18.

Altered Physiology

Conductive Hearing Loss

1 Impairment in the mechanism of conducting sound waves to the cochlea
   a Blockage of sound waves from outer ear, external canal, or middle ear (lack of loudness)
   b Tympanic membrane damage and scarring
   c Dislocation or disturbance of tiny ossicular bones in the middle ear
2 Often recognized in the school-age child.

Sensorineural Hearing Loss

1 Malfunction of inner ear apparatus or eighth cranial nerve — medically irreversible
   a Lack of loudness
   b Distorted sounds due to defect of cochlea or neural pathways to temporal lobe of the brain
   c Problems with discrimination of sound
2 Mixed hearing loss; both sensorineural and conductive hearing loss in some children.

Clinical Manifestations

Infant

1 Little or no interest in sounds of his environment
   a Does not blink at loud noise
   b Does not turn eyes toward sound of musical toy or mother's voice at 3 months of age
   c Does not turn towards whispered voice within 1 metre at 8-12 months of age
   d Hyperactivity or gesturing may increase

2 Lack of minimal vocalization
  a Does not coo or gurgle
  b May not smile
  c Babbling decreases after 6-8 months of age
3 Lack of neonatal reflex startle to noise 1-2 metres (3-6 feet) away.

Toddlers

1 Little or no vocalization
  a Sounds produced poorly
  b Will not repeat a word with single stimulus
  c Uses gestures to express needs
2 Little interest in environmental sounds
    Does not respond to name, doorbell, or telephone.

Preschool and School-age Child

1 Behavioural disturbances
  a Intense, constant activity
  b Temper tantrums
  c Inattentiveness
  d Slow learner
2 May show abrupt change in social or communicative behaviour

Sensorineural vs. Conductive Hearing Loss

1 Sensorineural
  a Child may talk more loudly than necessary.
  b Child may not respond to average loudness but responds to loud sounds.
  c When intensity of sound is increased above the threshold of sensitivity, child shows some type of response.
2 Conductive
  a Child has tendency to talk in relatively soft voice.
  b He hears better in a noisy environment.
  c Child can hear loud speech and sounds.

Diagnostic Evaluation

1 Otolaryngological examination (inspection of external ear and tympanic membrane) — to rule out involvement of conductive apparatus
2 Audiological examination — to establish the extent of hearing loss and to determine type of hearing aid needed
  a Observation of child's response to sounds calibrated for intensity and frequency
  b Objective measuring techniques of hearing loss, i.e. cortical audiometry

3   Hearing loss classification
Pure tone audiometry hearing threshold level:

0-25 dB	Normal hearing
26-40 dB	Mild hearing impairment
41-55 dB	Moderate hearing loss
56-70 dB	Moderately severe hearing loss
71-90 dB	Severe hearing loss
91+ dB	Profound hearing loss.

Complications

1   In childhood when there is a hearing disorder, there is a delay of speech and language development; thus, there is a loss of contact between the individual, his peers, and his environment.
2   Biological, behavioural, and social complications may result when there is a breakdown of the normal communicative process.
3   The seriousness of the total problem depends upon the nature and extent of auditory involvement and upon the age of onset and length of time before the hearing problem is detected.

Treatment

1   Conductive hearing loss
   a Surgical correction of defect
   b Hearing aid
2   Sensorineural hearing loss
   a Hearing aid
   b Special training
      (1) Language acquisition
      (2) Auditory training
      (3) Speech therapy
      (4) Perceptual motor training.

Nursing Objectives

The nurse may become involved with the child with impaired hearing in the hospital in three situations: (1) before diagnosis has been made when she may detect a hearing loss; (2) at the time of diagnosis; and (3) after diagnosis has been made when giving nursing care to the hospitalized child.

Detection: Early Care after Diagnosis

To be familiar with the normal pattern of language and learning development and the manifestations of hearing loss in the infant and child.

1   Knowing the stages of growth and development can be helpful in recognizing and suspecting hearing impairment in the individual child.
2   Be alert to and assess the child's response to auditory stimulation.
    a Does infant stop activity and listen to vocal sounds?
    b Does the child respond to his name?
    c Does the child have unusual visual alertness at age 1 year?
3   The critical period of learning or language development is from birth to 16 months.

To be familiar with the causes of hearing impairment and recognize from the history if the child may be in a high-risk area.

1   Ensure that follow-up hearing evaluation is planned.
2   Criteria for high risk of impaired hearing (see Aetiology, p. 582).

To record observations and report to paediatrician any suspicious behaviour by the infant or child that indicates possible hearing loss.

1   Early diagnosis is the key to successful habilitation and optimal development of the capabilities of the child. Early intervention is aimed towards the child's acquisition of heard and spoken language.
    a After 16 months of age, progress is more difficult.
    b If hearing loss occurs after the time of critical language development, rehabilitation is less difficult, as the groundwork for verbal communication has been established.
2   The impulse for learning spontaneous speech and acquiring most of the basic verbal skills as well as the structure on which mature use of language and speech is built is reached during the first 3-4 years of life.

To be familiar with community resources and the professional team involved.

1   Each child must be treated as an individual.
2   Knowing general philosophies and training techniques of the involved resource can be helpful.
    Help child to capitalize on assets and minimize limitations.

To be familiar with the guidelines and techniques of educating a child with impaired hearing.

1   The main mode of communication for the child with impaired hearing is visual, supplemented by auditory clues.
    a Educational task is to develop the child's understanding and expression of language.
    b Speech can be learned through a multisensory approach, using visual, tactile, kinesthetic and auditory stimulation.

2   The child with a less severe hearing loss uses auditory stimulation, supplemented by visual clues, as his main mode of communication.

Educational task is to develop adequate speech and language and the best use of residual hearing.

3   The three basic methods currently used in educating deaf children include:

a *Oral approach* — Emphasizes verbal communication, speech reading, and auditory training. Most useful when the child has some hearing.

b *Manual communication* — Sign language.

c *Total communication approach* — Combines sign language with auditory training and speech reading.

4   The newest concept in education is cued speech, which visually pinpoints a single sound being spoken by using a manual supplement to lip reading of hand shapes used near the mouth to make language sounds look different on the lips or hand.

5   Whatever method of education and communication is used, it is critical for parents to enter the educational process so that they can establish communication with their child.

To help the family cope with and accept a newly diagnosed hearing impairment in their child.

1   Encourage the paediatrician to have both parents present when he tells them the diagnosis. This allows the parents to support each other.

2   Do not focus all your attention on the child. Show your concern and interest in the parents.

3   Be aware that parents must be given time to adjust to this usually drastic and unexpected change in their lives before they can deal constructively with meeting the needs of the child.

4   At this time parents need general information — good literature that is specific to their child's problem.

Contact with other parents who have made successful adjustments to living with their hearing-impaired children can be helpful to parents.

To be aware of the problems facing the mother (and family) of a hearing-impaired child.
Offer them specific guidance in handling and caring for the child.

1   Problems encountered

a Lack of knowledge of principles of parenting methods that govern her child's development.

b Does not receive cues from her child that are familiar to most mothers.

c Does not get feedback from her child in speech (vocalization), emotional response, or achievement — all of which increase spontaneous mothering. Communicating limitations tend to restrict early mother-child relationships.

Child is not equipped to show his attachment to his mother.

d Parent must be in close contact with the child to control and regulate his behaviour.

e Her child is infantile in lack of impulse control and is unable to understand and order his world.

f Mother may show embarrassment because of her child's behaviour.

g There is a possible tendency to neglect or deny common childhood conflicts and/or problems.

h Frustration — feels she does not know how to help her child.

2   Specific guidance to offer mother:

a Allow and encourage her to communicate with her child through mime, gestures, and body language.

b Optimize auditory environment.

c Teach her how to talk to her child — to use verbal and nonverbal reinforcement of behaviour.

d Help her baby develop "watching behaviour" by rewarding him with pleasure and praise.

e Encourage her to look directly into the child's eyes when she talks to him.

f Help her to understand that her child is probably unable to express his anxieties; frustration lead to anger and sudden rage or temper tantrums. Help her to gain confidence in her own resourcefulness and care by anticipating child's random behaviour through her knowledge of its coincidence with certain situations.

g Teach her the stages of language development.

To foster continuous parental acceptance of the child and provide support for family.

1   Invite parents to become involved in the care of their hospitalized child as much as possible.

2   Help parents to understand the problems the child faces and will face as he gets older.

a Although hearing impairment does alter life's experience for the child, it does not limit intelligence or capacity for emotional response and normal growth and development.

b Child may not be able to participate in activities in which sounds and verbal commands are used.

c Often the referral agency will become very involved in supporting the family.

3   Help parents become aware of their importance in the success of the progress of the child.

a Parents have the most important educational influence on the child.

b Opportunities to use effective ways of stimulating child's awareness and understanding of speech occur daily in the home.

c The child needs the warmth and security of a family setting.

4   Help parents to understand what can be accomplished in their child's education to enable him to be a contributing member of society.

5   Stress the importance of close follow-up by the specialists caring for the child.

6   Help parents to understand the use and importance of the hearing aid their child is using.

a Most children with a hearing loss have enough residual hearing to respond to and/or recognize sounds with the use of an aid.

b Parents must be convinced of the value of the aid but not pay too much attention to it.

c Young child does not have much difficulty in adjusting to the hearing aid if the ear mould is comfortable and the sound amplification is not too unpleasant.

Place the aid on the child and have him wear it during waking hours.

d For the older child who has become used to the aid as a youngster, it is part of his body image and he is dependent upon the sound.

e Parents should be sensitive to child's reactions to the aid.

f Follow-up care is vital; a malfunctioning aid can cause the child to lose interest in its use.

7   Help shape healthy parental attitudes about their child and guide them through this difficult time.

a Prevent denial.

b Parents need sympathetic understanding during the time of diagnosis and immediately following when they are bewildered and grieving.

c Parental attitudes may be the primary factor in determining the success or failure of the child's progress.

8   Encourage the parents to write for literature from appropriate agencies.

Care of the Hospitalized Child who has a Hearing Loss

To interview the parents at the time of admission to learn as much as possible about the child and his activities at home.

1   What is the child's way of communicating his needs? How do parents communicate with the child?

2   Be aware of the child's schedule and activities at home.
     Know what activities he can or cannot do and what he likes to do.

3   Be aware of how parents discipline child and how they comfort him.

4   Does the child wear a hearing aid? When? Any special exercises or training that needs to be continued?

5   Share this information with nursing staff in the nursing care plan to assure continuity of care from home to hospital and to minimize fear and frustration in the child.

To attend to the child's needs according to the medical or surgical problem that required his hospitalization.

To plan and provide for the appropriate type of play programme and stimulation for the child.

1   Assess the child's level of development and growth and use information provided by parents.

2   Allow the child as much independence as possible in his care, but provide guidance as necessary — prevent boredom.

3   Encourage the development of the child's abilities.

To meet the emotional needs of the child with impaired hearing for closeness and belonging.

1 Place the child in a room with a friendly, outgoing child.
2 Plan frequent nurse-patient interactions.
   a Gentle touch
   b Games or activities he enjoys
3 Encourage parents, especially mother, to take an active part in his care, thus decreasing fear of desertion. Offer facilities to live in, if she or father is able to do so.
4 Be aware of coping behaviours seen in the child, including visual information gathering, avoidance, and comfort-seeking measures.

To offer continuous parental support.

1 Help parents to think of their child as a child first, then as a child with special needs.
2 Emphasize their importance in the habilitation of their child. Point out the value of the home environment in his development.
   a Talk about the daily routines.
   b Talk about mother's role in stimulating the child's interest in sounds and speech.
   c Encourage the use of hearing aids and the learning programme set up by specialists in hearing problems in children.
   d Residential placement may be considered when local facilities are nonexistent or when the home environment would be detrimental to the child's progress.
3 Encourage parents to talk about their fears, frustrations, and feelings in caring for the child at home.
   Initiate a social worker referral, if a social worker is not already involved from the special training centre.
4 Other members of the family must be considered.
   a This child does need special handling, but he does not need all the attention all the time.
   b Other members of the family should be included in his care, but they also have a life of their own and need as much parental attention as they would receive if this child were not present in the family.
   c Parents need time to themselves. They should be encouraged to go out alone together and to give time to their marriage.
5 Help the parents realize that even though progress of their child is long drawn-out, the child may be able to live a somewhat normal life in the community.
   a Are parents aware of and do they accept the short-term and long-term goals?
   b Is the child receiving special training in a local facility?

Useful Addresses

1 National Deaf Children's Society, 31 Gloucester Place, London W1H 4EA.
2 The Royal National Institute for the Deaf, 105 Gower Street, London WC1.
3 Deaf, Blind and Rubella Children's Society, 164 Cromwell Road, Coventry CB4 8AH.
4 The Royal National Institute for the Blind, 224-228 Great Portland Street, London W1N 6AA.
5 The Partially Sighted Society, Exhall Front School, Wheelright Lane, Coventry CV7 9HP.
6 The National Association for the Education of the Partially Sighted, Joseph Clarke School, Vincent Road, Highams Park, London E4 9PP.

FURTHER READING

Conditions of the Eye

Books
Chapman E K, *Visually Handicapped Children and Young People*, Routledge & Kegan Paul, 1978.
Frailberg S, *Insights from the Blind*, Souvenir Press, 1977.
Smith V Keen J (eds), *Visual Handicap in Children*, Spastics International, 1979.

Articles
Barkes J K, Colour vision and screening in children, *Journal of Maternal Child Health*, July 1979: 261-263.
Blass T *et al.*, Body movement and verbal encoding in the congenitally blind, *Perception and Motor Skills*, August 1974, 39: 279-293.
Mehta V, Growing up blind in a sighted world, *New Society*, 13 January 1983: 47-50
Morin S F Jones R L, Social comparison of abilities in blind children and adolescents, *Journal of Psychology*, July 1974, 84: 237-243.
Neu C, Coping with newly diagnosed blindness, *American Journal of Nursing*, December 1975, 75: 161-163.
Rose M H, Coping behaviour of physically handicapped children, *Nursing Clinics of North America*, June 1975, 10: 329-339.
Sonksen P, Sound and the visually handicapped baby, *Child*, November/December 1979: 413-420.

Conditions of the Ear

Books

Nolan M Tucker I, *The Hearing Impaired Child and the Family Souvenir Press*, 1981.
Bloom F, *101 Questions and Answers about Deaf Children: A Guide for Parents and Professionals*, Clare Books, 1983.

Articles

Bluestone C D Shurin P A, Middle ear disease in children, *Pediatric Clinics of North America*, May 1974, 21: 379-400.
Burton D, Family counselling, *Hearing (RNID)*, May 1980: 40
Hughes L A, *et al.*, Complications of tympanostomy tubes, *Archives of Otolaryngology*, 1974, 100: 151-155.
Kemker, F, Classification of auditory impairment, *Otolaryngology Clinics of North America*, February 1975, 8: 3-17.
Lesser S R Easser B R, Psychiatric management of the deaf child, *Canadian Nurse*, October 1975, 71: 23-25.
Linthicum F H, Evaluation of the child with sensorineural hearing impairment, *Otolaryngology Clinics of North America*, February 1975, 8: 3-17.
Martin V S, What it means to be the parent of a deaf child, *Otolaryngology Clinics of North America*, February 1975, 8: 59-67.

Blind and Deaf Children

Freeman P, *Understanding the Deaf/Blind Child*, Heinemann Medical, 1975.
General Nursing Council, *Aspects of Sick Children's Nursing: a Learning Package*, General Nursing Council, 1982, Units 45 and 46.

Books for Parents

Knowles S E Mogford K, *Hear and Say*, Toy Libraries Association, 1978.

Books for Siblings or for the Handicapped Child

Bloom F, *The Boy Who Couldn't Hear*, Bodley Head, 1977.
Nicholls A, *Sight*, Studio Vista, 1975.
Nicholls A, *Hearing*, Studio Vista, 1975.
Peter D, *Claire and Emma*, Black, 1976.
Peterson P, *Sally Can't See*, Black, 1976.

12

CONNECTIVE TISSUE DISEASE

JUVENILE RHEUMATOID ARTHRITIS

Juvenile rheumatoid arthritis (JRA) is a chronic, generalized, systemic disease that involves a wide spectrum of manifestations, including joint, connective tissue, and visceral lesions throughout the body.

Aetiology
1   The cause of juvenile rheumatoid arthritis is unknown.
    a Infection from an unidentified organism
    b Immune process.

Modes of Onset and Clinical Manifestations

Acute Febrile-Systemic (Still's Disease)
1   Highest incidence of onset is in children under 7 years of age; females are affected more often than males.
2   Initially joint involvement is variable — from no joint pain to generalized florid arthritis.
3   Systemic characteristics:
    a Irritability, anorexia, and malaise
    b Intermittent fever — one or two spikes a day over 38.9°C; occurrence of subnormal temperature between elevations; possible seizures
    c Rash consisting of small, discrete, pink macules with pale centres occurring on trunk and extremities
    d Hepatosplenomegaly
    e Generalized lymphadenopathy

f Anaemia

g Periorbital oedema

h Carditis — tachycardia (disproportionate to fever), tachypnoea, pericarditis, myocarditis

i Pleuritis or pneumonitis independent of carditis.

Polyarticular Onset

1 Highest incidence of onset is in child of 6-12 years; higher incidence in females than males.
2 Characterized by arthritis of more than four joints.
  a Acute onset is manifested by painful swelling of joints.
  b Insidious onset — minimal or no joint pain; however, child may wince on movement or may limp on walking.
  c Large joints most often involved are knees, wrists, ankles, and elbows.
  d Other areas often involved
    (1) Rheumatoid foot — metatarsophalangeal joints swollen and tender; pain in heel
    (2) Cervical spine — tenderness and restricted movement.
3 Systemic manifestation occurs less frequently than in acute febrile onset; may see low-grade fever and general lymphadenopathy.

Oligoarticular Onset

1 Highest incidence of onset is in children 1-6 years of age. Females are affected more often than males.
2 Characterized by arthritis of one, or up to four joints.
  a Child under 5 years may be listless and irritable, have low-grade fever, and fail to grow at normal rate.
  b Older child does not appear ill.
3 Systemic manifestations are few.
  a May see rash, low-grade fever, lymphadenopathy, and splenomegaly.
  b There is increased incidence of iridocyclitis.

Generalized Clinical Manifestations

Joints
(Changes may occur with or without systemic symptoms.)

1 Symptoms may develop gradually with progressive stiffness, swelling, and impaired motion of a joint or joints.
2 Symptoms may develop rapidly with sudden appearance of symptomatic arthritis in one or more joints.
3 Knees, ankles, feet, wrists, or fingers are usually involved initially.
4 Joints are swollen and warm.
5 Pain and stiffness of joint may appear before objective changes develop.

6   Limitation of motion of inflamed joints occurs.
7   Characteristic posture is one of guarding joints from movement; an anxious pained expression (with polyarthritis) is common.
8   Morning stiffness of joints following periods of inactivity occurs.
9   Atrophy and weakness of muscles near the affected joints may develop.
10   Skin over inflamed joints may be pigmented.
11   Chronically affected joints may become dislocated, deformed, or fused.
12   Subcutaneous nodules may appear over pressure points (knees, elbows, etc.).
13   Condition may ultimately affect any joint in the body (knees, ankles, wrists, feet, fingers, toes, shoulders, elbows, neck, jaw, hips, and sacroiliac joints are frequently involved).
14   Small, deformed feet result from foot involvement in early childhood.
15   Micrognathia (unusually small lower jaw), as a result of temporomandibular arthritis, is one hallmark of juvenile rheumatoid arthritis.
16   Spindling or fusiform changes of the fingers may occur.

Inflammation of the Eye (Unilateral or Bilateral)
Child may have no early symptoms. If symptoms occur late, child may develop irreversible eye damage, including scarring and adhesions of the iris and cataracts.
1   Redness
2   Pain
3   Photophobia
4   Decreased visual acuity
5   Nonreactive pupil.

Generalized Growth Retardation
1   During periods of remission, growth spurts may occur.
2   Treatment with long-term steroid therapy as well as the disease process may contribute to growth failure.

Altered Physiology

1   In early stages one or many joints show signs of inflammation.
2   The inflammation is initially localized in a joint capsule, primarily in the synovium. The tissue becomes thickened from congestion and oedema.
3   A characteristic inflammatory response develops in the form of a synovial proliferation which invades the interior of the joint.
4   The inflammatory tissue extends into the interior of the joint along the surface of the articular cartilage to which it may be adherent, so that it deprives the cartilage of nutrition.

5   By starvation and invasion, this inflammatory tissue slowly destroys the articular cartilage.
6   Synovial tissue eventually frees the joint space leading to narrowing, fibrous ankylosis and bony fusion.
7   Growth centres next to inflamed joints may undergo either premature epiphyseal closure or accelerated epiphyseal growth.
8   Tendons and tendon sheaths may develop inflammatory changes similar to the synovial tissues.
9   Inflammation of muscle may occur.
10 Rheumatoid nodules are uncommon in children.

Diagnostic Evaluation

(Of limited value.)

1   Elevated sedimentation rate
2   Leucocytosis
3   High total serum proteins
4   Positive creatine protein
5   High frequency of serum antinuclear antibodies with oligarticular onset
6   Possible alteration in serum proteins (increased alpha and gamma; decreased albumin)
7   Changes in bone, demonstrated by x-rays — initially nonspecific.

Treatment

The objectives of treatment are: to relieve joint inflammation and pain; to maintain and increase joint range of motion, muscle strength, and tone; to preserve total growth and development potential; and to support emotional outlook of patient and his family.

1   Although this is a painful disease of long duration, the outlook for remission is good.
2   There is no specific cure; treatment is supportive:
    a Drug therapy to reduce inflammation
    b Exercise programme to promote joint movement.

Complications

1   Bony deformities — crippling from progressive polyarthritis
2   Psychological and social reactions to this chronic illness
3   Iridocyclitis — leading to cataracts, glaucoma, or blindness
4   Pericarditis.

Nursing Objectives

To offer the patient and his parents realistic encouragement.

1   Although the response to medication is slow, the recovery is slow, and episodes of acute illness recur, the long-term outlook is generally good.
2   The child may be hospitalized during an acute attack and systemic illness.

To discuss with the parents and the child what they know about the disease and what they expect from treatment.

1   Determine what information has been given to them by the paediatrician.
2   The child and his family must understand the disease and treatment. This is a chronic disease and has an unpredictable course; however, compliance with prescribed treatment will minimize crippling from progressive polyarthritis and allow child to grow and develop to his potential.

To be an effective member of the special team caring for this patient and his family.

The team often includes paediatrician, rheumatologist, social worker, physiotherapist, occupational therapist, psychologist/psychiatrist, ophthalmologist, sick children's nurse, health visitor, and teacher.

To assist in the programme of physiotherapy in order to maintain or increase joint range of motion and muscle strength and tone.

1   The parents and child are instructed in the exercises. Encourage development of programme (with parental involvement) while patient remains in the hospital.
2   Night splints for the wrists and knees may be prescribed to do the following:
   a Give rest and relief of pain.
   b Prevent or correct deformity.
   c Maintain damaged joint in functional position.
   d Know proper application of splint and help patient to adjust to it.
3   A hot bath prior to the exercises and following long rest periods may make the exercises less painful.
4   Full range of motion exercises should be performed every day.
5   Orthopaedic surgery may be required to correct some deformities.

To provide the child with the freedom to engage in as much activity as he is able to tolerate.

1   Children will limit their own activity.
2   Those activities that produce overtiring or cause joint pain should be avoided.
3   Diversional activities should encourage movement based upon child tolerance.
4   Encourage the child to be as self-sufficient as possible.
5   Allow the child to make some decisions himself (e.g. when he prefers to do his exercises).
6   Limit the use of wheelchairs. Tricycles and pedal cars provide good modes of mobility and exercise.

To use the principles of proper body mechanics and posture whether the child is at rest or is active.

1 Provide firm mattress to prevent sagging joints.
2 Use thin pillow (not more than 5 cm thick) to prevent dowager hump. Do not place pillows under joints.
3 Child may attempt to protect joints by assuming a position of flexion to ease discomfort.

To administer medications which are utilized to treat juvenile rheumatoid arthritis. Know usage, side effects, and screening tests to be done during therapy.

1 Salicylates
   a Anti-inflammatory, analgesic, antipyretic
   b See 'Salicylates and Steroids,' under Rheumatic Fever, p. 606, for side effects.
2 Systemic steroids
   a Used in addition to salicylates when salicylates alone are not effective. Their use does not prevent complications of severe arthritis or influence ultimate prognosis.
   b See the reference to salicylates and steroids, under Rheumatic Fever.
   c Tuberculin test should be done prior to starting steroid therapy.
   d Monitor for glucosuria.

To educate and motivate parents and child in continuing programme of treatment at home.
Help parents to understand the needs of the child.

1 Extra rest — but not bed rest, which will contribute to contractures and muscle atrophy.
2 Programme of daily exercises — this can be adjusted to fit in with mother's or family's routine.
3 The child should attend school regularly and participate in ordinary school activities.
   a This participation will allow child to obtain social and scholastic achievement.
   b Teachers should be informed of child's condition and needs.
      (1) Child should get out of seat and walk around room every hour.
      (2) Desk and chair should properly fit child, i.e. when child is sitting with his back in the chair, his feet should be on the floor at right angles to legs; the seat should be deep enough to support thighs without pressure on popliteal arteries.
   c Recreation is important — swimming is a beneficial sport activity.
4 Compensate for activities of daily living — help child understand he must do as much for himself as possible.
   Adapt items he uses to make their use easier (e.g. lift toilet seat several centimetres).

5   Provide nutritionally balanced diet to eliminate obesity that puts additional weight on joints.

6   Do not force unnecessary restrictions upon child that can produce acute behavioural upsets and interfere with his social development.

7   This disease affects the whole family. Remind parents to devote time to other members of the family and to their marriage. Various agencies can provide pertinent literature and can direct family to helpful local resources.

8   The child needs continual follow-up after hospitalization. Inform the district nurse prior to discharge.

   a The health visitor/school nurse can assist in home management.

   b Social worker can assist in helping parents work out their emotions and seek financial assistance.

   c Ophthalmologist — must examine patient every 3-6 months for occurrence of iridocyclitis. Encourage parents to report any eye symptoms that the child may develop.

   d The physician must be consulted when any new symptoms occur, in an acute attack, or when progression is apparent, as well as for routine care.

HENOCH-SCHÖNLEIN PURPURA (ANAPHYLACTOID PURPURA)

Henoch-Schönlein purpura is a diffuse vascular disease resulting from inflammatory reaction around capillaries and arterioles involving the skin, intestines, joints, and kidneys.

Incidence and Aetiology

1   Slightly higher incidence in males than in females. Increased incidence of onset is between ages 3 and 7 years.

2   Possible cause is an allergic reaction to a variety of antigenic stimuli such as infection (e.g. by beta-haemolytic streptococci), allergens, insect bites, food, and drugs.

3   Cause is unknown.

4   Disease is usually self-limited.

Clinical Manifestations

1   Rash — sudden onset may precede or follow other manifestations.

   a Typical rash begins with itching, urticarial wheals and then proceeds to maculopapular erythematous lesions.

   b These lesions become less raised and more petechial or purpuric in character and do not fade with pressure.

   c Several stages of the rash may be present at one time.

d Rash appears primarily on buttocks, lower back, extensor aspects of arms and legs, and face.

2 Arthritis of knee and ankle joints develops; the condition is moderately severe, with painful swelling due to periarticular oedema. Movement is limited.

3 Local oedema — especially of scrotum

4 Colicky abdominal pain — from submucosal haemorrhage

5 Nausea and vomiting

6 Proteinuria

7 Microscopic haematuria.

Diagnostic Evaluation

1 Appearance of rash

2 Blood studies
  a Platelet count — normal
  b Erythrocyte sedimentation rate (ESR) — elevated
  c Anaemia possible
  d Azotaemia (with severe kidney involvement)
  e pH and prothromboplastin tests

3 Urine studies
  a Proteinuria
  b Microscopic haematuria
  c Casts

4 Stool — shows occult blood.

Complications

1 Colicky abdominal pain, related to vasculitis and oedema of the bowel: steroids may be used.

2 Intussusception

3 Acute nephritis or nephrotic syndrome.

Treatment

Treatment is primarily symptomatic and supportive

1 Encourage bed rest until child is able to ambulate and can do so without increasing oedema of feet.

2 Remove allergen if it is known.

3 Give possible antibiotic therapy if acute episode was preceded by infection.

4 Manage complicating abdominal or renal involvement:
  a Steroids (prednisone) may relieve abdominal symptoms and prevent intussusception.

b Immunosuppressive therapy (azathioprine or cyclophosphamide) may be given to stabilize persistent renal involvement.

Nursing Objectives

To offer the patient and his parents realistic encouragement.

The long-term outlook is good when renal involvement is minimal.

To assist child in expressing his feelings about illness and hospitalization.

1   Provide the child with an opportunity to openly discuss his feelings about illness and his situation when he is able to verbalize these feelings.
2   Provide child with the opportunity to express his feelings; utilize play as a method.
3   Allow child to make some decisions (appropriate for his age), and to become involved in planning his own care.
4   Consider his age and then allow and encourage parental participation.

To provide physical comfort for the child's painful and swollen joints.

Salicylates are found not to be particularly effective (see Juvenile Rheumatoid Arthritis, p. 594).

To observe for developing signs and symptoms of complications.

1   Renal
    a Record intake and output
    b Record relative density of urine
    c Observe colour and characteristics of urine
    d Observe development of or increase in oedema.
2   Intussusception — sudden onset
    a Paroxysmal abdominal pain
    b Currant jelly-like stools
    c Vomiting
    d Increasing absence of stools
    e Increasing abdominal distension and tenderness.

To observe and record child's general condition and the current status of the rash.

To be aware of the action and side effects of medications used in the treatment of anaphylactoid purpura.

See Juvenile Rheumatoid Arthritis, p. 594.

To encourage parents to return with child for follow-up.

ACUTE RHEUMATIC FEVER

Acute rheumatic fever is a systemic disease characterized by inflammatory lesions of connective tissue and endothelial tissue.

Aetiology

1   The exact pathogenesis is uncertain.
2   The most important factor in the aetiology of rheumatic fever is now accepted to be Group A beta-haemolytic streptococcus.
3   Most first attacks of rheumatic fever are preceded by streptococcal infection at an interval of several days to several weeks.
4   There appears to be an inherited tendency or family predisposition towards rheumatic fever.

Altered Physiology

1   The unique pathological lesion of rheumatic fever is the Aschoff body.
2   The basic changes consist of exudative and proliferative inflammatory reactions in the mesenchymal supporting tissue of the heart, joints, blood vessels, and subcutaneous tissues.
3   The inflammatory process involves all layers of the heart.
4   The inflammation may involve the leaflets and/or chordae tendinae of the heart valves, most frequently the mitral and/or aortic valves.

Clinical Manifestations and Diagnostic Evaluation

No single clinical or laboratory finding is characteristic of rheumatic fever. The diagnosis is based on a combination of manifestations characteristics of this disease and in the absence of other diseases which may mimic it.

1   For this reason, the modified Jones criteria are utilized.
2   The presence of two major criteria, or one major and two minor criteria together with evidence of a recent streptococcal infection indicates a high probability of the presence of rheumatic fever.

Major Manifestations

1   Carditis — manifested by significant murmurs, signs of pericarditis, cardiac enlargement, or congestive heart failure.
2   Polyarthritis — almost always migratory and manifested by swelling, heat, redness, and tenderness, or by pain and limitation of motion or two or more joints.
3   Chorea — purposeless, involuntary, rapid movements often associated with muscle weakness.
4   Erythema margination — an evanescent, pink rash.
    a The erythematous areas have pale centres and round or serpiginous (creeping eruption) margins.
    b They vary greatly in size and occur mainly on the trunk and proximal parts of the extremities, never on the face.
    c The erythema is transient, migrates from place to place, and may be brought out by the application of heat.
5   Subcutaneous nodules — firm, painless nodules seen or felt over the extensor surface of certain joints, particularly elbows, knees, and wrists, in the occipital region, or over the spinous processes of the thoracic and lumbar vertebrae; the skin overlying them moves freely and is not inflamed.

Minor Manifestations

1   *Clinical*
    a History of previous rheumatic fever or evidence of pre-existing rheumatic heart disease
    b Arthralgia — pain in one or more joints without evidence of inflammation, tenderness to touch, or limitation of motion
    c Fever — temperature in excess of 38°C.
2   *Laboratory*
    a Erythrocyte sedimentation rate — elevated
    b C-reactive protein — positive
    c Electrocardiographic changes — mainly P-R interval prolongation
    d Leucocytosis.

Supporting Evidence of Streptococcal Infection

1   Increased titre of streptococcal antibodies (antistreptolysin O, and ASO titre)
2   Positive throat culture for Group A streptococci
3   Recent scarlet fever.

Other Clinical Features

1   Abdominal pain
2   Rapid sleeping pulse (tachycardia out of proportion to fever)
3   Malaise
4   Anaemia

5   Epistaxis
6   Precordial pain.

Nursing Objectives

To become informed as to the child's symptomatology and the medical plan of care.

1   Discuss with the paediatrician his plan for medical treatment.
2   Make a baseline nursing assessment of the child's condition.
   a Determine from the child whether he is experiencing any pain or discomfort (also observe the child's facial expression as he moves since children may deny pain thinking they will be able to go home).
   b Describe the pain as to location, when it occurs, whether there is any heat, swelling, redness, or tenderness.
   c Examine the knees, elbows, wrists, occipital region, and spine for nodules; describe location.
   d Determine whether the child has any muscle weakness or rapid, purposeless movements.
   e Assess the child's emotional status.
   f Report any significant information to the paediatrician.

To initiate specific preventive teaching in order to prevent a recurrence or an additional case of the rheumatic fever within the family.

1   Have all family members screened for *Streptococcus* by referring them for throat cultures.
2   All persons with positive cultures should be treated.
3   Teach the specific symptoms of streptococcal infections.

To treat the precipitating streptococcal infection.

Administer antibiotics as prescribed by the paediatrician (generally intramuscular benzylpenicillin).

Nursing Alert: Before administering penicillin, elicit a history for possible drug allergy.

To evaluate the child for evidence of response to treatment or progression of disease.

1   Observe for the development or disappearance of any major or minor manifestations of the disease.
2   Monitor carditis by careful documentation of the child's pulse, respirations, and blood pressure.
   a The pulse should be counted for one full minute.
   b The sleeping pulse is a good indication of the extent of carditis. It should be obtained without waking the child.

To provide symptomatic management of the child's fever.
1   Refer to section on fever, p. 105.
2   Antipyretic drugs are usually withheld during the diagnostic period.

To suppress the rheumatic inflammatory process by administering appropriate medications.

1   Salicylates (generally prescribed for patients without carditis)
    a Observe for gastrointestinal upsets, ringing in the ears, headaches, bleeding, and disturbances in the mental state.
    b Administer milk or antacids with salicylates.
    c Report side effects promptly.
    d Aspirin therapy should be monitored by salicylate levels.
2   Steroids (generally prescribed for patients with carditis; as steroids are tapered, administration of salicylates is begun)
    a Prepare the child and his family for the expected side effects of steroid therapy:
        (1) Body appearance may change through rounding facial contour
        (2) Localized fat deposits
        (3) Appearance of acne or excessive hair
        (4) Weight gain with linear markings appearing in the stretched skin.
    b Mental and emotional disturbances may necessitate discontinuance of the medication.
    c Hypertension and the tendency to accumulate water and sodium within the tissues may result from steroid therapy.
        (1) Provide a low sodium diet
        (2) Weigh child daily — report sudden weight increases.
    d Steroids diminish the child's resistance to infection and may mask symptoms of infection.

Nursing Alert: Do not place a child with an infectious disease in the room with the child with rheumatic fever.
Restrict visitors and personnel with infectious diseases from contact with the child on steroid therapy.

    e A combination of steroid therapy and stress may lead to the development of gastric ulcers.
3   Administer medications punctually and at regular intervals to achieve constant therapeutic blood levels.
4   Report signs of increased rheumatic activity as salicylates or steroids are being tapered.

To alleviate the child's anxiety about the functioning of his heart, because anxiety utilizes energy and produces fatigue.

1   Give the child information about rheumatic fever in terms that he can understand, e.g. 'Rheumatic fever is a hard thing to understand because you can't see it. When you scratch yourself, you can see the mark, and you can

see the scratch heal. Rheumatic fever is something like that — only you can't see the healing because it happens to the tissue underneath the skin. (And sometimes it happens to the valves in the heart.)'

2   Continually reinforce the teaching and encourage the child to ask questions.
3   Assure the child that we know how to treat rheumatic fever.
4   Communicate information about the child's reactions to all staff members in order to provide consistent information.

To decrease the cardiac workload until the acute inflammatory reaction has subsided.

1   Explain to the child the need for rest (usually prescribed for 4-12 weeks, depending on the severity of the disease and paediatrician's preference).
2   Assure the child that bed rest will be imposed no longer than necessary.
3   Organize nursing care to provide periods of uninterrupted rest.
4   Explain to the child what procedures are going to be performed before they are performed. If possible, give explanations when parents are present. This will help to reassure the child that they know and understand.
5   Assure the child that his needs will be met. Ensure that he knows 'his' nurses.
6   Assist the child to resume activity very gradually once he is asymptomatic at rest and indicators of acute inflammation have become normal.
    a Allow the child to participate in decisions about such matters as timing his periods of activity.
    b Monitor the pulse rate carefully after periods of activity in order to assess the degree of cardiac compensation.

To provide frequent and comfortable changes in position to aid in relaxation and to prevent tissue breakdown.

1   Elevate the back of the bed and support the arms with pillows when child is dyspnoeic.
2   Position the legs in good body alignment — use a footboard.
3   When the joints are painful, move the child gently, supporting the extremity.
4   Provide meticulous skin care.

To provide nursing care for the child with congestive heart failure.

Refer to section on congestive heart failure, p. 390.

To provide safe, supportive care for the child with chorea.

1   Place the child in a bed with padded side rails, especially if uncontrolled body movements are severe.
2   Feed the child slowly and carefully because of uncoordinated movements of the head, mouth, and swallowing muscles. Avoid the use of sharp eating utensils.
3   Provide frequent feedings that are high in energy, protein, vitamins, and iron, because constant movements cause the child to burn energy at a rapid rate.
4   Spend time talking with the child even though his speech may be defective. If severe, utilize other methods of communication.

5   Administer sedation, if ordered.
6   Reassure the child about the cause of his instability, and tell him that his symptoms will subside.
7   Encourage positive parent-child relationships which may have been strained if the onset of symptoms was insidious (lack of concentration at school, mood swings, irritability, etc.).
8   Help the child regain his former skills once symptoms begin to subside.
    a Support the child during periods of ambulation.
    b Provide activities which require the use of large muscles and progress to materials which require fine coordination.

To assist the child to develop a realistic attitude towards his illness and encourage him to discuss his concerns.
1   Help him to realize the restrictions he must face and the fact that progress is slow.
2   Attempt to avoid negative connotations related to activity restriction. Emphasize what the child is allowed to do — that is, say 'You may be up in the chair for 2 hours every day', rather than 'You have to stay in bed all day, except for 2 hours'.
3   Help him cope with his fears that his playmates may ostracize him or pity him.
4   Alleviate his anxieties about keeping up with his class and school activities.
    Introduce the child to the hospital school teacher, so that education can continue according to the child's condition and activity.

To provide for diversional activity that will help the child feel a sense of achievement and satisfaction.
1   Initiate some long-term projects, e.g. growing bulbs or plants for the ward.
2   Refer to section on the hospitalized child, p. 63.

To help the child to maintain contact with his peers during hospitalization.
1   Encourage correspondence.
2   Maintain telephone contact — if possible.
3   Place with children of the same age, sex, and interests and preferably with a child with a long-term illness.

To assist the family to deal with the emotional and financial stresses caused by the illness and hospitalization.
1   Assess family's needs in this area and initiate a referral to a social worker if indicated. Financial help may be available towards fares for long-term visiting.
2   Refer to sections on family stress in paediatric illness (p. 64), and family-centred care (p. 66).

To prevent a recurrent attack of rheumatic fever by reinforcing the need for prophylactic antimicrobial therapy.

1   Penicillin is the drug of choice — either intramuscular benzathine penicillin every 28 days or oral phenoxymethylpenicillin (penicillin V) twice daily.
2   Continuous prophylaxis is recommended throughout the childhood years and well into adult life, often indefinitely.
3   Utilize creativity in recommending methods to remind families about administering medication.
    a The child should be taught to assume responsibility for his own medication at an early age so that it becomes habitual.
    b Some children profit from the use of a calendar or special chart. Others find is useful to associate their medication schedule with other routine tasks, such as brushing their teeth.
4   Be certain that the child receives his prophylactic medication on schedule during his hospitalization and during subsequent hospitalizations (including hospitalization for treatment of other illnesses).
5   When indicated, additional prophylaxis should be utilized for prevention of infective endocarditis.
    Antibiotic cover may be indicated prior to dental care and invasive procedures and treatments.

To begin to prepare for discharge with the parents in time that sufficient adjustments and preparation may be made.

1   The child should have a bed of his own and, preferably, a room of his own.
2   A responsible adult must be in the home to care for him.
3   Specific information as to:
    a Specifically what activity is allowed
    b When to administer medications, correct amounts — caution about specific side effects
    c Where to obtain the medication
    d Specific dietary instruction
    e Specific symptoms to report:
        (1) Pain
        (2) Malaise
        (3) Anorexia
        (4) Tachycardia (teach to take the pulse)
        (5) Tachypnoea
        (6) Weight gain — keep chart
    f Telephone number of paediatrician or hospital clinic
    g When to return to the clinic.
4   Initiate nursing referral to community nursing service — this should be done prior to discharge.

FURTHER READING

Books

Brimblecombe F Barltrop D, *Children in Health and Disease,* Baillière Tindall, 1978.
Hughes J G, *Synopsis of Pediatrics,* Mosby, 1984.
Jolly H, *Diseases of Children,* Blackwell Scientific, 1981.
Pahayi, G S, *Essential Rheumatology for Nurses and Therapists,* Baillière Tindall, 1980.

Articles

Ansell B, The early diagnosis of rheumatic diseases in children, *Practitioner,* January 1978: 42-48.
Calabro J J *et al.,* Juvenile rheumatoid arthritis: a general review and report on 100 patients observed for 15 years, *Seminars in Rheumatoid Arthritis,* February 1976, 5: 257-298.
Grossman B J Mukhopadhyag D, Juvenile rheumatoid arthritis, *Current Problems in Paediatrics,* October 1975, 5:3-65.
Hall M A Ansell B, Investigation and treatment of joint pain in childhood, *Journal of Maternal and Child Health,* April 1978: 114-123.

13

NEUROLOGICAL SYSTEM CONDITIONS

DIAGNOSTIC EVALUATION OF NEUROLOGICAL DISEASE

Radiological Procedures

Skull X-ray

Reveals configuration, density, vascular markings, and intracranial calcification and tumours.

Air Studies

A gaseous replacement of the fluid within the ventricles and subarachnoid systems serves as a contrast medium because air is less dense than fluid to Roentgen rays.

1 *Pneumoencephalogram* — withdrawal of cerebrospinal fluid and injection of air or other gas by means of a lumbar puncture.
   a Demonstrates ventricular system and subarachnoid space overlying the hemispheres and basal cisterns.
   b Useful in diagnosing degenerative cerebral atrophy and in detecting mass lesions at the base of the brain.
2 *Fractional pneumoencephalogram* — withdrawal of small amounts of fluid and injection of small amounts of air to visualize the ventricular system.
3 *Ventriculogram* — withdrawal of cerebrospinal fluid and injection of air or gas directly into the lateral ventricles through openings in the skull.
   a In the older child trephines (burr holes) are made through a scalp incision; ventricles are punctured by a special needle. A brain needle can be inserted into the ventricles of an infant through wide sutures or the fontanelle.
   b The cerebrospinal fluid is replaced with air, the cannulae are withdrawn, and the scalp wounds are closed.
   c If a lesion is present, there is a change in the size, shape, or position of the ventricular, subarachnoid, or cisternal spaces.

4 *Nursing management following pneumoencephalogram or ventriculogram*
  a Watch the patient for increasing intracranial pressure.
    (1) Disturbances of intracranial pressure may cause serious complications.
    (2) Prepare for ventricular tap and prompt decompression.
  b Take vital signs as frequently as clinical condition indicates and until stabilized.
  c Assess for complaints of headache, fever, and for signs of shock.
    (1) Keep child cool and quiet.
    (2) Give analgesics as directed — duration of headache depends on the speed with which the intracranial air is absorbed.
    (3) Nausea and vomiting may follow air studies.
    (4) Parenteral fluids may be necessary for first 24 hours.

Isotope Cisternography

Use of radioactive tracer injected into lumbar subarachnoid space. Useful in studying cerebrospinal fluid circulation, to locate cerebrospinal fluid leak, and to evaluate hydrocephalus, etc.

Cerebral Angiography

The x-ray study of the vascular system of the brain (cerebral circulation) by the injection of contrast material into a selected artery.

1 Contrast material may be injected into common carotid, vertebral, or subclavian artery, or arch of the aorta. Selective catheterization may be done via a femoral or brachial artery.
2 After injection of selected artery, x-rays are made of arterial and venous phases of circulation through brain and head.
3 Useful in demonstrating position of arteries, intracranial aneurysms, presence or absence of abnormal vasculature, haematomas, tumours.
4 Nursing support
  a *Before angiogram*
    (1) Withhold meal preceding test.
    (2) Patient may be given sedative before going to x-ray department — may help minimize intensity of burning sensation felt along course of injected vessel. A burning sensation, lasting for a few seconds, may possibly be felt behind the eyes, or in jaw, teeth, tongue, and lips.
    (3) Further sedation will be prescribed or anaesthesia given.
  b *Following angiogram*
    (1) Make repeated observations for neurological sequelae — motor or sensory deterioration, alterations in level of responsiveness, weakness on one side, speech disturbances, arrhythmias, blood pressure fluctuation.
    (2) Observe injection site for haematoma formation; apply an ice cap intermittently — to relieve swelling and discomfort.

(3) Evaluate peripheral pulses — changes may develop if there is haematoma formation at puncture site or embolization to a distant artery.

(4) Note colour and temperature of involved extremity.

Brain Scan

Following intake (oral or intravenous) of radiopharmaceutical, the radioactivity subsequently transmitted through the skull is scanned by a rectilinear scanner which prints out a picture based on the number of counts received from the brain as it scans (or a gamma camera, which prints out image without actually scanning, may be used; this is a more recent imaging device).

1   The child may be pretreated with Lugol's solution or potassium perchlorate to block the radiopharmaceutical uptake in the thyroid, salivary glands, choroid plexus, and gastrointestinal mucosa.

2   Brain scanning is useful in early detection and evaluation of intracranial neoplasms, stroke, abscess, follow-up of surgical or radiation therapy of brain.

3   This test is based on the principle that a radiopharmaceutical may diffuse through a disrupted blood-brain barrier into the abnormal cerebral tissue. (Normal brain tissue is relatively impermeable.) There is an increased uptake of radioactive material at the site of pathology.

4   *Nursing responsibility*
    a Explain to patient that he will be expected to lie quietly during the procedure.
    b This is a noninvasive procedure.

Computed Tomography

Computerized axial tomography (CAT) is an imaging method in which the head is scanned in successive layers by a narrow beam of x-rays. It provides a cross-sectional view of the brain and distinguishes differences in the densities of various brain tissues. A computer printout is obtained of the absorption values of the tissues in the plane that is being scanned. This same information is also shown on a cathode ray tube for additional radiological evaluation.

1   Lesions are seen as variations in tissue density differing from the surrounding normal brain tissue.

2   Abnormalities of tissue density indicate possible tumour masses, brain infarction, ventricular displacement; useful in patients with head trauma, suspected brain tumour, hydrocephalus.

3   May be done with intravenous contrast medium enhancement to more accurately define boundaries of certain lesions and indicate presence of otherwise undetectable lesions.

4   *Patient preparation*
   a Inquire about allergies and any previous adverse reaction to contrast agent.
   b See that a consent form has been signed.
   c No special preparation is required; this is a noninvasive technique that can be done on an outpatient basis.
   d Instruct the patient that he must lie perfectly still while the test is being carried out; he cannot talk or move his face as this distorts the picture.

Echoencephalography

The recording of echoes from the deep structures within the skull (generated by the transmission of ultrasound [high frequency] waves) to determine the position of midline structures of the brain and the distance from the midline to the lateral ventricular wall or the third ventricular wall.

1   Useful for detecting a shift of the cerebral midline structures caused by subdural haematoma, intracerebral haemorrhage, massive cerebral infarction, and neoplasms; can display dilation of ventricles; useful in evaluation of hydrocephalus.
2   Ultrasonic transducers are positioned over specified areas of the head; the echoes are imaged and stored on the oscilloscope.
3   *Nursing responsibilities*
   a There is no special patient preparation.
   b Explain that this is a noninvasive test and that some type of liquid (mineral oil) may be used to eliminate the air gap between the transducer and the head.

Myelography

The injection of contrast medium (gas or an opaque medium) into the spinal subarachnoid space by spinal puncture for radiological examination; outlines the spinal subarachnoid space and shows distortion of the spinal cord or dural sac by tumours, cysts, herniated intervertebral discs, or other lesions.

1   After injection of the contrast medium, the head of the table is tilted down and the course of the contrast medium is observed radioscopically.
2   Contrast material may be removed after test completion by syringe and needle aspiration; patient may complain of sharp pain down leg during aspiration if a nerve root has been aspirated against a needle point — needle point is rotated or an adjustment in needle depth is made.
   With newer water-soluble contrast agents a smaller needle can be used (less likely to produce headache).
3   *Nursing responsibilities*
   a *Before test*
      (1) Reinforce paediatrician's explanation of procedure; explain that it is usually not painful and that the x-ray table will be tilted in varying positions during the study.

(2) Omit the meal preceding myelography.

(3) Patient's legs may be wrapped with elastic compression bandages to eliminate hypotension during procedure.

(4) Patient may be given sedative prior to test to help him cope with a rather lengthy (2 hour) procedure.

b *Post-test*

(1) Instruct the patient to lie in prone position for several hours; he may be kept in bed in supine position (turning from side to side) for 12-24 hours.

(2) Encourage child to drink liberal quantities of fluid — for rehydration and replacement of cerebrospinal fluid and to decrease incidence of postlumbar puncture headache (thought to be due to escape of spinal fluid).

(3) Assess neurological and vital signs; note motor and sensory deviations from normal.

(4) Check child's ability to micturate.

(5) Watch for fever, stiff neck, photophobia, or other signs of chemical or bacterial meningitis.

(6) Head of bed may be elevated following procedure if all of the dye was not retrieved.

Lumber Epidural Venography

Percutaneous insertion of a catheter into the femoral vein; catheter is guided into ascending lumbar vein and/or internal iliac veins. Contrast medium is injected to opacify epidural venous plexus (fills epidural veins overlying disc spaces).

1 May reveal deviation or compression of the epidural veins due to herniated disc or tumour.

2 Useful in diagnosis of herniated lumbar discs not demonstrated by myelography.

3 *Nursing responsibilities*

   a *Before test*

     (1) Determine if patient has had any allergies to contrast material.

     (2) Check to see if consent form has been signed.

   b *After test*

   Observe site for haematoma formation.

Electroencephalography (EEG)

Records, by means of electrodes applied on the scalp surface (or by microelectrodes placed within brain tissue), the electrical activity which is generated in the brain.

1 Provides physiological assessment of cerebral activity; useful in diagnosis of the epilepsies and as a screening procedure for coma and organic brain syndrome; also used as an indicator of brain death.

2   Electrodes are arranged on the scalp to permit the recording of activity in various head regions; the amplified activity of the neurons is recorded on a continuously moving paper sheet.
  a For baseline recording the patient lies quietly with his eyes closed.
  b For activation procedures (done to elicit abnormal electrical activities) patient may be asked to hyperventilate for 3-4 minutes, look at a bright flashing light, or receive an injection of medication.
  c EEG may also be made during sleep and upon awakening.
3   Pharyngeal (electrode inserted through nose; rests on mucosa of pharyngeal roof) and sphenoidal (inserted transcutaneously with tips resting on sphenoid bone near foramen ovale) electrodes are used when epileptogenic area is inaccessible to conventional scalp preparation.
4   Patient preparation for routine recording.
  a Antiepileptic medication and tranquillizers may be withheld 24 hours before EEG — may alter EEG wave patterns.
  b Omit coffee, tea, or cola drinks in meal before test; do not omit meal.
  c Shampoo hair night before tests; omit hair sprays and hair dressings.
  d Reassure patient and parents that he will not receive an electrical shock, that the EEG takes approximately 45-60 minutes (more for a sleep EEG), and that the EEG is *not* a form of treatment or a test of intelligence or insanity.

Electromyography (EMG)

The introduction of needle electrodes into the skeletal muscles to study changes in electric potential of muscles and nerves leading to them. These are shown on an oscilloscope and amplified by a loudspeaker for simultaneous visual and auditory analysis and comparison.

1   Useful in determining the presence of a neuromuscular disorder; helps distinguish weakness due to neuropathy from that due to other causes.
2   *Nursing responsibilities*
  a No special patient preparation is required.
  b Explain to the patient that he will experience a sensation similar to that of an intramuscular injection as the needle is inserted into the muscle.

CEREBRAL PALSY

Cerebral palsy is a comprehensive diagnostic term used to designate a group of nonprogressive disorders resulting from malfunction of the motor centres and pathways, of the brain. Although there are varying degrees and clinical manifestations of cerebral palsy, it is generally characterized by paralysis, weakness, incoordination and/or ataxia. Cerebral palsy is a major cause of disability among children in the UK.

Aetiology

Antenatal Factors

1   Infection: rubella, toxoplasmosis, herpes simplex, cytomegalic inclusions and other viral or infectious agents
2   Maternal anoxia, anaemia, placental infarcts, abruptio placentae
3   Antenatal cerebral haemorrhage, maternal bleeding, maternal toxaemia, Rh or ABO incompatibility
4   Antenatal anoxia, twisting or kinking of the cord
5   Miscellaneous — toxins, drugs.

Perinatal Factors

1   Anoxia from any cause
    a Anaesthetic and analgesic drugs administered to the mother may cause anoxia in the infant's brain
    b Prolonged labour
    c Placenta previa or abruptio
    d Respiratory obstruction
2   Cerebral trauma during delivery
3   Complications of birth
    a 'Light for dates' babies, preterm and postmature infants
    b Hyperbilirubinaemia
    c Haemolytic disorders
    d Respiratory distress
    e Infections
    f Hypoglycaemia
    g Hypocalcaemia.

Postnatal Factors

1   Head trauma
2   Infections
    a Meningitis
    b Encephalitis
    c Brain abscess
3   Vascular accidents
4   Lead poisoning
5   Anoxia
6   Neoplastic and late neurodevelopmental defects.

Clinical Manifestations

Early Signs

May include one or more of the following:

1   Asymmetry in motion or contour
2   Listlessness or irritability
3   Difficulty in feeding, sucking, or swallowing
4   Excessive or feeble cry
5   Long, thin infants who are slow to gain weight.

Later Signs

May include one or more of the following:

1   Failure to follow normal pattern of motor development
2   Persistence of infantile reflexes
3   Weakness
4   Apparent preference for one hand before 12-15 months
5   Abnormal postures
6   Delayed or defective speech
7   Evidence of mental retardation.

Factors Influencing Symptoms and Degree of Involvement

(Range - from very mild to severe.)

1   Extent and location of cerebral lesion
2   Age at which interruption of brain development occurred
     Intellectual, language, and social skills which were acquired before damage can usually be retained
3   Status of reflex patterns.

Common Associated Findings

1   Seizures
2   Hearing deficiency
3   Visual defect
4   Perceptual disorders
5   Mental handicap
6   Language disorders.

Classification of Cerebral Palsy

Clinical Type

1   Spasticity — in 50-60% of patients
    a Generally appears before 6 months of age.

b Motor activity is impaired because of disharmony of muscle movements.

(1) Arms

(a) Child often holds his arm pressed against his body with the forearm bent at right angles to the upper arm and the hand bent against the forearm. The fist may be clenched tightly.

(b) Child with mild involvement may demonstrate an overextended appearance of the fingers and rotation of the wrists when he reaches for things.

(2) Legs — may be more (usually) or less involved than arms.

(a) Mild case may only be evident when the child walks, demonstrating wide-based gait (with arms outstretched.) The fingers may be alternately clenched and extended.

(b) Child with moderate involvement may demonstrate slow and laboured movements. Walking is jerky and unrhythmic. Balance is poor.

(c) Child with severe involvement may be unable to sit or walk unsupported.

(d) When both legs are involved, bilateral contractures may cause 'scissoring'. Child crosses his legs and points his toes.)

2   Dyskinesia — in 20-25% of patients

a Characterized by involuntary, extraneous motor activity; accentuated by emotional stress.

b Athetosis is the most common manifestation of this group.

(1) Any or all limbs may be involved.

(2) Characterized by uncontrollable, jerky, irregular, twisting movements of the extremities, especially the fingers and wrists, except when at rest or asleep.

(3) If legs are involved, child may walk in a writhing, lurching, stumbling manner with noticeable incoordination of the arms. When calm and well rested he may walk well.

3   Ataxia — in 1-10% of patients

a Characterized by inability to achieve balance or awkwardness in maintaining it, with associated gross and/or fine motor incoordination.

b Gait is often high-stepping, stumbling, or lurching.

c Nystagmus is common.

d Manifested in varying degrees depending on the pathology.

4   Mixed types — in 15-40% of patients

a Consists of various combinations of the above types.

b Athetosis combined with spasticity or rigidity and ataxia occur frequently.

Topographical Classification

1   Hemiplegia — findings are limited to one side of the body (35-40% of patients)

2   Diplegia — the legs are involved more than the arms (10-20%)
3   Paraplegia — the legs only are involved (10-20%)
4   Quadriplegia — all four extremities are involved (15-20%)
5   Monoplegia — only one limb is involved (rare)
6   Triplegia — three limbs are involved (rare).

Degree of Severity

1   Mild — impairment only of fine precision movement.
2   Moderate — gross and fine movements and speech are impaired, but child is able to perform usual activities of living.
3   Severe — inability to perform adequately the usual activities of daily living, i.e. walking, using hands, communicating verbally.

Diagnostic Evaluation

1   History, including antenatal and perinatal factors
2   Neurological examination
3   Laboratory data — pneumoencephalogram is helpful in some instances
4   Psychological testing to determine cognitive functioning
5   Psychosocial assessment, including family adaptation.

Prognosis

Factors influencing the prognosis include

1   Extent of the manifestations
2   Existence of associated defects, especially mental handicap
3   Ability of the family to cope and to see what is right and normal about their child
4   Type and availability of community resources.

Altered Physiology

Spastic Type

1   Defect in the cortical motor area or pyramidal tract causes abnormally strong tonus of certain muscle groups.
2   Attempt to move a joint causes muscles to contract and block the motion. Permanent contractures develop without muscle training.

Athetotic Type

Lesions of the extrapyramidal tract and basal ganglia cause involuntary, uncoordinated, uncontrollable movements of muscle groups.

Ataxia

Disturbances of balance result from cerebellar involvement.

Goal and Management

Goal

The goal is normality. The aim is to help each child reach optimal functional ability in adulthood. Broad aims of therapy include:

1 To gain optimal appearance and integration of motor function
2 To establish locomotion, communication, and self-help skills
3 To correct associated defects
4 To provide opportunities for education appropriate for the individual child's needs and capabilities.

Management

1 Requires comprehensive evaluation and intervention, including:
  a General health care
  b Correction or alleviation of specific neuromotor deficits and/or associated disabilities
  c Developmental enrichment experiences
  d Development of prevocational, vocational, and socialization skills
  e Emotional, behavioural, and social adjustments.
2 Requires coordination and integration of the contributions of numerous health care professionals.
3 The ability of the family to carry out both supportive and participant roles in rehabilitation is a key determinant of the success of any comprehensive management programme.

Nursing Management

Like other children, the child with cerebral palsy receives the bulk of his care at home and within his community. The nursing role is no longer confined to care within the hospital setting. Within the expanded role, nurses are involved in working with the family on household routine, integrating the child into the family unit, and helping to 'mainstream' the child into ordinary schools, recreational activities, social situations with the opposite sex, etc.

However, the child with cerebral palsy may experience several hospitalizations for diagnostic evaluation, orthopaedic management, and/or medical care. The nurse should consider the following guidelines when caring for the hospitalized child with cerebral palsy.

Nursing Objectives

To assist parents with initial coping and with long-range adaptation to the child's disability.

1   Encourage the parents to express their feelings about the child and his diagnosis and help them to deal with these feelings.
2   Introduce the concept that the child's potential in large part reflects the quality of parental adaptation.
3   Assist parents to appraise the child's assets so that they may capitalize on these positive features.
    a Early recognition of the extent of the child's handicap and realistic direction for obtainable goals are essential.
    b Help parents to recognize immediate needs and identify short-term goals which can be integrated into the long-range plan.
4   Encourage the parents to care for the child during his hospitalization so that they will feel secure about meeting his daily physical needs (feeding, exercise, braces, etc.).
    Refer to section on Family Centred Care, p. 66.
5   Introduce parents to members of the health team who will be involved with the child's care and management.
6   Begin parental teaching about the disability.
    a Provide parents with appropriate reading material. Encourage their questions and provide them with the information they need.
    b Refer to Parental Teaching, which follows this section on nursing objectives.
7   Assist parents in interpreting the child's diagnosis and needs to other family members, teachers, and friends.
8   Initiate appropriate referrals:
    a Health visitor
    b School nurse
    c Education authorities
    d Local branch of the Spastics Society
    e Parent groups.

To promote the attainment of developmental milestones as much as possible.

1   Evaluate the child's developmental level and then assist him to build one skill upon another. (Refer to sections on Growth and Development, p. 7, and the Hospitalized Child, p. 56.)
2   Provide for continuity of care from home to hospital.
    a Obtain a thorough history from the mother regarding the child's usual home routines, and use this in planning the child's care during hospitalization.
       (1) Feeding
       (2) Sleeping
       (3) Physiotherapy
       (4) Stage of growth and development

(5) Play

(6) Special interests, security objects, etc.

b Ask the parents to bring to the hospital any special devices or equipment which the child uses in his daily activities.

c Encourage the child's parents to participate in the child's care. (Refer to section on Family Centred Care, p. 66.)

3   Be alert for associated defects which could be corrected:

a Hearing

b Speech

c Vision

(1) Squinting

(2) Failure to follow objects

(3) Bringing objects very close to the face.

To provide emotional support to parents.

1   Acknowledge the numerous challenges of daily management and the changes in family life associated with caring for a child with cerebral palsy.

2   Allow the parent(s) to express frustrations they may feel because of the many demands placed on them, with few rewards.

3   Acknowledge parents' feelings of frustration and anger as legitimate and understandable.

4   Provide positive feedback for effective parenting skills and positive approaches to caring for the child.

5   Assist parents to deal with siblings' responses to the disabled child.

6   Assist parents to secure respite from the day-to-day care of the child, as appropriate.

To provide for the child's physical care needs.

1   Safety

a Evaluate the child's need for specific safety measures (suction machine, helmet, seizure precautions, etc.), and modify the environment as appropriate to ensure the child's safety.

b Select toys that are safe.

2   Nutrition

a Maintain a pleasant environment, free from distractions.

(1) Provide a comfortable chair.

(2) Serve the child alone, initially. After he begins to master the task of eating, he may enjoy eating with other children.

(3) Do not attempt feedings if the child is very fatigued.

b Encourage independence, but do not force the child.

(1) Find the eating position in which the child can do the most for himself.

(2) Allow the child to hold the spoon even if he has to be fed with another one.

(3) Stand behind the child and reach over his shoulder to guide the spoon from the plate to his mouth.

(4) Serve foods that stick to the spoon, like thick apple sauce, mashed potato, etc.

(5) Encourage finger foods that the child can handle alone.

(6) Provide appropriate special equipment for the child to use in feeding himself:

  (a) Spoon and fork with special handles
  (b) Plate and glass holders, etc.
  (c) Feeding chair.

(7) Disregard 'messy' eating.

  (a) Place newspapers around the feeding chair.
  (b) Use a large plastic 'pelican' bib or towel to protect the child's clothes.

c If the child must be fed, do so slowly and carefully. The child may have difficulty sucking and swallowing because he cannot control the muscles of his throat.

(1) Offer foods which the child likes.

(2) Cut solid foods into small pieces.

(3) Place the food on the back of the tongue for ease in swallowing.

3   Exercise

a Carry out appropriate exercises under the direction of the physiotherapist.

b Use appropriate appliances to facilitate muscle control and improve body functioning:

(1) Splints
(2) Casts
(3) Braces.

c Encourage active motions that are functionally useful.

d Use play (games, peg boards, puzzles, etc.) as techniques to improve coordination.

e Maintain good body alignment to prevent contractures.

4   Rest

a Avoid exciting events before rest or bedtime.

b Administer tranquillizing agents or anticonvulsants, etc., as prescribed by the paediatrician.

c Avoid stress and frustration during the child's programme of physiotherapy.

To ensure continuity of care.

1   Communicate with representatives of all of the disciplines involved with the child's management.

2   Communicate with community services already involved with the child and his family.

3 Formulate a consistent nursing care plan which is well coordinated with the plans and goals of related disciplines and meets the needs of the *entire* child and his family.
4 On discharge, send a report of the child's hospitalization, including a summary of nursing problems, to the health visitor/district nurse.

Parental Teaching

1 Instruct parent in all areas of the child's physical care.
2 Reinforce teaching done by physiotherapists. Assist parents to integrate therapy into play activities.
3 Assist parents to modify equipment and activities to facilitate home care.
4 Provide practical suggestions for feeding, holding, bathing, infant stimulation, etc.
5 The child needs regular medical and dental evaluations.
  a It is important for the child to receive his childhood immunizations.
  b He should be taken to the dentist every 6 months starting at the age of 2 years.
  c He may require some adaptations of his toothbrush in order to use it effectively.
    (1) The handle can be built up with sponge or a more sophisticated enlarging device.
    (2) Brushes with specially bent handles are available.
6 The child needs discipline in order to feel secure and relaxed.
    He should have realistic limits set, within which he can function successfully.

Agencies

1 The Spastics Society, 12 Park Crescent, London W1.
2 Friends of the Cheyne Centre for Spastic Children, 63 Cheyne Walk, London SW3.

HYDROCEPHALUS

Hydrocephalus is a condition of imbalance between the production of cerebrospinal fluid and its absorption over the surface of the brain into the circulatory system. It is characterized by an abnormal increase in cerebrospinal fluid volume within the intracranial cavity and by enlargement of the child's head.

Aetiology

1   Obstruction in the system between the source of cerebrospinal fluid production and the area of reabsorption (the obstruction may be partial, intermittent or complete)
    a The majority of cases are of this type.
    b Causes:
       (1) Congenital — aetiology largely unknown
       (2) Acquired
          (a) Meningitis
          (b) Trauma
          (c) Spontaneous intracranial bleeding
          (d) Neoplasms
2   Failure in the absorption system — cause unknown
3   Excessive production of cerebrospinal fluid — cause unknown (rare).

Types of Hydrocephalus

1   Noncommunicating hydrocephalus
       An obstruction is located within or at the outlets of the ventricular system, preventing any or all of the cerebrospinal fluid from leaving the ventricles and entering the subarachnoid space.
2   Communicating hydrocephalus
    a There is free communication between the ventricles and the subarachnoid space.
    b Abnormal reabsorption of the cerebrospinal fluid in the subarachnoid space occurs.
    c This is the most common form of hydrocephalus.

Altered Physiology

1   The ventricular system is greatly distended
2   The increased ventricular pressure results in thinning of the cerebral cortex and cranial bones, especially in the frontal, parietal, and temporal areas.
3   The floor of the third ventricle commonly bulges downwards, compresses the optic nerves, dilates the sella turcica, and often compresses the hypophysis cerebri.
4   The basal ganglia, brain stem, and cerebellum remain relatively normal but compressed.
5   The choroid plexus is usually atrophied to some degree.

Clinical Manifestations

1 May be rapid, or slow and steadily advancing, or remittent.
2 Clinical signs depend on the age of the child, whether or not the anterior fontanelle has closed, and whether the cranial sutures have fused.
   a Infants
      (1) Excessive head growth (may be seen up to 3 years of age)
      (2) Delayed closure of the anterior fontanelle
      Fontanelle may become tense and elevated above the surface of the skull.
      (3) Signs of increased intracranial pressure include:
         (a) Vomiting
         (b) Restlessness and irritability
         (c) High-pitched, shrill cry
         (d) Alteration in vital signs:
            Increased systolic blood pressure
            Decreased pulse
            Decreased and irregular respirations
         (e) Pupillary changes
         (f) Seizures (possible)
         (g) Lethargy
         (h) Stupor
         (i) Coma
      (4) Alteration of muscle tone of the extremities
      (5) Later physical signs
         (a) Forehead becomes prominent
         (b) Scalp appears shiny with prominent scalp veins
         (c) Eyebrows and eyelids may be drawn upwards, exposing the sclera above the iris
         (d) Infant cannot gaze upwards, causing 'sunset eyes'
         (e) Strabismus, nystagmus, and optic atrophy may occur
         (f) Infant has difficulty in holding head up
         (g) Child may experience physical and/or mental developmental lag.
   b Older children who have closed sutures
      (1) Signs of increased intracranial pressure include:
         (a) Headache
         (b) Vomiting
         (c) Lethargy, fatigue, apathy
         (d) Personality changes
         (e) Separation of cranial sutures (may be seen in children up to 10 years of age)
         (f) Double vision, constricted peripheral vision, sudden appearance of internal strabismus, pupillary changes
         (g) Alteration in vital signs similar to those seen in infants
         (h) Difficulty with gait

(i) Stupor
(j) Coma.

Diagnostic Evaluation

1 Radiological findings show the following:
   a Widening of the fontanelle and sutures
   b Erosion of intracranial bone.
2 Transillumination of the infant's head allows visualization of significant fluid collection.
3 Percussion of the infant's skull may produce a typical 'cracked pot' sound (MacEwen's sign).
4 Pneumoencephalography (introduction of air into the lumbar subarachnoid space) may show the following:
   a Dilated ventricles
   b Extent of the brain damage and the location of the obstruction.
5 Ventriculography (introduction of air into the lateral ventricles):
   Abnormalities are visualized in the ventricular system or the subarachnoid space.
6 Ophthalmoscopy may reveal papilloedema.
7 Isotopic encephalography (cisternography) may demonstrate abnormal absorption of cerebrospinal fluid.
8 CAT scan (computerized axial tomography) provides a noninvasive means of diagnosing some types of hydrocephalus by computer analysis of x-ray transmission data.

Prognosis

1 Prognosis is dependent on early diagnosis and prompt therapy.
2 The outcome of treatment depends on the time it is begun, the success of the surgical procedure, good follow-up care, and the child's innate motor and intellectual capabilities.
   a With improved diagnostic and management techniques, the prognosis is becoming considerably better. Many children experience normal motor and intellectual development.
   b The severity of neurological deficits is directly proportional to the interval between onset and the time of diagnosis.
3 Spontaneous arrest sometimes occurs as a result of natural compensatory mechanisms or rupture of the ventricle into the subarachnoid space.
4 A child with postmeningitic hydrocephalus might also undergo spontaneous remission following gradual disappearance of adhesions.
5 Approximately two-thirds of patients will die at an early age if they are not given surgical treatment.

Surgical Treatment

General Procedure

A tube with a one-way valve is inserted surgically to lead cerebrospinal fluid from the brain directly into the bloodstream or into some other body cavity. The valve most commonly used is the Spitz-Holter valve; Pudenz and Hakin valves can also be inserted.

Purpose

Procedure reduces the volume and thus the pressure of the cerebrospinal fluid within the ventricles.

Specific Surgical Procedures

1 Ventriculoperitoneal shunt
   a Diverts cerebrospinal fluid from a lateral ventricle or the spinal subarachnoid space to the peritoneal cavity.
   b A tube is passed from the lateral ventricle through an occipital burr hole subcutaneously through the posterior aspect of neck and paraspinal region to the peritoneal cavity through a small incision in the right lower quadrant.
2 Ventriculoatrial shunt
   a A tube is passed from the dilated lateral ventricle through a burr hole in the parietal region of the skull.
   b It is then passed under the skin behind the ear and into a vein down to a point where it discharges into the right atrium or superior vena cava.
   c The tube passes at one point through a one-way pressure sensitive system.
   d The valve or valves close to prevent reflux of blood into the ventricle and open as ventricular pressure rises, allowing fluid to pass from the ventricle into the bloodstream.

Complications

1 Need for shunt revision frequently occurs because of occlusion, infection, or malfunction.
2 Shunt revision may be necessary because of growth of the child. Newer models, which are not yet widely available, include coiled tubing to allow the shunt to grow with the child.
3 Shunt dependence frequently occurs. The child rapidly manifests symptoms of increased intracranial pressure if the shunt does not function properly.
4 Children with ventriculoatrial shunts may experience multiple pulmonary thromboses, with pulmonary hypertension and congestive heart failure occurring in later years.

Preoperative Nursing Objectives

To observe for and record disease progress.

1   Measure and record the head circumference daily.
    a Record the greatest circumference each time.
    b Measure the head at approximately the same time each day.
    c Use a centimetre measure for greatest accuracy.
2   Observe for evidence of increased intracranial pressure. Note especially:
    a Vomiting
    b Changes in vital signs
        (1) Increased systolic blood pressure
        (2) Decreased pulse
        (3) Decreased or irregular respirations
    c Pupillary changes
    d Change in level of consciousness.
3   Note especially these changes in appearance:
    a Increased head size, prominent forehead (noticeable over days or weeks)
    b 'Sunset' eyes
    c Opisthotonic positioning — occurs with brain stem herniation.

To provide adequate nutrition.

1   Feeding is often a problem, because the child may be listless, anorectous, and prone to vomiting.
2   Complete nursing care and treatments before feeding so that the child will not be disturbed after feeding.
3   Hold the infant in a semisitting position with head well supported during feeding. Allow ample time for burping.
4   Offer small frequent feedings.
5   Place the child on his side with his head elevated after feeding to prevent aspiration.

To assist with diagnostic procedures.

1   Be familiar with the procedure which is being performed. (See diagnostic tests.)
2   Explain the procedure to the child and his parents at their levels of comprehension.
    a Make certain that they understand what will happen before and after as well as during the procedure.
    b Play is frequently helpful for explaining the procedure to a young child.
3   Administer prescribed sedatives.
    a Give the sedative exactly at the prescribed time to ensure its effectiveness.
    b Organize activities so that the child is permitted to rest after administration of the medications.

Nursing Alert: Sedatives are contraindicated in many cases because of increased intracranial pressure. If administered, the child should be observed very closely for evidence of respiratory depression.

4   Apply protective measures to limit motion as necessary. (See section on paediatric procedures: restraints, p. 115, and positioning for a lumbar puncture, p. 148.)

5   Observe the child closely following the procedure :

    a Leaking of cerebrospinal fluid from the sites of subdural or ventricular taps.

    These tap holes should be covered with a small piece of gauze or cotton saturated with collodion.

    b Reactions to the sedative, especially respiratory depression

    c Changes in vital signs indicative of shock

    d Signs of increased intracranial pressure which may occur if air has been injected into the ventricles.

To provide supportive nursing care as indicated by the child's condition.

(Without treatment, the child becomes more helpless as head size increases.)

1   Prevent pressure sores and the development of contractures.

    a Place the child on a sponge rubber or sheepskin pad or an alternating pressure mattress to keep his weight evenly distributed.

    b Keep the scalp clean and dry.

    c Turn the child's head frequently; change his position every 2 hours.

    (1) When turning the child, rotate his head and body together to prevent strain on the neck.

    (2) A firm pillow may be placed under the head and shoulders for further support when lifting the child.

    d Provide meticulous skin care to all parts of the body.

    (1) Observe the skin for evidence of pressure sores.

    (2) Pressure sores on the head are a frequent problem.

    e Give passive range of motion exercises to the extremities, especially the legs.

2   Keep the eyes moistened if the child is unable to close his eyelids normally. This prevents corneal ulcerations and infections.

3   Provide for the child's emotional needs of love and affection.

    a Hold and cuddle the infant as much as possible.

    b Play with the child according to his mental development.

To provide emotional support to the parents.

1   Encourage parents to visit and to participate in the child's care as much as possible. Provide facilities for parents to be resident, if they are able to do so.

2   Encourage the parents to talk about the child's problem and how they feel about it.

3   Provide parents with appropriate information concerning the defect. Answer their questions directly and honestly. Correct any misconceptions that they may have such as fear that the child's head may burst.

Postoperative Nursing Objectives

To provide immediate, supportive nursing care.

1   Monitor the child's temperature, pulse, respiration, blood pressure, and pupillary size and reaction every 15 minutes until fully reactive; then monitor every 1-2 hours.
2   Avoid hypothermia or hyperthermia.
    a Provide appropriate blankets or covers as indicated by body temperature.
    b An incubator may be used for an infant.
    c An older child may profit from use of the hypothermia blanket.
3   Aspirate mucus from the nose and throat as necessary to prevent respiratory difficulty.
4   Turn the child every 2 hours.
5   Use a nasogastric tube on free drainage if necessary for abdominal distension.
    a This is most frequently used when a ventriculoperitoneal shunt has been performed.
    b Measure the drainage and record the amount and colour.
6   Give frequent mouth care to prevent dryness of the mucous membranes.
7   Observe for pallor or mottled condition of the skin, coldness, or clamminess of the body and decreased level of consciousness.
8   Administer prescribed prophylactic antibiotics.

To allow for optimal draining of cerebrospinal fluid through the shunt.

1   Pump the shunt and position the child as directed by the surgeon.
    a If pumping is prescribed, carefully compress the valve the specified number of times at regularly scheduled intervals.
    b Report any difficulties in pumping the shunt to the surgeon.

To prevent the development of pressure sores on the skin overlying the valve in patients with ventriculovenous shunt.

1   Place cotton behind and over the ears under the head dressing.
2   Avoid positioning the child on the area of the valve or the incision until the wound is well healed.

To maintain fluid and electrolyte balance.

1   Accurately measure and record total fluid intake and output.
    An external collecting device rather than an indwelling catheter should be used to measure urine output whenever possible, as this reduces the danger

of an infection ascending from the bladder to the spinal canal. (See procedure for urine collection, p. 141.)

Elevate the head of the bed slightly, if the infant's condition permits, to prevent backflow of urine.

2 Administer intravenous fluids as prescribed. (See procedure, p. 155.)
3 Begin oral feedings once the child is fully recovered from the anaesthetic and displays interest.
   a Begin with small amounts of 5% dextrose and water.
   b Gradually introduce formula.
   c Introduce solid foods suitable to the child's age and tolerance. (Refer to section on nutrition, p. 36.)
   d Encourage a high protein diet.

To observe for signs of complications.

1 Increased intracranial pressure indicates shunt malfunction. (Refer to listing of symptoms under clinical manifestations.)
2 Dehydration may be manifested in the following ways:
   a Sunken fontanelle (without additional signs of dehydration, this may only indicate a successful shunt)
   b Decreased urine output, increased relative density.
   c Diminished skin turgor and dryness of mucous membranes
   d Lethargy
3 Infection may be manifested by:
   a Fever (temperature normally fluctuates during the first 24 hours after surgery)
   b Purulent drainage from the incision
   c Swelling, redness, and tenderness along the shunt tract.

To provide continued emotional support to the parents.

1 Begin discharge planning early. (See Parental Teaching, below.)
2 Accompany all instructions with reassurance necessary to prevent the parents from becoming anxious or fearful about assuming the care of the child.

   Relay the success that other mothers have had in dealing with similar infants.
3 Encourage the parents to treat the child as normally as possible, providing him with appropriate toys and love.
4 Help the parents with problems of assisting siblings and grandparents to deal with the child's needs.
5 Initiate appropriate referrals
   a Social worker
   b Health visitor
   c Parent groups.

Parental Teaching

1 Parents should be given complete explanations of the disease, the surgery, and the changes that the surgery produced.
2 Physical nursing care
  a Special attention should be directed towards specific techniques of supportive nursing care, for example:
    (1) Turning
    (2) Skin care
    (3) Play
    (4) Exercises to strengthen the child's muscles
  b Feeding techniques and patterns
  c Pumping of shunt, if ordered by the surgeon.
3 Symptoms of increased intracranial pressure, shunt malfunction, infection, and dehydration must be treated.

  Parents should be taught not only to recognize these complications (refer to prior listing of signs of complications) but also to report them immediately to the paediatrician.
4 Illnesses which cause vomiting and diarrhoea or which prevent an adequate fluid intake are a great threat to the child who has had a shunt procedure. The parents should be instructed regarding:
  a Prevention of such illnesses
  b Early recognition of warning symptoms
  c Necessity of seeking immediate medical care so that the child can receive intravenous therapy to replace fluid and electrolyte loss.
5 The child's emotional needs should be stressed. Parents should be encouraged to treat the child as normally as possible. Generally, few restrictions need to be placed on his daily activities.
6 If appropriate, refer to section on mental handicap for additional areas of parent teaching. See p. 683.

Agencies

The Association for Spina Bifida and Hydrocephalus, 22 Upper Woburn Place, London WC1 10 EP.

SPINA BIFIDA

Spina bifida refers to a malformation of the spine in which the posterior portion of the laminae of the vertebrae fails to close. Several types of spina bifida are recognized of which the following three are the most common (Figure 13.1):

1 *Spina bifida occulta,* in which the defect is only in the vertebrae. The spinal cord and meninges are normal (Figure 13.1 [b]).

2   *Meningocele*, in which the meninges protrude through the opening in the spinal canal, forming a cyst filled with cerebrospinal fluid and covered with skin (Figure 13.1 [c]).

3   *Meningomyelocele* (or myelomeningocele), in which both the spinal cord and cord membranes protrude through the defect in the laminae of the spinal canal. Meningomyeloceles are covered by a thin membrane (Figure 13.1 [d]).

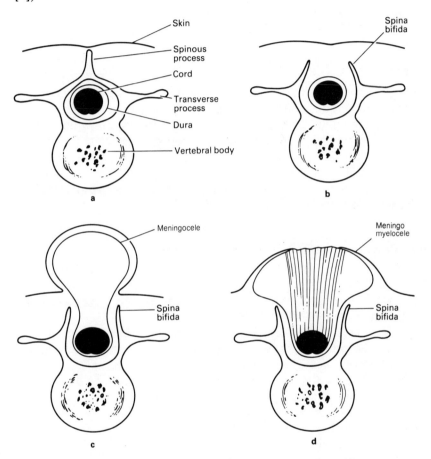

Figure 13.1 Spina bifida: (a) normal canal with spinous processes projecting posteriorly; (b) spina bifida without involvement of the meninges or spinal cord; (c) meningocele showing the spina bifida and meningeal involvement; (d) meningomyocele defect showing spina bifida, meningeal deficiency and exposed nervous tissue. (From Young D G Martin E J, *Young and Weller's Baby Surgery*, HM&M, 1979, with permission.)

Aetiology

1   Unknown but generally thought to result from genetic predisposition triggered by something in the environment.
2   Involves an arrest in the orderly formation of the vertebral arches and spinal cord that occurs between the fourth and sixth weeks of embryogenesis.
    Theories of causation:
    (1) There is incomplete closure of the neural tube during the fourth week of embryonic life.
    (2) The neural tube forms adequately but then ruptures.

Incidence

1   Geographical distribution and incidence vary widely, throughout the UK.
2   Most common developmental defect of the central nervous system.
3   More common in Caucasians of Celtic origin than in nonwhite population.
4   Condition may have other congenital anomalies associated with it.
5   Women who have had surgery for spina bifida in infancy have a 3-5% risk of having children with a neural tube defect.
6   The recurrence risks for parents who have had one or two affected children are about 5% and 10-12%, respectively.

Altered Physiology and Clinical Manifestations

Spina Bifida Occulta

1   Most common type; may occur in as many as 10% of otherwise normal children.
2   The bony defect may range from a very thin slit separating one lamina from the spinous process to a complete absence of the spines and laminae.
3   A thin fibrous membrane sometimes covers the defect.
4   The spinal cord and its meninges may be connected with a fistulous tract extending to and opening on to the surface of the skin.
5   Most patients have no symptoms.
    a They may have a dimple in the skin or a growth of hair over the malformed vertebrae.
    b There is no externally visible sac.

Meningocele

1   An external cystic defect can be seen in the spinal cord, usually in the centre line.
    a The sac is composed only of meninges and filled with cerebrospinal fluid.
    b The cord and nerve roots are usually normal.
2   The defect may occur anywhere on the cord. Higher defects (from thorax and up) are usually meningoceles.

3   There is seldom evidence of weakness of the legs or lack of sphincter control.
4   Surgical correction is necessary to prevent rupture of the sac and subsequent infection.
5   Hydrocephalus may be an associated finding and may be aggravated after surgery for a meningocele.
    a Occurs in about 9% of patients.
    b Usually not associated with the Arnold-Chiari malformation.
6   Prognosis is good with surgical correction.

Meningomyelocele (Myelomeningocele)

1   Most common type of open spinal defect.
    Occurs four to five times more frequently than meningocele.
2   A round, raised, and poorly epithelialized area may be noted at any level of the spinal column. However, the highest incidence of the lesion occurs in the lumbosacral area.
3   The lesion contains both the spinal cord and cord membranes. A bluish area may be evident on the top because of exposed neural tissue.
4   The sac may leak *in utero* or may rupture after birth, allowing free drainage of cerebrospinal fluid. This renders the child highly susceptible to meningitis.
5   Prognosis
    a Influenced by the site of the lesion and the presence and degree of associated hydrocephalus.
    Generally, the higher the defect, the greater the extent of neurological deficit and the greater the likelihood of hydrocephalus.
    b In the absence of treatment, most infants with meningomyelocele die early in infancy.
    c Surgical intervention is most effective if it is done early in the neonatal period, preferably within the first 2 hours of life.
    d Even with surgical intervention, infants can be expected to manifest associated neurosurgical, orthopaedic, and/or urological problems.
    e New techniques of treatment, intensive research, and improved services have increased life expectancy and have greatly enhanced the quality of life for most children who receive treatment for the defect.

Common Clinical Problems Associated with Meningomyelocele

Neurological Problems

1   Arnold-Chiari malformation
    a Associated malformation of the brain stem and downward displacement of the cerebellar tonsils and the fourth ventricle occur.
    b Causes a block in the flow of cerebrospinal fluid through the ventricles and leads to failure in the reabsorption mechanism of cerebrospinal fluid.

c Produces significant hydrocephalus in approximately two-thirds of children with meningomyelocele.

2   Loss of motor control and sensation below the level of the lesion

These conditions are highly variable and depend on the size of the lesion and its position on the cord. For example:

a A low thoracic lesion may cause total flaccid paralysis below the waist.

b A small sacral lesion may cause only patchy spots of decreased sensation in the feet.

Mobility and Orthopaedic Problems

1   Contractures may occur in the ankles, knees, and/or hips. Hips may be pulled out of the sockets.

a Nature and degree of involvement depends on size and location of lesion.

b Occurs because some threads of innervation do get through. One side of a hip, knee, or ankle may be innervated and the opposing side may not be. The unopposed side then becomes pulled out of position.

2   Clubfeet are a common accompanying anomaly.

This anomaly is thought to be related to a position of paraplegic feet in uterus.

3   Scoliosis is common in later years.

a Occurs in approximately 50% of patients.

b Caused by the congenital lesion in the spinal column.

4   Ambulation and ability to be upright are possible through various types of bracing and equipment.

Extent of bracing will depend on extent of sensory and motor loss. Children with low sacral lesions can ambulate with small, short, leg braces. Older children with significant loss may choose to use a wheelchair.

Urological Problems

1   Almost all lesions affect the sacral nerves which innervate the bladder. The bladder fails to respond to normal messages that it is time to micturate, and simply fills and overflows. Usually the bladder does not empty completely, causing two sets of problems:

a Susceptibility to urinary tract infections because of constant stasis.

b Incontinence, because the bladder is never completely empty and fails to receive signals to micturate.

2   Management

a Children must be followed routinely with intravenous pylography, micturating cystoureterogram, urine culture and sensitivity. Urea and creatinine levels must be measured to assess renal status.

b Urinary diversions (ileal loop) have been done in the past for infection and continence management.

(1) Some boys wear external penile devices.

(2) The newest technique of management is clean, intermittent self-catheterization which has been very effective. Children can generally be taught to catheterize themselves by the age of 6-7 years. Parents can catheterize younger children.

(3) Research is currently being done to develop mechanical sphincters and electrical bladder-stimulating pacemakers.

c Medications

(1) Antibiotics such as nitrofurantoin, sulphafurazole, cetrimoxazole (Septrin) and ampicillin are used periodically or prophylactically to prevent urinary tract infections.

(2) Medications such as imipramine hydrochloride (Tofranil) and ephedrine sulphate are used to help children retain their urine until it can be micturated at one time (rather than to dribble continuously). When self-catheterization is used in conjunction with medication many children can stay dry for 3-4 hours at a time.

d Dietary recommendations

Adequate fluid intake is essential to maintain good urinary flow.

e The ability to stay dry for reasonable time intervals is one of the greatest factors in enhancing self-esteem and positive body image.

Bowel Problems

1   Faecal incontinence and constipation are promoted by poor innervation of the anal sphincter and bowel musculature.
2   To compensate for decreased sensation, children are placed on a toileting schedule and are taught to push. Medications such as stool softeners, suppositories or Microlax enemas may be utilized to help determine scheduling.
3   Remaining unconstipated is essential to any type of faecal control. High-bulk, high-roughage and/or high-fluid diets as well as medications may be used to increase bulk or soften stool.

Skin Problems

1   Areas of decreased sensation have a tendency to break down. Braces and shoes should be checked frequently for rubbing.
2   During hospitalization, the nurse should be particularly watchful for areas of skin breakdown. The use of air mattresses, sheepskin, and other similar materials may help to prevent skin breakdown in bedridden children.

Dietary Problems

1   Many children become overweight because of activity limitations, and a tendency for parents and family to be overindulgent with sweets.
2   Dietary control is necessary to prevent obesity.

Developmental Problems

1   Most children have average intellectual ability despite hydrocephalus.
    a There may be an organic origin of the higher incidence of learning disabilities.
    b Most children are able to learn in a 'mainstreamed' normal school, provided they are able to overcome other barriers (architectural and attitudinal).
2   The most significant problems are secondarily handicapping conditions which develop when a child has a disability of this degree. (Refer to section on family stress in paediatric illness, p. 56.)
3   Disabled children need exposure to all activities and to rules and regulations of the nondisabled.

Prevention and Treatment of Meningomyelocele

Antenatal Detection

Antenatal detection is now possible through amniocentesis and measurement of alpha-fetoprotein. This testing should be offered to all women at risk (women who are affected themselves or have had other affected children).

Surgical Intervention

1   Procedure
    Laminectomy and closure of the open lesion and/or removal of the sac can usually be done soon after birth.
2   Purpose
    a To prevent further deterioration of neural function
    b To minimize the danger of rupture and infection, especially meningitis
    c To improve cosmetic effect
    d To facilitate handling of the infant by parents and nurses.

Multidisciplinary Follow-up for Associated Problems

1   A coordinated team approach will help maximize the physical and mental potential of each affected child.
    a A group of health care personnel (including a neurologist, neurosurgeon, orthopaedic surgeon, urologist, paediatrician, nurse, social worker, health visitor, and physiotherapist) should be available to the child and family.
    b A continuing, stable relationship with one person on the health care team who is coordinating efforts for the child is of great benefit.
2   Numerous neurosurgical, orthopaedic, and urological procedures and operations may be necessary to help the child to achieve his maximum potential.

Preoperative Nursing Objectives for Initial Surgery in the Neonatal Period

To prevent leakage of cerebrospinal fluid or rupture of the sac or lesion.

1 Position the infant on his abdomen.
   a Avoid placing the infant on his back, because this would cause pressure on the sac.
   b Check the position of the child at least once every hour.
2 Do not place a nappy or other covering directly over the sac.
3 A doughnut-shaped sterile padding must be placed around the sac.
4 Observe the sac frequently for evidence of irritation or leakage of cerebrospinal fluid.

To prevent infection.

1 Infection of the sac
   a This is most commonly caused by contamination by urine and faeces.
   b Keep the buttocks and genitalia scrupulously clean.
      (1) Keep the infant's head higher than his buttocks.
      (2) Whenever possible, keep buttocks exposed.
   c A sterile gauze nonadherent pad or towel or a sterile, moistened dressing may be applied according to the surgeon's preference.
      When the sterile covering is used, it should be changed frequently to keep the area free of exudate and to maintain sterility.
2 Infection of the bladder and urinary tract
   a Infection is frequently caused by stasis of urine.
   b Express or Credé bladder with each nappy change.
      (1) Apply firm, gentle pressure to the abdomen, beginning in the umbilical area and progressing towards the symphysis pubis.
      (2) Continue the procedure as long as urine can be manually expressed.
   c Encourage fluid intake to dilute the urine.
   d Administer prescribed prophylactic antibiotics.

To prevent deformities and ulcerations of lower extremities.

1 Maintain the infant in the prone position with hips only slightly flexed to decrease tension on the sac.
2 Place a foam rubber pad covered with a soft cloth between the infant's legs to maintain the hips in abduction and to prevent or counteract subluxation. A nappy roll or small pillow may be used in place of the foam rubber pad.
3 Allow the baby's feet to hang freely over the pads or mattress edge to prevent aggravation of foot deformities.
4 Change the infant's position when permissible to relieve pressure.
5 Provide meticulous skin care to all areas of the body — especially ankles, knees, tip of nose, cheeks, and chin.
6 Provide passive range of motion exercises for those muscles and joints which the infant does not use spontaneously.

7   Use a foam or fleece pad to reduce pressure of the mattress against the infant's skin.

To provide adequate nutrition and hydration.

1   Hold the infant for feedings if permissible. This provides the needed position change and affection and facilitates feeding.
     Position the infant in such a way that pressure on the back is eliminated. This may be accomplished by holding the infant in normal feeding position with elbow rotated to avoid touching the sac. Alternatives include feeding the infant on his side or while he is prone on the nurse's lap.
2   The child who must be fed in the prone position should have his head turned to one side and tilted upward.
3   Stop the feeding frequently so that the baby can rest and air can be expelled.
     a These infants cannot always be burped in the same way as normal babies.
     b Small, frequent feedings may be necessary.
4   Monitor the infant's weight pattern to ensure adequate gain.

To provide normal infant stimulation.

1   Establish eye contact with the infant by sitting at the cot with your face at the level of his.
2   Provide appropriate toys, such as bright mobiles or musical toys.
3   Refer to section on Growth and Development, p. 7.

To monitor neurological status and observe for signs of complications.

1   Hydrocephalus
     a Irritability
     b Feeding difficulty, vomiting, decreased appetite
     c Increased head circumference
     d Tense fontanelle
     e Temperature fluctuations
     f Decreased alertness
2   Infection
     a Oozing of fluid or pus from the sac
     b Fever
     c Irritability or listlessness
     d Convulsions
     e Concentrated or foul-smelling urine
3   Record the following:
     a Frequent vital signs
     b Behaviour of the infant
     c Activity of the legs
     d Degree of continence
     e Evidence of urine retention or faecal impaction

f Daily head circumference

g Evidence of complications.

To provide initial emotional support to the family.

1 Encourage parents to talk about their child and how they feel about the defect.

2 Provide them with basic information about the condition. Answer their questions simply and directly. Reinforce medical interpretations.

3 Encourage them to become involved with the child's care from the beginning.

    a Demonstrate techniques for holding and feeding the child and for providing routine care.

    b Emphasize what is *normal* and *well* about their infant.

4 Initiate communication with appropriate members of the multidisciplinary team which manages infants with these problems.

For nursing management of the infant with hydrocephalus or clubfoot, refer to Hydrocephalus, p. 625, and Clubfoot, p. 712.

Postoperative Nursing Objectives

To prevent postoperative complications.

1 Shock

    a Keep the infant warm by placing him in an incubator or under radiant warmer.

    b Maintain infant in a prone, level position for a few postoperative days.

2 Respiratory problems

    a Periodically change infant's position if permitted by his condition and by the extent of surgery.

    b Have oxygen available if necessary.

    c Report abdominal distension which may interfere with breathing and feeding.

3 Nutritional problems

    a The infant may be fed intravenously for several days or may be fed via nasogastric tube if he is unable to take oral feedings (see procedures for intravenous therapy, p. 155, and nasogastric feeding, p. 130).

    b Apply previously stated principles when bottle-feeding the infant.

4 Infection

    a Keep the surgical dressing clean and dry.

    b Observe the dressing frequently for drainage.

    c Apply previously stated principles to prevent infection.

    d Administer prescribed antibiotics.

5   Nursing observations — record the following:
  a Frequent measurements of temperature, pulse, and respiration
  b Colour
  c Neurological status
  d Evidence of abdominal distension
  e Condition of dressing
  f Evidence of infection
  g Degree of continence
  h Behaviour of the infant
  i Evidence of hydrocephalus.

To continue appropriate preoperative nursing activities.

1   Once the infant's back is well healed, he may be placed in a supine position for brief periods, which are gradually increased as the skin tolerates it.
2   The infant may also be positioned on his side at no more than a 45° angle for brief periods. This position, however, has the disadvantage of placing the hips in flexion and reduces the desirable use of the arms.
3   Special positioning may be requested by the orthopaedic surgeon or the physiotherapist.
4   Nappies may be worn once the back is well healed.

To provide continued emotional support to the family.

1   Encourage continued participation by parents in the infant's care.
2   Facilitate communication and interaction with appropriate members of the multidisciplinary team.
     It is essential that open lines of communication exist between team members and the staff that provides daily care for the infant. This ensures that families receive consistent information and facilitates continuity of care.
3   Foster the goal of helping the child to become as independent as possible.
     a Emphasize rehabilitation which makes use of the normal parts of the body and minimizes the disabilities.
     b Focus on immediate planning in such areas as ambulation and bowel and bladder management.
4   Begin discharge teaching early. (See below.)
5   Provide support for dealing with the usual problems of a newborn baby. Answer questions related to feeding, diet, bathing, problems of growth and development, and discipline.

Parental Teaching

1   Prepare parents to feed, hold, and stimulate their infant as normally as possible.

Include information related to the management of the usual neonatal problems such as bathing, feeding, formula preparation, and sleeping. (Refer to section on Growth and Development, p. 7.)

2   Teach parents any special techniques which may be required for the infant's physical care. Examples:
   a Methods of holding and positioning the infant
   b Techniques of feeding
   c Care of the incision
   d Provision for adequate elimination:
      (1) Procedure for bladder expression
      (2) Administration of prescribed prophylactic antibiotics
      (3) Signs of constipation and alleviation of the problem through diet regulation
   e Physiotherapy exercises
   f Skin care
      (1) General measures for avoiding pressure sores, such as frequent position changes
      (2) Perineal care
         (a) Frequent nappy changes
         (b) Careful laundering of nappies
         (c) Application of protective ointments
      (3) Daily inspection of the skin for such changes as reddened areas and bruises.

3   Safety
   The child with decreased sensation in the extremities should be protected from prolonged pressure, from burns or trauma due to bath water that is too warm, and from contact with hot or sharp objects.

4   Familiarize parents with signs of associated problems, especially signs of increased intracranial pressure or shunt malfunction and signs of infection.
   Instruct parents to notify the paediatrician if a problem does occur.

5   Be certain that a mechanism is developed for the family to receive continued support and teaching following discharge. Ensure referral is made to family health visitor.

Agency

The Association for Spina Bifida and Hydrocephalus, 22 Upper Woburn Place, London WC1 10EP.

BACTERIAL MENINGITIS

Bacterial meningitis is an inflammation of the meninges which follows the invasion of the spinal fluid by a bacterial agent.

Aetiology

1 The proportion of cases due to a specific organism varies from year to year; there is also considerable geographical difference.
2 The most common organisms causing bacterial meningitis in different age groups are:
   a Birth to 2 months
   (1) *Escherichia coli*
   (2) *Streptococcus*, Group B
   (3) *Staphylococcus*
   b 2 months to 3 years
   (1) *Haemophilus influenzae*
   (2) *Diplococcus pneumoniae*
   (3) *Neisseria meningitidis*
   c 3-16 years
   (1) *Diplococcus pneumoniae*
   (2) *Neisseria meningitidis*.

Altered Physiology

1 Bacterial meningitis is almost always preceded by an upper respiratory infection, which is complicated by bacteraemia.
2 Bacteria in the circulating blood then invade the spinal fluid.
3 Bacterial meningitis may occur as an extension of a local bacterial infection such as otitis media, mastoiditis, or sinusitis.
4 Bacteria may also gain direct entry through penetrating wound, spinal tap, surgery, or anatomical abnormalities.
5 The infective process results in inflammation, exudation, and varying degrees of tissue damage in the brain.

Clinical Manifestations

1 Signs and symptoms are variable, depending on the patient's age, the causative agent, and the duration of the illness when diagnosed.
   a Infants less than 1 month of age display the following symptoms:
   (1) Irritability
   (2) Lethargy
   (3) Vomiting
   (4) Lack of appetite
   (5) Seizures
   (6) High-pitched cry
   b Infants up to 2 years of age manifest symptoms similar to those of the young infant and in addition may have:
   (1) Fever
   (2) Tenseness of the fontanelle

(3) Neck rigidity

(4) Positive Kernig's and/or Brudzinski's signs

    (a) Kernig's sign

      With the child in the supine position and knees flexed, the leg is flexed at the hip so that the thigh is brought to a position perpendicular to the trunk. An attempt is then made to extend the knee. If meningeal irritation is present, this cannot be done and attempts to extend the knee result in pain.

    (b) Brudzinski's sign

      Spontaneous flexion of the lower limbs following passive flexion of the neck.

c Children over 2 years of age:

  (1) Common initial symptoms

    (a) Vomiting

    (b) Headache

    (c) Mental confusion

    (d) Lethargy

  (2) Later symptoms

    (a) Neck rigidity within 12-24 hours after onset

    (b) Positive Kernig's and/or Brudzinski's sign

    (c) Seizures

    (d) Progressive decline in responsiveness.

2 Onset may be insidious or fulminant.

3 Petechiae or purpura may develop.

  a Characteristic skin lesions are most often observed in cases of meningococcal or *Pseudomonas* infection.

  b Haemorrhagic rashes may occur in any child with overwhelming bacterial sepsis because of disseminated intravascular coagulation.

4 Septic arthritis suggests either meningococcal or *Haemophilus influenzae* infection.

Diagnostic Evaluation

1 Diagnosis is usually established by performance of a lumbar puncture and examination of the cerebrospinal fluid.

  a Elevated cerebrospinal fluid pressure

  b High cell count with mostly polymorphonuclear cells

  c Low glucose level

  d Elevated protein level (may also be normal)

  e Gram stain and cultures positive — to identify the causative organism

2 Additional laboratory studies

  a Complete blood count (total white blood cell count is often increased, with a shift to the left)

  b Platelet count

c Urinalysis
d Blood, urine, and nasopharyngeal cultures
e Serum electrolytes — often demonstrate hyponatraemia and hypochloraemia
f Serum glucose
g Blood urea nitrogen (BUN) and creatinine
h Tuberculin skin test
i Skull and chest x-rays.

Treatment

1 Intravenous administration of the appropriate antibiotics to promote rapid destruction of the bacteria and to suppress the emergence of resistant strains
2 Recognition and treatment of hyponatraemia
3 Supportive management of the comatose child or the child with seizures
4 Appropriate prophylactic treatment provided for contacts when indicated

Complications

1 Seizures
2 Cerebral oedema
3 Subdural effusion
4 Hydrocephalus
5 Cerebral infarction or abscess
6 Diffuse residual effects, including slowed development.

Nursing Objectives

To practise measures which will prevent the transmission of infection in the nursery.

1 Place the child in isolation until at least 24 hours after initiation of antibiotic therapy.
2 Practise careful handwashing technique — to serve as a model of good technique.
3 Personnel with infection should avoid contact with infants.
   a Seek medical care for infection. (Cultures should be taken.)
   b Remain out of the nursery.
   c Wear a mask when it is necessary to enter the nursery.
4 Teach parents and other visitors proper handwashing and gown technique.
5 Maintain sterile technique when procedures demanding this technique are performed.
6 Identify close contacts or high-risk children who might benefit from meningococci vaccination.

To assess the child for evidence of disease progression or response to therapy.

1 Determine baseline data at admission. Include the following information:
   a Weight
   b Head circumference
   c Vital signs
   d Blood pressure
   e Neurological status
   f History related to present illness
   g Usual behaviour and feeding patterns.
2 Monitor vital signs, blood pressure, and neurological status at frequent intervals.
3 Monitor intake and output continuously.
4 Monitor weight and head circumference at least daily.
5 Observe for and report the appearance or disappearance of any of the previously listed clinical manifestations.
   a Be especially alert for vague symptoms which appear early in the course of meningeal irritation in infants:
   (1) Lethargy
   (2) Irritability
   (3) Poor feeding or refusal to feed
   (4) Weight loss
   (5) Temperature changes.
   b Be consistent in planning for the care of infants to provide a means by which these early symptoms may be detected:
   (1) Accurate charting of the infant's previous behaviour
   (2) Assigning the same nurse to care for an infant on successive days.

To administer the prescribed antibiotic therapy to control the infection.

1 Administer medications at the specified time to achieve optimal serum levels.
2 Since medications are generally administered intravenously for 2-3 weeks, restrain the child in a functional position which safeguards the integrity of the intravenous infusion.
3 Observe medication sites for evidence of infiltration or development of tissue irritation.
4 Be aware of the actions, proper dilution, and side effects of specific medications.
5 Be aware of drug interactions and incompatibilities.

To observe for evidence of complications of the disease.

Report the following:

1 Decreased respirations, decreased pulse rate, increased systolic blood pressure, visual disturbances, pupillary changes, or decreased responsiveness, which may indicate increased intracranial pressure

2   Decreased urine volume and increased body weight, which may indicate inappropriate secretion of antidiuretic hormone

3   Sudden appearance of a skin rash and bleeding from other sites, which may indicate disseminated intravascular coagulation

4   Persistent or recurring fever, bulging fontanelle, signs of increased intracranial pressure, focal neurological signs, seizures, or increased head circumference which may indicate subdural effusion

5   Hearing disturbances and apparent deafness.

To provide for the nutritional needs of the patient.

1   During the acute phase of the illness, the patient may be unable to take or tolerate oral feedings.

a Carefully monitor the administration of intravenous fluids.

b Provide nasogastric feedings if necessary (see section on feeding methods, p. 130).

c Provide for the sucking needs of the infant by offering a dummy.

2   Initiate oral feedings as soon as the patient's condition improves.

a Infants

(1) Begin by offering small feedings and observe for the following responses:

(a) Vomiting

(b) Abdominal distension

(c) Infant's interest in feeding and ability to suck

(d) If the infant tires with feeding.

(2) Supplement oral feedings with nasogastric feedings if necessary.

(3) Gradually increase amount of feeding.

(4) Resume regular feeding schedule based on infant's ability to tolerate it.

(5) Hold the infant for feedings as soon as his condition warrants it.

b Older children — refer to section on nutrition, p. 36.

3   Carefully monitor the child's weight to ensure that energy needs are being met.

To provide a supportive environment during the stage of irritability.

1   Reduce the general noise level around the child and shield child from sudden loud noises.

2   Organize nursing care to provide for periods of uninterrupted rest. Disturb only when necessary.

3   Keep general handling of the child at a minimum. When necessary, approach the child slowly and gently.

4   Maintain subdued lighting as much as possible.

5   Speak in a low, well-modulated tone of voice to reduce anxiety.

To provide therapeutic care for the child who experiences seizures.

(See section on Seizures, below.)

To provide therapeutic care for the febrile child.

(See section on Fever, p. 105.)

To observe for episodes of apnoea and initiate measures to stimulate respiration.

1 Observe the infant closely for apnoea or have the infant placed on a respiratory monitor.
2 Stimulate infant when apnoea does occur.
   a Slap on feet and provide more vigorous stimulation if necessary.
   b When spontaneous respiration does not occur within 15-20 seconds, apply hand resuscitator or perform mouth-to-mouth resuscitation.
3 Report frequent periods of apnoae to paediatrician.
4 Record length of apnoea episode and response to stimulation on nursing record.

To provide supportive care for the child during the convalescent phase of illness.

1 Record disappearance of symptoms and indications that the child is returning to his normal state.
2 Provide for the emotional needs of the child. (Refer to section on the Hospitalized Child, p.56.)
3 Encourage parental visiting and family-centred care.
4 Note any evidence that the child is developing sequelae of the illness, such as deafness, brain abnormality, or hydrocephalus.

Parental Support and Teaching

1 Encourage parents and siblings to visit the child.
   a Encourage their participation in the child's care.
   b Provide them with an opportunity to express their concerns.
   c Answer questions they may have regarding the infant's progress and care.
2 Discuss symptoms parents should watch for as signs of possible complications.
3 Give specific instruction regarding medications to be administered at home.

CONVULSIVE DISORDERS (SEIZURE DISORDERS, EPILEPSY)

Convulsive disorder is a term used to encompass a number of varieties of episodic disturbances of brain function. Convulsions should not be regarded as one specific disease, but as a symptom of an underlying disorder. They are relatively common in children, being more prevalent during the first 2 years than at any other time in life.

Aetiology

1 Idiopathic
2 Antenatal factors
   a Genetic predisposition
   b Congenital structural anomalies
   c Fetal infections
   d Maternal diseases
3 Perinatal factors
   a Trauma
   b Hypoxia
   c Jaundice
   d Infection
   e Prematurity
   f Drug withdrawal
4 Postnatal factors
   a Primary infection of the central nervous system
   b Infectious diseases of childhood with encephalopathy
   c Head trauma
   d Circulatory diseases
   e Toxic encephalopathy
   f Allergic encephalopathy
   g Metabolic encephalopathy
   h Degenerative diseases
   i Cerebral neoplasms
   j Renal disease.

Altered Physiology

1 The basic mechanism for all seizures appears to be prolonged depolarization causing brain cells to become overactive and to discharge in a sudden, violent, disorderly manner.
2 This paroxysmal burst of electrical energy spreads to adjacent areas or may jump to distant areas of the central nervous system. A seizure results.
3 The biochemical basis of seizures is incompletely understood.
4 Some seizures appear to occur under the influence of a triggering factor.
   a In the adolescent, the onset of menstruation
   b Nonsensory factors, such as hyperthermia, hyperventilation, metabolic disorders, sleep deprivation, emotional disturbances, and physical stress
   c Sensory factors, such as those related to vision, hearing, touch, the startle reaction, and those that are self-induced.

Clinical Manifestations

Grand Mal Epilepsy

1 Onset
  a Onset is abrupt.
  b May occur at night.
  c An aura occurs in about one-third of epileptic children prior to a grand mal seizure.
2 Tonic spasm
  a The child's entire body becomes stiff.
  b He usually loses consciousness.
  c The face may become pale and distorted.
  d His eyes are frequently fixed in one position.
  e His back may be arched with his head held backward or to one side.
  f His arms are usually flexed and his hands clenched.
  g If standing, the child falls to the ground.
  h He may utter a peculiar, piercing cry.
  i The child may be incontinent and may bite his tongue or cheek. (This occurs because of sudden forceful contraction of his jaw and abdominal muscles.)
  j He is often unable to swallow his saliva.
  k Breathing is ineffective and cyanosis results if spasm includes the muscles of respiration.
  l The pulse may become weak and irregular.
3 Clonic phase
  a Characterized by twitching movements which follow the tonic state.
  b Usually start in one place and become generalized, including the muscles of the face.
4 Duration
  a Varies.
  b Usually, convulsions cease after a few minutes and consciousness returns.
5 Postconvulsive state of child
  a Usually is sleepy or exhausted.
  b May complain of headache.
  c May appear to be in a dazed state.
  d Often performs relatively automatic tasks without being able to recall the episode.
6 Secondary symptomatology
  a Represents the patient's response over a long period of time to the injurious attitudes of other people towards the child and the diagnosis.
  b Child develops a self-image consistent with his perception of how others view him.

7   Electroencephalogram (EEG)
   a Definite abnormalities can usually be demonstrated in the interval between seizures.
      (1) Random spike discharges
      (2) Diffuse high-voltage slow waves
      (3) Pattern abnormal for child's chronological age
   b Multiple high-voltage spike discharges are demonstrated during the seizure.
   c Asymmetries between the two hemispheres and diffuse slowing may be observed after the seizure.

Status Epilepticus

1   Refers to grand mal seizures which occur in series without the patient's regaining consciousness between attacks.
2   Transient postictal (i.e. period following seizures) signs and symptoms include ataxia, aphasia, and mental sluggishness.
3   Irreversible brain damage may occur secondary to prolonged cellular hypoxia.
4   This condition should be treated as a medical emergency.

Petit Mal Epilepsy

1   Onset — occurs most frequently in children from 3 years of age through to adolescence.
2   Clinical signs
   a Loss of contact with the environment for a few brief seconds:
      (1) The child may appear to be staring or daydreaming.
      (2) If reading or writing, the child will suddenly discontinue the activity and may resume it when the seizure has ended.
   b Minor manifestations include rolling of the eyes, nodding of the head, and slight quivering or jerking of the trunk and limb muscles.
3   Duration — usually less than 30 seconds.
4   Frequency — varies from one or two per month to several hundred each day.
5   Precipitating factors may include hyperventilation, fatigue, hypoglycaemia, and stress.
6   Postconvulsive state
   a Child appears normal.
   b Is not aware of having had a convulsion.
7   Electroencephalogram (EEG)
      Has characteristic three-per-second spike and wave pattern during the seizure.

Focal Seizures

1   Psychomotor
   a Common in childhood; highest incidence in children over 3 years of age.

b Seizure discharge usually originates in the temporal lobe and may be referred to as 'temporal lobe seizures' or epilepsy.

c Clinical signs

(1) Symptoms of irritability or gastric upset may precede the onset of a seizure by hours or days.

(2) Aura, if present, often includes bad odour or taste.

(3) Most common motor symptom is drawing or jerking of the mouth and face.

(4) Perceptual alterations may occur.

(5) Dysphagia or aphasia may be present.

(6) May demonstrate tonic posturing or a desire to urinate.

(7) May perform coordinated but inappropriate movements repeatedly in a stereotyped manner (e.g. clutching, kicking, picking at clothes, walking in circles, chewing, licking, spitting).

(8) Consciousness may be impaired but is rarely completely lost.

d Duration — brief, usually from 30 seconds to 5-10 minutes.

e Postconvulsive state — child may be confused after an attack but usually has no memory of what happened.

2 Focal motor (Jacksonian seizures)

a Clinical signs

(1) Sudden jerking movements occur in a particular area of the body, such as the face, thumb, or toe.

(2) Seizure begins in one area of the body and spreads to adjacent areas on the same side in a fixed progression.

(3) Consciousness may or may not be disturbed.

b Prognosis

Seizures may become more extensive as the child matures, leading to grand mal seizures.

3 Focal sensory (rare in children)

Sensations occur, such as numbness, tingling, and coldness in the part of the body controlled by the area of the brain cell overactivity.

Infantile Myoclonic Fits (Massive Myoclonic Spasms)

1 These fits are peculiar to infants; they are second in incidence only to grand mal fits in this age group.

2 Peak incidence is in children between 3 and 6 months; onset after 2 years of age is rare.

3 Clinical signs

a Sudden, forceful, myoclonic contractions involving the musculature of the trunk, neck, and extremities.

(1) Flexor type — infant adducts and flexes his limbs, drops his head, and doubles upon himself; Salaam attacks.

(2) Occasionally of the extensor type — infant extends neck, spreads arms out, and bends body backward in a position described as 'spread eagle'.

b A cry or grunt may accompany severe attack.

c Infant may grimace, laugh, or appear fearful during or after the attack.

4   Duration — momentary (usually under 1 minute).

5   Frequency — varies from a few attacks per day to hundreds per day.

6   EEG — random, high-voltage slow waves and spikes suggestive of a diffuse disorganized state, known as hypsarrhythmia.

7   Prognosis

a Usually this type of fit disappears spontaneously after child reaches 4 years of age.

b The spasm may gradually diminish in frequency and severity and then cease.

c Subsequent grand mal or other types of seizure may develop.

d Mental handicap usually accompanies this disorder.

Prognosis

1   General prognosis depends on type and severity of seizure disorder, coexisting mental handicap, organic disorders, and the type of medical management.

a Medically treated seizures

(1) Spontaneous cessation of seizures may occur.

(2) Drugs may be gradually discontinued when the child has been free from attacks for an extensive period and his EEG pattern has reverted to normal.

b Nontreated epilepsy

Seizures tend to become more numerous.

2   Mental development

a Convulsive episodes do not in themselves usually cause irreversible brain damage.

b Hypoxia during seizures can cause mental handicap.

c Epileptic children with normal mentality can be expected to maintain it with proper control of seizures.

Children with petit mal and essentially normal EEG patterns generally have a more favourable prognosis for normal mentality than do children with grand mal or psychomotor seizures.

Chemotherapy

General Principles Related to the Administration of Medications

1   Selection of the most effective drug(s) depends upon correct identification of the clinical seizure type.

2   A desirable drug level is one which will prevent attacks without producing drowsiness or unsteadiness.

3   Dosages are adjusted according to blood level and clinical signs.

4   Accurate timing is essential to prevent seizures.
This is especially true when there is a tendency for the child to have convulsions at a certain period each day.
5   Enteric coated tablets which have a delayed effect should be used for children who are prone to attacks during sleep.
6   Most anticonvulsants are available in liquid form as well as in capsules or tablets. Anticonvulsive syrups should be prescribed for infants and young children.
7   It may take several months to find the best combination of medications and the best dosages of each to control the child's seizures.
8   Total control of symptoms may not be achieved in every patient.
9   Dosage adjustment may be required from time to time because of the child's growth.
10 Duration of therapy should be prolonged. Medication is usually not discontinued until at least 3-4 years after the last attack.
11 Weaning from medication should always be gradual, with stepwise reduction of dosage and withdrawal of one drug at a time.

Common Drugs Used for the Control of Seizures in Children

1   Phenobarbitone (Luminal)
    a Dosage
       (1) An initial loading dose is usually given intramuscularly or intravenously for an acute, ongoing seizure, because it takes from days to weeks to achieve therapeutic blood levels by the oral route alone.
       (2) The dosage is reduced for maintenance therapy and is generally administered orally.
    b Indications and advantages
       (1) Drug of choice for initial trial
       (2) One of the safest anticonvulsant drugs
       (3) Relatively inexpensive
    c Untoward effects
       (1) Excitement, hyperactivity
       (2) Rash
       (3) Gastrointestinal symptoms
       (4) Dizziness, ataxia
       (5) Aggravated psychomotor seizures
       (6) Drowsiness
    d Toxic effects (rare, except in overdose, accidental ingestion)
       Respiratory, circulatory, or renal depression
    e Contraindications
       (1) Severe hepatic or renal dysfunction
       (2) Hypersensitivity
2   Phenytoin sodium (Epanutin)
    a Route — oral

b Indications and advantages

(1) Does not produce excessive drowsiness

(2) Safest drug for the management of psychomotor epilepsy

(3) Often used with phenobarbitone

c Untoward effects

(1) May accentuate petit mal seizures

(2) Hypertrophy of the gums

Daily gum massage is an important aspect of nursing care for a patient taking phenytoin sodium (Epanutin)

(3) Hirsutism

(4) Rickets

(5) Nystagmus

d Toxic effects — (rare, except in overdose, accidental ingestion)

(1) Blood dyscrasias

(2) Liver damage

3   Ethosuximide (Zarontin)

a Route — oral

b Indications and advantages

(1) Used for petit mal seizures

(2) Occurrence of blood dyscrasia is less common following administration of ethosuximide than with trimethadionel (Troxidone) — the other medication frequently used to control petit mal seizures.

c Untoward effects

(1) Drowsiness

(2) May increase grand mal seizures

(3) Dermatitis

(4) Gastrointestinal symptoms

(5) Dizziness and 'glare' when looking at bright objects, sometimes necessitating the use of tinted glasses.

(6) Ataxia

d Toxic effects

(1) Blood dyscrasias

(2) Psychiatric symptoms

e Contraindications

Hepatic or renal disease

4   Primidone (Mysoline)

a Route — oral

b Indications and advantages

(1) Used alone or with other anticonvulsants to control grand mal, psychomotor, or focal seizures.

(2) May control grand mal seizures not responsive to treatment by other anticonvulsant therapy.

c Untoward effects

(1) More common

(a) Ataxia

      (b) Vertigo
   (2) Occasional
      (a) Gastrointestinal symptoms
      (b) Fatigue
      (c) Diplopia
      (d) Nystagmus
      (e) Skin eruption

d Toxic effects
   (1) Megaloblastic anaemia may occur as a rare idiosyncratic response to the drug.
   (2) Drowsiness in breast-fed infants of primidone-treated mothers indicates that breast feeding should be discontinued.

e Contraindications
   (1) Patients who are hypersensitive to phenobarbitone
   (2) Patients with porphyria

5   Diazepam (Valium)

a Route — oral, intravenous, or intramuscular

b Indications and advantages
   (1) Intravenous or intramuscular diazepam is indicated in the treatment of status epilepticus and severe recurrent convulsive seizures.
   (2) Oral diazepam may be used adjunctively in maintenance therapy for convulsive disorders.

c Special precautions
   (1) If administered intravenously, give slowly over 3 minutes. Avoid intra-arterial administration or extravasation.
   (2) Administer intravenously with caution to children with limited pulmonary reserve, because of the possibility that apnoea and/or cardiac arrest may occur.
   (3) Tonic status epilepticus has been precipitated in patients treated with intravenous diazepam for petit mal seizures.
   (4) Concomitant use of barbiturates, alcohol, or other central nervous system depressants may potentiate the action of diazepam with increased risk of apnoea.
   (5) Administer with caution to children with compromised renal function.

d Untoward effects
   (1) More common
      (a) Ataxia
      (b) Drowsiness
      (c) Fatigue
      (d) Venous thrombosis and phlebitis at injection site
   (2) Less common
      (a) Gastrointestinal symptoms
      (b) Confusion, depression
      (c) Headache
      (d) Tremor

(e) Vertigo
(f) Incontinence or urinary retention
(g) Visual disturbances
(h) Skin rash
(i) Anxiety
(j) Sleep disturbance
(k) Neutropenia
(l) Jaundice
e Toxic effects
(1) Somnolence
(2) Confusion
(3) Diminished reflexes
(4) Hypotension
(5) Coma
(6) Apnoea
(7) Cardiac arrest.

Nursing Objectives

To control the seizures.

Administer medications as ordered.

To protect the child from injury during a convulsive episode.

1   Preventive measures
   a Remove hard toys from the bed.
   b Keep a padded tongue blade immediately available to put between the child's teeth to prevent him from biting his tongue.
   c Pad the sides of the cot.
   d Have a suction machine available to remove secretions during a seizure.
   e Have an emergency oxygen source in the room in case of sudden respiratory difficulty.
2   Emergency actions
   a Clear the area around the child if he is not in bed.
   b Do not restrain him.
   c Loosen the clothing around his neck.
   d Turn the child on his side so that saliva can flow out of his mouth.
   e Place a small, folded blanket under the head to prevent trauma if the seizure occurs when the child is on the floor.
   f Place a padded tongue blade between the teeth to prevent damage to the tongue and cheeks and to facilitate respiration if tonic-clonic activity is noted in the face and jaw.
      If the teeth have clamped shut, do not attempt to force them open.
   g Suction the child and administer oxygen as necessary.

h Do not give anything by mouth.

i Place the child in bed after the seizure if he is not already there.

To record accurately the seizures, include the following:

1 Behaviour before the seizure, aura
2 Types of movements observed
   a Tonic
      (1) Body becomes stiff
      (2) Muscles in a state of constant contraction
   b Clonic
      Twitching, jerking motions
3 Time seizure began and ended
4 Site where twitching or contraction began
5 Areas of the body involved
6 Movements of the eyes and changes in pupil size
7 Incontinence
8 Amount of perspiration
9 Respiratory changes
10 Colour change — pallor, cyanosis, flushing
11 Mouth — teeth clenched, movement, tongue bitten, foaming at the mouth
12 Apparent degree of consciousness during the seizure
13 Behaviour after the seizure
   a Degree of memory for recent events
   b Types of speech
   c Coordination
   d Paralysis or weakness
   e Sleeping after the attack
   f Pupil reaction
   g Vital signs.

To observe the child for recurrent seizures.

1 Place the child where he can be watched closely.
2 Monitor vital signs and assess neurological status frequently.
3 Check the child frequently. Report:
   a Behaviour changes
   b Irritability
   c Restlessness
   d Listlessness.

To provide emotional support to the child's parents.

1 Describe completely any examinations, evaluations, treatments that the child is receiving:
   a EEG
   b Pneumoencephalogram

    c Blood studies

    d Medications.

2   Provide information regarding the disease itself.

    a Orientation should be a continuing process.

    b Too much information at one time is undesirable.

    c Points of emphasis:

      (1) Epilepsy is *not* contagious, is seldom dangerous, and does *not* indicate insanity or mental handicap.

      (2) Most children with epilepsy have infrequent seizures and with medications these can be completely controlled.

      (3) The child may have normal intelligence and can live a useful and productive life.

      (4) The child's medication is not addicting when used as prescribed. It should in no way influence his mental ability or personality or cause him to become a drug addict.

      (5) It is impossible to predict accurately the possibility of the convulsive disorder appearing in siblings or offspring of the affected child.

    d Refer the family to appropriate community resources and services.

      (1) Social worker

      (2) Health visitor

      (3) School nurse

      (4) Psychiatrist

      (5) Parent groups

      (6) Voluntary agencies.

    e Provide the parents with appropriate literature.

3   Observe the parent-child reaction for evidence of rejection or overprotection.

    Offer reassurance and praise for achievements in dealing with the child's problems.

4   Prepare parents for the fact that it may take several months of regulating drug dosages before adequate control is obtained.

To minimize anxiety during the child's hospitalization.

1   Rationale

    The therapeutic value of anticonvulsant drugs is decreased if the child has more anxiety than he can handle.

2   Explain the diagnostic and treatment plan to the child in a manner that he can understand.

    a The use of play is very effective in explaining things to younger children and in allowing them to express their feelings.

    b The older child should be encouraged to ask questions and to talk about his experience.

3   Allow the child as much normal activity as possible.

    Allow him to be dressed if desired.

4   If the child does have a seizure, stay with him and remain calm.
    a Stay with the child after a convulsion and reassure him and his parents that he is all right.
    b Help the child to adjust to reality if he has difficulty remembering the episode.
    c Older children may require intervention to deal with guilt and embarrassment secondary to incontinence and the loss of body control.
    d Maintain a quiet environment if the child has had a long convulsive period.
5   Provide diversion appropriate for the child's age.
    Play equipment should be such that it will not cause injury during a seizure.
6   Avoid unnecessary stimulation.

Parental Teaching

1   The child should have as normal an environment as possible.
    a Attendance at an ordinary school with healthy children should be encouraged.
        (1) Contact should be made with the school nurse who can help the child's teacher understand his disease, emergency treatment of seizures, etc.
        (2) Child should be allowed to participate in organizations and outside activities with limited restrictions.
            (a) Each child must be treated individually; the kind of activity depends on the degree of control.
            (b) Generally, children with seizure disorders should not be allowed to climb in high places or swim alone.
            (c) Responsible adults should be made aware of the child's disease.
        (3) Child should not be made to feel that he can never be left alone.
        (4) He needs to be disciplined as a normal child.
        He should not gain attention directly or indirectly by having seizures.
2   The child should be given appropriate information regarding his diagnosis and treatment. He is less confident of his body and his control over it and therefore less confident of himself.
    a He should be included in conferences with the paediatrician.
    b He needs an opportunity to ask questions which should be answered honestly.
    c He should be aware of his restrictions and helped to deal with them.
    d He should gradually be given responsibility for taking his own medications faithfully.
    e He should be encouraged to wear a medic-alert bracelet.
3   The older child and adolescent should be helped to achieve independence.
    a He should be given the opportunity for privacy to discuss his diagnosis with his paediatrician.

b He should be allowed to use his own judgement in his daily activities.

c He should be helped to develop realistic educational and career goals.

(1) The assistance of a social worker or psychiatrist may be invaluable during this period.

(2) Genetic counselling may be indicated in some cases.

(a) People with epilepsy can marry and have children.

(b) There is no proof that epilepsy is hereditary although there may be a tendency to transmit a low convulsive threshold.

(c) The decision to marry must be based on the individual's own feelings of security and self-confidence and his ability to assume the responsibility of marriage.

(3) Counselling regarding such matters as securing a driver's licence and obtaining life, health, and motor vehicle insurance should be available, when of age.

d Any fantasies that 'there is nothing wrong with me' or the refusal to take medications require prompt intervention.

4   Factors which may precipitate a convulsive episode should be avoided.

a The seizures should be treated matter-of-factly. A calm, reassuring attitude is essential during and after a seizure.

The attitude of adults when the child has a seizure influences the attitude of other children towards him.

b The child should be kept in optimal physical condition with special attention to the status of his teeth and eyes and to the prevention of infection.

c Excessive fatigue, overhydration and hyperventilation should be avoided.

d Irregular, fluctuating schedules are detrimental. A routine of daily living should be encouraged.

5   Medical care and supervision to control convulsions are essential.

Instructions regarding medical and nursing care should be stressed.

(1) Administration of medications

(2) Emergency care during a seizure

(3) Observations

(a) Signs of impending seizure

(b) Behaviour during and after the seizure

(4) Diet

Ketogenic diets are no longer widely used, except in difficult cases.

6   Parents should be referred to appropriate support groups for help in dealing with their feelings, concerns, and problems related to their child.

Agencies

British Epilepsy Association, New Wokingham Road, Wokingham, Berkshire.

FEBRILE CONVULSIONS

Febrile convulsions refer to seizures which occur in the context of a febrile illness in a previously normal child. The seizures are brief and generalized. They should be distinguished from focal or prolonged seizures which occur in a child with an underlying seizure disorder that is exacerbated by fever.

Aetiology

1　Accompany intercurrent infections — especially viral illness, tonsillitis, pharyngitis, and otitis.
2　Appear to occur in a familial pattern, although exact pattern of inheritance is incompletely understood.

Incidence

1　Febrile convulsions occur in approximately 2.5% of all children.
2　The vast majority of first febrile seizures occur in children between the ages of 6 months and 3 years of age.
3　Febrile seizures are unusual after 5 years of age.

Clinical Manifestations

1　Most febrile convulsions consist of generalized tonic-clonic seizures.
2　Seizures generally last less than 20 minutes.
3　Fever is usually high — over 38.8° rectally.
4　Seizures usually occur near the onset of fever rather than after prolonged fever.

Diagnostic Evaluation

1　Measures are directed towards delineating the cause of any seizure as precisely as possible so that its implications and prognosis may be discussed with the parents.
2　Diagnostic methods include:
　　a Physical examination with special attention to neurological status
　　b Transillumination of the skull
　　c Cerebrospinal fluid examination
　　d Complete blood count and urinalysis
　　e Cultures of nasopharynx, blood, or urine as appropriate to determine cause of fever
　　f Blood sugar, calcium, and electrolyte levels
　　g Electroencephalogram (EEG)
　　　　(1) Similar to that found during and after a grand mal seizure
　　　　(2) Abnormality frequently persists for as long as a week after the seizure

(3) Interseizure record — normal

h Skull films at time of first seizure.

Prognosis

1   The likelihood of seizure recurrence is about 40-50% for a second febrile seizure and about 15% for a third seizure.
2   Approximately 30% of recurrences occur within 6 months of the first seizure; 50% occur within 13 months; all occur within 30 months.
3   Factors influencing recurrence rate:
a The younger the child at the time of the first seizure, the greater the risk for additional febrile seizures.
b Girls may be more likely than boys to have a recurrent febrile convulsion.
c Children with a positive family history of febrile convulsions have a greater risk of recurrent febrile convulsions.
4   The risk of development of nonfebrile convulsions is relatively low (about 3%). At risk are those children who demonstrate the following characteristics:
a Multiple febrile seizures during one day
b Prolonged febrile seizures
c Persistent electroencephalographic abnormalities
d Central nervous system infections.

Nursing Objectives

To assess and reduce fever.

Refer to section on Fever, p. 105.

To intervene appropriately during and after the febrile convulsions.

Refer to first four objectives in previous section, p. 660.

Parental Teaching

1   Remain calm and efficient if the child has a seizure in the presence of his parents.
2   Reinforce realistic, reassuring information such as:
a A convulsion does not necessarily imply that the underlying disease is a serious one.
b Children rarely die in seizures.
c The prognosis depends on the cause of the convulsion.
(1) A single febrile seizure is not indicative of later chronic epilepsy.
(2) Children who have a tendency to develop febrile convulsions usually lose it as they grow older.

(3) Occasional, brief convulsions have no adverse effects on the child's ultimate development.

3   Discuss and demonstrate emergency management of seizures.

4   Stress that medical evaluation is indicated as soon as the child develops fever.

Prompt administration of antipyretic measures is necessary when the child is febrile.

5   Reinforce medical instructions regarding anticonvulsant therapy.

a The advisability of long-term anticonvulsant medications in normal children with simple febrile convulsions is currently controversial. Recommendations vary with paediatrician preference.

b Intermittent therapy with phenobarbitone during febrile episodes is apparently of no value because of the length of time required to achieve therapeutic serum levels of the drug.

SUBDURAL HAEMATOMA

Subdural haematoma refers to an accumulation of fluid, blood, and its degradation products within the potential space between the dura and arachnoid (subdural space). Subdural haematomas are classified as acute, subacute, or chronic, depending on the time period between injury and the onset of symptoms.

Aetiology

1   Direct or indirect trauma to the head:
   a Birth trauma
   b Accidental causes
   c Purposeful violence, as in the battered child syndrome (see p. 771).
2   Meningitis

Classification*

1   Acute
   a Syndrome presents as an acute problem within 3 days from the time of presumed injury.
   b Condition often associated with other intracranial injuries. This connection increases the mortality rate associated with this type of subdural haematoma.

Note: Classification does not imply any basic differences in the disease process but refers only to the duration of the lesion before it becomes manifest. The classification varies slightly among several sources.

c May occur at any age.

d It is the least common type of subdural haematoma.

2   Subacute

Syndrome presents within 4-14 days from the time of presumed injury.

3   Chronic

a Syndrome presents at 2-4 weeks or more from the time of presumed injury.

b Most common type of subdural haematoma in children.

c Represents 20% of childhood head injuries.

d In 85% of cases children are 1 year of age or less.

e In 80% of cases children have bilateral involvement.

f In children over 2 years, subdural haematomas are most frequently unilateral.

g It may be difficult or impossible to obtain a history of trauma, since the precipitating episode often appears relatively insignificant and may pass unnoticed or be quickly forgotten.

Altered Physiology

1   Trauma to the head causes tearing of the delicate subdural veins, resulting in small haemorrhages into the subdural space. (Bleeding may be of arterial origin in cases of acute subdural haematoma.)

2   As the blood breaks down, there is an increased capillary permeability and effusion of blood cells and protein into the subdural space.

3   The breakdown products of blood stimulate the growth of connective tissue and capillaries largely from the dura.

4   A membrane is formed which usually extends frontally and laterally over the hemispheres, surrounding the clot.

5   Fluid accumulates within the membrane and increases the width of the subdural space.

6   Further haemorrhages occur.

7   The lesion enlarges, expanding the skull and, if unrelieved, ultimately causes cerebral atrophy or death from compression and herniation.

8   The lesion may arrest spontaneously at any point.

9   Further bleeding may occur into an already existing sac and may increase symptoms.

10   In long-standing subdural haematoma, the fluid may disappear, leaving a constricting membrane which prevents normal brain growth.

Clinical Manifestations

Acute

1   Often present with continuous unconsciousness from the time of injury, but child may present with a lucid interval.

2   Ensuing manifestations include deterioration of level of consciousness, evidence of progressive hemiplegia, and signs of brain stem herniation (pupillary enlargement, changes in vital signs, development of decerebrate state, and respiratory failure).

Chronic

1   Insidious onset.
2   Symptoms are variable and are related to the age of the child.
   a Infants
     (1) Early signs
       (a) Anorexia
       (b) Difficulty feeding
       (c) Vomiting
       (d) Irritability
       (e) Low grade fever
       (f) Retinal haemorrhages
       (g) Failure to gain weight
     (2) Later signs
       (a) Enlargement of the head
       (b) Bulging and pulsation of the anterior fontanelle
       (c) Tight, glossy scalp with dilated scalp veins
       (d) Stabismus, pupillary inequality, ocular palsies (rare)
       (e) Hyperactive reflexes
       (f) Seizures
       (g) Retarded motor development
   b Older children
     (1) Early signs
       (a) Lethargy
       (b) Anorexia
       (c) Symptoms of increased intracranial pressure:
          Vomiting
          Irritability
          Increased blood pressure
          Decreased pulse
          Decreased or irregular respirations
          Headache
     (2) Later signs (may occur immediately if bleeding takes place rapidly)
       (a) Convulsions
       (b) Coma.

Diagnostic Evaluation

1   Complete blood count — anaemia of blood loss; low serum protein level.
2   X-ray — satural separation in infants.

3   Transillumination of the skull in infants — increased.
4   Lumbar puncture — may contain red blood cells, a slight excess of white cells, and increased protein. Procedure may be risky with increased intracranial pressure.
5   Bilateral subdural taps — fluid of any sort in excess of 1-2 ml or with a protein content significantly higher than that of the cerebrospinal fluid obtained at the same time.
6   Electroencephalogram may be abnormal.
7   Carotid angiography shows defect.
8   Cranial computed tomography (CCT scan) is the procedure of choice for screening children with suspected subdural haematoma.

Complications

1   Mental handicap
2   Ocular abnormalities
3   Seizures
4   Spasticity
5   Paralysis.

Treatment

1   Acute subdural haematoma
    Requires evacuation of the clot through a burr hole or craniotomy.
2   Chronic subdural haematoma
    a Repeated subdural taps are done to remove the abnormal fluid.
    (1) In infants, the needle can be inserted through the fontanelle or suture line.
    (2) In older children, burr holes into the skull are necessary before the needle can be inserted.
    (3) The subdural taps may be the only treatment required if the fluid disappears entirely and symptoms do not recur.
    (4) Concurrently, treatment is instituted to correct anaemia, electrolyte imbalance, and malnutrition.
    b Shunting procedure may be indicated if repeated taps fail significantly to reduce the volume or protein content of the subdural collections. Shunting is generally to the peritoneal or pleural cavities.

Prognosis

1   Treatment is usually successful when the diagnosis is made early — before cerebral atrophy and a fixed neurological deficit have occurred. In such cases, subsequent development is normal.

2   Prognosis is dependent on the effect of the initial trauma on the brain as well as the effect of continued fluid collection.
3   Mortality in massive, acute subdural bleeding is very high, even if promptly diagnosed.

Nursing Objectives

To assess the child's neurological status in order to help evaluate the effectiveness of treatment or to identify disease progress.

Observe for and document the following:

1   General behaviour — especially irritability, lethargy, and evidence of personality changes.
    It is important to obtain a thorough history from the child's parents regarding his normal behaviour and level of functioning so that abnormalities can be more easily recognized.
2   Appetite and feeding difficulties, including vomiting.
3   Signs of increased intracranial pressure.
    a Vital signs, including pulse, respiration, and blood pressure should be monitored frequently.
    b Be alert for:
    (1) Increased systolic blood pressure
    (2) Increased pulse pressure
    (3) Decreased pulse or irregularities
    (4) Changes in respiratory rate or difficulty breathing.
4   Level of consciousness.
    Describe findings explicitly. The following 'levels' may be useful as guidelines:
    a Alert and responds immediately and appropriately to visual, auditory, and tactile stimuli.
    b Lethargic, drowsy, and inactive but can be aroused to an alert state.
    c Lethargic and dull; responds with vigorous stimulation, but quickly returns to lethargic state.
    d Can be aroused only to a very low level of response with vigorous stimulation.
    e Moderate coma with rudimentary physiological or psychomotor responses.
    f Totally nonresponsive, even to deep pain stimuli.
5   Pupillary changes — especially dilated pupil, double vision, lack of response to light, alterations in visual acuity, and decreased integrity of eye movements.
6   Convulsions.
7   Motor function, including ability to move all extremities.
    The ability to grasp should be checked and compared bilaterally.

To observe for signs of complications.

1   Infection
    a Record temperature frequently.
    b Report purulent drainage from the site of the subdural tap.
2   Recurrent bleeding
    Note rapid changes in vital signs indicating shock or increased intracranial pressure.
3   Paralysis.

To avoid additional increase in intracranial pressure.

1   Maintain a quiet environment.
2   Avoid sudden changes in position.
3   Organize nursing activities to allow for long periods of uninterrupted rest.
4   Administer laxatives or suppositories to prevent straining during a bowel movement.

To assist with subdural taps.

1   Wrap the infant or young child in a mummy restraint. (See procedure on protective devices to limit motion, p. 115.)
2   Hold the child securely to avoid injury caused by sudden movement.
3   Apply firm pressure over the puncture site(s) for a few minutes after the tap has been completed to prevent fluid leakage along the needle tract.
4   Observe the child frequently after the procedure for:
    a Shock
    b Drainage from the site of the tap
    (1) Note whether this is serious drainage or frank blood.
    (2) Reinforce the dressing, if present, to prevent contamination of the wound.

To provide adequate nutrition.

Apply principles stated in the section on hydrocephalus, p. 625

To provide supportive care to the child in coma.

1   Keep the child's eyes well lubricated to prevent corneal damage.
2   Suction the child as necessary to remove secretions in the mouth and nasopharynx.
3   Provide frequent mouth care.
4   Maintain adequate nutrition and hydration through nasogastric feedings. (Refer to procedure, p. 130.)
5   Carefully regulate fluid administration to avoid danger of rapidly increasing intracranial pressure.
6   Measure urine output and record relative density.
    Observe for bladder distension (indicates fluid retention). Express (Credé) bladder or utilize indwelling catheter if child is unable to micturate.

7   Administer suppositories or enemas as necessary to prevent constipation and impaction.
8   Change the child's position frequently and provide meticulous skin care to prevent hypostatic pneumonia and pressure sores.
9   Prevent contractures.
    a Apply passive range of motion exercises to all extremities.
    b Place pillows appropriately to support the child's body in good alignment.
    c Use a footboard for the older child.
10 Have emergency equipment available for cardiopulmonary resuscitation, respiratory assistance, blood transfusion, subdural tap, etc.
11 Avoid discussing the child's condition near the bedside. Even though comatose, the child may be able to hear.
12 Observe for the development of the following complications:
    a Respiratory problems (infection, aspiration, obstruction, atelectasis)
    b Fluid and electrolyte imbalance
    c Infection (urinary or central nervous system)
    d Bladder and gastrointestinal distension.

To care for the child with a craniotomy.

See section on the postoperative care of the child with a brain tumour, p. 743.

To provide for the child's emotional needs.

1   Hold and cuddle the infant as much as possible according to his condition.
2   Provide diversion according to the child's age.
    a Infants — mobiles or musical toys
    b Older children — quiet games, reading, etc.

To provide emotional support to the parents.

1   Encourage as much parental participation in the child's care as possible.
2   Reassure the parents that the prognosis is favourable and adequate treatment is being provided.
3   Avoid blaming the parents for the child's injury.
    a Attempt to alleviate their guilt feelings if present.
    b Refer the parents to a social worker.
    c Inform family health visitor prior to discharge.

Parental Teaching

Reinforce explanations in the following areas:

1   The condition
2   The causes of the child's specific symptoms
3   The need and rationale for treatment
4   Postoperative and recovery expectations

5   Signs of recurrent bleeding
6   Safety measures to prevent accidents in the future.

REYE'S SYNDROME

Reye's syndrome is a children's disease which has been clinically characterized as a nonspecific 'encephalopathy and fatty degeneration of the viscera, mainly affecting the liver, brain, and kidney'.

Aetiology and Incidence

1   Unknown
2   Most consistent single factor is an antecedent viral infection
    a Mean age of onset is $3\frac{1}{2}$ years.
    b Condition very rare.
3   Related viruses include: adenovirus, Coxsackie, herpes simplex and zoster, influenza A, retrovirus, and polio type I.
4   Other controversial possibilities (contributors):
    a Genetic make-up of individual child that increases his susceptibility
    b Environmental factors — incidence higher in suburban-rural areas
    c Clinical — salicylates.

Altered Physiology

1   Liver — enlarged and bright yellow; fatty infiltration in the form of small lipid droplets; mitochondria are large and swollen with some decrease of enzymatic activity, particularly for ammonia detoxification.
2   Brain — cerebral oedema with small ventricles, possible neuronal necrosis, findings consistent with hypoxia, inflammatory reaction absent, grossly enlarged mitochondria; and pervasive watery blebs.
3   Kidney — fatty degeneration of loop of Henle and proximal convoluted tubules with a few lipid droplets in distal tubular cells.
4   Heart — fatty accumulation in fibres; bundle of His, and bundle branches.

Clinical Manifestations

Nursing Alert: Early diagnosis is critical because of the rapidly fatal course of the disease.

1   Prodromal illness (see aetiology) that may be improving
2   Sudden pernicious vomiting — fever usually not present
3   Irrational behaviour
4   Altered sensorium — from mild lethargy to progressive stupor and coma

5   Hyperventilation, tachypnoea
6   Hepatomegaly.

Diagnosis

1   General condition and appearance of child:
    History of prodromal illness — mild upper respiratory infection or other infection with sudden development of pernicious vomiting, presence of other symptoms.
2   Differential diagnosis — acute toxic encephalopathy, hepatic coma, hepatitis, meningitis, or encephalitis. History to rule out ingestion of medications or toxic materials.
3   Laboratory — essential to obtain: elevated serum glutamic-oxaloacetic transaminase (SGOT) level; prolonged prothrombin and partial prothrombin times; serum glucose decreased.
4   Laboratory — optional: acid-base imbalance; increased fatty acids (fatty acidaemia without ketoanaemia); elevated uric acid; normal or slightly elevated serum bilirubin jaundice.
5   Lumbar puncture — done if cerebrospinal fluid is needed to rule out other diagnoses. If symptoms of increased intracranial pressure exist, the performance of a lumbar puncture is to be avoided to prevent rapid decompression and herniation of the brain.
6   Liver biopsy — usually done; however, the biopsy may not be done unless evidence is insufficient to make a definite diagnosis (shows microvesicular fatty degeneration of liver).

Medical and Nursing Management

1   Because this is a multisystem disease, it must be emphasized that:
    a Intracerebral integrity is of utmost priority, and if the brain can be supported through the course of the illness, the chances of the other organs running their course uneventfully are very high and are of less concern.
    b The multidisciplinary team must have a leader who initiates, coordinates, and supervises *all* activities and medical planning. It may be the physician, neurosurgeon, endocrinologist, or the attending paediatrician. However, it should be the person with the knowledge and capability of monitoring and directing care 24 hours a day.
2   Treatment is supportive by maintaining adequate levels of circulating glucose and cerebral perfusion while preventing or controlling IICP (increased intracranial pressure).

Nursing Intervention

1   During the acute phase of the disease, the child should be cared for in an intensive care unit.

2   Refer to:
   a Respiratory procedures, p. 174
   b Cardiopulmonary resuscitation, p. 199
   c Assisting with obtaining blood for gas analysis, p. 139
   d Intensive care, p. 73
   e Intravenous therapy, p. 155
   f Increased intracranial pressure, p. 630
   g Care of the comatose patient, p. 672
   h Nasogastric tube procedures, p. 130
   i Catheter procedure, p. 163.
3   Be aware of the medical plan of treatment being used, and be alert to the rapidity of the course of the disease. Particularly important factors:
   a Note and report immediately any changes in the child's status or stage of progression (see clinical manifestations).
   b Therapy is directed at maintaining normal intracranial pressure and adequate cerebral perfusion.
   c Protect the child from complications that may result from the comatose condition or life-saving medical intervention.
   d Maintain fluid and electrolyte balance.
   e Before any procedure is done for the child, consider the effects on his intracranial pressure.
4   Support parents during the time that the child may be in the intensive care unit.
   a Prior to the first visit, explain in detail what the child will look like. Accompany the parents when they first visit their child. Since this may be traumatic, do not force them to maintain lengthy contact with the child.
   b Address parental concerns and answer questions regarding:
      (1) How they should react to their child
      (2) Amount of parental participation that is beneficial
      (3) Fears and fantasies during lengthy periods when they are unable to visit child
      (4) Concerns for other children and other family members, and their reactions to the illness
      (5) Technical questions.
   c Provide the parents with the phone number of the intensive care unit.
   d Make sure parents have a comfortable place to sleep if they elect to stay at the hospital.
   e Help the family express their feelings about what has happened and how it is affecting them.
      (1) Assess how they are coping; their family support systems.
      (2) Initiate referrals to appropriate agencies, i.e. the family health visitor.
      (3) The lack of knowledge and rapid course of the disease from a mild to a critical illness may be difficult for parents to understand. They may have extreme feelings of guilt, and blame themselves or others for not recognizing the seriousness of the illness sooner. They may have other

children at home with similar prodromal viral infection who may be experiencing guilty feelings about the ill sibling.

5 Provide psychological and emotional support to the child.

a Although the child may be heavily sedated, comatose, or paralysed from muscle relaxants, he perceives in varying degrees what is happening to him and to his environment.

b Explain procedures to the child while they are being done.

c Conversations about the child, his condition, or other children should take place away from the sick child.

d Encourage parents to bring in a favourite toy or security object.

e Show a constant awareness of any activity, noise, etc., that increases or changes intracranial pressure.

f When a sedated or comatose child awakens, he may be disoriented and have no memory of previous events. Provide explanations and reassurance as appropriate.

g Parental separation may increase anxiety; offer residential accommodation to parents.

6 Post-transfer to paediatric nursing unit:

a Once the child is alert, his condition stable, and he is recovering, he should be transferred to the regular paediatric unit.

b The child recovering from Reye's syndrome without any neurological sequelae should recover fairly rapidly. Provide support as needed.

c When the child has experienced sequelae or complications, attention to his physical manifestations will be needed, i.e. special physiotherapy. A multidisciplinary team approach to treatment will continue to provide for a coordinated approach to care.

d The child and his family will continue to need emotional support during this period.

e A critical role of the nurse is to educate herself, other members of the staff, and the community about Reye's syndrome:

(1) Learn to recognize the symptoms that may lead to a diagnosis of the illness.

(2) Be prepared for the course of the illness, from a mild disease to one that is life-threatening.

(3) Support parent groups and other community groups to educate parents about Reye's syndrome, and to seek medical consultation when symptoms may indicate the disease.

Parents' Support Group

National Reye's Syndrome Foundation of the UK, 55 High Street, Banbury, Oxfordshire OX16 8JJ.

FURTHER READING

Books

Bickerstaff E R, *Neurology*, Hodder & Stoughton, 1978.
Farmer T (ed.), *Paediatric Neurology*, Harper & Row, 1975.
Hayward R, *Essentials of Neurosurgery*, Blackwell Scientific, 1980.
Jabbour T *et al.*, *Pediatric Neurology Handbook*, Medical Examination Publishing, 1976.
Levin D C *et al.*, *A Practical Guide to Pediatric Intensive Care*, Mosby, 1979.
McCormick W Bell W, *Increased Intracranial Pressure in Children*, Saunders, 1978.
O'Donohue N V, *Epilepsies of Childhood*, Butterworth, 1979.
Scipien G *et al.*, *Comprehensive Pediatric Nursing*, McGraw-Hill, 1979.
Swainman K Wright F, *The Practice of Pediatric Neurology*, Vols 1 & 2, Mosby, 1979.
Till K, *Paediatric Neurosurgery*, Blackwell Scientific, 1975.
Ward F Bower B D, *A Study of Certain Social Aspects of Epilepsy in Childhood*, Spastics International, 1978.

Articles

Altschuler A *et al.*, Even children can learn to do clean self-catheterization, *American Journal of Nursing*, January 1977, 77: 97.
Barnes N D Roberton N R C, Fits, faints and funny turns, *Update*, February 1979: 379-389.
Braney M, The child with hydrocephalus, *American Journal of Nursing*, 1973, 73: 828.
Brett E M, Epilepsy and convulsions in children, *Nursing Mirror*, August 1978: 20-22.
Cass A S, Urinary tract complications in myelomeningocele patients, *Journal of Urology*, January 1976, 115: 102.
Dorer A, Problems of teenagers with spina bifida, *Physiotherapy*, June 1977: 190-193.
Epstein B, The cerebral palsied child, *Update*, July 1979: 127-134.
Geddes N, Intermittent catheterization for patients with spina bifida, *Canadian Nurse*, June 1978: 34-35.
Geddes N Hendry J, Living with a congenital anomaly: spina bifida, *Canadian Nurse*, June 1978, 29-33.
Hosking G, Topics in child neurology — epilepsy, *Nursing Mirror*, March 1980: 22-25.
Lorber J Zachary R, Spina bifida — to treat or not to treat, *Nursing Mirror*, September 1978: 13-9.
Lyon R *et al.*, Intermittent catheterization rather than urinary diversion in children with myelomeningocele, *Journal of Urology*, March 1975, 113: 109.
National Child Development Study — Epilepsy in Childhood, *British Medical Journal*, January 1980, 207.
Till K, Cerebellar tumours in children, *Journal of Maternal and Child Health*, October 1978, 326 -89.
Tyrell J, The young adult with spina bifida, *Journal of Maternal and Child Health*, July 1984: 208-212.
Weeks H L, What every ICU nurse should know about Reye's syndrome, *Maternal and Child Nursing*, July/August 1976: 231-238.

Wright E G, Reye's syndrome, in *Current Practice in Pediatric Nursing,* Vol 3 (P L Chinn and K B Leonard, eds), Mosby, pp 206-221.

Books for Parents

Lorber P, *Your Child with Spina Bifida,* ASBAH 1981.
Lorber P, *Your Child with Hydrocephalus,* ASBAH, 1981.

Books for Siblings of Child with Spina Bifida

White P, *Janet at School,* Black, 1978.

14

THE MENTALLY HANDICAPPED CHILD

MENTAL HANDICAP

A person who is mentally handicapped does not develop in childhood as quickly as other children nor attain the full mental capacities of a normal adult.*

Aetiology

General

1 Congenital lack of brain cells
2 Later destruction of cells originally present.

Prenatal Factors

1 Heredity
2 Fetal irradiation
3 Infection — maternal or fetal
4 Kernicterus due to Rh or ABO incompatibility
5 Anoxia
6 Cranial anomalies
   a Hydrocephalus
   b Craniosynostosis
7 Chromosomal abnormalities
8 Disorders of metabolism.

Antenatal Factors

1 Anoxia
   a Maternal
   b Placental
   c Respiratory obstruction

* Definition of mental handicap: from White Paper on *Better Services for the Mentally Handicapped.* Cmnd 4683, HMSO, 1971.

2 Breech delivery with delay in delivery of the head
3 Cerebral injury
   a Trauma
   b Cephalopelvic disproportion
   c Precipitate delivery
   d Preterm delivery
4 Infection
5 Intracranial haemorrhage.

Postnatal Factors

1 Central nervous system infection
2 Brain injury, haemorrhage, or tumour
3 Cerebral degenerative disease
4 Anoxia
5 Poisoning
6 Vascular disorders
7 Social and cultural factors.

Unknown

1 No identifiable organic or biological cause for 65-75% of handicap in children.
2 Suspected causes include sociocultural or environmental deprivation or poverty.
3 Generally, these children are more mildly handicapped than children with associated organic and physical defects.

Incidence

Present information suggests that the number of people needing special mental handicap services in England ranges from 2.9 to 3.4 per 1000 population.

Classification

1 In the past, the IQ score has been used to separate handicapped children into educational potential divisions:
   a Mildly handicapped (educable) — IQ 55-75
   b Moderately handicapped (trainable) — IQ 25-55
   c Severely handicapped — IQ below 25.
2 It is now known that although the IQ score may be helpful in assessing and planning for handicapped children, low IQ itself is not sufficient to make a diagnosis of mental handicap.
3 Both intellectual level and adaptive behaviour level (the effectiveness or degree with which the individual meets the standards of personal independence and social responsibility expected of his age and cultural

group) should be considered when one makes the classification. A person's IQ performance does not remain constant for life.

4 Scales have been developed for measuring and classifying adaptive behaviour based on the following expectations:

a *Infancy and early childhood*
(1) Sensory-motor skills development
(2) Communication skills (including speech and language)
(3) Self-help skills
(4) Socialization

b *Childhood and early adolescence*
(1) Application of basic academic skills in daily life activities
(2) Application of appropriate reasoning and judgement in mastery of environment
(3) Social skills, group activities

c *Late adolesence and adult life*
Vocational and social responsibilities and performances.

5 Only those children who demonstrate deficits in both intellectual level and adaptive behaviour should be classified as mentally handicapped.

Clinical Manifestations

1 Developmental delay — failure to meet normal motor, mental, and/or social milestones for age

2 Physical
a Approximately 75% of handicapped individuals have no obvious physical stigma.
b Mentally handicapped children have a greater percentage of sensory defects, language disorders, neuromuscular impairment, seizures, and physical anomalies than the general population.

Diagnostic Evaluation

1 Diagnosis is difficult and is most reliable when the determination is made by a comprehensive team that offers medical, psychological, social, and educational examinations.

2 Care must be taken to ensure that no child is mislabelled as mentally handicapped.

Prognosis

1 Factors which influence the prognosis:
a Degree of handicap
b Existence of additional, physical defects
c Family and community resources available to help the child to use his mental resources

2 Factors which favour improvement in intelligence:
   a Modification of the environment to eliminate stress and deprivation
   b Improvement in learning opportunities
   c Increased social acceptance
   d Early intervention
3 The prognosis is best for the mildly handicapped child without a coexistent physical defect.

Nursing Objectives

To support parents during the initial period of diagnosis.

(Refer to section on family stress and coping with serious or chronic illness in childhood, p. 66.)

1 Provide time for the parents to comprehend the extent of their problem and to mobilize their resources to work on its solution.
   a When parents appear ready, offer counselling and verbal support at a slow pace, one step at a time.
   b Be sensitive to clues concerning the type of support that is most helpful to each family.
2 Encourage both parents to talk about the diagnosis and how they feel about it.
   a The parents' reaction will be individually determined by such factors as the nature of the diagnosis, the manner in which the family is told of the diagnosis, the perceived attitude of health professionals, the parents' previous life experiences, their attitudes towards the mentally handicapped, their marital relationship, and their personal aspirations.
   b Expect attitudes of guilt, shame, and self-pity; feelings of grief, hostility, and ambivalence; expressions of denial; thoughts that they might be unable to care for the child.
   c Provide privacy for discussions.
   d Express sympathetic understanding of the family's problems and show acceptance of their attitudes.
   Reassure them that many parents react to the diagnosis with grief and sorrow.
3 Assure the family that their child has had the benefit of the best diagnostic procedures and has been given any treatment that is indicated.
4 If appropriate, initiate a referral to a social worker, a psychiatrist, or any other professional who may assist the family to deal with their immediate reactions and may plan for the child's long-term care.
   Many parents benefit from the continuous or intermittent support of a variety of health professionals.
5 Communicate a genuine concern for the parents as individuals and an understanding of the responsibilities they have outside the hospital, i.e. care of other children, work, etc.

To foster acceptance of the child by his parents and family, and to increase feelings of self-worth and self-confidence in parents.

1   Serve as a role model by interacting with the child in a manner which conveys acceptance, respect, and love.

2   Help parents to develop a fundamental understanding of what has happened to their child and what this means in terms of his future development.

   a Clarify and support medical speculations regarding the cause of the handicap.

   (1) Genetic counselling is indicated, especially in familial types of handicap.

   (2) Answer parental questions sensitively but directly.

   (3) Provide explanations in terms they can understand.

   (4) Avoid vague generalities, such as 'the child is slow,' and demoralizing words, such as 'moron' or 'imbecile'.

   b Provide as much specific information as possible.

   Parents have the right to know what diagnostic tests have been done, what positive or negative conclusions have been made, what uncertainties remain, and what general prognosis can be made.

3   Involve both parents in the child's care so that they may gain a realistic concept of his ability.

   a Point out the child's areas of strengths and weaknesses and show how these can be considered in his management.

   b Emphasize the *well* part of the child and that he has the same needs as a normal child for love and security.

4   Include the family as soon as possible with other members of the health team in planning for the child's future care.

   a The plan should be based on the degree of the child's handicap, the reaction of the family to the diagnosis, and the availability of community resources.

   b The family should be supported in the decisions they make.

   c The family should be guided to make decisions for the child's care which will allow for maximum utilization of his capabilities.

5   Discuss with parents their plans for dealing with the siblings of the handicapped child.

   a Adequate explanations and information should be given to siblings early to avoid any misconceptions later.

   b Siblings often need help in explaining the handicapped child's abnormality to their friends.

   c Caution parents to guard against intense sibling rivalry; the other children often feel neglected because of the amount of time devoted to the handicapped child.

6   If appropriate, initiate a referral to the health visitor or community nurse for the mentally handicapped for assistance with planning and implementing home care.

To provide mental and motor stimulation.

1 Assess the child's functional level of development, and define and implement plans to help him achieve the next developmental tasks. (Refer to section on growth and development, p. 7.)

2 Play is an essential part of the child's care.
   Select toys on the basis of functional level, not on the age group for which they were intended.

3 Expose the child to a variety of materials and toys which stimulate all of his senses.
   a Equipment such as rocking chairs, musical instruments, record players, blocks, art materials, and simple picture books are indispensable.
   b Toys should be accessible for the child to use when he desires.

4 An educational specialist or play worker may be able to provide invaluable guidance in this area.

To teach the child basic skills with the long-range goal of developing independent behaviour at the highest level possible according to the child's potential.

1 Determine the child's care plan according to his individual areas of strengths and weaknesses and coordinate it with the plans of the related health professionals.

2 Because a handicapped child has a limited attention span, present a smaller amount of material to him at a slower rate and over a longer period of time than to a normal child.

3 Provide organized, consistent, and repetitive experiences.

4 Employ techniques of positive reinforcement.
   a Give rewards for positive responses so that the probability of recurrence of that response will be strengthened.
   Rewards should be given consistently and immediately after the approved response.
   b Do not reward unacceptable behaviours.

5 Break complex behaviours down into small steps which the child can easily achieve.
   a This is very important in the areas of feeding, dressing, and toilet training.
   b Do not expect the child to transfer learning from one situation to another.

6 Base expectations for the child on his mental ability, *not* on his chronological age.

7 Maintain a relaxed learning environment.

To reduce destructive behaviour and encourage that which is socially acceptable.

1 Establish a routine of daily living so that the child knows precisely what is expected of him.

2 Employ consistent discipline.

a Use language that the child understands so that he can comprehend his misdeed.

b When punishment is necessary, i.e. not giving a reward, it should follow the misdeed immediately.

3   Provide immediate reinforcement for positive behaviours and ignore undesirable behaviours.

To prepare the mentally handicapped individual so that he may cope successfully (within his potential) with the problems and adjustments of adult life.

1   Help parents identify areas of home responsibilities which may be delegated to the handicapped child.

2   In the child's early learning activities, provide habits which are essential to his later vocational life:

a Getting to places on time

b Cooperating

c Focusing and holding attention on the task at hand

d Establishing acceptable interpersonal relationships.

3   Help the child to develop a set of attitudes and behaviours that will motivate him to work.

4   Identify attainable occupational goals early in the child's educational experience.

Early education should tie into later social and vocational programmes.

To be aware of nursing activities associated with hospitalization of a child previously diagnosed as mentally handicapped.

1   Apply all of the previously outlined principles.

2   Obtain a thorough nursing history from the parent and/or child regarding the child's usual home routines:

a Feeding

b Sleeping

c Toilet habits

d Learning activities

e Play

f Vocabulary

g Discipline.

3   Utilize the information obtained to develop a nursing care plan which provides for continuity of care from home to hospital in order to maintain the child's sense of security and minimize his regression.

Counsel the mother that some regression can be anticipated as with normal children who require hospitalization.

4   Encourage parental participation to the extent that it is therapeutic for both the child and the parent(s).

5   Provide a safe environment according to the child's needs.

a This environment is best determined by observing the child and from information obtained during the admission interview.

b If possible, use the type of bed with which the child is familiar.

c Remove any objects that are potentially injurious to the child.

6 Whenever possible, assign consistent nursing personnel to care for the child.

7 Explain procedures to the child using communication methods appropriate for his level of cognitive development.

To help modify existing social attitudes towards the mentally handicapped.

1 Assess and work through your own feelings about the handicapped, including personal attitudes and defences which are used to avoid personal involvement in the care of handicapped children and their families.

2 Utilize opportunities to influence the attitudes of other hospitalized children and their families.

a Serve as a role model in your own interactions with handicapped children.

b Encourage hospitalized children to socialize with the handicapped child during play or other activities, and help them to understand and accept the child.

c Provide opportunities for other parents to discuss their feelings about the mentally handicapped and to ask questions. Correct any misconceptions they may have.

3 Support community activities for the mentally handicapped.

Parental Teaching

1 The child may require more medical supervision than the normal person. Regular dental care is also essential.

a The child is often more susceptible to infections.

b He may eat poorly.

c He may be underweight or overweight.

d He may have poor motor coordination.

e He often has speech and language problems.

2 Secondary handicaps such as visual or hearing problems should be treated.

3 The child's environment has a great influence on his behaviour, growth, and development. It should provide experiences which contribute to a positive self-concept of a person who is loved, wanted, valued, and respected.

4 Parents need to be helped to recognize their child's methods of communicating so that they can respond to his needs.

5 Parents should be assisted to identify learning readiness in their child in order to help him achieve his maximum level of development without subjecting him to unnecessary experiences of failure and frustration.

6 Practical, tangible suggestions relative to everyday living should be offered to the parents:

a Selection of toys

b Techniques of feeding

c Patterns for toilet training

d Methods of discipline.
7 Special precautions may be necessary to provide a safe environment for the child.

His delayed motor, intellectual, and social development make him more vulnerable to the usual childhood accidents.
8 The child should have the opportunity of participating in social, religious, and recreational activities.

a Organizations should be selected in which the probability of success is the highest.

b The parent should discuss the situation with the group leader and the leader should have an opportunity to meet the child so that both child and leader can assess each other.
9 Available literature should be offered to parents; they should also be made aware of community resources:

a Primary health care centres

b Day care centres

c Nursery groups

d Special schools

e Parent groups

f Volunteer organizations

g Specialized diagnostic facilities

h Recreational programmes

i Vocational training

j Residential situations

k National associations.
10 Parents need to know that they are important as people. They each should be encouraged to lead a normal life. They should be helped to feel that they are not their child's only resource, but that others care and are willing to help.

Agencies

1 The Association for Spina Bifida and Hydrocephalus, 22 Upper Woburn Place, London WC1 10EP
2 British Epilepsy Association, New Wokingham Road, Wokingham, Berkshire
3 Friends of the Cheyne Society for Spastic Children, 63 Cheyne Walk, London SW3 5NA
4 National Society for Mentally Handicapped Children, 117-123 Golden Lane, London EC1Y ORT
5 The Spastics Society, 12 Park Crescent, London W1N 4EQ.

DOWN'S SYNDROME

Down's syndrome is a chromosomal abnormality involving an extra chromosome (number 21), characterized by a typical physical appearance and mental handicap.

Aetiology

Trisomy 21

1 The abnormality is an error in cell division.
   a Both number 21 chromosomes in the pair instead of just one of the pair migrate to one daughter cell during meiosis.
   b 47 chromosomes are present in the new individual rather than the normal 46.
   c There are three number 21 chromosomes, thus extra genetic material.
2 Occurrence is associated with advanced maternal age.
   a Risk is increased after maternal age of 35.
   b Recurrence in the same set of parents is rare, but dependent upon maternal age.
3 This form of Down's syndrome is not inherited.

Translocation

1 Chromosome number 21 attaches to another chromosome, usually the 13 — 15 group.
2 This abnormal attachment occurs in the parent.
   a Parent passes on to the offspring an extra dose of chromosome 21, plus a normal chromosome 21.
   b The child with this type of Down's syndrome has 46 chromosomes.
3 This form of Down's syndrome is inherited.
   In most cases it is a fresh occurrence, and for chromosomally normal parents there is small risk of a future child with Down's syndrome. In one-third of the cases, one parent is a balanced translocation carrier; thus, there is risk of recurrence.

Altered Physiology

1 The normal person, without Down's syndrome, has 46 chromosomes (23 pairs).
   a One pair of chromosomes is sex-determining.
   b 22 pairs of chromosomes are non-sex-determining and are called autosomes.
2 The individual with Down's syndrome has an extra chromosome — number 21. He carries extra genetic material.

3   Abnormalities that are present at birth occurred during fetal growth.
   a Normal fetal growth has been interfered with.
   b This interference affects mainly the heart, brain, eyes, hands, and general growth.

Clinical Manifestations

1   Physical stigmata recognized at birth:
   a Marked hypotonia and floppiness
   b Joint hyperextension or hyperflexibility
   c Tendency to keep mouth open with tongue protruding; high, arched palate; furrowed tongue
   d Brachycephaly with relatively flat occiput
   e Eyes slant upward and outward with internal epicanthal folds
   f Excess skin on back of neck
   g Flattened nasal bridge and flat facial profile
   h Small ears, often incompletely developed
   i Spade-like hands; there is inward curving of distal phalanx of fifth finger; simian crease
   j Short, broad feet; there is a wide separation between first and second toe (plantar furrow)
   k Small male genitalia
   l Absence of Moro reflex. (Response to sudden loud noise, causing body to stiffen and arms to go up and out, then forward and towards each other. Thumb and index finger will assume 'C'-shape.)
2   Complications most likely to be present at birth;
   a Congenital cardiac defects, especially atrial septal defect
   b Duodenal stenosis and other intestinal obstruction
3   Later findings in the child (up to 1 year of age):
   a Slow intellectual development (IQ 20-75; mean: 50)
   b Slow motor development.

Complications

1   Recurrent infection of upper respiratory tract
2   Skin infections
3   Complications secondary to physical anomalies present at birth:
   a Eye problems — strabismus; error in refractions
   b Elevated leucocyte enzymes
     (1) Small percentage of affected children born with fatal leukaemia
     (2) Leukaemia — acute type developing in first 2-3 years
4   Serious behavioural problems.

Diagnostic Evaluation

Chromosomal analysis (karyotyping) will show how the third chromosome, number 21, is attached to another autosome in translocation or nondisjunction.

Nursing Objectives — Newborn

To establish and maintain adequate nutrition to allow for growth and development.

1 The diet is calculated according to infant's needs.
2 Due to poor muscle tone and protruding tongue, the infant may be a poor eater with a weak and ineffective suck.
 a Provide with appropriate teat so that minimal sucking effort is needed to feed.
 b Allow adequate time for feeding. Do not allow the infant to become overly tired.
 c Note and report poor eating and insufficient sucking.

To observe carefully for any signs of physical complications that may occur with Down's syndrome. Record and report them immediately.

1 Intestinal obstruction (duodenal stenosis)
 a Observe for abdominal distension and its association with feeding.
 b Note vomiting — what is vomited and when.
  (1) Bile-stained vomit indicates lower tract obstruction.
  (2) Partially digested milk indicates upper tract obstruction.
 c Note absence of stools.
2 Congenital cardiac defect
 a When taking vital signs, note any irregularity of the heart rate. Murmurs may not be evident to the untrained ear. Note any respiratory distress or laboured respirations.
 b Note any cyanosis and when it occurs — with crying, feeding, or all the time.
 c Be particularly alert to the infant tiring easily during feeding.

To provide a safe environment for the infant.

1 Infant is usually very floppy due to poor muscle tone. When handling the infant, support him well with a firm grasp.
2 Position infant in such a manner that if vomiting should occur he will not aspirate.
 a If he is on his abdomen, be certain that he can turn his head to the side.
 b Prop him with a nappy roll so that position will be maintained.
 c This infant is not usually very active; thus, his position will need to be changed frequently.

To provide proper stimulation according to the child's age.

1   Be aware that this infant needs stimulation from the very start to begin to help him develop to his potential. Develop a plan of stimulation so that your activity and actions lead towards this goal.

    a Babies with Down's syndrome who are quiet and undemanding tend to be understimulated, so they do not reach their full potential.

    b Begin a programme of mental stimulation early — one that can be continued at home.

        (1) Programme should include exercises built around existing reflexes; these can reduce hypotonia.

        (2) Encourage exercises to develop eye-hand coordination and later finger-thumb grasp.

2   Offer positive and effective sensory stimulation.

    Hold and fondle infant, especially during feeding.

3   When the infant is awake, the adult face in his visual field is good stimulation and should interest him for a few seconds.

4   The gentle sound of talking or music can provide a pleasant auditory experience. The infant should stop activity and listen.

To encourage parental participation in caring for and handling the infant and to foster acceptance of the child by his parents and family.

1   Provide opportunities for the parents to learn all aspects of caring for their baby. The basic needs of the baby with Down's syndrome are the same as those of other infants.

    Emphasize the need for parents to appreciate the child for his unique attributes; he can be lovable and can be enjoyed as a person, but he demands special attention.

2   All the support and help given the parents during hospitalization will make home care easier. Early intervention and support should strengthen and support the parental role.

    a Encourage paediatrician to have both parents present, possibly with the infant, when he tells them of child's diagnosis. In this way they can turn to each other for support.

    b Make special efforts to involve the father. Respond to his needs — he may require special attention, support, and guidance.

    c Adaptation by both parents is critical for the continual improvement of the child's functioning and to foster optimal growth and development.

    d Encourage parents to tell siblings about their 'special' baby early. Openness with the family can provide mutual support and communication.

    e Help parents to be honest in their thoughts and emotions over the baby.

    f Help parents to accept the fact that their child has Down's syndrome and to accept the child for himself.

3   Assist parents in learning what Down's syndrome is and how it alters a child's mental and physical development.

a Provide appropriate literature. (See bibliography for some suggestions.)
b Inform them of local or national organizations.
c Alert parents to some common physical deviations that occur with Down's syndrome and the consequent effect of these deviations on behaviour. If possible, provide an adjusted timetable of development which takes into account the child's handicap.
4   Initiate referral to health visitor, prior to discharge home, who will be helpful to the family in planning home care and providing support.
5   Initiate social work referral. The social worker can help parents to better understand their family situation and their feelings about their child.
6   Invite parents to join a group of parents who have children with Down's syndrome. Counselling can also alleviate the parent's loss of self-concept and feeling of self-worth.
7   Be aware of problems that new parents of a Down's syndrome baby may encounter:
a Grief for the loss of the expected normal child
b Poor communication with the baby's paediatrician
c Difficulty in telling family and friends.
8   Emphasize the infant's need for love, affection, consideration, and individual attention.

To work effectively with parents.

To accomplish this, health professionals relating to parents must:

1   Recognize and understand their own feelings about the infant.
2   Have an objective approach to each family situation.
3   Discuss all information with both parents.

The Older Child

The older child with Down's syndrome is usually admitted to the hospital because of some medical complication, such as an acute respiratory infection.

To interview the parents thoroughly at the time of admission to learn as much as possible about the child and his activities at home.

1   What is the child's vocabulary? What words or sounds does he use for elimination, certain foods, etc.?
2   Be aware of the child's schedule and activities at home.
a This patient usually functions better in a familiar environment. He may react adversely to the new situation.
b Know what activities the child can or cannot do and what he likes to do.
3   Be familiar with the child's eating habits and pattern.
a Give him foods he likes and avoid foods he dislikes.
b Adjust his mealtimes to those he is used to as much as possible and know at which mealtime he eats best.

4 Be aware of how parents discipline the child.
5 Incorporate this information into nursing care plans to assure continuity of care from home to hospital to minimize fear and frustration in the child.
6 Plan the child's day according to what he is used to as much as possible.

To attend to the child's needs according to the medical problem that required his hospitalization.

To provide a safe environment for the child according to his needs.

1 This can best be judged by observing the child and by obtaining information during the parental interview.
2 If possible, use the type of bed the child is familiar with.
3 Remove any objects which might be injurious to the child should he play with them.

To plan and provide for the appropriate type of play programme and stimulation for the child.

1 Assess the child's level of growth and development and consider this in the plan.
2 Do not try to teach the child new or different things as he may react adversely to the newness.
3 Allow the child as much independence as possible in his care, but provide guidance as necessary.
4 Permit the development of the child's abilities. Minimize frustrating situations.

To foster continuing parental acceptance of the child and to provide support for them.

1 Invite parents to care for their child as much as they can. Rooming-in may be advisable.
2 Help the parents to understand why the child behaves as he does.
3 Encourage parents to talk about their feelings or problems they have with the child. Re-emphasize the need for parents to appreciate their child for his unique attributes and special characteristics, such as sociability and sensitivity to feelings of others.
4 Initiate a teaching programme for the child and his parents early. Continued educational experiences are vital. Offer the family available literature and help its members to become familiar with community resources.
   a Parents can provide positive and effective sensory training.
   b Help child to socialize with other children and provide an environment that will stimulate him mentally.
5 Allow parents to continue to maintain what other responsibilities they may have outside the hospital, i.e. other children, work.
   Do not insist they stay at the hospital and attend only to this child.

Parental Teaching

Parental teaching is one very important aspect in the nursing care of a child with Down's syndrome, especially in the following areas:

1. The environment has an influence on the rate of the child's progress in performance, behaviour, growth, and development.

    a The role of the parents is critical. A nurturing and loving environment gives the child the best chance to develop to his full potential.

    b Encourage the entire family to be included in the child's care.

    c The child will usually be lovable and quiet, affectionate, and socially responsive if he is loved and if individual attention is given to his specific needs.

    d Patience and understanding must be developed by parents and family.

2. The child learns best in the play situation.

    a The child is slower at learning and will require more time to learn each new skill.

    b The child tends to mimic, which later results in learning.

    c He may have a sensitivity to rhythmic stimulation and usually likes music.

    d Social development is more advanced than the level of mental development.

3. Provide a safe environment.

    Because he may be less sensitive to heat, cold and pain, attention should be directed towards eliminating these hazards.

4. Help parents to understand that in spite of signs of slow mental growth, the child can make steady progress. In early life, the child with Down's syndrome should not be stereotyped in behaviour. His behaviour is similar to the norm when mental age is considered. Help parents not to lower their expectations.

    a The child needs a great deal of repetition in all areas of learning.

    b He usually has a good memory, can acquire a fairly large vocabulary and can learn to spell. Arithmetic may be more difficult for him.

    c Speech may lag behind walking by 1-2 years. He may encounter trouble in pronouncing certain words. Stammering may occur if the child is under pressure.

    d Parents need help in learning to recognize the child's readiness to learn these skills.

    e A general decrease of IQ score occurs with increasing age and should be an expected occurrence because of the increasing verbal and abstract content of test materials at the higher mental age.

5. The child's motor development is slow. The degree of hypotonia probably greatly influences the early motor development; genetic potential and environmental stimulation of the child also influence motor development.

    a Encourage motor coordination. It will take time for the child to learn to sit. At age 5 or 6 years, he may still walk like a 2-year-old child. Toilet training can generally be accomplished.

b The child's liking for music and sense of rhythm can be used to help develop motor coordination.

c He may always have trouble with fine motor skills.

d Encourage child to do as much for himself as he can.

6 Precautionary measures should be taken.

a Discuss the importance of good nutrition for growth. Supply available literature for a balanced diet appropriate for age.

b Obtain prompt treatment for any medical problems that may occur. This child is particularly prone to infection. Good nutrition, proper exercise, appropriate dress, and good general hygiene can help prevent infection.

c The child with Down's syndrome needs discipline. Limits need to be set so he knows what he can or cannot do.

7 Other members of the family must be considered.

a The child should not be thought of as a sick child, but as a child who needs special handling to promote his individual growth and development. But he does not need all the attention all the time.

b The family should be included in his care, but its members also must have lives of their own and as much parental attention as they would receive if the child were not present in the family.

c Parents need time to themselves. They should be encouraged to go out alone together and to give time to their marriage.

d Encourage parents to be open with the family and to discuss concerns. Children are sensitive to parental distress. Lack of communication can create and increase parental isolation and can cause unrealistic concerns.

e Sibling reactions generally reflect the parents' reactions toward the child with Down's syndrome.

f Assist parents to assess their family situation to promote healthy family relationships. Do the following situations exist?

(1) Are older siblings frequent caretakers of the child with Down's syndrome?

(2) Is there excessive parental attention to afflicted child at expense of other siblings?

(3) Do the parents show hostility towards the child?

(4) Are there excessive expectations of other children?

(5) Is the family dominated by the destructiveness or overactivity of child with Down's syndrome?

8 Future in society

a The child with Down's syndrome should go to school. He learns by copying. Have parents discuss the child's problem with the school nurse, the teacher, and other adults who have close contact with the child.

b Education enables the child with Down's syndrome to be productive to some extent in society, to have a fuller life, and to take pride in his accomplishments. Such children can learn routine housework, gardening, or farming. They can run errands, learn to obey traffic rules, and ride on buses.

c Help parents to discuss their feelings or plans regarding continued home care or placement in an institution.

Agencies

1   Down's Babies Association, Queenbourne Community Centre, Ridgacre Road, Quinton, Birmingham
2   See also list on p. 688.

FURTHER READING

Books

Apley J, *Care of the Handicapped Child,* Heinemann Medical, 1978.
Brooks B, *Teaching Mentally Handicapped Children: Practical Activities,* Ward Lock Educational, 1979.
Cunningham C, *Down's Syndrome: An Introduction for Parents,* Human Horizon Series, 1982.
General Nursing Council, *Aspects of Sick Children's Nursing: A Learning Package,* General Nursing Council, 1982, Study Units 40-44.
Jeffree D McConkey R, *Let Me Speak,* Human Horizons Series, 1976.
Perkins E *et al., Helping the Retarded,* British Institute of Mental Handicap, 1980.
Robinson N Robinson H, *The Mentally Retarded Child, A Psychological Approach,* McGraw-Hill, 1976.
Scipien G *et al., Comprehensive Pediatric Nursing,* McGraw-Hill, 1979.
Simon A B, *Modern Management of Mental Handicap,* MTP, 1980.

Articles

Ayer S, Handicapped children in the community, *Nursing Times,* 12 September 1980: 66-69.
Berry R, Behavioural principles, *Nursing Times,* August 1978: 1327-1330.
Bowers M, Working with preschool mentally handicapped children, *APEX,* June 1980: 22-24.
Brimblecombe F, The Honeylands project, *Journal of Maternal and Child Health,* September 1977: 361-366.
Bromley D Lister T, What the parents want, *Health and Social Services Journal,* February 1980: 225-226.
Burden R L, Measuring the effects of stress in the mothers of handicapped children, *Child Care, Health and Development,* March/April 1980: 111-125.
Bushby S, Training the mentally handicapped: the reinforcers, *Nursing Mirror,* 18 September 1980: 18-20 and 25 September 1980: 22-24.
Cowper-Smith F, Active leisure for the handicapped, *Nursing Times,* May 1977: 774-776.
Cunningham C C Sloper T, Parents of Down's syndrome babies; their early needs, *Child Care, Health and Development,* September/October 1977: 325-47.

Erickson M P, Talking with fathers of young children with Down's syndrome, *Children Today*, November/December 1974, 3: 22-25.

Evans B, Blissymbolics, *World Medicine*, August 1978: 35-36.

Harris J, Working with parents of mentally handicapped children on a long term basis, *Child Care, Health and Development*, March/April 1978: 121-130.

Kiernan C, The hands say it all, *Nursing Mirror*, 25 September 1980: 16-20.

Kirrell H G, Self mutilation in the retarded child, *Nursing Times*, November 1979: 2023-2024.

Mental handicap: progress, problems and priorities: a review of mental handicap services in England since 1971, DHSS, 1980.

Mortimore F, Making movement fun, National Society for Mentally Handicapped Children, 1977.

Oliver A, Dancing for the mentally handicapped, *Social Work Service*, 1978: 40.

O'Neil S, Behaviour modification: towards a human experience, *Nursing Clinics of North America*, June 1975, 10: 373-381.

Patullo A, The socio-sexual development of the handicapped child — a preventive care approach, *Nursing Clinics of North America*, June 1975, 10: 361-373.

Pueschel S Murphy A, Counselling parents of infants with Down's syndrome, *Postgraduate Medicine*, December 1975, 58: 90-95.

Scudamore R, Down's syndrome — learning, *Community Outlook/Nursing Times*, October 1979: 320-328.

Scully C, Something to bite on: dental care for mentally handicapped children, National Society for Mentally Handicapped Children, 1976.

Smith B Phillips C J, Identification of severe mental handicap, *Child Care, Health and Development*, May/June 1978: 195-203.

Stowitschek J Hofmeister A, Parent training packages, *Children Today*, March/April 1975, 4: 23-25.

Wordsworth E, Helping parents help each other, *Community Care*, August 1979: 22-23.

For Parents

Carr J, *Helping you Handicapped child*, Penguin, 1980.

Cunningham C Sloper P, *Helping your Handicapped Baby*, Human Horizon Series, 1978.

McCormack M, *A Mentally Handicapped Child in the Family*, Constable, 1978.

For Siblings

Grollman S H, *More Time to Grow*, Beacon Press, 1977.
Laser H, *Don't Forget Tom*, Black, 1974.
Sobel H L, *My Brother, Steven, is Retarded*, Gollancz, 1978.

15

ORTHOPAEDIC CONDITIONS

FRACTURES

Generally, nursing care of the child with a fracture is similar to that of an adult. The child is usually hospitalized only for application of a cast (see procedure for cast care, p. 228) or to be placed in traction (see procedure for traction, p. 220). The nurse should be aware of the following principles concerning fractures in paediatrics.

General Considerations

1   Bones do not fracture as easily in children as in adults.
    Bones are softer and more pliable.
2   Greenstick fractures in normal bones are unique to children.
    a The bone breaks at one cortex and bends at the other.
    b There is no complete loss of bony continuity.
    c The younger the child, the more likely he is to sustain a greenstick fracture.
    d The radius, ulna, clavicle, or long bone in the hand are most likely to sustain a greenstick fracture.
3   Comminuted fractures are less common in paediatric patients.
4   Injuries of the epiphyseal plate are unique to children.
    a The epiphyseal plate is weaker than normal tendons, ligaments, or joint capsule.
    b Injury resulting in a torn ligament or dislocation in the adult is more likely to produce a separation of the epiphysis in a child.
    c The lower radial epiphysis is more frequently separated than any other.
    d This type of injury may cause growth disturbance.
5   Fractures in paediatric patients heal more readily than those in adults.
    a The younger the child, the more rapidly the fracture unites.
    b The thick periosteum and abundant blood supply make nonunion rare.
6   End-to-end apposition of fracture surfaces is not essential in paediatric patients.

a The long bones may be allowed to unite with side-to-side apposition in children up to 11-12 years of age.

b Subsequent moulding will produce a normal bone by the end of growth.

7   Following injury, the limbs in children are likely to swell much more rapidly and the swelling to disappear more quickly than in an adult.

8   Function is usually restored rapidly and sometimes spontaneously following injury in children.

Common Fractures in Children

Fracture of the Clavicle

Cause

1   Compression of the shoulders during delivery of a baby
2   Transmitted force caused by falling on an outstretched hand, elbow, or side of the shoulder
3   Direct force (rare).

Treatment

1   Immobilization with a figure of eight bandage or plaster of Paris cast.
2   Complete fixation by supporting the limb in a triangular sling suspended from the opposite shoulder.
     This treatment is helpful if the child demonstrates associated torticollis.

Healing Time

1   Younger children: 3-4 weeks
2   Older children: 5-6 weeks.

Fracture of the Neck of the Humerus

Cause

1   Indirect force from a fall on an outstretched hand
2   Direct force by blow or fall on the lateral aspect of the shoulder.

Treatment

1   Minimal displacement
     Immobilization of the shoulder and upper limb in a collar and cuff sling with application of external splint.
2   Considerable displacement of bone fragments
     a Open operation under anaesthesia may be needed.

b Immobilization of the shoulder and upper arm initially in shoulder spica, then with collar and cuff sling.

Healing Time

1 Minimal displacement: 3-4 weeks
2 Considerable displacement: 4-6 weeks.

Fractures of the Shaft of the Humerus

Cause

1 Birth injury — most common long bone to be fractured at that time
2 Direct force, such as a fall on the side of the arm
3 Indirect force, such as throwing a ball, grabbing a child's arm to prevent a fall, and pulling an arm in and out of a sleeve roughly.

Treatment

1 Reduction of the fracture
2 Immobilization
   a Young children
   (1) Application of collar and cuff sling with a hanging plaster or gutter splints.
   (2) If union fails (in a small percentage of children only), bone grafting will be required.
   b Older children or adolescents
   (1) A shoulder spica cast is used for an unstable fracture.
   (2) Skeletal traction and suspension of the forearm and hand are indicated if the local skin and soft tissue conditions do not permit skin traction.
   (3) A hanging cast may be used for an older adolescent.
      (a) This type of cast permits the child to be ambulatory and active.
      (b) Erect position should be maintained as much as possible during the day.
      (c) The child should sleep in a semirecumbent position.
      (d) There should be no support at the elbow.
      (e) Pressure from clothing or anything that might compress the arm against the body must be avoided as it interferes with traction.

Healing Time

4-6 weeks.

Supracondylar Fracture of the Humerus

Cause

Fall on an outstretched hand with hyperextension of the elbow (most common type of elbow fracture in children and adolescents).

Treatment

1 Should be managed as an acute emergency because of the danger of neuro-vascular complications: Volkmann's ischaemic contracture.
2 Fracture reduced by direct traction and manual pressure on displaced fragment.
3 Application of collar and cuff sling with elbow flexed to just above a right angle.
4 Circulation must be carefully assessed at regular intervals.

Healing Time

1 3-6 weeks.
2 Several months may be required for complete restoration of function.

Complications

1 Malunion and changes in carrying angle
2 Vascular complications
   The extremity should be observed for pallor, pain, absent pulse, paresthesia, and paralysis.

Fractures of the Distal Third of the Radius and Ulna

Cause

1 Fracture may result from indirect force, such as falling on an outstretched hand.
2 Bones may break at different levels, and each fracture may be complete or greenstick.

Treatment

1 Greenstick fracture
   a Closed reduction if the degree of angulation exceeds 30° in infants or 15° in children
   b Immobilization in a long arm cast
2 Complete fracture
   a Reduction under anaesthesia
   b Immobilization in an above-elbow cast.

Healing Time

4-6 weeks.

Fractures Involving the Distal Radial Physis

Cause

1   Indirect force by falling on an outstretched hand
2   Most common physical injury.

Treatment

1   Closed reduction
2   Immobilization in a long arm cast.

Healing Time

3-4 weeks.

Femoral Shaft Fracture

Cause

1   Major force, either direct or indirect, such as that sustained in motor vehicle accidents or falls from a height
2   Requires treatment as serious injury because of the blood loss and potential shock which may accompany the primary trauma.

Treatment

1   Infants and children under 2 years of age
    a Gallow's or Bryant's traction for 2-3 weeks until the fracture is stable
    b Occasionally immobilization in a hip spica cast may be required.
2   Older children and adolescents
    Reduction and fixed traction until fracture is stable. Traction is usually with a Thomas splint. Sometimes internal traction is required, e.g. with a Küntscher intramedullary rod.

Healing Time

3-12 weeks, depending on the child's age and the type of fracture.

Complications

1   Discrepancy in limb length
2   Angular deformities of the femoral shaft.

Fracture of the Tibia or Fibula

Cause

1 Direct force
2 Indirect rotational twisting force.

Treatment

1 Closed reduction
2 Immobilization in a long leg cast — during the final weeks of healing, partial weight-bearing in a walking cast may be permitted.

Healing Time

3-6 weeks, depending on the age of the child and the type of fracture.

OSTEOMYELITIS

Osteomyelitis is an infection which may involve all parts of a bone.

Aetiology

1 Pathogenic bacteria commonly associated with osteomyelitis
   a *Staphylococcus aureus* — responsible for the majority of cases (up to 90%)
   b Streptococcal organisms
   c *Salmonella*
   d *Proteus*
   e *Pseudomonas*
2 Identifiable primary lesions
   a Furunculosis
   b Impetigo
   c Vaccinations
   d Infected chicken-pox
   e Burns
   f Infected scratches, pimples, or boils
   g Nose or throat infections
   h Abscessed teeth
3 Preconditions favouring development of osteomyelitis in children
   a Bone regions that have suffered trauma
   b Bone that suffers from low oxygen tension of sickle cell anaemia.

Incidence

1 Most frequent occurrence between 5-14 years of age
2 More frequent in males than in females.

Altered Physiology

1 Infection starts in the soft, medullary tissues.
2 This causes hyperaemia, changes in the capillary permeability and oedema of the tissue.
3 Granulocytic leucocytes infiltrate the area and are destroyed by bacteria, liberating a proteolytic enzyme which causes tissue necrosis.
4 The inflammatory reaction causes thrombosis of vessels, producing irregular areas of bone ischaemia.
5 Pus forms and spreads toward the diaphysis and extends through the cortex of the bone.
6 A subperiosteal abscess is formed with elevation of the periosteum.
7 There is further interference of blood supply to the bone shaft.
  a Vascular supply may remain sufficient to maintain life of bone tissue:
    (1) New bone is created.
    (2) Bone healing occurs.
  b Vascular supply may be diminished below that which is necessary to maintain life of bone tissue.
    (1) Bone dies and becomes inert.
    Small pieces of dead bone may be completely destroyed by granulation tissue from contiguous living tissue.
    (2) Large pieces of dead bone cannot be completely destroyed.
      (a) Central residual remains as a sequestrum composed of cancellous or cortical bone or a combination.
      (b) New bone is laid down beneath the elevated periosteum and tends to form an encasement (involucrum) around the sequestrum.
      (c) The involucrum is punctured by numerous channels through which pus may escape from the inside.
      (d) Pockets of infection are walled off in which organisms can lie dormant for long periods of time.
      (e) Chronic sinuses may form which eventually reach the surface and drain.
      (f) Drainage continues until infection quiets once more.
      Channels become plugged up with granulations and remain closed until the pressure of the pus builds up and causes the sinuses to reopen or reach the surface via new channels (chronic osteomyelitis).
      (g) Complete healing takes place only when all of the dead bone has been destroyed, discharged, or excised.

Clinical Manifestations

Onset

1 Usually abrupt
2 May be altered when osteomyelitis follows an infection which has been treated by antibiotics.

Initial Symptoms

1 Pain in the involved area
2 Fever
3 Malaise.

Later Symptoms

1 Swelling and redness over the affected bone
2 Weakness
3 Irritability
4 Generalized signs of sepsis.

Common Sites of Infection in Children

1 Large, cylindrical bones of the extremities
   a Femur
   b Tibia
   c Humerus
   d Radius
2 Primary focus is usually in the metaphysis of a bone at the end of the area of most rapid growth
   a Knee region
   b Lower end of the femur
   c Upper end of the tibia.

Diagnostic Evaluation

1 Leucocytosis.
2 Blood culture — usually positive.
3 Sedimentation rate usually elevated.
4 X-rays show:
   a Progressive findings
      (1) Periosteal reaction
      (2) Areas of radiolucency secondary to bone destruction
      (3) Evidence of the formation of involucrum (reactive, living bone).
   b Progress of the disease not seen on x-ray for at least 5 days in small children; as long as 8-10 days in older children.
5 Tomography may reveal bone changes at an early stage.

Treatment

1 Intravenous administration of antimicrobial therapy
2 Immobilization of the affected extremity
3 Surgical decompression of the infected bony area may be necessary with insertion of drains.

Prognosis

1 Mortality rate markedly improved with the advent of antibiotics
2 Depends on early institution of appropriate therapy and adequate continuation.

Nursing Objectives

To treat the infection with antibiotic therapy.

1 Administer intravenous antibiotic as prescribed by the paediatrician or orthopaedic surgeon.
   a Administer medication exactly on schedule in order to maintain consistent blood levels.
   b Monitor intravenous infusion carefully, if instituted.
   (1) Notify paediatrician if infiltration is suspected, so that the intravenous infusion can be restarted.
   (2) A venous cutdown is often necessary, especially for a small child.
   (3) A constant infusion pump may be helpful if the infusion rate is slow.
   (4) A heparin lock may be useful, because it allows the child to be more active between medication doses.
2 Be alert for evidence of drug reactions.

To increase the child's comfort.

1 Administer analgesics as ordered by the paediatrician.
2 Rest the affected extremity.
   a Traction or splints may be used to reduce pain and prevent contractures in the soft tissues.
   b Avoid excessive handling of the infected extremity, because this is very painful and may spread infection.
   (1) Bed clothes should be changed only when necessary.
   (2) When it is necessary to move the extremity, support the joints above and below the affected part as well as the area itself.
   (3) Move the extremity in a smooth, unhurried, and gentle manner.

To protect other patients and personnel from the infectious organism.

1 Isolate children with draining wounds.
2 Utilize careful handwashing procedure.
3 Utilize strict aseptic technique when performing irrigations, changing dressings, and handling drainage.

To facilitate wound healing.

Maintain adequate nutrition and hydration.

1 Offer abundant fluids according to the child's preference.

2 Provide a diet which is rich in protein and vitamin C.
3 Offer child a choice of known favourite foods.
4 Refer to section on nutrition, p. 36.

To observe for evidence of response to treatment or progress of disease.

1 Monitor the child's temperature at frequent intervals and record the pattern.
   Notify the paediatrician of a sudden increase in temperature.
2 Monitor and record the extent of swelling, redness, pain, and limitation of movement in the affected extremity.
3 Monitor and record the amount and nature of drainage if the infection has been drained.

To provide emotional support to the parents.

1 Parents often feel guilty if they did not recognize early signs of the disease.
2 Assist parents to express and deal with their feelings.
   Refer to social worker if appropriate.
3 Refer to section on family-centred care, p. 66.

To assist the child to maintain many of his normal activities during the lengthy hospitalization.

1 Allow the child to be dressed in normal clothes even when on bed rest.
2 Encourage the child to attend playroom activities, even if he must be moved in his bed.
3 Plan nursing care programme which allows time for hospital school activities to ensure that ongoing education is maintained.
4 Encourage visiting by family and friends.

To provide for continuity of care following the child's discharge from the hospital.

1 Encourage parents to participate in all aspects of the child's care during hospitalization.
   a Parents should be instructed and should have an opportunity to practise (under nursing supervision) all procedures which will be required at home. (Procedures often include changes of dressing, application of a splint, or use of appliances such as crutches.)
   b The child should not be discharged until both the parents and the nurse are satisfied with the parents' level of competence.
2 Instruct parents to observe for evidence of complications, such as deformity, stiffness of joints, fracture, and disease recurrence.
3 Refer to community nursing service if appropriate.

CONGENITAL DISLOCATION OF THE HIP

Congenital dislocation of the hip refers to a malposition of the head of the femur in the acetabulum. The head of the femur is usually dislocated posterosuperiorly. Dislocation may be either partial or complete and may be either unilateral or bilateral.

Aetiology

1   Unknown
2   Possible.causes
  a Abnormal development of the joint caused by:
    (1) Fetal position
    (2) Genetic factors
  b Abnormal relaxation of the capsule and ligaments of the joint caused by hormonal factors
  c Environmental factors such as breech delivery.

Altered Physiology

1   Acetabulum tends to be shallow and extremely oblique.
2   Head of the femur tends to be smaller than normal.
3   Ossification centres are delayed in appearance.

Incidence

1   More common in female infants than in males.
2   Recurrence risk among siblings is greater when one child in the family has been affected.

Clinical Manifestations

(May not be observed until 1-2 months of age)

1   Asymmetry of the gluteal folds with deeper creases apparent on the affected side.
2   Limited ability to abduct the hip when the infant is lying on his back with his knees and hips flexed to 90°.
      Normally, the hips will abduct at least 65°.
3   Trendelenburg's sign.
      Pelvis drops on the normal side if the child stands on his abnormal leg.
4   Apparent shortening of the thigh.
5   Knee joint on the affected side appears higher than the normal joint.
6   Delayed walking.
7   Limp.
  a Trunk dips when the child puts weight on his involved leg.
  b Waddling gait is observed in children with bilateral dislocation.

Diagnostic Evaluation

1 Barlow's test
   a With the infant on a firm surface, the examiner grasps the symphysis pubis in front and the sacrum in back with one hand. The second hand grasps the thigh on the side of the hip being tested.
   b Slight outward pressure is applied over the proximal thigh by the thumb while longitudinal pressure is applied in an effort to dislocate the hip out of its socket.
   c Sensation of abnormal movement indicates a dislocation.
2 Ortolani's test
   a The examiner positions his hands in the same manner as for Barlow's test.
   b The thigh is brought away from the midline of the body into a position of abduction.
   c A sensation or sound of a clicking or jerking into place may be detected with reduction of the head into the socket.
3 X-ray data (helpful only after the age of 4-5 months, when the hip bones are sufficiently developed)
   a Upper end of the femur does not point into the acetabulum.
   b Poor development of the acetabulum.

Treatment

1 Varies with age and extent of the defect.
2 Early stages
   a Reduction by gentle manipulation
   b Splinting the hip in abduction by means of double or triple nappies, an abduction splint, or a cloth harness
3 Later stages
   a Preliminary traction
   b Closed reduction
   c Immobilization in a hip spica cast or splint
4 Older child
   a Preliminary traction
   b Possible need for open reduction or osteotomy
   c Immobilization in a hip spica cast.

Prognosis

1 Depends on the age of the child when the condition is diagnosed.
2 Delay in diagnosis prolongs treatment and may preclude formation of a normal hip.

Nursing Management

Generally, nursing care of the child with congenital dislocation of the hip is provided by the mother at home supported by the primary health care team with visits to the orthopaedic outpatient clinics. This regime combines to keep hospital inpatient stay to the minimum. Nursing activities during hospitalization are those related to the child's care when he is in traction or after application of a hip spica cast (refer to p. 220). In addition, the following considerations are important:

1   If the child is to be treated with an abduction splint, explain its purpose and demonstrate its application to the parents.

   a Allow parents to practise application of the splint with nursing supervision.

   b Clarify with parents the times that the splint is to be worn and how long it can be removed for bathing, dressing, nappy changes, etc.

   c Demonstrate handling of the child in such a way that the hips are kept abducted.

2   Encourage family-centred care (refer to p. 66).

CONGENITAL CLUBFOOT (TALIPES EQUINOVARUS)

Congenital clubfoot refers to a deformity in which the affected foot and leg have a clublike appearance. Talipes equinovarus is one of the most common congenital deformities of the foot, occurring in approximately one in 1000 live births.

Aetiology

1   Exact cause unknown.

2   Evidence indicates a mixed genetic and environmental causation.

3   Tends to recur in families already having one affected child.

4   Males are affected twice as often as females.

Pathophysiology

1   Pathological anatomy

   a Inversion and abduction of the forepart of the foot

   b Inversion of the heel

   c Equinus fixation of the foot in plantar flexion at the ankle and subtalar joints.

2   Soft tissue changes are adaptive in nature, conforming to the skeletal deformity.

    The soft tissues on the medial and posterior aspect of the foot and ankle are shortened.

Clinical Manifestations

1 Varies in severity from a mild deformity to one in which the toes touch the medial side of the lower leg.
   a Rigid type
      (1) Very severe deformity
      (2) Corrected only minimally by passive manipulation
      (3) Usually accompanied by moderate atrophy of the leg.
   b Flexible type
   The condition can be readily corrected to neutral position by passive manipulation.
2 Deformity increases progressively, and contractures become more rigid if the deformity is untreated.
   a Child bears weight on the lateral border of the foot.
   b Ambulation is difficult and gait is awkward.
   c Callosities and bursae may develop over the lateral side of the foot.

Diagnostic Evaluation

1 Diagnosis is determined by clinical manifestations.
2 X-ray valuable for the following:
   a Determination of the degree of varus and equinus deformity
   b Demonstration of the deranged mechanics of the hindfoot
   c Accurate assessment of the amount of correction obtained with treatment.

Treatment and Nursing Management

1 Passive stretching exercises to manipulate the foot into normal position
   a Technique of manipulation should be demonstrated to the nurse and parents by the physiotherapist, because there are many variations in the manner of performing the manipulation.
   b The foot should be grasped well below the malleoli with one hand while the ankle is held rigid and stable with the other hand to avoid displacement of the epiphysis.
   c The midfoot should not be stretched by forced dorsiflexion of the forefoot, or a 'rocker-bottom' foot will result.
   d The corrected position should be maintained to the count of 10.
   e The exercises should be continued for 10-15 minutes several times each day.
   f Manipulation should be done before feeding, because it may cause some discomfort for the baby.
2 Adhesive strapping
   a The foot is held in corrected position by adhesive strapping.
   The adhesive is applied only to the outer side of the leg and ankle to

prevent obstruction of circulation or of further correction by manipulation.

b Manipulation exercises should be continued before each feeding.

c The strapping may be changed or reinforced by an additional layer of adhesive tape if necessary.

3   Manipulation and casting

a A plaster of Paris cast is applied from the toes to the groin with the knee flexed.

Casts are changed frequently; with each cast change the foot is manipulated to obtain further correction.

b Once the deformity is fully corrected, the foot is held in an overcorrected position in a solid cast for 3-6 weeks.

(1) Parents should be instructed in cast care. (Refer to p. 228.)

(2) Parents should be alerted that if the foot portion of the cast becomes thin or worn, the cast should be reapplied.

4   Denis Browne splint

a The splint is composed of a flexible horizontal bar attached to a pair of footplates.

(1) The infant's feet are attached to the footplates by means of special shoes or adhesive tape.

(2) The desired position of the foot is controlled by positioning the abduction bar and the footplates.

(3) The infant provides his own corrective manipulation of his normal activity.

b Parents should be instructed in the following details of care:

(1) Application and removal of the splint

(2) Times the splint is to be worn

(3) Protection of the feet by socks

(4) Skin care

(5) Use of splint key to tighten the shoes against the bar if they become loose.

5   Continued treatment

a Treatment is continued until the child is able to walk normally and until the wear on several pairs of shoes demonstrates that there has been no recurrence of deformity.

b Foot is held in an overcorrected position at night by means of bivalved casts or a Denis Browne splint.

c A prewalker clubfoot shoe with valgus strap may be prescribed for the infant's use during the day.

d An older child may require special shoes which promote walking in the overcorrected position.

e Passive stretching exercises are continued.

6   Indications for surgical measures

a Failure of conservative methods to correct the deformity.

b In older children severe and rigid deformities which will obviously not respond to nonsurgical measures.

PERTHES DISEASE

Perthes disease is an aseptic necrosis of the capital femoral epiphysis secondary to ischaemia.

Aetiology

Unknown.

Incidence

1 Males between the ages of 4-10 years of age are most frequently affected.
2 Condition tends to recur in families.

Clinical Manifestations

(May be intermittent initially.)

1 Synovitis causing limp and pain in the hip
2 Referred pain to the knee, inner thigh, and groin
3 Limited abduction and internal rotation of the hip
4 Mild to moderate muscle spasm
5 Atrophy of the muscles of the mid and upper thigh
6 Bilateral involvement is infrequent.

Altered Physiology

Stage I (Avascularity)

1 Spontaneous interruption of the blood supply to the upper femoral epiphysis occurs.
2 Bone-forming cells in the epiphysis die and bone ceases to grow.
3 Slight widening of the joint space occurs.
4 Swelling of the soft tissues around the hip occurs.

Stage II (Revascularization)

1 Growth of new vessels supplies the area of necrosis; both bone resorption and deposition take place.
2 The new bone is not strong, and pathological fractures occur.
3 Abnormal forces on the weakened epiphysis may produce progressive deformity, including lateral epiphyseal fracture and extrusion of the femoral head laterally from the acetabulum.

Stage III (Reossification)

1 The head of the femur gradually reforms.

2   Nucleus of the epiphysis breaks up into a number of fragments with cyst-like spaces between them.
3   New bone starts to develop at the medial and lateral edges of the epiphysis which becomes widened.
4   Dead bone is removed and is replaced with new bone which gradually spreads to heal the lesion.

Stage IV (Postrecovery period)

1   Without treatment
    a Head of the femur flattens and becomes mushroom shaped.
    b Incongruity between the head of the femur and the acetabulum persists.
    c Degenerative changes develop later in life.
2   Complete recovery
    a Head of the femur remains spherical.
    b Acetabulum appears normal.
    c Width of the neck of the femur is normal.

Diagnostic Evaluation

X-ray findings are related to the stage of the disease.

1   Incipient period
    a Swelling of the capsular shadows about the hip
    b Widening of the joint space
    c Demineralization of the femoral metaphysis in the neck
    d Evidence of growth cessation of the proximal femoral epiphysis
2   Period of necrosis
    Increased density of the femoral head is observed in addition to the above changes.
3   Regenerative period
    a Radiolucent areas — indication of revitalization of the femoral head
    b Considerable flattening and widening of the femoral head
    c Regeneration of the femoral head occurring until the head is filled in completely.

Treatment

(Depends on type of involvement)

1   First goal — to restore full range of motion of the hip joint by alleviating synovitis and muscle spasm
    Bed rest with or without traction
2   Second goal — to locate the femoral head deep in the acetabulum, thereby protecting it while revascularization and growth occur
    a Abduction spica

b Abduction splint

c Patten bottom splint

d Femoral osteotomy

e Full activity and full weight-bearing are feasible only if the first stage of the disease is clearly over and there has been minimal involvement of the femoral head

3 Final goal — to return to weight-bearing

a Justified only when there have been no new dense areas in the femoral head for 2 months

b The child must have full range of motion at the hip joint

c There must be evidence that reconstruction is taking place in the femoral head.

Prognosis

1 Depends on the stage at which the disease was diagnosed and treatment was instituted.

a Treatment is more effective when it is begun early in the disease.

b Treatment is considered successful if the contour of the hip joint allows normal function after resolution of the disease.

2 The disease may be present for 2-4 years, after which time it spontaneously resolves.

3 Limitation of motion and incongruity of joint surfaces may result if treatment is ineffective; condition may lead to degenerative joint disease in later life.

Nursing Objectives

To care for the child requiring traction or a spica cast.

Refer to relevant procedures, pp. 220 and 228.

To evaluate the home and provide guidance to the family regarding the child's home care.

1 This guidance is important, because treatment may be continued in the home for an extended period.

2 Consult with the primary health care team to arrange for support services to child and family.

3 Encourage family participation in the child's care so that members can become familiar with the details of his management. (Refer to section on family-centred care, p. 66.)

4 A firm mattress is necessary, together with a bed cradle.

To enable the child to participate in as many normal activities of life as possible.

1 Plans must be made for continuing education.

2   Diversion is an extremely important consideration.
3   Play should include exercise for uninvolved extremities.
4   Special activities with peers should be arranged.

To provide emotional support to the child and his family because of the long-term nature of the illness.

1   Provide the family with frequent opportunities to express their feelings and concerns.
    Techniques of therapeutic play should be used with the child.
2   Point out even small indications of the recovery process.
3   Introduce the family to other families with similarly affected children, if available.

Patient and Parental Education

1   General techniques of home nursing
    a Bathing and skin care
    b Maintenance of good muscle tone, proper body alignment and prevention of contractures
    c Provision for elimination
    d Nutritional considerations
    e Bedmaking
    f Special equipment (e.g. traction, casts)
2   Pathology of the disease and rationale of treatment
    a Reinforce medical explanations and clarify interpretations as necessary.
    b Allow the child to view his own x-rays with his parents, to increase his knowledge of the disease.
    c Emphasize that complete recovery can occur only with strict adherence to the treatment regimen.
3   Necessity of regular medical follow-up for evaluation of the child's progress.

STRUCTURAL SCOLIOSIS

Structural scoliosis is a lateral curvature of the spine characterized by a defect in the bones and surrounding tissues of the spine.

Classification

1   According to the spinal segment involved
    a Thoracic
    b Lumbar
    c Thoracolumbar
2   According to age group

a Infantile — birth to 3 years
b Juvenile — 4-9 years
c Adolescent — 10 years to cessation of growth (usually found in females, with a right thoracic curve most common).

Aetiology

1 Idiopathic
   a Accounts for 80% of cases
   b Possible familial incidence
2 Congenital
   a Failure of vertebral formation
   b Failure of segmentation
3 Neuropathic — results from conditions such as poliomyelitis, cerebral palsy, paralysis, and neurofibromatosis
4 Myopathic — associated with conditions such as muscular dystrophy and myopathies
5 Osteopathic — results from conditions such as fractures, bone disease, arthritis, and infection
6 Trauma such as fractures, burns, thoracoplasty
7 Irritative phenomena such as spinal cord tumour or nerve root irritation
8 Miscellaneous — Marfan's syndrome, postirradiation, metabolic, nutritional, or endocrinic factors.

Clinical Manifestations

1 Presenting complaints
   a Poor posture
   b One shoulder higher than the other
   c Hemline hanging unevenly
   d One hip that seems more prominent
   e Crooked neck
   f Lump on back
   g Waistline uneven
   h One breast appearing larger
2 Visualization of deformity
3 Occasionally back pain

Note: It is very rare for scoliosis to cause any discomfort before middle age, yet the earlier scoliosis of the spine is treated, the better the long term results. Screening programmes by school nurses to detect this condition at an early stage are now routinely being carried out in some schools.

Pathophysiology

1   Lateral flexion of a scoliotic spine causes the trunk to shift away from the midline, altering the centre of gravity and causing shortening of the spine.
2   Simultaneously, the spine rotates on its longitudinal axis, contributing to many of the clinical manifestations.
3   The vertebrae become permanently wedge-shaped.
4   The scoliosis is increased by additional factors:
    a The weight of the trunk itself.
    b The muscles on the concave side, being contracted, have a mechanical advantage over the lengthened muscles on the convex side.
    c Disturbed forces on active growing vertebral elements bring about structural changes in the bone.
5   Changes occur in the shape of the rib cage.
    a The thoracic cavity narrows.
    b The ribs do not move in a plane which allows normal expansion of the lungs.
6   Untreated scoliosis may cause back pain, degenerative arthritis, and disturbances in cardiopulmonary function in later life.

Diagnostic Evaluation

1   Detailed history from patient, parent, and other family members
2   Thorough examination of the back with patient first in the forward bent position and then standing erect
3   Assessment of the neurological status of the lower limbs
4   Inclusion of clinical photographs in the record for future reference
5   X-ray of the spine to identify and measure primary and compensating curves
6   Pulmonary function studies for children who require surgery to predict risk of postoperative respiratory complications
7   Intravenous pyelography for children with congenital scoliosis because of a high evidence of associated renal anomalies.

Treatment

1   Milwaukee brace and exercises
    May eliminate the need for surgery or may prevent a curvature from becoming worse.
2   Casts — used preoperatively to correct a curvature or postoperatively to maintain correction
    a Localizer cast — utilizes cephalopelvic traction as well as pressure directly over the major curves to provide correction
    b Cotrel's EDF (elongation, derotation, and flexion) cast — used to correct the rib lump of severe thoracic curves

3   Traction — used preoperatively to stretch out soft tissue structures or correct spinal curvature
     a Cotrel traction — used for soft tissue stretching around moderate curves
     b Halofemoral and halopelvic traction — used to correct severe and resistant curves
     The child may be returned to traction postoperatively.
4   Surgery
     a Harrington instrumentation and posterior spinal fusion
        (1) Indications:
           (a) Thoracic curves of 40-70°
           (b) Double major curves
           (c) Paralytic scoliosis in which the whole spine is involved, necessitating fusion from the upper thoracic spine, possibly to the sacrum
        (2) A plaster of Paris jacket is usually required for 6 weeks-1 year postoperatively to maintain correction depending on the age of the child and the type of scoliosis.
     b Dwyer instrumentation and anterior spinal fusion
        (1) Indications:
           (a) Severe lumbar or thoracolumbar lordosis
           (b) Problems such as myelomeningocele that preclude a posterior approach
           (c) When maximum correction is essential
           (d) For effective derotation of rotated spines
           (e) When previous posterior approaches have failed
        (2) A plaster of Paris jacket is usually required postoperatively for 3-4 months to maintain correction.

Prognosis

Best when curve is mild at the time of initial diagnosis and effective treatment is initiated early.

Nursing Objectives

To care for the child who is using a Milwaukee brace.

1   Educate the child and parents concerning the brace and supplemental exercise programme.
     a Clarify goals of therapy with the family.
     b Exercises are prescribed to increase muscle strength of the torso to counteract the effects of splinting and to assist actively in correcting the abnormal curves and rib deformities.
     c Offer incentives for compliance with the recommended treatment programme.

2   Prevent break in tissue integrity.
   a Provide meticulous skin care to areas in contact with the brace.
   b Use a smooth-fitting vest or stockinette under the brace to protect the skin.
   c Examine skin surfaces for evidence of pressure areas.
   d Have brace adjusted if skin breakdown occurs because of improper fit.
3   Assist child and family to modify normal activities such as bathing and dressing to accommodate the brace.
   a Clothing must be loose or must be purchased in larger sizes to fit over the outside of the appliance.
   b Hair washing can be facilitated by wheeling a stretcher bed up to a sink, or by having the patient lie with the head extended over the side of the bed above a washbasin. Shampoo spray attachement fitted on to the taps will make the procedure easier.

To care for the child in Cotrel traction.

Refer to section on traction, p. 220.

To care for the child in halopelvic/femoral traction.

Refer to section on traction, p. 220.

To prepare the child for surgical correction (spinal fusion).

1   Explain to the child and his parents the nature of the care immediately before surgery, the anaesthesia, postoperative care, and appearance.
2   Introduce the child and his parents to a nurse from the intensive care unit if the child will be transferred there postoperatively.
3   Have the child practise aspects of the anticipated therapy, such as deep breathing and other respiratory routines, leg exercises, logrolling, use of the Stryker frame or CircOlectric bed, and use of the fracture bedpan.

To provide postoperative care to the child following spinal fusion.

1   Observe for signs of hypotension.
   a Monitor fluid balance.
   b Maintain blood pressure at desired level; report changes.
2   Observe wound for bleeding, haematoma, or infection.
   a Maintain aseptic technique when caring for the wound.
   b Report any redness, swelling, drainage, or heat in the incisional area.
3   Relieve pain.
   a Identify causes of pain through discussion with patient and through observation.
   b Administer analgesic therapy as ordered by the surgeon.
4   Maintain tissue integrity.
   a Turn patient as ordered. (Usually patient is turned by logrolling at 2-hour intervals.)

b Provide skin care with each turning manoeuvre.

c Use sheepskin under pressure areas.

5   Prevent respiratory complications.

Utilize breathing exercises, blow bottles, and/or intermittent positive pressure to increase respiratory exchange.

6   Observe for neurological deficits.

Assess neurological status regularly, including dorsiflexion, mobility of legs, perineal sensation, and bladder function.

7   Observe for evidence of urinary retention which may develop as an effect of anaesthesia, neurological trauma, hypovolaemia, or drugs.

a Maintain careful record of intake and output.

b Notify surgeon if patient does not micturate within 8 hours following surgery.

c Care for the urethral catheter if present.

8   Observe for signs of paralytic ileus.

Note hypoactive and hyperactive bowel sounds, nausea, vomiting, or abdominal pain as diet is gradually increased.

9   Prevent development of thrombophlebitis.

a Have patient do leg exercises.

b Observe for leg swelling, redness, or pain upon dorsiflexion; also note chest symptoms such as dyspnoea, chest pain, or haemoptysis.

10   Prevent displacement of the rod or hook.

a Do not lift patient under the axillae.

b Use turning sheet.

c Instruct patient not to lift hands over head.

11   Maintain adequate nutrition and hydration.

a Be aware of normal requirements for size and age.

b Evaluate nutritional value of diet and provide appropriate supplements.

12   Provide a safe environment for the patient.

a Place the bed so that it is not easily jolted.

b Be certain that all equipment is in good working order and that all staff are familiar with its use.

To care for the child following application of a jacket cast.

1   Observe for evidence of compromised circulation.

Report changes in colour, sensation, temperature of extremities, respiratory compromise, or abdominal distress.

2   Prevent potential trauma.

a Help patient to accept the realities of limited activity by providing safe alternatives.

b Facilitate patient's getting in and out of bed by use of a hospital bed.

c Teach patient safe methods of becoming mobile.

3   For additional information related to cast care, refer to section on casts, p. 220.

To provide emotional support to the child.

1   Allow the child to continue as many of his normal activities as possible.
   a Continue schooling.
   b Encourage peer and sibling visiting or telephone contact.
2   Provide diversional activities.
   a Assess patient's interests and provide things that he can do within the limits of his position.
   b Use prism glasses, mirrors, bedboards and easels.
   c Bring others into the patient's room or bed area and transport the patient in his bed to the recreation room as soon as his condition allows.
   d Establish a regular routine of care in nursing plan that allows flexibility for special treats and events.
3   Be sensitive to the patient's concerns about body image and intervene appropriately.
   a Many adolescent girls express concerns that the cast will prevent growth or change the shape of their breasts, or that menstruation will temporarily cease while they are in the cast.
   b Patients may feel vulnerable because of the restrictions imposed by casts or traction.
4   Provide as much privacy as possible especially during bathing, toileting, and cast changing.
5   Refer to section on the hospitalized adolescent, p. 65.

To prepare the patient and family for discharge.

1   Have patient and family practise cast care during hospitalization.
2   Demonstrate techniques of personal hygiene, including such matters as special skin care and hair washing.
3   Assist patient to develop an exercise programme within limitations but adequate to maintain muscle tone after consultation with the physiotherapist.
4   Provide dietary instructions, including basic nutritional needs for age and necessary modifications because of immobilization.
5   Provide assistive devices to facilitate physical care needs.
6   Prearrange home equipment with available services.
7   Provide continuity by liaison with the community nursing service.
8   Arrange for transportation and/or social service assistance if needed.

RICKETS

Rickets can occur as a result of:

1   Lack of vitamin D
2   Insufficient intake of calcium and phosphorus in the diet
3   Lack of sunshine.

Incidence

Uncommon, but may be seen in the children of immigrant families in cities, e.g. Glasgow or London. The most active signs of rickets appear in children between 6 months and 2 years of age.

Clinical Manifestations

1 Pallor and anaemia. Lethargy but sometimes restlessness.
2 Muscles generally soft and flabby. Rickets may be seen in fat babies as well as undernourished ones.
3 Craniotabes — thinning of the suture line. The skull becomes thickened and bossed.
4 Bones of the legs bend, giving rise to either knock-knees or bow legs.
5 Delayed closure of fontanelles.
6 Harrison's sulcus to form rickety rosary and pigeon chest. Dentition is delayed.
7 Tetany or convulsions in more serious states.

Clinical Evaluation

1 X-ray
2 Plasma inorganic phosphate reduced. Alkaline phosphatase raised.
3 Low plasma calcium with children showing signs of tetany.

Treatment

1 Daily administration of 1000-5000 i.u. of vitamin D will produce healing of bone.
2 Suitable diet, according to age of child and parents' religious faith, should contain sufficient protein, calcium, and phosphorus (see p. 36).
3 Orthopaedic correction of any deformity if necessary.

Parental Support and Education

The primary health care team, i.e. health visitor, general practitioner, social worker, will need to provide support and guidance concerning the child's development, environment and nutritional state. Advice on nutrition may also be sought from the hospital dietician.

GENUVALGUM (KNOCK-KNEE)

Knock-knee is extremely common in childhood, often associated with overweight. Rickets, however, should always be excluded.

As the child begins to bear weight on everted ankles, the weight causes knock-knees to develop as a compensatory factor.

Treatment

Shoes build up on the 'turned-in' or valgus edge of the foot will often provide the cure for the knock-knee and the valgus ankles in about 5 years. In severe cases night splints may be prescribed, rarely osteotomy may be required.

FURTHER READING

Books

Blockley N J, *Children's Orthopaedics — Practical Problems*, Butterworth, 1976.
Ferguson A, *Orthopedic Surgery in Infancy and Childhood*, Williams and Wilkins, 1975.
Roaf R Hodkinson L J, *Textbook of Orthopaedic Nursing*, Blackwell Scientific, 1980.
Scipien G *et al.*, *Comprehensive Pediatric Nursing*, McGraw-Hill, 1979.

Articles

Anon., Children's feet, *Proceedings of the Royal Society of Medicine*, 1974, 70: 375-377.
Davis S Lewis S, Managing scoliosis: fashions for the body and mind, *American Journal of Maternal and Child Nursing*, May/June 1984: 186-187.
Dickson R A, Screening for scoliosis, *British Medical Journal*, 4 August 1985: 269-270.
Dunwoody C J Pais M, Scoliosis (review), *Nursing*, September 1983: 24-25.
Fixsen J, The management of congenital dislocation of the hips, *Journal of Maternal and Child Health*, August 1979: 300-304.
Fixsen J, Congenital dislocation of the hip and club foot in the young child, *Health Visitor*, August 1983: 281-283.
Fixsen J Valman H B, ABC (ages 1-7): limp in children, *British Medical Journal*, 19 September 1981: 780-781.
Hall M A Ansell B M, Investigation and treatment of joint pain in childhood, *Journal of Maternal and Child Health*, April 1978: 114-123.
Harrold A J, Problems in congenital dislocation of the hip, *British Medical Journal*, April 1977: 1071-1073.
Hooper G, Spinal disorders in childhood, *Nursing Mirror*, 30 October 1980: 16-18.
Mitchell G, Disorders of the hip, *Nursing Mirror*, 13 November 1980: 26-28.
O'Brian J P van Akkervecken P R, School screening for scoliosis, *Practitionery*, November 1977: 739-742.
Place M J *et al.*, Effectiveness of neonatal screening for congenital dislocation of the hip, *Lancet*, July 1978: 249-250.
Mein S, Congenital dislocation of the hip: a mother's experience, *Health Visitor*, August 1983: 288-289.
Smith C, Nursing the patient in traction, *Nursing Times*, 18 April 1984: 36-39.
Sodha U, Congenital scoliosis, *Nursing Times*, 28 August 1980: 1524-1525.
Walker G, Joint pain in children, *Modern Medicine*, June 1980: 27-31.

16

PAEDIATRIC ONCOLOGY

GENERAL CONSIDERATIONS

Incidence
1 Cancer is the leading cause of death from disease in children from 1 to 14 years of age.
2 Cancer affects approximately 10 per 100,000 children annually.

Types

Types of Cancer in Children
1 Leukaemia
2 Cancer of the central nervous system
3 Lymphoma
4 Neuroblastoma
5 Rhabdomyosarcoma
6 Wilms' tumour
7 Bone tumour
8 Retinoblastoma.

Less Common Central Nervous System Neoplasms
1 Craniopharyngiomas
2 Cerebral tumours
3 Optic nerve gliomas
4 Pineal tumours.

Warning Signals of Cancer in Children
1 Marked change in bowel or bladder habits; nausea and vomiting for no apparent cause

2   Bloody discharge of any kind; failure to stop bleeding in the usual time
3   Presence of swelling, lump, or mass anywhere in the body
4   Any change in the size or appearance of moles or birthmarks
5   Unexplained stumbling in the child
6   Generally run-down condition
7   Unexplained pain or persistent crying of an infant or child.

Principles of Treatment

1   Surgery
2   Radiation therapy
   a Prepare the child and his family for the procedure.
   b Do not wash off any marks placed by the radiologist to indicate the area to be treated.
   c Initiate comfort and support measures when the child demonstrates any side effects of treatment:
      (1) General malaise and headache
      (2) Nausea and vomiting
      (3) Diarrhoea
      (4) Anorexia
      (5) Skin irritation and breakdown
      (6) Lethargy.
3   Chemotherapy
   a Be aware of the chemotherapeutic agents most frequently used to treat childhood cancer, their side effects, and precautions for administration. Refer to Table 16.1, p. 739.
   b Care for the child who develops side effects of chemotherapy.
      (1) Prepare the child and his family for the possible side effects of the chemotherapeutic agents he is receiving.
         Explain to the child that the medicine is to help him feel better but that when he first begins to take the medicine he may feel sicker. By explaining this prior to the development of the symptoms, the child will be more trusting and less frightened.
      (2) Nausea and vomiting
         (a) Administer antiemetics as prescribed.
         (b) Plan activities and meals according to the medical schedule.
            Many children prefer to receive chemotherapeutic agents that cause nausea and vomiting during the evening so that they can sleep through the hours of greatest nausea.
         (c) Carefully observe the sleeping child who is prone to vomiting. Position him in a manner which prevents aspiration.
         (d) Offer foods and fluids which are most appealing to the child (e.g. warm tea, carbonated beverages, soups).
         (e) Record the nature of the nausea and vomiting.

(f) Report any prolonged or delayed nausea or vomiting which may be an indication that the medication should be withheld or that the dosage should be reduced.

(3) Anorexia

(a) Create a pleasant eating environment that is free of sights, sounds, and odours that cause nausea or that discourage or distract the child.

(b) Encourage the child to eat in the playroom with other children.

(c) Give good mouth care prior to eating.

(d) Provide frequent small meals.

(4) Extreme fluctuations in appetite

Be aware that this is temporary and that, eventually, normal eating patterns will be established. Reassure parents of this fact.

(5) Gastrointestinal mucosal cell damage causing stomatitis, gastro-intestinal ulceration, rectal ulceration, diarrhoea, or bleeding

(a) Provide meticulous oral hygiene. Local anaesthetics may be prescribed for painful mouth ulcers.

(b) If diarrhoea or rectal ulcers occur, keep the skin clean and dry to prevent maceration and secondary infection.

(c) These signs of toxicity are generally indications for temporary discontinuation of therapy or a reduction of dosage.

(6) Alopecia

(a) Assist the family in obtaining wigs or caps in preparation for hair loss.

(b) Reassure the child and family that the hair will grow back, although it might be of a different colour and texture.

(7) For side effects and nursing interventions associated with specific drugs refer to Table 16.1.

Prevention

1   Children and adults should be educated regarding the hazards of known carcinogens, especially cigarette smoking, and excessive exposure to sunlight or radiation.

2   Female adolescents should be instructed concerning the method of breast self-examination. Males should be taught to do testicular self-examination. Periodic examinations should be encouraged for cancer screening.

3   Parents should be taught the warning signals of childhood cancer.

ACUTE LYMPHOBLASTIC LEUKAEMIA

Acute lymphoblastic leukaemia is a primary disorder of the bone marrow in which the normal marrow elements are replaced by immature or undifferentiated blast cells. When the quantity of normal marrow is depleted below the level necessary to maintain peripheral blood elements within normal ranges, anaemia, neutropaenia, and thrombocytopaenia occur.

Incidence and Classification

1 Acute leukaemia is the most common malignancy in children. Approximately 420 children under the age of 15 years are likely to develop acute leukaemia annually in the UK.
2 Acute leukaemia is classified according to the cell type involved.
  a Approximately 85% of paediatric cases are of the acute lymphoblastic leukaemia (ALL) type.
  b The remainder are primarily cases of acute myeloblastic leukaemia (AML).
3 The clincal pictures of ALL and AML are similar, but the response of the child to therapy is markedly different.
  The percentage of children achieving remission is smaller with AML (approximately 60-65% as compared to 90-95% with ALL), and the mean survival time is shorter with AML.
4 The peak incidence of ALL among white children is 5-6 years, and the range of incidence is predominantly during the preschool period.
  This variation in age incidence is not observed in children of nonwhite racial groups.

Aetiology

1 The exact cause of acute leukaemia is unknown.
2 Environmental causes, infectious agents (especially viruses), genetic factors, and chromosomal abnormalities are suspected in some cases.

Clinical Manifestations

1 Manifestations depend on the degree to which the bone marrow has been compromised and the location and extent of extramedullary infiltration.
2 Presenting symptoms:
  a Increasing lethargy
  b General malaise
  c Persistent fever of unknown cause
  d Recurrent infection
  e Prolonged bleeding following simple surgical procedures (e.g. dental extractions and tonsillectomy)
  f Tendency to bruise easily
  g Pallor
  h Enlarged lymph nodes
  i Abdominal pain due to organomegaly

j Bone and joint pain
k Headache and vomiting (with central nervous system involvement)
3 Presenting symptoms may be isolated or in any combination or sequence.

Altered Physiology

1 Acute lymphocytic leukaemia results from the growth of an abnormal type of nongranular, fragile leucocyte in the blood-forming tissues, particularly in the bone marrow, spleen, and lymph nodes.
2 The abnormal cell has little cytoplasm and a round, homogeneous nucleus which resembles that of a lymphoblast.
3 Normal bone marrow elements may be displaced or replaced in this type of leukaemia.
4 The changes in the blood and bone marrow result from the accumulation of leukaemic cells and from the deficiency of normal cells.
   a Red cell precursors and megakaryocytes from which platelets are formed are decreased, causing anaemia, prolonged and unusual bleeding, and tendency to bruise easily.
   b Normal white cells are markedly decreased, predisposing the child to infection.
   c Leukaemic cells may infiltrate into lymph nodes, spleen, and liver, causing diffuse adenopathy and hepatosplenomegaly.
   d Expansion of marrow or infiltration of leukaemic cells into bone results in bone or joint pain.
   e Invasion of the central nervous system by leukaemic cells may cause headache, vomiting, cranial nerve palsies, convulsions, and coma.
5 The bone marrow is hyperplastic with a uniform appearance due to the presence of leukaemic cells.

Diagnostic Evaluation

Physical Findings

1 Pallor, especially of the mucous membranes
2 Scattered petechiae and ecchymoses
3 Generalized lymphadenopathy
4 Enlarged liver and spleen
5 Unexplained bruising
6 Continued bone and joint pain
7 Fever.

Laboratory Evaluation

1 May have altered peripheral blood counts. Blood studies may show the following:

    a Low haemoglobin, red cell count, haematocrit, and platelet count
    b Decreased, elevated, or normal white cell count
2 Stained peripheral smear and bone marrow examination show large numbers of lymphoblasts and lymphocytes.
3 Lumbar puncture — to determine if there is central nervous system involvement.
4 Renal and liver function studies — to determine any contraindications or precautions for chemotherapy.

Complications

1 Infection — most frequently occurs in the lungs, gastrointestinal tract, or skin
2 Haemorrhage — usually due to thrombocytopaenia
3 Central nervous system involvement
4 Bony involvement
5 Testicular involvement
6 Urate nephropathy.

Treatment

Supportive Therapy

To control disease complications such as hyperuricaemia, infection, anaemia, and bleeding. These children are best treated in special centres for their care and management.

Specific Therapy

To eradicate malignant cells and to restore normal marrow function.

1 Chemotherapy is utilized to achieve complete remission with restoration of normal peripheral blood and physical findings.
2 At present there is no universally accepted standard therapy for the treatment of children with acute leukaemia, but most centres have similar protocols which utilize the same drugs alone or in combination (refer to Table 16.1).
3 Components of therapy:
    a Induction — course of therapy designed to achieve a complete remission
    b Consolidation — period of intensive chemotherapy begun after remission to further reduce the number of leukaemic cells
    c Central nervous system prophylaxis — treatment begun early in the course of the illness to destroy leukaemic cells that have infiltrated the central nervous system. It generally consists of cranial irradiation and intrathecal methotrexate.

d Maintenance or continuation therapy — to maintain remission and to continue reducing the number of leukaemic cells

e Reinduction or reinforcement therapy — to increase the duration of the remission

f Relapse therapy

g Extramedullary disease therapy.

4   Trials are currently in progress in the UK to determine the best combinations of drugs to achieve the longest remissions with the least immunosuppression.

5   Two modes of therapy — bone marrow transplantation and immunotherapy — are currently under investigation and may hold promise for the future.

Prognosis

1   Uncertain.

2   The life span of children with ALL has been lengthened.

3   Some children have achieved continuous remission.

4   The first relapse from complete remission can be considered a poor prognostic indicator of further long-term survival.

5   Many children not in continuous remission survive 5 years or more.

6   The term 'cure' is difficult to define, because later relapses still occur after long remissions.

7   Prognosis appears to be related to the child's age and white blood count on diagnosis, and the exact cell type of the leukaemia.

Nursing Objectives

To provide emotional support to the parents when the diagnosis of leukaemia is made known to them.

1   Be available to the parents when they feel that they want to discuss their feelings.

2   Kindness, concern, consideration, and sincerity towards the child and his parents help to serve as a source of consolation.

3   Contact the family's clergyman or the hospital chaplain if the parents desire this.

4   Utilize the services of a social worker (if available) in helping the family work out their feelings.

5   Avoid discussing life expectancy in terms of the time element — offer the hope that therapy will be effective and will prolong life.

6   Allow the parents to participate in the child's care so that they will feel that they are actually doing something for the child. This also helps the family feel more secure if they plan to take the child home to care for him. (Refer to section on family-centred care, p. 66.)

7   Assess family dynamics and coping mechanisms and plan intervention accordingly. (Refer to sections on family stress in paediatric illness, p. 68, and family developmental tasks, p. 67.)

To give skilful, supportive care in the early stages of treatment and to sustain life until antileukaemic agents have had a chance to become effective.

1   Initiate nursing activities associated with anaemia. (Refer to p. 346.)
2   Provide adequate hydration.
   a Maintain parenteral fluid administration.
   b Offer small amounts of oral fluids if tolerated.
   c Record and report vomiting if this occurs.
3   Observe renal function carefully
   a Measure and record urinary output.
   b Check relative density.
   c Observe the urine for any evidence of gross bleeding.
4   Provide a highly nutritious diet if the child can tolerate it.
   a Determine the child's likes and dislikes.
   b Offer small, frequent meals.
   c Offer supplemental feedings which are high in kilojoules and protein.
   d Encourage parents to assist at mealtime.
   e Allow the child to eat with a group at a table if his condition allows this.
5   Protect the child from sources of infection.
   a Family, friends, personnel and other patients who have infections should not be visiting or caring for the child.
   b Do not place a child with an infection in the room with a child with leukaemia.
   c Reverse barrier nursing may be utilized (a protective technique that provides the child with protection from those people with whom he has contact — gowns and masks are worn by any person with whom the child has contact; also gloves and theatre caps depending on local procedure).
      Explain to both the child and his parents the purpose of this protective technique.
   d Observe the child closely and be alert to signs of impending infection.
      (1) Observe any area of broken skin or mucous membrane for signs of infection.
      (2) Report any febrile incidents.
   e Teach preventive measures at discharge (i.e. handwashing, isolation from children with communicable disease).

To be alert for the symptoms of haemorrhage which may occur when the platelet count is diminished or may appear as side effects of antileukaemic therapy.

1   Record vital signs and report any changes which may be indicative of haemorrhage:
   a Tachycardia
   b Lowered blood pressure

c Pallor

d Diaphoresis

e Increasing anxiety and restlessness.

2 Give careful oral hygiene since the gums and mucous membranes of the mouth bleed easily.

　a Use a soft toothbrush.

　b If the child's mouth is bleeding or painful, clean the teeth and mouth with a moistened cotton swab.

　c Use a nonirritating rinse for the mouth.

　d Apply petroleum jelly to cracked, dry lips.

3 Observe for gastrointestinal bleeding:

　a Haematemesis

　b Tarry stools or bloodstained stools.

4 Move and turn the child gently since haemarthrosis may occur and cause movement to be very painful.

　a Handle the child in a gentle manner.

　b Turn frequently to prevent pressure sores.

　c Place the child in proper body alignment, in a position comfortable for him.

　d Allow child to be out of bed in a chair if this position is more comfortable for him.

5 Avoid intramuscular injections if possible.

6 Handle catheters as well as drainage and suction tubes carefully to prevent mucosal bleeding.

7 Protect the child from injury by monitoring his activities and environmental hazards.

8 Be aware of emergency procedures for control of bleeding:

　a Careful application of local pressure so as not to interfere with clot formation

　b Administration of blood and blood components (refer to section on anaemia, p. 347).

To prepare the child for diagnostic and treatment procedures.

1 Utilize knowledge of growth and development to prepare the child for such procedures as bone marrow aspirations, blood transfusions, and chemotherapy. (Refer to section on the hospitalized child, p. 58.)

2 Provide a means for talking about the experience. Play, storytelling, or role-playing may be helpful.

3 Convey to the child an acceptance of his fears and anger.

To control hyperuricaemia which may occur because of rapid cell turnover and tumour lysis.

1 Administer allopurinol as prescribed to neutralize the effects of uric acid on the kidney.

2 Provide liberal oral and/or intravenous hydration.

3   Administer sodium bicarbonate or acetazolamide (Diamox) as ordered to alkalize the urine.

4   Collect urine specimens to monitor urinary excretion of uric acid.

To be aware of the chemotherapeutic agents and the side effects of these agents which are capable of inducing remissions in children with acute leukaemia.

1   Induction — Usually includes a combination of vincristine and prednisone. A third drug, such as 6-mercaptopurine, L-asparaginase, daunorubicin, adriamycin, or cytosine arabinoside, may be added.

2   Maintenance — Usually includes methotrexate, used in alternating sequence with the same drugs used to induce remission. Also includes periodic CNS prophylaxis.

3   Reinduction — Remissions can often be reinduced using the same initial drugs or with other agents.

4   Refer to Table 16.1.

To provide symptomatic care for the child who develops side effects of chemotherapy.

1   Prepare the child and his family for the possible side effects of the antileukaemic agents he is receiving.

Explain to the child that the medicine is to help him feel better but that when he first begins to take the medicine he may feel sicker. By explaining this prior to the development of symptoms, the child will be more trusting and less frightened.

2   Nausea and vomiting

   a Administer antiemetics as prescribed.

   b Plan activities and meals according to the medical schedule.

   Many children prefer to receive chemotherapeutic agents that cause nausea and vomiting during the evening so that they can sleep through the hours of greatest nausea.

   c Carefully observe the sleeping child who is prone to vomiting. Position him in a manner which prevents aspiration.

   d Offer foods and fluids which are most appealing to the child (e.g. warm tea, soft or 'fizzy' beverages, soups).

   e Record the nature of the nausea and vomiting.

   f Report any prolonged or delayed nausea or vomiting which may be an indication that the medication should be withheld or that the dosage should be reduced.

3   Anorexia

   a Create a pleasant eating environment that is free of sights, sounds, and odours that cause nausea or that discourage or distract the child.

   b Encourage the child to eat in the playroom with other children.

   c Give good mouth care prior to eating.

   d Provide frequent small meals.

4　Extreme fluctuations in appetite

Be aware that this is temporary and that, eventually, normal eating patterns will be established. Reassure parents of this fact.

5　Gastrointestinal mucosal cell damage causing stomatitis, gastrointestinal ulceration, rectal ulceration, diarrhoea, or bleeding

a Provide meticulous oral hygiene. Local anaesthetics may be prescribed for painful mouth ulcers.

b If diarrhoea or rectal ulcers occur, keep the skin clean and dry to prevent maceration and secondary infection.

6　Answer parental questions related to such matters as home management, the purpose of periodic tests, treatments and clinic visits, side effects of medications, and indications for medical intervention.

7　Facilitate communication with the outpatient clinic nurse who may interact with the child during the entire course of illness.

8　Initiate appropriate referrals (e.g. to social worker, parent group, clergy, health visitor, and school nurse).

To observe for the possibility of CNS involvement.

Report changes in behaviour or personality: persistent nausea and vomiting, headache, lethargy, irritability, dizziness, ataxia, convulsions, or alteration in state of consciousness.

To provide supportive nursing care to the child receiving cranial irradiation.

Refer to section on radiation therapy, p. 728.

To provide pain relief.

1　Position the child so that he is most comfortable. Water beds and beanbag chairs are often helpful.

2　Administer medications on a preventive schedule before pain becomes severe. Individualize medication schedule for each patient.

3　Manipulate the environment as necessary to increase the child's comfort and minimize unnecessary exertion.

To provide emotional support to the child.

1　Provide for continuity of care.

2　Encourage family-centred care (refer to p. 66).

3　Prepare the child for potential changes in his body image (alopecia, weight loss, wasting, etc.) and help him cope with related feelings.

4　Facilitate play activities for the child and utilize opportunities to communicate with him through play.

5　Maintain some discipline, placing calm limitations on unacceptable behaviour.

6　Provide appropriate diversional activities.

7   Encourage independence and provide opportunities which allow the child to control his environment.

8   Avoid exposing the child to activities that he will be unable to accomplish.

To provide continued emotional support to the parents throughout the course of hospitalization.

1   Assist parents to feel comfortable on the unit.

2   Provide guidelines concerning how parents and the treatment team can work together most profitably.

3   Encourage parental participation in care — to the extent that they feel comfortable.

4   Suggest tasks that the parents may do to reduce their feelings of helplessness and anxiety.

5   Provide for continuity of care so that parents are able to establish trusting relationships with a few nurses.

6   Assist parents to deal with anticipatory grief.

7   Assist parents to deal with other family members, especially siblings and grandparents and friends.

8   Encourage parents to discuss concerns about limiting their child's activities, protecting him from infection, disciplining him, and having anxieties about the illness.

9   Answer parental questions related to such matters as home management, the purpose of periodic tests, treatments and clinic visits, side effects of medications, and indications for medical intervention.

10   Facilitate communication with the clinic nurse and/or clinical specialist who may interact with the child during the entire course of illness.

11   Initiate appropriate referrals (e.g. to social worker, parent group, clergy, and community health nurse).

To provide supportive care to the terminally ill or dying child.

(Refer to section on care of the dying child, p. 89.)

Table 16.1 Drugs commonly used in the treatment of childhood leukaemia

Drug/category	Administration	Side effects/toxicity	Specific nursing implication
Prednisone: adrenocorticosteroid	Oral	Increased appetite, weight gain, fluid retention, hypertension, Cushing's syndrome, striation, growth arrest, immunosuppression, psychosis, gastrointestinal tract ulceration.	1 Avoid excessive sodium intake. 2 Observe for evidence of gastrointestinal bleeding. 3 Protect from infection.
Vincristine (Oncovin): periwinkle alkaloid	Intravenous	Alopecia, constipation, peripheral neuropathy, hyponatraemia, mild myelosuppression. Stomatitis, nausea, and vomiting. Dysuria, polyuria. Causes chemical irritation on extravasation.	1 Use different needles to withdraw and inject. Check patency of intravenous line with saline flush before injecting. Inject cautiously, observing for signs of infiltration. Follow injection with saline flush. 2 Observe for constipation; report condition promptly. Keep well hydrated. Administer laxatives or stool softeners as ordered. 3 Alter activities appropriately if weakness of hands, feet, or legs occurs or if patient becomes easily fatigued. 4 Prepare children and parents for the possibility of numbness and tingling of fingers and toes.
Adriamycin: antibiotic	Intravenous	Nausea, vomiting and diarrhoea, alopecia, stomatitis, myelosuppression, cardiotoxicity, red urine. Causes chemical irritation on extravasation.	1 Utilize the same precautions when administering this medication as vincristine. ECG may be performed predose because of the side effect of cardiotoxicity.

Table 16.1 (continued)

Drug/category	Administration	Side effects/toxicity	Specific nursing implication
L-Asparaginase: enzyme	Intravenous, intramuscular	Hypersensitivity reaction, nausea and vomiting, lethargy, somnolence, fever, hepatotoxicity, coagulopathy, pancreatitis, hyperproteinaemia.	1 Observe for hypersensitivity Have adrenaline, hydrocortisone, chlorpheniramine (Piriton) and resuscitation equipment available. 2 Observe for confusion, irritability, convulsions, and other neurological signs. 3 Do not shake vial. 4 Use clear solution only.
Daunomycin: antibiotic	Intravenous	Cardiotoxicity, myelosuppression, nausea and vomiting, abdominal pain, fever, skin rash, red urine. Cause chemical irritation on extravasation.	1 Utilize the same precautions when administering this medication as those followed by vincristine. ECG may be performed predose because of cardiotoxicity.
6-Mercaptopurine: antimetabolite; purine antagonist	Oral, intravenous	Nausea and vomiting, myelosuppression, anorexia. dermatitis, mucous membrane ulceration, hepatotoxicity, abdominal pain and diarrhoea.	1 Dosage should be reduced to one-third of the usual dosage if a child is receiving allopurinol, since this drug inhibits the degradation of 6-mercaptopurine.
Methotrexate: antimetabolite folic acid antagonist	Oral, intravenous, intramuscular, intrathecal	Nausea, vomiting, and diarrhoea, mucosal ulceration, myelo-supression, pneumonitis, osteoporosis, hepatotoxicity, hyperpigmentation, cystitis.	1 Avoid side effects of meningeal irritation during intrathecal by diluting the drug in a preservative, free vehicle, bringing temperature and filtering through an 0.22 micrometre Millipore filter. 2 Do not enter vial twice for intrathecal use.

3 Method of intrathecal injection:

a A lumbar puncture is performed.

b A volume of spinal fluid equal to the volume of drug to be injected is removed.

c Without aspiration, the medication is injected in a continuous infusion (15-30 seconds/10 ml of solution).

d The stylet is reinserted and the needle is removed.

e The child may be required to remain in the Trendelenburg position for 30 minutes after the injection to ensure optimal circulation of the medication throughout the central nervous system.

Cyclophosphamide (endoxane): alkylating agent

Oral or intravenous

Alopecia, nausea and vomiting, myelosuppression, haemorrhagic cystitis, mucous membrane ulceration, immunosuppression, infertility, hyperpigmentation. Alteration in taste.

1 To prevent exposure of the bladder to chemical irritants, maintain liberal hydration for 48 hours after weekly dose and then continuously when given daily. Have the child empty his bladder frequently after the drug is administered, including at least once during the night.
2 Protect child from infection.
3 Try to give well-flavoured foods because of taste alteration.

Table 16.1 (*continued*)

Drug/category	Administration	Side effects/toxicity	Specific nursing implication
Cytosine arabinoside (Ara-C): antimetabolite; pyrimidine antagonist	Intravenous, intramuscular, subcutaneous, or intrathecal	Nausea and vomiting, myelosuppression, mucous membrane ulcerations, hepatotoxicity, immunosuppression.	1 Anticipate severe nausea and vomiting during or soon after administration. 2 May require premedication with antiemetics. 3 Protect child from infection. 4 Do not enter vial twice for intrathecal use.

Agencies

1   Leukaemia Society, 45 Craignor Avenue, Queens Park, Bournemouth.
2   Leukaemia Research Fund, 48 Great Ormond Street, London WCl.

BRAIN TUMOURS

Brain tumours are expanding lesions within the skull; they account for 10-15% of the malignant tumours which occur in children.

Aetiology

The aetiology of brain tumour is unknown.

Clinical Manifestations

(Signs and symptoms are directly related to the location and size of the tumour.)

1   Headache
    a May occur at any time, but usually is more severe in early morning hours.
    b May be intermittent and disappear for days or weeks — may be due to yielding of the sutures
2   Nausea or vomiting
    a May occur at any time, but frequently occurs in early morning hours.
    b Vomiting may be projectile
3   Visual disturbances
    a Nystagmus
    b Diplopia
    c Blurred vision
    d Loss of peripheral vision
    e Significant loss of visual acuity
4   Muscular problems
    a Lack of balance
    b Incoordination
    c Deficits in muscle functioning — eyes, face, extremities
    d Paralysis
    e Spasticity
5   Behavioural changes
    a Arrest or regression in development
    b Irritability or lassitude
    c Lack of attentiveness
    d Deterioration in school performance
    e Personality changes
    f Loss of sphincter control
    g Disturbances in sleep and eating patterns

6 Slow cerebration
   a Child answers questions after a considerable delay
   b Child appears to talk slowly
   c Child responds to any stimulus in a slow manner
7 Seizures — usually focal, psychomotor, or generalized.

Diagnostic Evaluation

(Determined by the type of tumour that is suspected; usually includes many or all of the following procedures):

1 Thorough neurological examination
   a Fundoscopic examination
   b Tests for cerebral function (level of consciousness, orientation, intellectual performance, mood, behaviour, etc.)
   c Assessment of cranial nerves
   d Tests for cerebellar function (e.g. balance and coordination)
   e Evaluation of the motor system — especially muscle size, tone, strength, and abnormal muscle movements
   f Evaluation of the sensory system
   g Assessment of reflexes
2 Electroencephalogram — of limited value, but possibly useful when seizures are manifested
3 Skull x-ray
4 Computed tomography (EMI scan or CAT scan)
   a Safe, noninvasive procedure using a combination of sophisticated electronic and computer technology.

Treatment

1 Surgery is performed to determine the type of the tumour, the extent of invasiveness, and to excise as much of the lesion as possible.
2 Radiation therapy is usually initiated as soon as the diagnosis is established and the surgical wound healed.
3 Chemotherapy is used to induce remissions in recurrent brain tumours, especially astrocytomas and medulloblastomas. The role of chemotherapy for treatment of primary tumours is currently being investigated. Commonly used drugs include nitrosoureas, vincristine, methotrexate, procarbazine, and steroids.

Prognosis

1 Prognosis is improved in cases involving early diagnosis and adequate therapy.

2 Prognosis is related to completeness of surgical removal, extent of invasion, and rate of tumour growth.
3 Approximately 50% of children with brain tumours will survive more that 1 year.
4 Five-year survivors are increasing, especially in children with medulloblastoma or higher-grade astrocytoma.

Cerebellar Astrocytoma

Cerebellar astrocytoma is a slow-growing, often cystic type of tumour of the cerebellum.

Incidence

1 Cerebellar astrocytomas account for approximately 25% of brain tumours in children.
2 The peak incidence occurs at 5-8 years of age.

Clinical Manifestations

Insidious onset and slow course.

1 Evidence of increased intracranial pressure — especially headache, visual disturbances, papilloedema, and personality changes.
2 Cerebellar signs — ataxia, dysmetria (inability to control the range of muscular movement), nystagmus.
3 Behavioural changes.

Pathophysiology

1 The tumour produces slowly increasing intracranial pressure.
2 Condition classified according to its malignancy — from Grade I (least malignant) to Grade IV (most malignant).

Treatment

Surgical removal — the tumour can usually be removed with few sequelae.

Medulloblastoma

Medulloblastoma is a highly malignant, rapidly growing tumour usually found in the cerebellum.

Incidence

1   Medulloblastomas account for nearly 20% of brain tumours in children.
2   The peak incidence occurs in children from 2 to 6 years of age.
3   About 75% of medulloblastomas occur in males.

Clinical Manifestations

1   Similar to manifestations of cerebellar astrocytoma, but condition develops more rapidly.
2   The child may present with unsteady gait, anorexia, vomiting, and early morning headache and later develop ataxia, nystagmus, papilloedema, and drowsiness.

Pathophysiology

1   The tumour grows rapidly and produces evidence of increased intracranial pressure progressing over a period of weeks.
2   As the tumour grows, it seeds along cerebrospinal fluid (CSF) pathways.

Treatment

1   Surgical decompression of posterior fossa (complete removal is rarely possible)
2   Radiation of site, cerebrum, and spinal canal
3   Chemotherapy
4   Shunt to relieve CSF obstruction.

Brain Stem Glioma

Brain stem glioma is a tumour of the brain stem. It accounts for approximately 10% of brain tumours in children.

Incidence

1   Brain stem gliomas occur almost exclusively in children.
2   The peak age at onset is 5-8 years.

Clinical Manifestations

1   Cranial nerve palsies
    a Strabismus
    b Weakness, atrophy and fasciculations of the tongue
    c Swallowing difficulties

2 Hemiparesis
3 Cerebellar ataxia
4 Signs of increased intracranial pressure (rare).

Altered Physiology

1 Through its growth this type of tumour interferes early with the function of cranial nerve nuclei, pyramidal tracts, and cerebellar pathways.
2 Tumour usually demonstrates rapid growth and recurrence.

Treatment

1 Surgical removal is not possible.
2 Radiation of site may produce temporary improvement.

Care of the Child Undergoing Surgery for Brain Tumour

Nursing Objectives

To assess the child's neurological status in order to help locate the site of the tumour and the extent of involvement; to identify signs of disease progress.

1 Obtain a thorough nursing history from the child and his parents — particularly data related to normal behavioural patterns and presenting symptoms.
2 Perform portions of the neurological examination as appropriate.
   Assess muscle strength, coordination, gait, and posture.
3 Observe for the appearance or disappearance of any of the clinical manifestations previously described. Report these to the physician and record each of the following in detail:
   a Headache — duration, location, severity
   b Vomiting — time occurring, whether or not projectile
   c Convulsions — activity prior to seizure; type of seizure; areas of body involved; behaviour during and after seizure.
4 Monitor vital signs frequently, including blood pressure and pupillary reaction.
5 Monitor occular signs.
   Check pupils for size, equality, reaction to light, and accommodation.
6 Observe for signs of brain stem herniation — should be considered a neurosurgical emergency.
   a Attacks of opisthotonos
   b Tilting of the head; neck stiffness
   c Poorly reactive pupils

d Increased blood pressure; widened pulse pressure
e Change in respiratory rate and nature of respirations
f Irregularity of pulse or lowered pulse rate
g Alterations of body temperature.

To provide the parents and child with emotional support during the very stressful preoperative period.

1 Assess the family unit and its coping mechanisms. (Refer to sections on family stress in paediatric illness, family developmental tasks, and family-centred care, p. 66.)
2 Allow parents to ask questions and encourage them to discuss their fears and concerns.
    Many parents feel quilty for not seeking help earlier because they either did not recognize or dismissed symptoms.
3 Deliver nursing care to the child in a manner that provides support.
    a Assume a gentle, concerned attitude towards both parents and child.
    b Make the child as comfortable as possible.
4 Utilize knowledge of growth and development to provide emotional care for the child. (Refer to section on the hospitalized child, p. 58.)
5 Prepare child and parents for what to expect during hospitalization (e.g. nursing routines and diagnostic tests).

To provide appropriate nursing care for the child undergoing diagnostic tests.

1 Prepare the child and parents for each procedure.
2 If ordered, administer preliminary sedative on time. (If child is not adequately sedated, completion of the test may be impossible.)

To prepare the child and parents for surgery.

1 Refer to section on preparation for surgery, p. 83.
2 Determine surgeon's plans regarding shaving the head, bandages, and other procedures, and prepare the child accordingly.
    a Encourage the child to express his feelings regarding the threat to his body image.
    b Reassure the child that he will be able to wear a wig or hat after recovery.
3 Prepare parents for the postoperative appearance of their child and for the fact that he might be comatose immediately following surgery.
4 If appropriate, introduce the child and his family to intensive care nursing personnel and arrange a tour of the unit.

To provide an adequate diet for the child preoperatively.

1 Re-feed the child when he vomits. (Vomiting is usually not associated with nausea.)
2 Allow the child to participate in the choice of foods and drinks.
3 Maintain intravenous hydration if indicated.

To provide care for the child during the immediate postoperative period.

(This is usually provided in an intensive care unit.)

1   Position the child according to surgeon's orders — usually on his unaffected side with his head level.
      Raising the foot of the bed may increase intracranial pressure and bleeding.
2   Check the dressing for bleeding and for drainage of cerebrospinal fluid.
3   Monitor the child's temperature closely.
      a A marked rise in temperature may be due to trauma, to disturbance of the heat-regulating centre, or to intracranial oedema.
      b If hyperthermia occurs, utilize appropriate measures to reduce it. (Refer to section on fever, p. 105.)
      Temperature should not be reduced too rapidly.
4   Observe child closely for signs of shock, increased intracranial pressure, and alterations in level of consciousness.
5   Assess the child for oedema of the head, face, and neck.
      a Oedema may inhibit respirations and impair circulation of lacrimal secretion.
      b Apply cold compresses to the affected areas, being careful not to dampen the dressing.
      c Apply methylcellulose drops to the eyes to prevent corneal damage.
6   Carefully regulate fluid administration in order to prevent increased cerebral oedema.
7   Change the child's position frequently and provide meticulous skin care to prevent hypostatic pneumonia and pressure sores.
      a Move the child carefully and slowly, being certain to move the head in line with the body.
      b Support paralysed or spastic extremities with pillows, rolls, or other means.
8   Avoid discussing the child's condition in his presence, even if he appears to be unconscious, as hearing is often the first sense to return. The child should be spoken to in the same manner as preoperatively.
9   Have emergency equipment readily available for cardiopulmonary resuscitation, respiratory assistance, oxygen inhalation, blood transfusion, ventricular tap, and other potential emergency situations.
10   Continue to support parents, who may be very frightened and upset by the appearance of their child and necessary emergency procedures.

To provide care for the child during the convalescent phase.

1   Maintain adequate nutrition and hydration.
      a Encourage the child to eat increasingly larger meals.
      b Provide tube feedings if the child is unable to eat.
2   Allow and encourage the child to regain his independence as his condition improves.

3   Facilitate the return of normal parent-child relationships.
    a Parents may tend to be overprotective.
    b Help parents to see the child's increasing capabilities and encourage them to foster independence.
4   Make provisions for play activities.
    a Allow the child to meet and play with other children.
    b Provide the child with quiet play activities when it is necessary to encourage rest.
    c Be careful that the child does not hit his head or fall until he is completely healed.
        A head dressing, football helmet, or wig may be used to prevent trauma should the child fall.
5   Assist the child to adjust to his altered body image.
    a Utilize stocking caps, surgical caps, head scarves, hats, or wigs as appropriate.
    b If the child's hair has not been totally shaved, it may be combed so that the area of baldness is not evident.
    c Reassure the child that his hair will grow back.

To care for the child receiving radiation therapy.

Refer to section on radiation therapy, p. 728.

To care for the child receiving chemotherapy.

Refer to section on chemotherapy, p. 728.

To prepare the child and his family for discharge.

1   Provide parents with written information regarding the child's needs — medications, activity, care of incision, follow-up appointments, etc.
2   Initiate a referral to the family health visitor to reinforce teaching and to maintain therapeutic support for the family.
3   Encourage the parents to contact the child's teacher and the school nurse before the child returns to school so that they can prepare his classmates for his return and help them to deal with their feelings.
4   Provide parents with the phone number of the nursing unit so that they may call if questions occur to them after discharge.

To provide supportive care to the terminally ill child.

Refer to section on the dying child, p. 89.

WILMS' TUMOUR

Wilms' tumour is a malignant renal tumour.

Aetiology

1 The aetiology of Wilms' tumour is not known.
2 Current evidence implicates unknown genetic factors.

Incidence

1 Wilms' tumour is the most common neoplasm involving the retroperitoneal space in children.
2 It constitutes approximately 30% of all paediatric renal masses and 4% of all childhood tumours.
3 75% of cases occur before the child is 5 years of age.
4 Average age at time of diagnosis is 3 years.

Clinical Manifestations

1 A firm, abdominal mass is usually the presenting sign; it may be on either side of the abdomen or flank. (It is frequently observed by the parents.)
2 Abdominal pain, which is related to rapid growth of the tumour, may occur. As the tumour enlarges, pressure may cause constipation, vomiting, abdominal distress, anorexia, weight loss, and dyspnoea.
3 Less common: hypertension, fever, haematuria, anaemia.
4 Associated anomalies:
   a Hemihypertrophy
   b Anirida (absence of the iris)
   c Genitourinary anomalies.

Pathophysiology

1 Wilms' tumour has a capacity for very rapid growth and usually grows to a large size before it is diagnosed.
2 The effect of the tumour on the kidney depends on the site of the tumour.
3 In most cases, the tumour expands the renal parenchyma, and the kidney becomes stretched over the surface of the tumour.
4 The covering of the tumour may be very thin and easily torn.
5 The tumour is often exceedingly vascular, soft, mushy, or gelatinous in character.
6 Wilms' tumours present various histological patterns from patient to patient.
7 The neoplasms metastasize early, either by direct extension or by way of the bloodstream. May invade perirenal tissues, lymph nodes, the liver, the diaphragm, abdominal muscles, and the lungs. Invasions of bone and brain are less common.

8   Staging of Wilms' tumour is done on the basis of clinical and anatomical findings. It ranges from Group I (tumour is limited to the kidney and is completely resected) to Group IV (metastases are present in the liver, lung, bone, or brain). Group V includes those cases in which there is bilateral involvement either initially or subsequently.

Diagnostic Evaluation

1   Abdominal x-ray
2   Intravenous pylography — to demonstrate the tumour and to assess the status of the opposite kidney
3   X-ray of chest, skull, long bones — to identify metastases
4   Urinalysis
5   Bone marrow examination — for tumour cells
6   Blood chemistries, especially serum glutamic-oxaloacetic transaminase (SGOT), blood urea nitrogen (BUN), lactic dehydrogenase (LDH), uric acid, and alkaline phosphatase.

Treatment

1   Determined by the stage of the tumour.
2   Includes a combination of surgery, radiation therapy, and chemotherapy.

Prognosis

1   Guarded.
2   High cure rate associated with early diagnosis and optimal treatment. A survival rate of 50% has been reported with localized disease.
3   Prognosis best in children who are less than 18 months old and whose tumour is classified as Group I.

Nursing Objectives

To support the family and the child at the time the diagnosis is made.
1   Discuss with the paediatrician what specific information has been given to the parents.
2   Provide the parents with the opportunity to express their concerns.
3   Provide the parents with a place where they may have some privacy when they wish to be alone.
4   Convey a compassionate attitude to the parents in talking with them, and assure them that their child's needs will be met.
5   Refer to sections on family stress in paediatric illness, and family-centred care, p. 66.

To exercise caution in the manipulation of the child in order to avoid inadvertently increasing the danger of metastasis.

1 Bathe the child carefully, avoiding manipulation of the abdomen.
2 Hold the child carefully to prevent abdominal pressure.
3 Communicate the need for this caution to all staff members.
4 Place a sign on the child's bed to reduce indiscriminate palpation.

To explain to the child and his parents the elements of preoperative and postoperative care.

1 Utilize knowledge of growth and development to plan a teaching programme for the child that will include diagnostic tests, preoperative care, and postoperative care. (Refer to section on the hospitalized child, p. 58.)
2 Involve the parents in the teaching plan and encourage them to support the child at this time.

To provide preoperative and postoperative care for the child.

1 Refer to section on the child undergoing surgery, p. 83.
2 Many children require gastric suction postoperatively to prevent distention or vomiting.
   a Refer to Guidelines: Nasogastric Intubation, p. 179.
   b Monitor gastric output accurately and replace it with appropriate intravenous fluids as prescribed by the physician.
   c When oral feedings are resumed, begin with small amounts of clear fluids.
3 Continue to avoid abdominal manipulation, because cells may have escaped locally from the excised tumour.

To care for the child receiving radiation therapy.

1 Radiation therapy is given to the tumour bed postoperatively to render nonviable all cells that have escaped locally from the excised tumour. It is usually indicated for all children with Wilms' tumour except those under 18 months of age with Stage I disease.
2 Alterations in the growth and development of bones, joints, and musculature may occur as a result of radiation therapy.
3 Be aware that acute skin reactions occasionally occur when dactinomycin is given concomitantly with or follows administration of radiation therapy.
4 Refer to section on radiation therapy, p. 728.

To care for the child receiving chemotherapy.

1 Chemotherapy is initiated postoperatively to achieve maximal killing of tumour cells.
2 The usual chemotherapeutic agents employed are dactinomycin, vincristine, and adriamycin.
3 Prepare the child and his family for chemotherapy.
4 Refer to section on chemotherapy, p. 728.

To provide diversional therapy for the child.

Provide the child with the opportunity for play as his condition permits.

To provide supportive care appropriate for the dying child when the tumour metastasizes and the child's condition deteriorates.

See section on the dying child, p. 89.

FURTHER READING

Books

Alexander M Brown M, *Pediatric History and Physical Diagnosis for Nurses*, McGraw-Hill, 1979.
Communication and Cancer Education, Alpha Publications, 1981.
Petrillo M Sanger S, *Emotional Care of Hospitalized Children*, 2nd edn, Lippincott, 1980.
Pochedly C (ed.), *Clinical Management of Cancer in Children*, Edward Arnold, 1976.
Pochedly C (ed.), *Paediatric Cancer Therapy*, Pitman Medical, 1979.
Psychological and Social Aspects of Childhood Malignancy, Annales Nestlé, 1983, 41 (2).
Scipien G *et al.*, *Comprehensive Pediatric Nursing*, McGraw-Hill, 1979.
Spinetta J Deasy-Spinetta P, *Living with Childhood Cancer*, Mosby, 1981.

Articles

Anon., Childhood cancers, *Nursing Mirror*, August 1980, Supplement.
Banner J H Mott M G, Sex and prognosis in childhood acute lymphoblastic leukaemia, *Lancet*, July 1978; 128 -29.
Eiser C Lansdown R, Retrospective study of intellectual development in children treated for acute lymphoblastic leukaemia, *Archives of Diseases in Childhood*, July 1977: 525-529.
Ferguson J, Late psychologic effect of a serious illness in childhood, *Nursing Clinics of North America*, March 1976, 11: 83-95.
Gaddy D S, Nursing care in childhood cancer, *American Journal of Nursing*, March 1982: 415-421.
Hayes V Knox J E, Reducing hospital-related stress in parents of children with cancer, *Canadian Nurse*, 1983, 79: 10-24.
Innes E L, Leukaemia in children — progress and problems, *Nursing Times*, March 1979, paediatric news supplement.
Martinson L, The child with leukaemia: parents help each other, *American Journal of Nursing*, July 1976, 76: 1120-1122.
Menkens J, All for one: a team approach to the care of children with cancer, *Nursing Mirror*, November 1984: 35-37.
Mitchell-Heggs *et al.*, A symposium on cancer in children, *Nursing Mirror*, April 1977: 48-64.
Pearson D, Cancer in children, *Update*, May 1978: 1169-1180.

Robotham A, Children with leukaemia, *Nursing Times*, 16 February 1983: 28-29.

Ross D M Ross S A, Stress reduction procedures for the school-aged hospitalized leukaemic child, *Paediatric Nursing*, November/December 1984: 393-395

Stevens M M *et al.*, Adolescent health — I: coping with cancer, *Australian Family Physician*, 1983, 12: 2.

Till K, Cerebellar tumours in children, *Journal of Maternal and Child Health*, October 1978: 326-332.

17

SPECIAL PAEDIATRIC PROBLEMS — POISONING, NONACCIDENTAL INJURY, GENETIC COUNSELLING

POISONING

Ingested Poisons

Poisoning by ingestion refers to the oral intake of a harmful substance which, even in a small amount, can damage tissues and disturb bodily functions. In the paediatric population, poisoning is often caused by the ingestion of medications as well as toxic household substances such as furniture polish, paraffin, paint remover, disinfectants, and bleach. Fatal accidental poisoning in children is relatively uncommon, accounting for 20-30 deaths yearly in England and Wales. However, the number of poisoning incidents resulting in admission to hospital has increased to 30,000 per annum. Most commonly involved are children aged 1-4 years.

Aetiology
1 Improper or dangerous storage
2 Poor lighting — causes errors in reading
3 Human factors
   a Failure to read label properly
   b Failure to return poison to its proper place
   c Failure to recognize the material as poisonous.

Clinical Manifestations
1 Gastrointestinal symptoms (common in metallic, acid, alkali and bacterial poisonings)
   a Anorexia
   b Abdominal pain
   c Nausea
   d Vomiting

    e Diarrhoea and/or intestinal cramping
2   Central nervous system symptoms
    a Convulsions — common in poisoning due to ingestion of central nervous system stimulants such as strychnine
    b Coma — common in poisoning due to ingestion of central nervous system depressants such as alcohol, atropine, chloral hydrate, barbiturates
    c Dilated pupils — common in poisoning due to atropine, nicotine, cocaine, ephedrine
    d Pinpoint pupils — common in poisoning due to opiates
3   Skin symptoms
    a Rashes
    b Burns
    c Eye inflammation
    d Skin irritation
    e Stains around the mouth or lesions of the mucous membranes
    f Cyanosis — cyanide and strychnine poisoning
4   Cardiopulmonary symptoms
    a Dyspnoea
    b Cardiopulmonary depression or arrest.

Diagnostic Evaluation

Analysis reveals presence of toxic substances in:

1   Blood
2   Urine
3   Gastric washings
4   Vomitus.

Nursing Objectives

To assist the family by telephone management.

1   Calmly secure and record the following information:
    a Name, address, and telephone number of caller
    b Age and condition of the child
    c Name of the ingested product, approximate amount ingested, and time of ingestion.
2   Instruct the caller regarding appropriate emergency actions; dial 999 for emergency ambulance, or take child by car to nearest hospital with accident and emergency department.
3   Instruct parents to save vomitus, unswallowed liquid or pills, and the container, and then to bring them to the hospital as aids in identifying the poison.

To identify the poison.

1   Determine the nature of the ingested substance from the child's history or by reading the label on the container.
2   If necessary, call the nearest poison control centre to identify the toxic ingredient and obtain recommendations for emergency treatment.
3   Save vomitus and urine output for analysis.

To remove the poison from the body.

1   Induce vomiting if no contraindications present, e.g. alteration in level of consciousness or if poisoning due to caustics, acids, or paraffin.
     a Administer syrup of ipecacuanha according to the directions on the label: 10 ml (children aged 6-18 months) or 15 ml (older children) with warm water (200 ml) or fruit juice.
Note: Do not use tincture of ipecacuanha; it is much stronger than the syrup and is itself a poison.
     b Keep the child active, walking about the room or use a rocking horse for motion.
     c If no vomiting occurs after 20-30 minutes, repeat dose of syrup of ipecacuanha.
     d Rarely there is no vomiting after second dose. These children should be given a gastric lavage.

Nursing Alert: Do not induce vomiting if:
1   **The child is convulsing, semiconscious, or comatose.**
2   **Poison if known to be a strong acid or alkali, strychnine, or a hydrocarbon (e.g. lighter fluid, petrol, paraffin, paint remover, nailpolish remover). Strong acids or alkalis may damage the oesophagus for a second time during vomiting, and hydrocarbons cause severe pneumonia if aspirated.**

2   Administer gastric lavage. This is indicated when vomiting is contraindicated, when vomiting is impossible because of the child's condition or when induction of vomiting has been unsuccessful.
     a The child should be well wrapped and secure in a blanket and, whenever possible, held by a parent in the prone or left lateral position.
     b A cuffed endotracheal tube may be inserted prior to lavage to protect the child from aspiration.
     c Use the largest size tube that can be passed orally — preferably one with a double lumen.
     d Aspirate the stomach, keep aspirate.
     e Lavage with small repeated introductions and withdrawals of either normal saline, half-normal saline, special lavage solution or 50 ml or 1.4% sodium bicarbonate solution until about 500 ml of solution has been used.
     f Do not leave a large amount of solution in the child's stomach.
     g Be aware of the dangers associated with lavage:
         (1) Oesophageal perforation may occur in corrosive poisoning.

(2) Gastric haemorrhage
(3) Impaired pulmonary function resulting from aspiration
(4) Cardiac arrest
(5) Convulsions — may result from stimulation in strychnine ingestion.

To reduce the effect of the poison by administering an antidote.

1   An antidote may either react with the poison to prevent its absorption or counteract the effects of the poison after its absorption.
2   Not all poisons have specific antidotes.
3   Information regarding appropriate antidotes for specific poisons is available through all poison control centres and in many paediatric textbooks.
    Antidotes for the most common poisons should be listed in the accident and emergency department of the hospital.
4   Effectiveness of the antidote usually depends on the amount of time which elapses between ingestion of the poison and administration of the antidote.
5   Activated charcoal absorbs all poisons except cyanide.
    Administer orally, after vomiting has occurred, in a dose of 5-10 grams per gram of ingested poison in 177-237 ml of water.

To eliminate the absorbed poison.

1   Force diuresis
    a Administer large quantities of fluid either orally or intravenously.
    b Carefully monitor intake and output.
2   Assist with kidney dialysis which may be necessary if the child's own kidneys are not functioning effectively.
3   Assist with exchange transfusion if this method is indicated for removing the poison.

To observe the child for progression of symptoms and to provide supportive care should these develop.

1   Central nervous system involvement
    a Observe for: restlessness, confusion, delirium, convulsions, lethargy, stupor, coma.
    b Administer sedation with caution — in order to avoid depression and masking of symptoms.
    c Avoid excessive manipulation of the child.
    d See nursing care of the child with seizures, p. 660.
    e See nursing care of the unconscious patient, p. 672.
2   Respiratory involvement
    a Observe for: respiratory depression, obstruction, pulmonary oedema, pneumonia, tachypnoea.
    b Have an artificial airway available.
    c Be prepared to administer oxygen and provide artificial respiration.

    d Other nursing concerns:

      (1) Nursing care of the child on a ventilator, p. 191

      (2) Procedure for administration of oxygen, p. 186

      (3) Procedure of cardiopulmonary resuscitation, p. 196.

3   Cardiovascular involvement

    a Observe for: peripheral circulatory collapse, disturbances of heart rate and rhythm, cardiac failure.

    b Maintain intravenous therapy of saline and glucose solution, plasma or blood. See procedure for the administration of intravenous fluids, p. 155.

    c Be prepared for cardiac arrest. See procedure for cardiopulmonary resuscitation, p. 196.

4   Gastrointestinal involvement

    a Observe for: nausea, pain, abdominal distention, and difficulty in swallowing.

    b Maintain intravenous therapy to replace water and electrolyte loss.

    c Offer a diet which is easily swallowed and digested.

      (1) Begin with clear liquid.

      (2) Progress to full liquids, soft foods, and then a normal diet as the child's condition improves.

5   Kidney involvement

    a Observe the child for decreased urine output.

    Record urine output exactly.

    b Observe for hypertension.

    c Insert indwelling catheter if necessary for urinary retention.

    d Administer appropriate amounts of fluids and electrolytes.

    e See nursing care of the child with renal failure, p. 477.

6   General considerations

    a Maintain adequate kilojoule (calorie), fluid, and vitamin intake.

    Oral fluids are preferable if they can be retained.

    b Avoid hypo- or hyper-thermia.

      (1) Control of body temperature is impaired in many types of poisoning.

      (2) Monitor the child's temperature frequently.

    c Observe closely for infection.

      (1) This is especially important in ingestion of paraffin or other hydrocarbons, which cause chemical pneumonitis.

      (2) Isolate the patient from other children, especially those with respiratory infections.

      (3) Administer antibiotics as ordered by the paediatrician.

To provide emotional support for the child and his family.

1   Remain calm and efficient while working rapidly.

2   Discourage anxious parents from inappropriately handling, caressing, and overstimulating their child.

3   Counsel parents who often feel guilty about the accident.
    a Encourage parents to talk about the poisoning.
    b Emphasize how their quick action in getting treatment for their child has helped.
    c Discuss ways that they can be supportive to their child during his hospitalization.
    d Do not allow prolonged periods of self-incrimination to continue.
    Refer the parents to a social worker for assistance in resolving these feelings if necessary.
4   Involve the young child in therapeutic play to determine how he views the situation.
    a The child often sees nursing measures as punishments for his misdeed involving the poisoning.
    b Explain the child's treatment and correct his misinterpretations in a manner appropriate for his age.

To help prevent further poisoning episodes.

1   Initiate patient and parental teaching once the acute episode is over.
2   Notify family health visitor of any child admitted with accidental poisoning if possible before discharge home.
    A home assessment should be made so that underlying problems are recognized and appropriate help is provided.

Patient and Parental Teaching

Prevention

1   Information concerning poison prevention should be available on any hospital paediatric unit.
    a Many free booklets and posters are available from the Health Education Council and the Royal Society for the Prevention of Accidents.
    b Teaching may be done with any parent regardless of the reason for the child's hospitalization.
2   General precautions for parents to observe:
    a Keep medicines and poisons out of the reach of children.
    b Provide locked storage for highly toxic substances.
    c Do not store poisons in the same area as foods.
    d Be certain all containers are properly marked and labelled. Keep medicines, drugs, and household chemicals in their original containers.
    e Do not discard poisonous substances in receptables where children can reach them.
    f Teach children not to taste or eat unfamiliar substances.

g Medications

    (1) Clean out medicine cabinets periodically.

        (a) Dispose of old medications in containers out of the reach of children.

        (b) Prescription medications should be discarded when the illness for which they were prescribed has run its course.

        (c) Keep medications in 'child-proof' containers that are securely closed.

    (2) Read all labels carefully before each use.

        (a) Follow exact directions on the label.

        (b) Never take a drug from an unlabelled bottle.

    (3) Do not give medicines prescribed for one child to another child.

    (4) Never refer to drugs as sweets or bribe children with such inducements.

    (5) Never give or take medications in the dark.

h Never puncture or burn aerosol containers.

i Store lawn and garden pesticides in a separate place under lock and key outside of the house.

j Know where nearest telephone is to make emergency call for the ambulance service.

Emergency Actions for Parents

1   Suspect poisoning with the occurrence of sudden, bizarre symptoms or peculiar behaviour in toddlers and children.

2   Call 999 emergency telephone service for ambulance. Give all relevant information about the child, his condition, and the substance he took.

3   Maintain an adequate airway in a child who is convulsing or who is not fully conscious.

4   Dilute the poison.

    a For ingestion of alkali (household toilet cleaner, bleach, ammonia) administer citrus juice or water.

        (1) One or two glasses for children under 5 years.

        (2) Up to 1 litre for anyone over 5 years.

    b For acidic substances (toilet bowl cleaner, rust remover, etc.) administer milk.

        (1) One or two glasses for children under 5 years.

        (2) Up to 1 litre for anyone over 5 years.

    c If nature of substance is unknown (whether acid or alkali), give water or milk.

Nursing Alert: Be careful not to administer such large quantities of fluid that the poison is forced through the pylorus.

5   Make the child vomit if so directed. Do not induce vomiting if any of the following occurs:

a Child is unconscious or convulsing.

b Ingested poison was a strong corrosive such as lye or drain cleaner.

c Ingested poison contains petrol, paraffin, or other petroleum distillates.
   Vomiting may be induced by placing child over knee and touching the back of the throat with a finger to stimulate the gag reflex.

6   Transport the child promptly to the nearest accident and emergency department.
   a Wrap the child in a blanket to prevent chilling.
   b Bring the tablet container and any vomitus or urine to the hospital with the child.

7   Avoid excessive manipulation of the child.

8   Act promptly but calmly.

9   Do not assume the child is safe simply because the vomiting shows no trace of the poison or because child appears well. The poison may produce a delayed reaction or may have reached the small intestine, where it is still being absorbed.

Agency

Child Accident Prevention Committee, Faculty of Clinical Science, School of Medicine, University College, Gower Street, London WC1.

LEAD POISONING

Lead poisoning (plumbism) is a disease in young children that results from the consumption of lead in some form. Each year it causes the death of some children and leaves others with chronic neurological handicaps, mental handicap, and/or behavioural problems. Lead is a cumulative poison.

Aetiology

1   Ingestion of substances containing lead
   a Toys, furniture, windowsills, household fixtures, and plaster painted with lead-containing paint may be ingested.
   b Lead toys
   c Oil paints
   d Acidic juices or foods served in pottery made with lead glazes
   e Paints used in newspapers, magazines, children's books, matches, and playing cards
   f Water from lead pipes
   g Fruit covered with insecticides
   h Dirt containing lead fallout from automobile exhaust
   i Antique pewter, particularly when used to serve acidic juices or foods
   j Lead weights (curtain weights, fishing sinkers)

2   Inhalation of fumes containing lead (less common cause in children)
   a   Motor fuel
   b   Burning storage batteries
   c   Dust containing lead salts
3   Children of Asian families may be exposed to lead sulphate used as a cosmetic (surma).

Altered Physiology

1   Lead salts are absorbed by the blood from the respiratory tract or the intestines.
2   A large portion of the absorbed lead enters the portal circulation and is excreted by the liver.
3   Lead that reaches the systemic circulation is deposited in soft tissues, causing damage primarily to the nervous system, the blood, and the kidneys.
   a   Nervous system
     (1) Brain — oedema, vascular damage; destruction of brain cells, causing convulsive disorders; neurological deficits; learning difficulties
     (2) Peripheral nerve palsies
   b   Blood
     (1) Increases in the concentration of haemoglobin precursors in body fluids
     (2) Inhibition of a number of steps in the biosynthesis of haem, thus reducing the number of red blood cells, increasing fragility, and reducing half-life
   c   Kidneys
     Injury to the cells of the proximal tubules, causing abnormal excretion of amino acids, protein, glucose, and phosphate
4   Lead is slowly transferred from soft tissues to bone.
   a   It is deposited in insoluble form with calcium.
   b   The deposition causes increased thickness and density of long bones.
   c   Decalcification is associated with the release of lead from bone.

Epidemiological Factors

1   Slums and old neighbourhoods are high-risk areas because of old, deteriorating housing.
2   Pica (a habit of eating nonfood items such as paint chips, often involving a craving type of behaviour) is a common precondition.
   a   Poisoning associated with pica is a chronic process.
   b   Clinical manifestations appear after 3-6 months of fairly steady lead ingestion.

Incidence

1 Highest in children between 1 and 6 years of age, especially those between 1 and 3 years
2 High in children from poor, deprived families
3 No significant difference in sex
4 High among siblings
5 Symptomatic lead poisoning usually occurs in the summer months
6 Recurrence rate is high.

Clinical Manifestations

1 Gastrointestinal symptoms
   a Vomiting
   b Vague abdominal pain
   c Colic
   d Constipation
   e Loss of appetite
   f Weight loss
2 Central nervous system symptoms (common in children)
   a Falling, clumsiness, loss of coordination
   b Irritability
   c Dispositional changes
   d Convulsions with or without local paralysis
   e Drowsiness, coma
   f Peripheral nerve palsies
3 Haematological symptoms
   a Anaemia
   b Pallor
4 Cardiovascular symptoms
   a Hypertension
   b Bradycardia
5 Symptoms depend on the amount of lead in the soft tissues and blood:
   a Onset is insidious
   b Usually progresses from mild to severe manifestations as the lead slowly accumulates
   c Infants and toddlers may present severe manifestations initially
   d Symptoms may be intermittent for several months.

Diagnostic Evaluation

1 Increased serum lead levels
   Abnormal lead concentrations in the blood is the only certain index of excessive exposure (normal range 0-1.8 μmol/1). A haematocrit should be

done with each lead level so that a correction factor can be applied for anaemia.

2   Increased excretion of urine.
3   Anaemia with basophilic stippling of the blood cells seen on the smear. Elevated blood protoporphyrin. Fluorescence of red blood cells may be observed under ultraviolet light.
4   Urinary excretion of coproporphyrin.
5   Increased density at the epiphyseal line seen on x-ray examination of the bones.
6   Flat plate of abdomen — may reveal radio-opaque material if lead has been ingested during the preceding 24-36 hours.
7   Increased protein without an increase in the number of cells in the cerebrospinal fluid. The fluid may be under pressure in children with lead encephalopathy.
8   Mild glycosuria.

Prognosis

1   Improving with increased emphasis on prevention and screening.
2   Children with central nervous system involvement have a poor prognosis for normal development. Residual effects on the nervous system are permanent and progressive.

Late symptoms of mental retardation may appear 3-9 years after treatment. Specific intellectual defect may interfere with the child's progress at school.

Nursing Objectives

To collect a urine specimen as a diagnostic tool.

A 24-hour specimen is more accurate than a single micturated specimen. (See section on specimen collection, p. 144)

To prevent absorption of lead.

1   Induce vomiting or administer enemas if radio-opaque lead particles are observed on abdominal x-rays. This is only used with acute lead poisoning which is less common than chronic lead poisoning.

2   Make certain that all sources of lead are removed from the child's environment, including the hospital environment.

To increase excretion of lead from the body.

1   Administer appropriate chelating agents (refer to Table 17.1).
    a Action — Repeat with lead to form nontoxic compounds which are excreted by the body.
    b Dosage — Depends on individual drug, child's weight, severity of poisoning, prior history, and whether or not other chelating agents are being used simultaneously.

To provide supportive care to the child with encephalopathy.

1   Observe for:
    a Rising blood pressure
    b Papilloedema
    c Slow pulse
    d Convulsions
    e Unconsciousness
2   See section on neurological problems, p. 671.
3   Diuretics, e.g. mannitol (2.5 g/kg body weight by intravenous infusion) or dexamethasone (a corticosteroid) may be ordered to reduce cerebral oedema.
4   Plan nursing care around periods when medications must be given.

To observe for factors associated with lead poisoning.

1   Pica
    a Observe and record the child's eating habits and food preferences.
    b Report any attempted eating of nonfood substances.
    c Provide regular meals and make mealtime a pleasurable time for the child.
    d Discourage oral activity and substitute activity that contributes to play, social skills, and ego development.
    e Refer the family for additional social or psychiatric casework if indicated to reduce the psychological or cultural factors which result in pica in the child.
2   Strained parent-child relationships
    Record when family members visit as well as the nature of their interaction with the child.

Table 17.1 Chelating agents used to treat lead poisoning in children

	Calcium EDTA (ethylenediaminetetra-acetic acid, Versenate)	Dimercaprol (BAL)
Route of administration	CaEDTA is most usually given intravenously in a 5% dextrose infusion in four divided doses per 24 hours over a period of 5-7 days.	Intramuscular injection.
Excretion of lead	Urinary excretion increased 20-50 times.	Urinary and faecal output increased. Produces greater total excretion than calcium EDTA alone.
Untoward reactions	Rash, vomiting, tetany, lethargy, transient fever.	1 Symptoms begin within 10-15 minutes after injection of BAL and subside within 1-2 hours. 2 Symptoms: Increased lacrimation, salivation, sweating, nausea and vomiting, headache, pain in teeth, burning sensation of lips, mouth, throat; tachycardia, increased blood pressure, muscular ache, fever.

Toxic reactions	*Renal toxicity* 1 Do not administer to dehydrated patients. 2 Check urine daily for protein and blood. *Transient hypercalcaemia* 1 Monitor serum calcium.	*Renal toxicity* 1 Encourage fluids to maintain adequate excretion of the lead via the urine. 2 Check urine daily for protein and abnormalities of urinary sediment.
Special considerations/ precautions	1 Usual course of treatment is 5 days. A second course of therapy may be necessary after an interval of 2 days if signs and symptoms of lead poisoning persist or if serum level remains elevated.	1 Often given in combination with calcium EDTA. In children with very high lead levels, BAL is often given initially in order to lower the blood level before calcium EDTA is given, which may actually raise the blood lead level temporarily when therapy is initiated. 2 Monitor vital signs for 15 minutes after giving BAL, because of the potential for causing tachycardia and increased blood pressure. 3 Do not administer iron to children receiving BAL, since BAL forms a toxic complex with iron.

Note: D-Penicillamine as a chelating agent has the advantage of being effective when given orally. It is, however, unsuitable for those children with high blood lead levels.

To provide the child with social and motor stimulation.

1   Provide and encourage activities that will help the child to learn and progress from his present developmental state. (Refer to section on growth and development, health maintenance, p. 7.)
2   Initiate appropriate referrals in cases of obvious developmental delays. Such referrals may be to such professionals as psychologists, psychiatrists, and specialists in early child education.
3   Share the results of developmental testing with the parent(s) and discuss ways to provide stimulation for the child at home.

To provide emotional support to the parent(s)

1   Utilize sensitivity in interviewing and teaching to avoid causing or increasing guilt feelings about the poisoning and to establish a positive, trusting relationship between the family and the health care facility.
2   Explain the treatment and its purpose.

To prevent re-exposure of the child to lead.

1   Instruct parents regarding the seriousness of repeated exposure to lead.
2   Initiate a referral to the family health visitor to determine if exposure to lead is continuing and to provide continuing support to the family.
3   Advise parents to require landlord to remove lead paint from the walls; assist them with this process.
    a Refer the parents to the housing authority.
    b Do not allow the child in the home while lead paint is being removed.
4   When it is impossible to eliminate lead hazards from the home:
    a Scrape loose or chipped paint and plaster from the window sills, woodwork, mouldings, etc., and tape the areas with masking tape or contact paper.
    b Remove all crumbling plaster and replaster or cover the area with wallboard or contact paper.
5   Make certain that the family is able to provide close supervision of the child or assist them to make arrangements to ensure that the child is adequately supervised at home.

To participate in the prevention of lead poisoning.

1   Initiate and support educational campaigns in schools, clinics, libraries, and news media to alert parents and children to hazards and symptoms of lead poisoning.
2   Provide in clinics, waiting rooms, and other appropriate settings literature stressing the hazards of lead, sources of lead, and signs of lead intoxication.

3 Inquire about the presence of pica in all children under 6 years of age.
4 Screen siblings of known cases immediately.
5 Screen all children from high-risk areas.
6 Provide follow-up to all children suffering from lead poisoning as well as to those in the early stage of undue lead absorption to prevent their becoming poisoned.

Patient or Parental Teaching

Parent education is an extremely important part of the nursing care of a child with lead poisoning. It should include the following points of emphasis:

1 Long-term medical follow-up is essential.
  a Residual lead is liberated gradually after treatment.
    (1) May result in the renewal of symptoms.
    (2) May increase serum lead to a dangerous level.
    (3) Additional damage to the central nervous system may become apparent for several months (after discharge from the hospital).
  b Acute infections must be recognized and treated promptly. (These may reactivate the disease.)
2 Re-exposure to lead must be prevented.
3 Siblings and playmates should be screened for lead poisoning.
4 Literature stressing the causes and prevention of lead poisoning should be provided.

NONACCIDENTAL INJURY (THE BATTERED CHILD — ABUSE AND NEGLECT)

Child abuse and neglect refers to 'a child who is suffering from physical injury (inflicted upon him by other than accidental means), or sexual abuse, or malnutrition, or suffering physical or emotional harm or substantial risk thereof by reason of neglect. Reporting of neglect shall take into account the accepted child rearing practices of the culture of which he or she is part.'

1 Child abuse and neglect includes the following conditions:
  a Battering — physical injury
  b Nutritional neglect — deliberate omission of adequate nutrition. 'Failure to thrive' results when child's weight is below the third percentile for age and sex and child has no predisposing physical abnormality

c Drug abuse — intentional administration of harmful drugs
d Medical neglect — intentional omission of basic preventive-medicine practices or specific treatment for medical problems
e Sexual abuse — sexual assault or molestation
f Safety neglect — intentional omission of safety precautions appropriate for age of child
g Emotional abuse — scapegoating, belittling, humiliating, lack of mothering
h Child neglect — lack of providing the child with basic needs of survival: shelter, clothing, stimulation, development of trust, etc.

Aetiology

Child abuse is not a uniform phenomenon with one set of causal factors, but a multidimensional phenomenon. The phenomenon may be related to:

1   The combined presence of three factors — special kind of child, special kind of parent, special circumstances of crisis:
    a Psychopathology of the abuser
    b Cultural, social, and economic factors
    c Specific child characteristics, i.e. preterm infant separated from mother at birth before bonding has begun to develop, debilitated child needing special care.

Contributing Factors

1   Incidents of child abuse may develop as a result of disciplinary action taken by the abuser who responds in uncontrolled anger to real or perceived misconduct of the child. Parents may confuse punishment with discipline. 'Good parenting' may be equated with physical contact to eradicate undesirable child behaviour.
2   Incidents of child abuse may develop from a general attitude of resentment or rejection on the part of the abuser towards the child.
3   Atypical child behaviour (e.g. hyperactivity) may provoke the abuser. This may be child-initiated or child-provoked abuse.
4   Incidents of child abuse may develop out of a quarrel between the caretakers. The child may come to the aid of one parent, may find himself in the midst of the quarrel, or may object to the quarrel.
5   The abuser may be a stern, authoritarian disciplinarian.
6   The abuser may be under a great deal of stress because of life circumstances (debt, poverty, illness) and may thus resort to child abuse. Crisis and stress may be ongoing. The abuser may have a low frustration tolerance level and may not have a well-developed means of coping with stress in general.
7   The abuser may be intoxicated with alcohol or drugs at the time of the abuse.

8 Child abuse may occur while the mother is out of the home and the child is left in the care of a babysitter or boyfriend.

9 Lack of early mothering, inappropriate mother-child bonding, and punitive treatment as a child may contribute to child neglect.

10 Specific characteristics evident in many abusing parents include:

a Low self-esteem — a sense of incompetence in role; unworthiness; unimportance

b Unrealistic attitudes and expectations of child; little regard for child's own needs and age-appropriate abilities

c Fear of rejection — a deep need to feel wanted and loved, but a feeling of rejection when love is not obvious. A crying infant may elicit a feeling of rejection

d Inability to accept help — isolation from the community; loneliness

e Unhappiness due to unsatisfactory relationships; may look to child for satisfaction of own emotional needs

11 The abused or neglected child may be seen by the parent as 'special'. The preterm infant or one having a serious illness and separated from his mother for the first weeks of life may have resulted in failure of emotional bonding. Parents perhaps could not provide special care to the child because of their own psychological variables or situation.

Clinical Manifestations

Physical Characteristics Utilized as an Index of Suspicion

1 Child usually under 3 years of age. School-age child is also subject to abuse, however

2 General health of the child indicates neglect (nappy rash, poor hygiene, malnutrition)

3 Characteristic distribution of fractures (scattered over many different parts of body)

4 Disproportionate amount of soft tissue injury

5 Evidence that injuries occurred at different times (healed and new fractures, resolving and fresh bruises)

6 Cause of recent trauma in question

7 History of similar episodes in past

8 No new lesions occurring during the child's hospitalization

9 The child may develop behaviours through interaction with parents and peers that place him at risk for abuse.

Injuries or Types of Abuse that may Occur

1 Bruises, welts (most common)

2 Abrasions, contusions, lacerations (most common)

3 Wounds, cuts, punctures

4   Burns (cigarette, radiator, etc.), scalding
5   Bone fractures (including skull)
6   Sprains, dislocations
7   Subdural haemorrhage or haematoma
8   Brain damage
9   Internal injuries
10   Drug intoxication
11   Malnutrition (deliberately inflicted)
12   Freezing, exposure
13   Whiplash-type injury
14   Eye injuries
15   Periorbital injuries.

Possible Characteristics of the Child Suspected of Being Abused or Neglected

1   May show a wide range of reactions — may be either very withdrawn or overactive. Child may be anxious, tense, or nervous. The child subjected to violence over a long period commonly exhibits, even when quite young, an apprehensive anxious demeanour and expression known as 'frozen awareness' or 'frozen watchfulness'.
2   Avoids physical contact with parents; does not look to parents for comfort; shows distinct preference for one parent, while fearfully withdrawing from the other.
3   Is fearful, constantly alert for danger; seeks information as to what is going to happen next; is mistrustful of environment.
4   May show unusual affection for strangers or may be overly fearful of adults and avoid any physical contact with them.

Identifying Behaviour Common in Abusing or Neglecting Parent(s)

(Be aware that not all abusing parents exhibit these behaviours.)

1   Anxiously volunteers information or withholds information.
2   Gives an explanation of the injury that does not fit the condition or gets story confused concerning the injury.
3   Shows inappropriate reaction to severity of injury.
4   Becomes irritable about questions being asked.
5   Seldom touches or speaks to child; does not respond to him. May be critical of child or indicate unreal expectations of him.
6   Delays seeking medical help; refuses to sign consent for investigation and diagnosis. Frequently changes hospitals or doctor.
7   Shows no involvement in care of the hospitalized child; does not inquire about child.
8   The problem of abuse is a total family problem — family dysfunction.

Nursing Objectives

To inspect every child's body upon admission to the hospital for evidence of abuse.

1   Describe on nursing record all bruises, lacerations, etc., as to location and state of healing. Look carefully at areas generally covered with clothing, i.e. buttocks, underarms, behind knees, bottom of feet. Be alert for abuse of school-age child. Most often the child's injury is not severe enough to require medical attention, but the child may be hospitalized for some other medical problem.
2   Discuss with the paediatrician the case of any child suspected of being abused.
      Every nurse is morally responsible to report any situation where child abuse is suspected.

To be prepared to care effectively for the sexually assaulted child.

1   Sexual abuse should be suspected when the young, prepubital child presents with:
   a Trauma not readily explained
   b Gonorrhea, syphilis, or other sexually transmitted infections
   c Blood in urine or stool
   d Painful urination or defaecation
   e Penile or vaginal infection or itch
   f Penile or vaginal discharge
   g Report of increased, excessive masturbation
   h Report of increased, unusual fears.
2   Establish a relationship with the child based upon mutual respect, empathy, and sensitivity.
   a The child may be extremely calm or hysterical. He may verbally express a desire to talk about the incident. Take into consideration the different ways emotions are expressed by children at different developmental stages.
   b Consideration of the child's emotions in conjunction with a good relationship may encourage the child to express his feelings either verbally or through drawings or play.
   c Prepare the child both physically and psychologically for the necessary physical and pelvic examination.
   d Talk with the child without the presence of the parents, especially when incest is possible.
3   Document any physical findings — bruises, abrasions, telltale secretions in mouth or pharynx, on hair or skin, in and around buttocks, clothes.
   a Collect any necessary specimens for identification of organisms, sperm, or semen.
   b Take colour photographs.
4   Participate in the therapeutic approach.
   a Talk with the child and parents alone. Be honest with the mother.

b Prevent sexually transmitted disease, pregnancy, and tetanus. Prophylactic treatment should be given for penile penetration of any orifice.
c Support the parents who may have feelings of guilt, anger, and helplessness. Explain to them the extent of trauma and educate them regarding paediatric gynaecology; allow them to air their feelings. Support their parental role in handling the child (i.e. allow child to talk about or play out the incident, but do not force it).
d Encourage compliance with the treatment selected for the child, parents, and family (i.e. group counselling, psychiatry).

5   Participate in the case conference of the multidisciplinary team.

To observe and record pertinent information regarding the parent-child relationship.

1   Do the parents visit the child? Do parents become involved in caring for child?
2   How does the parent(s) respond to the child? Does the parent talk to the child, touch him, hold him, play with him?
3   How does the child react to the parent? Is he excited with the parent arrives? Does he appear frightened and withdrawn? Does he cry when the parent leaves?
4   What does the parent expect of the child? Are his expectations appropriate for child? Is there role-reversal between parent and child?

To obtain a thorough nursing history in order to establish a nursing care plan that is individualized to meet specific needs of the child.

1   Information should be obtained relating to the child's sleeping habits, toilet habits, favourite foods and eating habits, favourite toy or security objects, play habits and favourite playmate, names and ages of siblings, nickname, previous hospital experience, developmental assessment, and persons who will visit child.
2   Care and good judgement must be used in obtaining this information from parents, because they undoubtedly have already been asked many questions by many people. Use case notes already obtained to eliminate repetition.
3   Obtaining a nursing history in a nonthreatening, nonjudgemental manner can convey to parents that you have a genuine interest in caring for their child, and that you respect the knowledge they have as parents of their child. Getting the history will also allow you to assess the parents' knowledge and expectations of their child and will set a positive atmosphere for a continued relationship.

To provide for the child a milieu to reduce trauma similar to that of any hospitalized child placed in the strange and frightening environment of the hospital by implementing the principles of emotional support. (see p. 56.)

The child must be treated as an individual. He may need extra help in the following areas:

1 Having ambivalent feelings toward his parent or parents
2 Overcoming his low self-image and the fear that something is wrong with him
3 Fearing future abuse upon his return home
4 Satisfying his strong need for attention, affection, and having a trusting relationship with an adult
5 Learning alternative ways of expressing his needs and feelings.

To foster a trusting relationship with the child who may be fearful of adults.

1 Assign one particular nurse to care for the child over a period of time. Select the right nurse for the right patient. When going off duty, a colleague should be introduced to the child by an assigned nurse. Utilize the 'granny scheme' if available.
2 Make no threatening moves towards the child. The child will indicate his readiness and awareness of the environment by his verbal or facial expressions.
3 Touch the child gently.
4 Provide nonthreatening physical contact (hold the child frequently and cuddle him). Pick him up and carry him around; encourage any exploration of your face, hair, etc.
5 Enlist the cooperation of volunteers to provide additional mothering.
6 Provide appropriate opportunities for play.
7 Set limits for him.

To come to grips with your own feelings of anger, disgust, and contempt for the parents.

It may help to do the following:

1 Realize that most abusing parents do love their child and want the best for him in spite of their ambivalent feelings for him.
2 Understand the dynamics of child abuse and neglect. This crisis is due to the stress the parents are unable to cope with and to the deprivations they have themselves suffered in their past.
3 Focus on the needs of the parents rather than on the injuries of the child. Treatment is aimed at helping parents reach their maximum potential as parents.
4 Expect repeated rejection from the parents who lack self-esteem and trust.
5 Understand that these parents are often difficult to like under ordinary conditions. They are experiencing terror, guilt, and remorse; they are fearful and yet expect criticism and condemnation.

To foster a relationship with the parents that will encourage them to accept guidance and will help in dealing with the problem.

1   Assume a nonjudgemental attitude that is neither punitive nor threatening.
2   Refrain from questioning them about the incident of abuse. (The suspected abuser will be interviewed by the paediatrician, the social worker, and the authority who investigates the case.)
3   Include parents in the hospital experience — i.e. orient them to the unit and to any procedure to be done to the child. Serve as role model in the management of the child's behaviour as well as their own. Try to give the parents as much information as possible about the care of their child. Listen to what they are saying.
4   Refrain from challenging all the information they may give.
5   Express appropriate concern and kindness. Remain objective yet empathetic. This will help foster the parents' self-respect and improve their self-image and dignity.

To foster a healthy mother-child relationship.

1   Build a relationship by working with the mother's strengths rather than her weaknesses. Use compliments as positive reinforcement.
2   Serve as a role model of appropriate methods of child care in areas such as feeding, bathing, and play.
3   Provide the mother with psychological support and reinforcement for appropriate mothering behaviours she does exhibit.
4   Work with the mother in planning for the child's future care.
5   Determine in what areas the mother needs help: Does the baby cry a lot? How does this make her feel? How does she comfort him? When she is alone, is there someone she can call for help? Does she feel the child understands what she expects of him?
6   By forming a helping relationship with the mother, the nurse will strengthen the protective ability of the mother and bind her to her child.

To teach the parents about normal growth and development.

(See section on growth and development, p. 7.)

1   Give specific information and examples as to the type of behaviour to expect at the various stages of development. Point out in a nonthreatening way normal behaviour exhibited by their child.
2   Give specific information on dealing with this behaviour.
3   Serve as role model and teacher; minimize intensity when parents become threatened.

To teach the parents how to use discipline without resorting to physical force.

1   Discipline must be consistent. Offer suggestions for alternative ways of handling undesirable behaviour.

2 Rewards may be used for acceptable behaviour (e.g. a trip to the zoo, staying up later than usual for a special TV show, a special treat).

3 Rewards are withheld for unacceptable behaviour.

To support the parent and the child if a decision is made to have the child removed from the home.

1 The decision is made for the safety and protection of the child.

2 The parents are afforded the opportunity to have counselling to help them learn to deal with their problem.

3 The child must be prepared for his removal from the home and placement plans. He must be allowed time to work through his feelings.

To support the parents and child in preparation for discharge to home.

1 Both parents and child (if age is appropriate) need to know and understand any specific instructions relative to injury and follow-up care.

2 Parents need to be made aware of the most common posthospitalization behaviour children may have. (See p. 56.)

3 Make known to parents your continued concern and your availability as a source of help. Stress need for follow-up care. Help them to use community resources available, i.e health visitor, day-nurseries, voluntary agencies.

To be aware of the child who has the potential for being abused and to provide anticipatory guidance towards prevention of abuse.

1 The preterm infant, the hyperactive child, the chronically ill child, the mentally handicapped child, the child who requires a great deal of care and confines the mother to the home, the child involved in a disturbed mother-infant bond all have the potential for being abused.

2 Encourage early participation of mother (parents) in the care of the child during hospitalization.

3 Prepare the mother for the fact that the child does require a great deal of care, but encourage her to find outlets for her frustrations.

4 Provide her with the name and telephone number of someone at the hospital to whom she can look for help (e.g. social worker).

5 Initiate a referral to the health visitor before discharge home.

To be aware of the entire scope of nursing responsibilities in dealing with the abused and neglected child.

1 Case finding — identify the potential (or suspected) abused and neglected child. Be a participating and contributing member of the multidisciplinary team in treating and evaluating the abused child and his family.

2 Nurse-parent relationships — develop therapeutic, trusting relationships that will help parents develop to their full potential.

3 Support community assistance programmes to help parents overcome isolation.

4   Support public re-education to enhance the parenting capabilities of every man and woman: preparation for parenthood at school, preparation for specific family situations during antenatal care for both parents.

To be aware that the goal of treatment of the parents is to assure the physical and emotional safety of the child.

1   It is estimated that 90% of abusing parents can be rehabilitated.
2   Treatment is offered to help parents to do the following:
   a Understand and redirect their anger
   b Develop an adequate parent-child relationship
   c See their child as an individual with his own needs and differences
   d Enjoy their child
   e Develop realistic expectations of their child
   f Decrease their use of criticism
   g Increase their own sense of self-esteem and confidence
   h Establish supportive relationships with others
   i Improve economic situation (if appropriate)
   j Show progress towards physical, emotional, and intellectual development.

Agency

National Society for the Prevention of Cruelty to Children, 1 Riding House Street, London W1.

GENETIC COUNSELLING

Genetic counselling is the process of providing families with information about hereditary and congenital disorders. It involves determining the risk of occurrence or recurrence, interpreting the findings, and assisting the family in making a reasonable decision.

Indications for Antenatal Diagnosis of Genetic Disorders

1   Increased risk of chromosomal disorders
   a Advanced maternal age — woman 35 years of age and older
   b Parent known to be a carrier of chromosomal disorder
   c Previous pregnancy resulting in child with chromosomal disorder
2   Known risk for significant metabolic disorders
3   Known risk for significant sex-linked genetic disorders
4   Willingness to consider termination of the pregnancy if an abnormal fetus is detected.

Antenatal Diagnosis of Genetic Disorders

Amniocentesis

1   Method of obtaining amniotic fluid of a pregnant woman by inserting a needle transabdominally through the uterus.
2   Examination is made of amniotic fluid, amniotic fluid cells, and cultured amniotic fluid cells.
3   Procedure done at 13-16 weeks gestation.

X-ray, Roentgenography

1   Useful in diagnosing anencephaly, hydrocephaly, achondroplasia, and osteogenesis imperfecta congenita.
2   Many diagnoses are established only in the last trimester.
3   Risk of radiation exposure to fetus is high if done prior to third trimester.

Amniography-Fetography

1   A technique of intra-amniotic injection of a contrast material which opacifies the fluid and displaces the fetal soft tissue parts.
2   Useful in diagnosing soft tissue and gastrointestinal malformations.

Ultrasonography

1   Used in conjunction with other laboratory studies in diagnosing malformations of the central nervous system.
2   Used to determine the size of the fetus and the fetal head.

Fetoscope

Visualization of fetus *in utero* by endoscopic instruments.

Diagnostic Studies Performed from Amniocentesis

Amniotic Fluid

1   Steroid levels
2   Enzyme studies
3   Mucopolysaccharide determinations
4   Alpha-fetoprotein levels.

Amniotic Cells

1   Enzyme studies
2   Sex chromatin and Y-body flourescence.

Amniotic Fluid Cells, Cultured

1   Cytogenetic studies (karyotype)
2   Enzyme studies
3   Autoradiographic studies
4   Histochemistry.

Major Genetic Disorders

See Table 17.2.

Goals of Genetic Counselling

1   To provide clients with information about the genetic defect in question.
2   To communicate to clients the risk of transmitting the defect to subsequently conceived children.
3   To enable individuals and couples to make informed decisions regarding marriage and/or parenthood (e.g. having children, adopting children, continuing or terminating an existing pregnancy).
4   To provide psychological support to assist clients with their decision-making process and the necessary reordering of their lives.
5   To reduce the number of individuals affected by genetic disease.
6   To alert other health professionals involved with the family of the possibility of genetic disease in family background.

Nursing Objectives Related to Genetic Counselling

To identify families who need genetic counselling and to whom the service should be offered.

1   Be alert to information in the family history which would indicate referral for genetic counselling.
2   Be aware of evidence of deviation from normal growth and development and of other abnormalities (e.g. a single umbilical artery, low-set ears, or defects of the genitalia) which may indicate genetic problems.
3   Offer the opportunity for counselling to any family that has a child with a known genetic problem.

To assist families to acquire sufficient and correct information about the genetic problem in question.

1   Be aware of specialist units for genetic counselling.
2   Be knowledgeable about the types of genetic disorders and their probability of occurrence (see Table 17.2), genetic principles, and genetic diagnostic methods.

To serve as a liaison between the genetic counsellor and the family.

1 Prepare parents for the experience of counselling. Help them know what to anticipate to lower their anxiety level and to make the counselling sessions a better experience.
2 If possible, attend the counselling session. This facilitates reinforcement of information and makes it easier to answer questions adequately.
3 Assess the family's need for additional counselling sessions, and initiate these if the need is recognized.

To help families handle the information received and to guide them in coping with this crisis in their lives.

1 Utilize interviewing skills to facilitate discussion regarding parental feelings Consider such factors as timing and privacy.
2 Alleviate parental feelings of guilt and shame.
   a If a recessive trait is involved, both parents may blame themselves. A parent who is a carrier of a dominant anomaly may blame himself, and the other parent may blame him as well even if she (or he) does not outwardly express these feelings.
   b Emphasize that a person has no choice or responsibility in acquiring the genes that cause the problem.
   c Reassure parents that information gathered is important for determining an accurate diagnosis and the nature of inheritance; assure them that it will be kept confidential.
   d It may be helpful to inform parents that many other people have hidden, recessive genes.
3 Anticipate parental questions and areas of difficulty and conflict.
   a Many parents are afraid to ask questions. They may fear that they will sound stupid; they may not know what to ask — much less how to ask questions.
   b Listen carefully for parental areas of unanswered or unasked questions.
   c Help parents formulate questions. Utilize statements such as, 'Many parents have questions about _____.'
   d Be available to parents when they have something to ask.
   e Listen carefully to parent's questions and answer them whenever possible.
4 Remain objective.
   a Be aware of personal feelings about specific genetic disorders.
   b Come to terms with any emotional difficulties of your own related to genetic disorders and to issues such as abortion.
   c Avoid letting personal reactions affect your attitude towards counselling and behaviour towards family.
   (1) If the nurse avoids the situation, parents are tacitly given professional sanction to do the same thing.

Table 17.2 Common genetic disorders

Types	Incidence	Risk	Discussion
Chromosomal disorders			
1 Autosomal abnormalities			
Down's syndrome (Trisomy 21) (see p. 689)	1 in 600 live births; varies with maternal age; meiotic nondisjunction	Insufficient data	Chromosomal disorders result from:
	Young mother: 1 in 1000 live births	Spontaneous abortion rates are high (10-60%)	1 Failure of a chromosome to separate at cell division (nondisjunction), causing loss or gain of genetic material.
	Mother over 35: 1 in 300 live births		2 Cell division error causing a chromosomal imbalance or rearrangement of genetic material. Error is associated with major structural changes.
			Most of the variations and abnormalities are directly transmitted to offspring from parent.
2 Monosomy (autosomal)	Product of conception rarely survives		
3 Sex chromosome abnormalities			
Klinefelter's syndrome (XXY abnormality)	1 in 400 male live births		

Turner's syndrome (X abnormality, also monosomy sex chromosome, applies to phenotype female with genotype 45,XO)	1 in 2500-3000 female live births	

Mendelian disorders — single gene

1 Autosomal dominant

Achondroplasia, classic	1 in 10 000 live births	Usually sporadic occurrence. Affected parent has a 50% chance of having affected off-spring with each pregnancy	Mendelain inheritance: a single deleterious gene can cause multiple anomalies or isolated malformations.
Skeletal disorders (e.g. syndactyly)			

2 Autosomal recessive

Sickle cell anaemia	1 in 625 live births of black races	Risk of affected parent affected offspring is 25% per pregnancy; 50% carrier state	
Cystic fibrosis	1 in 2500 live births of Caucasians		
Tay-Sachs disease	50 live births per year (occurs mainly in Jewish children)		Carrier can be identified.

(continued)

Table 17.2 Common genetic disorders (*continued*)

Types	Incidence	Risk	Discussion
Inherited metabolic disorders (e.g. galactosaemia)			
3 Sex-linked recessive Glucose-6-phosphate dehydrogenase (G6PD) deficiency	12% of male live births in black races 24% of female live births in black races	If affected male reproduces, offspring will be as follows: males are normal; females are carriers	Sex-linked disorders occur mainly in males, although the female is the carrier. Most sex-linked disorders are recessive.
Haemophilia, classic Duchenne's muscular dystrophy	1 in 10 000 male live births	Unaffected female carrier offspring: 50% male affected; 50% male normal; 50% female carrier; 50% female normal	
4 Sex-linked dominant (rare) Vitamin D-resistant rickets		Transmitted from affected male to all female offspring; male offspring are normal; affected female — 50% of all offspring will be affected	

Multifactorial-polygenic disorders

Neural tube defects (mylomeningocele)	1 in 250-500 live births in the UK	Risk varies with racial background and geographical area. Recurrence risk is usually 2-7% but is related to outcome of previous pregnancies	Polygenic disorders are probably the result of several deleterious genes combined with environmental factors.
Cleft clip and cleft palate	1 in 1000 live births		These disorders are difficult to prove, because they are mainly the result of slight variations at multiple gene loci.
Pyloric stenosis	1 in 200 male live births 1 in 1000 female live births		

(2) A nurse who conveys the impression that she cannot cope with the fact of genetic disease is unlikely to convey assurance that a family should be able to cope with the consequences of the disease.

5   Reinforce information about the genetic disorder, probability, possible interventions to correct the defect or minimize the disability, self-care goals, and limitations requiring adaptation.

   a Frequently parents do not understand the meaning of the risk ratio quoted to them, or they may attach too much or too little importance to it.
   b Be certain that parents understand specifically what the predictions imply.

6   Clarify understanding of all family members.

   Have both parents present for discussions as frequently as possible to prevent misinterpretations and distortions from being passed from one to the other. Include grandparents and siblings as appropriate.

7   Assist parents to evaluate the total situation and to see the ramifications of any decision they may make.

   Assess realistically the expected burden to the parents, the child, and society; have them evaluate their capacity for dealing with the situation and expected problems.

8   Provide psychological support to allow parents to make and carry out decisions.

   a Parents who decide against having children should be given information about family planning methods and sterilization.
   b Parents who elect pregnancy should be informed about appropriate techniques of antenatal diagnosis of genetic disorders.
   c Parents who elect adoption should be given the opportunity for additional advice when the adoption is being undertaken.

To assure continued and comprehensive nursing care for the affected child and the family.
Communicate and liaise with other health care professionals and where indicated voluntary agencies to ensure continuity of care.

To provide information regarding known genetic risk factors to the general public.

1   Support the concept of premarital counselling.
2   Support antenatal counselling to increase awareness of potential hazards of infections such as rubella, to the impact of drugs on the fetus, and to pollution of water and foodstuffs by pesticides and fertilizers.

FURTHER READING

Poisoning

Books
Pacoe D J, Grossman M, *Quick Reference to Pediatric Emergencies*, 2nd edn, Lippincott, 1978.
Proudfoot A T, *Diagnosis and Management of Acute Poisoning*, Blackwell Scientific, 1981.
Valman H B, *Accident and Emergency Paediatrics*, Blackwell Scientific, 1976.

Articles
Craft A W Nicholson A, The management of poisoning in children, *Nursing Times*, June 1975, 71: 977-979.
Croft H Frenkel S, Children and lead poisoning, *American Journal of Nursing*, January 1975, 75: 2181-2184.
David O, Low lead levels and mental retardation, *Lancet*, December 1976, 1376-1379.
Fraser N C, Accidental poisoning deaths in British children, 1958-77, *British Medical Journal*, 26 June 1980: 1595-1598.
Healy M A Aslam M, The lead sandwich syndrome, *Nursing Times*, 9 September 1981: 1598-1600.
Henry J Volans G, ABC of poisoning: problems in children, *British Medical Journal*, 25 August 1984: 486-489.
Hodges S, Chronic lead poisoning: a problem of childhood, *Maternal and Child Health*, October 1983: 428-432.
Klein M Schlageter M, Non-treatment of screened children with intermediate blood levels, *Pediatrics*, August 1975, 56: 298-302.
Lawther Report, *Lead and Health: Report of the Working Party on Lead in the Environment*, HMSO, 1980.
McLean W, Child poisoning in England and Wales: some statistics on admission to hospital 1964-1976, *Health Trends*, February 1980: 9-12.
Rinear C Rinear E, Emergency! Part 3: on the spot care for burns, aspirations and poisoning, *Nursing*, April 1975, 5: 40-47.
Vale J A, Paediatric poisoning, *Prescriber's Journal*, June 1978: 67-74.
Wright B, Poisoning in children, *Nursing Mirror*, 19 October 1983: 18-20.
Wynn M Wynn A, Lead and the unborn, *New Society*, April 1980: 104-105.

Child Abuse

Books
Borland M (ed.), *Violence in the Family*, Manchester University Press, 1976.
Cooke J V Bowles R T, *Child Abuse — Commission and Omission*, Butterworth, 1980.
Creightons S J Owtram P J, *Child Victims of Physical Abuse*, NSPCC, 1977.

Helfer R E Kempe C H (eds), *Helping the Battered Child and His Family,* Lippincott, 1972.

Helfer R E Kempe C H, *The Battered Child,* University of Chicago Press, 1982.

Henry C Kempe C H, *Child Abuse,* Fontana, 1978.

Battye J Deakin M, Surveillance reduces baby deaths, *Nursing Mirror,* April 1979: 38-40.

Black J A Hughes F, Legal aspects of child injury or neglect, *British Medical Journal,* October 1979: 910-912.

Beswick K *et al.,* General practice and child abuse, *Journal of Maternal and Child Health,* March 1979: 74-78.

Cater J I Easton P M, Separation and other stress in child abuse, *Lancet,* May 1980: 972-974.

Chamberlain N, The nurse and the abusive parent, *Nursing,* October 1974, 4: 72-76.

Corey E J *et al.,* Factors contributing to child abuse, *Nursing Research,* July/August 1975, 24:293-305.

Dingwall R, Defining child mistreatment, *Heath Visitor Journal,* July 1983: 249-251.

Fraiberg S *et al.,* Ghosts in the nursery, *Journal of the American Academy of Child Psychiatrists,* Summer 1975, 14: 387-421.

Harris J, The harm done to children, *Community Care,* September 1978: 21.

Holt K, The damaged child, *Update,* September 1978: 629-636.

Hutchings J *et al.,* Child abuse, *Journal of Community Nursing,* January 1979: 14-15.

Kauffman C Neill K, Care of the hospitalized abused child and his family: nursing implications, *Maternal and Child Nursing,* Spring 1976, 1: 117-123.

Kempe C H, Approaches to preventing child abuse, *American Journal of Diseases in Childhood,* September 1976, 130: 941-947.

Lynch A, Child abuse in the school age population, *Journal of School Health,* March 1975, 45: 141-148.

McCauley M A, Burns, bruises may lead to total family counselling, *American Nurse,* October 1975, 5: 6.

Melville J, A parent's lifeline, *New Society,* September 1978: 567-568.

Musanandara T, Communication between workers: the key in cases of child abuse, *Health Visitor,* August 1984: 233.

Roberts J *et al.,* Postneonatal mortality in children from abusing families, *British Medical Journal,* July 188: 102-104.

Roberton D *et al.,* Unusual injury: recent injury in normal children and children with suspected non-accidental injury, *British Medical Journal,* 8 November 1982: 1399-1340.

Roth F, A practice regimen for diagnosis and treatment of child abuse, *Child Welfare,* April 1975, 54: 168-173.

Smith S M Hanson R, Interpersonal relationships and child-rearing practices in 214 parents of battered children, *British Journal of Psychiatry,* December 1975: 513-525.

Trowell J, Emotional abuse of children, *Health Visitor Journal,* July 1983: 252-255.

Violence to Children: Response to the First Report from the Select Committee on Violence in the Family, HMSO, 1978.

Genetic Counselling

Books

Milunsky A *et al.*, *Prevention of Genetic Disease and Mental Retardation*, Saunders, 1976.
Nyhan W L Sakati N O, *Genetic and Malformation Syndromes in Clinical Medicine*, Yearbook Medical, 1976.
Siggers D C, *Prenatal Diagnosis of Genetic Disease*, Blackwell Scientific, 1978.
Vaughn V C *et al.*, *Nelson's Textbook of Pediatrics*, 11th edn, Saunders, 1979.
Whaley L F Wong D C, *Nursing Care of Infants and Children*, Mosby, 1979.

Articles

Baraitser M, Who needs genetic counselling? *Update*, February 1980: 373-381.
Carter C O, Recent advances in genetic counselling, *Nursing Times*, October 1979: 1795-1798.
Culliton B J Waterfall W K, Antenatal diagnosis, *British Medical Journal*, December 1979: 1488-1489.
Holms L B, Current concepts in genetics: congenital malformations,
New England Journal of Medicine, July 1976, 295: 204-207.
McCance K L, Genetics: implications for preventative nursing practise, *Journal of Advanced Nursing*, September 1983: 359-363.
Milunsky A, Current concepts in genetics: prenatal diagnosis of genetic disorders, *New England Journal of Medicine*, August 1976, 295: 377-380.
Seller M J, Genetic counselling and reproductive patterns, *Midwife, Health Visitor and Community Nurse*, April 1982: 135-139.

INDEX

abdominal device, restraining, 119, 224
abdominal hernia, 223, 461-3
    inguinal, 461-2
    irreducible, 462
    nursing care, 462-3
    strangulated, 462
    treatment, 462-3
    umbilical, 461
abdominal paracentesis, 492-3
accidents, 48-56
achrondoplasia, 784
acidosis, in diabetes mellitus, 540, 541
adenoidectomy, 574-8
    indications, 574-5
    nursing care, 575-7
    parent teaching, 577-8
adolescent (13 years onwards)
    concept of death, 91, 93
    hospitalized, 43, 65-6
    impact of hospitalizations on
    development of, 65-6
    nutritional requirements of, 42-3
    safety, 55-6
adrenaline, 199
adriamycin, 736, 739, 753
age and physical characteristics, birth-
    adolescence, 9-27
air studies of central nervous system,
    611-2
allergic reactions to foods, 37, 38, 39, 42
allopurinol, 735
ambiguous genitalia, 507-8
amniocentesis, 781
amniography-fetography, 781

ampicillin, 496, 639
anaemia 343-51, 480
    clinical manifestations, 344
    in glomerulonephritis, acute, 480
    of infection, 345, 346, 350
    see also individual anaemias
anaesthesia, post-operative recovery from,
    85-7
anencephaly, 263
anaphylactoid purpura *see* Henoch-
    Schönlein purpura
angiography, cerebral, 612-3
ankle dorsiflexion, 244
anomalous venous return, 369
aorta, coarctation of, 368, 371-3, 398, 403
aortic valve stenosis, 366, 367, 369, 399,
    403
aplastic anaemias, 343, 345
appendicitis, 463-5
    complications, 465
    nursing care, 464-5
    Ara-C (cytosine arabinoside), 736-742
arm recoil, 8, 244
armboard restraint, 158, 159
Arnold-Chiari malformation, 637-8
arterial pressure, monitoring, 82
arteriovenous shunt, 216-9
arthritis, 29
artificial respiration, 200-5
L-asparaginase, 736, 740
asthma, 318-327
    anxiety, relief of, 322
    breathing habits, proper, 324-5
    classification, 318

complications, 320
drugs, 323
nursing objectives, 321-7
parent attitudes, 325-6
prevention, 324-7
treatment, 321
astrocytoma, cerebellar, 744, 745, 746
ataxia, 619, 620
atelectasis, 33, 85
athetosis, 619, 620
atopic eczema, 523-8
complications, 525
nursing objectives, 525-8
parent support, 527-8
treatment, 525
atrial septal defect, 368, 369, 370, 374-6, 398
atropine, 199
auditory blink reflex, 7,8
autosomy, 783, 784, 785

Babinski's sign (reflex), 7, 14
bacterial endocarditis, 370, 371, 383
bacterial meningitis, 645-51
complications, 648
nursing objectives, 648-51
in otitis media, 580
parent support and teaching, 651
treatment, 648
BAL, (dimercaprol) 768, 769
Barlow's test, 711
battered child see non-accidental injury
BCG (Bacillus Calmette-Guérin) vaccine, 44, 45
behavioural patterns, birth-adolescence, 9-26
types, 745-747
benzathine penicillin, 609
belt device, 116 (fig), 118
bicarbonate and fluid & electrolyte balance, 154, 483
biliary tract obstruction, 440
bilirubin, in newborn, 275-82
bilirubin-albumin capacity, plasma, 276
bladder control, 18
bladder, ectopic, 499-501
suprapubic aspiration, 142-4
Blalock-Hanlon procedure, 381

Blalock-Taussig shunt, 378, 403
blind child, 561-8
community resources, 568
early care, 562-6
hospital care, 566-8
blindness, 561-8
legal definition, 562
blood,
administration of, 347
collection of, 139-41
blood pressure measurement, 74, 81, 99, 102-5
body fluids as percentage of body weight, 150
bone marrow aspiration, 735
bone marrow invasion by leukaemia and tumors, 343, 727-731
bone marrow transplantation, 733
bone tumours, 727, 279-38, 743
bottle feeding, 36, 37, 125-8
bottle-mouth syndrome, 48
bowel fistula, 162
Bradford frame, 520
brain damage, 33
brain scan, 613
brain stem gliomas, 746-7
brain tumors, 727, 732, 743-50
nursing care, 747-50
breast feeding, 36, 120-5, 261
breathing exercises, 178-9
bronchiolitis, 307, 314-5
bronchopneumonia, 31
Browne's splint, 714
Brudzinski's sign, 34, 647
bullous impetigo, 528
burns, 162, 515-23
calculation of surface area, 517 (fig)
complications, 518
nursing objectives, 518-23
treatment, 223, 517

calamine lotion, 31
calcium and fluid and electrolyte balance, 152
calcium chloride, 199
calcium EDTA, 768, 769
calcium intake, 42
calories, standard basal, 155
cancer, 162, 727-54

treatment of 728-9
candidal nappy dermatitis, 535-7
candidiasis, oral, 535-7
carbimazole, 558
cardiac arrest, 199
cardiac catheterization, 394-6
cardiac massage, external, 201-5
cardiac monitoring, 81, 196, 197
cardiac surgery, nursing care in, 396-400
cardiopulmonary resuscitation, 199-205
casts, 228-236
    Cotrel's E.D.F., 720, 722
    localizer, 720
    spica, 229, 232-6, 702, 704, 711, 717
    for scoliosis, 720
cataract, 29, 569-70
catheterization, 73, 130, 131, 132, 133,
    137, 145, 155, 156, 158, 163, 164, 165,
    166, 168, 169, 179, 180, 181, 182, 188,
    206, 211, 212, 213, 394-6
cell-mediated immunodeficiency disorders,
    44
central nervous system, cancers of, 727,
    732, 737
central venous pressure, monitoring, 82,
    210, 211, 212
cerebral angiography, 612-3
cerebral (brain) tumours, 727, 732, 743-50
cerebral palsy, 616-25
    classification, 618-20
    nursing objectives, 621-5
cervical adenitis, 35
cervical oesophagostomy, 423
chemotherapy of tumours, 728, 729, 733,
    734, 735, 736, 740-2, 744, 746, 750,
    753
chest drainage, 82
chest physiotherapy, 174-83
chickenpox, 30-1
child abuse and neglect *see* non-accidental
    injury
child
    concept of death, 91, 92
    dying, 89-95
    undergoing surgery, 83-87, 747-50
childhood accidents, 48-56
childhood diseases, 28-35
chlorothiazide, 550

chorea, 604, 607
chromosomes, 689
circumcision, 505
cleft lip, 410-7, 786
cleft palate, 410-7, 786
clove-hitch device, 119-20
clubbing of fingers, 384
coarctation of aorta, 368, 371-3, 398, 403
coeliac disease, 429-35
    crisis, 430
    nursing objectives, 432-4
    treatment, 431-2
coeliac sprue, 439
cognitive development, 9-17, 19-26
colic, 37
colostomy, 446, 450-1, 453-4
coma, child in, 672-3
computer aided tomography (CAT),
    613-4, 628, 744
congenital clubfoot (talipes equinovarus),
    712-4
congenital dislocation of hip, 709-712
congenital heart disease, 366-90
    common malformations, 366-70
    congestive heart failure in, 388-9, 391
    congestive heart failure, 390-4, 480
    complications, 392
    nursing objectives, 392-4
conjunctival haemorrhages, 33
constipation, 37
continuous positive airway pressure, 191-6
contraindications for immunization, 44-5
convulsions, 33
convulsive disorders (seizure disorders,
    epilepsy), 651-64
    nursing objectives, 660-3
    recording seizures, 661
    treatment, 656-660
    types, 653-6
    focal seizures, 654-5
    grand mal, 653-4
    infantile myoclonic fits (massive
    myoclonic spasms), 655-6
    petit mal, 654
    status epilepticus, 654
Coombs test, 277
corticosteroids, 29, 31
cough, assisting patient to, 177-8, 501-2

cow's milk protein sensitivity, 439
cranial irradiation, 732, 737
craniopharyngiomas, 727
cretinism *see* hypothyroidism
cri-du-chat syndrome, 263
Crigler-Najjar syndrome, 275
crossed extensor reflex, 7, 9
croup, 307, 316-7
croupette, 189-90, 307
Crutchfield tongs, 220
cryptorchidism, 506-7
cultural differences and nutrition, 42
cupping, 176-7
cyclophosphamide, 488, 741
cystic fibrosis, 334-40, 439, 784
    complications, 336
    nursing objectives, 336-9
    treatment, 335-6
cytomegalovirus, 263
cytosine arabinoside, (Ara-C), 736, 742

dactinomycin, 753
daunomycin, 740
deafness *see* hearing, impaired
De Lange's syndrome, 263
Dennis Browne's splint, 714
dental care, 46-8
dental caries, 47, 48, 407-10
dental plaque, 47
development and growth, 7-27
developmental assessment scoring scheme
    246-247 (figs)
dextrose, 199
diabetes insipidus, 548-52
    nephrogenic, 548
    nursing objectives, 550-551
diabetes mellitus, 539-48
    acidosis in, 540-1
    coma, 540
    complications, 540
    diet, 541-2, 547
    insulin administration, 542-4
    urine testing, 544-5
dialysis, 206-16
    types, 206-7
    see also haemodialysis; peritoneal
    dialysis
diarrhoea, 436-8, 441-5

complications, 442
    nursing objectives, 442-4
diazepam (Valium), 659-60
digoxin, 199
dimercaprol (BAL), 768, 769
diplegia, 620
diptheria, 30-3
    immunization against, 11, 12, 20, 44
    vaccine, 44
discharge of infant from intensive care,
    planning for, 79-80
disodium cromoglycate, 323
disaccaride intolerance, 439
diuretics, 489
Down's syndrome, 689-97, 783
    complications, 690
    nursing objectives, 691-7
Duchenne's muscular dystrophy, 785
ductus arteriosus, patent, 255, 367-9, 370,
    373-4, 379, 398, 403
dwarfism, genetic, 263
Dwyer instrumentation, 721
dying child, care of, 89-95
dying, emotional stages of, 90 (fig)
dyskinesia, 619

ear conditions, 578-90
echoencephalgraphy, 614
ectopic bladder, 499
Eisenmenger's complex, 376-7
elbow device, 118
electrical and mechanical equipment and
    safety, 50
electrocardiogram (ECG), 81, 210, 211,
    212
electroencephalography (EEG), 615-6,
    654, 656, 744
electrolyte and fluid balance in children,
    149-55, 156-62, 163-8, 426, 440, 484,
    632, 633
electromyography (EMG), 616
emergency precautions and safety, 50-1
emotional development, 9-15
emphysema, 33
encephalitis, 29, 31
endoxana (cyclophosphamide), 741
enema, 113-4
enterobiasis, 474-5

Epanutin (phenytoin sodium), 657-8
epiglottis, 316-7
epilepsy *see* convulsive disorders
epispadias, 504
erythroblastosis fetalis, 277-8
ethnic minority groups, health-illness
    behaviour in, 87-8
ethosuximide (Zarontin), 658
evanthema subitum, 22-3
exchange transfusion, 73, 168-72, 172
    (fig)
eyes, 21, 562-74
    defects requiring surgery, 568-74
    nursing management of child requiring
    surgery, 571-74
    trauma, 570-1
failure to thrive syndrome, 282-6
    nursing objectives, 284-6
Fallot's tetralogy, 368-9, 377-9, 387,
    398-9, 403
falls, prevention of, and safety, 50
family centred care, 66-70
febrile convulsions, 665-7
febrile infection, acute and immunization,
    44
feeding, infant and nutrition, 37-8, 120-39
feeding patterns from birth to adolescence,
    36-43
fetoscope, 781
female pseudohermaphroditism, 507-8
fever, 105-9
    nursing management, 105-9
fever reduction by tepid water sponge
    technique, 107-9
fires and safety, 50
fluid and electrolyte balance, 149-55
fluid requirements of infant, 126
fluoride, 47
folic acid deficiency anaemia, 343, 350
fontanelle, closure of anterior, 14, 15
fontanelle, closure of posterior, 10
Fontan's operation, 383
food allergies, 37, 38, 39, 42
Forchheimer's spots, 28
Fowler's position, 166, 321
fractures, 700-5
    clavicle, 701
    comminuted, 700

femur, 704
fibula, 705
greenstick, 700, 703
humerus, 701-3
radius, 700, 703-4
tibia, 705
ulna, 700, 703-4

gag reflex, 261
galactosaemia, 785
gantrisin (sulpafurazole), 496
gastrostomy feeding, 134-6
genetic counselling, 780-8
genuvalgum, 725-6
German measles, 28-9
gestational age, neurological assessment,
    244
Glenn procedure, 383
glioma, brain stem, 746-7
glomerulonephritis, acute, 477-85
    complications, 479-80
    nursing objectives, 480-4
    patient/parent teaching, 484-5
glucose-6-phosphate dehydrogenase
    deficiency, 343, 785
gluten-induced enteropathy *see* coeliac
    disease
grasp reflex, 261
great vessels (arteries), transposition of,
    368-9, 379-82, 399
growth and development, 7-27
growth spurt, 24, 25

haemarthrosis, 359, 361
haemodialysis, 207, 216
haemolytic anaemias, 343, 346, 350
haemolytic disease of newborn, 343
haemophilia, 358-64, 785
    complications, 359
    nursing objectives, 360-3
haemorrhagic varicella, 31
Hakin valve, 629
Harrington instrumentation, 721
Harrison's sulcus, 725
head control, lack of in newborn, 8
head lag, 245
health visitor, 304, 750
health visitor, paediatric liason, 77

hearing impaired, 582-90
  conductive hearing loss, 583-4
  detection: early care, 586-9
  nursing objectives, 585-90
  sensorineural hearing loss, 583-4
hearing, impaired and the rubella
  syndrome, 29-31
heart murmur, 29
heel to ear manoeuvre, 244-5
hemiplegia, 619
Henoch-Schonlein purpura (anaphylactoid
  purpura), 600-2
hepatitis, 469-72
  type A, 469-72
  type B, 469-72
hepatocellular jaundice, 472
herniotomy, 463
heroin withdrawal syndrome, 293-8
herpes simplex, 263
Hirschsprung's disease, 445-54
  nursing care, 447-54
Hollister U Bag, 145, 146
hospitalized child, 56-87
  education, 72-3
  emotional and social needs, 56-7
  family-centred care, 66-70
  play for, 70-72
  story telling to, 71-2
hyaline membrane disease see respiratory
  distress syndrome
hydrocele, 505-6
hydrocephalus, 625-34
  types, 626
  nursing care, 631
  nursing objectives, 630-4
  with spina bifida, 537, 642-3
  surgical treatment, 629
  shunts for, 629
  valves for, 629
hyperalimentation (total parenteral
  nutrition), 73, 82, 162-8, 165 (fig)
  follow-up phase, 163-8
hyperbilirubinaemia, 250, 273-82
hyperglycaemia, 168
hypermagnesaemia, 273-5
hypernatraemia, 255
hypertension, 35
hypertensive encephalopathy, 479-80, 483

hyperthyroidism, 556-9
hypertonic saline test, 551
hypertrophic pyloric stenosis, 425-8, 786
hypertrophic subacute stenosis, 368
hypocalcaemia, 254, 273
hypoglycaemia, 84, 168, 253-4, 271, 274
hypomagnesaemia, 273-5
hyponatraemia, 255
hypoplastic anaemias, 345
hypospadias, 503-4
hypothyroidism, 552-6
  acquired (juvenile), 552
  congenital (cretinism), 552
hypoxia, 254-5
hypsarrhythmia, 656

ileal conduit (ileoloop), 511-3
ileostomy, 450-2
imaginary companion, child's, 19, 20
immunization, 11, 12, 20, 23, 44-6, 51,
  106
immunoglobulin, 29, 31, 45
immunosuppressive drugs, 488
immunosuppressive therapy, 29, 44
immunotherapy, 733
imperforate anus, 457-61
  nursing care, 459-61
impetigo, 528-30
  bullous, 528
  nursing objectives, 529-30
incubator, 190
incubator with oxygen, 190
infant, of addicted mother, 293-8
infant (3 months-1 year)
  artificial feeding, 125-128
  breast feeding, 120-5
  and death, 92
  of diabetic mother, 271-5
  energy requirements, 126
  feeding and nutrition, 36-8, 120-39
  fluid requirements, 126
  formula, 36, 37, 123, 127
  hospitalized, 38, 58-60
  impact of hospitalization on
  development of, 58-60
  intensive care of, 77-80
  intramuscular injections for the,
  112

oral medication, administering to, 110
post-mature, 268-71
safety, 51-2
weight gain expectation, 125
see also newborn; preterm infant; small for gestational age infant
infective endocarditis, 374-5, 403-4
inguinal hernia, 461-2
insulin, 542-4
intensive care, neonatal infant requiring, 73-5
intensive care nursery, 73-80
admission of preterm infant, 245, 248-9
newborn requiring, 75
nursing in, 73-5, 80
intensive care unit, paediatric, 81-3
nursing in, 81-2
physical care of the child, 81
intestinal obstruction, 466-9
nursing management, 467-9
intracranial pressure, monitoring, 82
intramuscular injections, 111-3
intrathecal methotrexate, 732
intravenous fluid therapy, 155-62, 159 (fig)
cutdown method, 156-62
needle method, 156
intrauterine growth retarded infant *see* small for gestational age infant
intussusception, 454-7
nursing care, 455-7
involucrum, 706
iridocyclitis, in juvenile rheumatoid arthritis, 598
iron deficiency anaemia, 39, 343, 344-5
nursing management, 348-50
iron, preparations of, 348-50
isoprenaline, 199
isotope cisternography, 612, 628

jacket device, 116 (fig), 117-118, 721, 723
jaundice, 472-3
in newborn 275-82
erythroblastosis fetalis and, 277-8
kernicterus, 279-80
nursing objectives, 280-2
phototherapy, 280-2
physiologic, 276-7

juvenile rheumatoid arthritis, 594-600
acute febrile systemic onset (Still's disease), 594-5
nursing objectives, 598-600

Kahn's criteria of tremulousness and irritability, 294
kernicterus, 279-80
Kernig's sign, 34, 647
kidneys, 477-493
Klinefelter's syndrome, 783
knock-knee, 725-6
Koplick's spots, 28
Küntscher intramedullar rod, 704
Kussmail breathing, 211

Landau's sign (reflex), 7, 10, 14, 16
laryngeal diptheria, 32
laryngitis, 29
acute, 316
laryngospasm, 183
late childhood *(9-12 years)*
lead poisoning (plumbism), 763-71
chelating agents, 768-9
nursing objectives, 766-7, 770-1
prevention, 770-1
leg recoil, 244
leukaemia, 29, 31, 343, 690, 727, 729-43
acute lymphoblastic, 729-738, 743
acute myeloblastic, 730
chemotherapy for, 728, 729, 732, 733, 734, 735, 736, 740-2
nursing objectives, 733-8
lice, 532-3
light for dates infant *see* small for gestational age infant
lignocaine, (xylocaine), 200
Logan bow, 413, 414
lordosis, 21
Lucey-Driscoll syndrome, 275
lumbar epidural venography, 615
lumbar puncture, 148-9
Luminal (phenobarbitone), 657, 667
lymph nodes, enlargement of, 28, 32, 730
lymphadenopathy, cervical, 30, 34
Lymphoma, 727

MacEwen's sign, 628

maculopapules, 28
magnesium and fluid and electrolyte balance, 152
malabsorption syndromes, 345, 350, 439-41
male pseudohermaphroditism, 508-9
Marfan's syndrome, 719
mastoiditis, 580-1
measles, 28-31
    vaccine, 44-5
methylthiouracil, 558
mechanical ventilation, 170-4
mechonium ileus, in cystic fibrosis, 324, 325
Meckel's diverticulum, 465-6
meconium ileus, in cystic fibrosis, 334-5
medications, administration of, 109-13
    intramuscular injections, 111-3
    oral, 110-1
medulloblastoma , 745-6
megaloblastic anaemias, 345, 350-1
meningitis, 35, 581
meningocele, 635 (fig), 637-7
meningoencephalitis, 31
meningomyelocele, 635 (fig), 637-40, 785
    nursing objectives, 641-5
mental handicap, 680-97
    classification, 681-2
    community resources, 688
    nursing objectives, 683-7
mentally handicapped child, 683-8
    hospitalized, 686-7
6-mercaptopurine, 736, 740
methadone withdrawal syndrome, 293-8
methotrexate, 350, 736, 740
middle childhood (5-9 years)
milk allergy, 37
Milwaukee brace, 720-2
monoplegia, 620
monosaccaride intolerance, 439
monosomy, 783, 784
Moro reflex, 7
motor development, 9-19, 21, 24, 26
motor vehicles and safety, 49
mummy device, 116 (fig), 117
mumps, 30-1
Mustard procedure, 382, 399
myocarditis, 31, 400-3

nursing objectives, 402-3
myelography, 614-5
myringotomy, 579, 581

nappy dermatitis, 435-7
nasal diptheria, 32
nasogastric feeding, 73, 130-33, 132 (fig)
nasojejunal feeding, 136-9
naxolone, 200
neck-righting reflex, 7, 13
neonatal infants (0-4 weeks)
    impact of hospitalization on development, 58
    intensive care of, 73-5
    nutrition of, 36, 37
nephrotic syndrome, 485-93
    nursing objectives, 487
neural tube defects, 785
neuritis, 31
neuroblastoma, 727
neurologic disease, diagnostic evaluation, 611-6
newborn child, (birth-3 months), 13
    growth and development of, 9-14
    reflexes of, 7-8, 9, 10, 11, 12, 13
nitrofurantoin (Furadantin), 497, 639
nitrosoureas, 744
non-accidental injury (battered child, child abuse and neglect), 771-80
    nursing objectives, 775-80
non-paralytic polio, 34
non-respiratory diptheria, 32
NPO, nil per os, 84
nurse, role of and childhood accidents, 48-9
nursing in intensive care units, realities of, 80
nutrition, and infant feeding, 37-8, 120-39
nutrition, birth-adolescence, 36-43

obesity, development of, 42
oesophageal atresia, 134, 162, 418-25
omphalocele, 162
oncology, paediatric, 727-54
ophthalmia neonatorum, 248
optical blink reflex, 7
optic nerve gliomas, 727
orchiopexy, 506

orchitis, 31
Ortolani's test, 711
osteogenesis imperfecta, 263
osteomyelitis, 705-9
    nursing objectives, 708-9
ostitis media, 578-82
    nursing objectives, 580-2
oxygen hood, 190
oxygen tent, 189
oxygen therapy, 73, 82, 186-9
oxyuriasis, 474-5

packed cells, 347
paediatric dosage calculation, 110
paediatric intensive care units, 81-3
palmar grasp reflex, 7, 12
pancreatic insufficiency and bone marrow
    failure, 439
parachute reflex, 8
paralytic ileus, 466
paralytic polio, 34
paraplegia, 620
Paul's tubing, 145, 146
pediculosis, 532-3
D-penicillamine, 769
penicillin, 31, 35
penicillin G, 35
penicillin, in prevention of rheumatic
    fever, 605, 609
percussion, 176-7
perineal urethrostomy, 504
peritoneal dialysis, 206-16
    nursing management, 208-16, 211 (fig)
    nursing responsibilities, 210
peritonsillar abscess, 35
Perthes' disease, 715-8
    nursing objectives, 718
pertussis, 32-3
pertussis, immunization against, 11, 12,
    44-5
    vaccine, 44-5
pharyngeal diptheria, 30
phenobarbitone (Luminal), 657, 667
phenytoin sodium (Epanutin), 657-8
phimosis, 502
phosphate and fluid and electrolyte
    balance, 152
photophobia, 29

phototherapy, 74, 280-2
pica, 764
pineal tumours, 727
piperazine, 474
plantar grasp, reflex, 7, 13
play
    associative, 18
    in hospitals, 70-2
    interactive, 18
    parallel, 16, 18
    patterns of, 23-5
    programmes for the hospitalized child,
    70-1
    stimulation of, 9-19
Pneumocystis carinii, 307, 312-5
pneumoencephalogram, 611, 628
pneumonia, 29, 31, 33, 35
pneumonia, bacterial, 307, 310-1
    influenzal, 312-3
    mycoplasma, 307, 314-5
    staphylococcal, 310-1
    streptococcal, 310-1
    viral, 307, 312-3
poisons, 756-71
    emergency action, 770-1
    identification, 758
    nursing objectives, 757-63, 766-7,
    770-1
    see also lead poisoning
poisoning ingestions and safety, 50, 761-3
poliomyelitis, 34-5
    vaccine, 44-5
poliomyelitis, immunization against, 11,
    12, 20, 44-5
polycythaemia, 265, 270, 276
popliteal angle, in preterm infant, 244
positive end expiratory pressure (PEEP),
    193
postive-supporting reflex, 7, 10
postural drainage, 174-7
posture, in preterm infant, 244
potassium abnormalities, 153-4
potassium and fluid and electrolyte
    balance, 152, 153, 154, 155, 483, 484
prednisone, 736, 740
pregnancy and rubella, 28, 29, 44, 263
pre-school child (3-5 years) 17, 20

concept of death, 91-2
growth and development of, 18-20
hospitalized, 61-3
impact of hospitalization on
development of, 61-3
nutritional requirements, 40-1
safety, 53-4
pre-term infant, 239-262
admission to nursery, 245, 248-9
anoxia at birth, 254-5
apnoeic episodes, 251, 299-304
complications, 243, 248-9, 253-6
diagnostic evaluation, 243
digestive system, 241-2
eyes, 243
family relationships fostered, 260-2
feeding, 128
first 24-28 hours of life, 249-56
growing (older), 256-61
and hyperalimentation, 162
infection prevented, 252-3
intracranial haemorrhage, 255
liver function, 242-3
nervous system, 242
neurological criteria assessment
techniques, 243-5
nursing objectives, 245, 248-9
nutrition, 258-9
ophthalmia neonatorum prophylaxis,
248
patent airway maintained, 245, 248
pathophysiology, 241-243
periodic breathing, 251
psychological needs, 259
renal function, 242
respiratory system, 241
sodium disturbance, 255
square window, 244
thermal stability, 242, 248, 251-2
ventral suspension, 245
vitamin K$_1$ administered, 248
primidone (Mysoline), 658-9
procarbazine, 744
propranolol, 199
protective measures to limit movement
(restraints), 104-8
pseudohermaphroditism, 507-8
psychosocial development, 15-20, 23,

25-7, 40, 77, 79
puberty, 24, 25, 26, 43
Pudenz valve, 629
pulmonary stenosis, 368, 370-1
pulse rate, 99, 100-2
pupillary reflexes, 7
pure red cells, 343
purpura, 29
pyloric stenosis, 786
Pyrantel embonate, 474
Pyrvinium embonate, 474

quadriplegia, 620

radiation therapy, 728, 732, 737, 746,
750, 753
Rammstedt's operation, 426
Rashkind procedure, 381
Rastelli procedure, 382
recoil of arm reflex, 8
rectal prolapse, 33
reflexes, 7-8, 9, 10, 11, 12, 13, 14, 16
renal vein thrombosis, 271
respiratory arrest, 199
respiratory disorders, 307-40
nursing objectives, 307-9
respiratory distress and subdural tap, 149
respiratory distress syndrome (hyaline
membrane disease), 243, 250, 254,
327-34
nursing objectives, 331-4
respiratory monitoring, 81, 196-7
respiratory paralysis, 35
respiratory rate, 99, 102
restraints, 115-120, 116 (fig)
retinoblastoma, 727
retrolental fibroplasia, 243
reverse barrier nursing, 734
Reye's syndrome, 674-7
rhabdomyosarcoma, 727
rheumatic fever, acute, 35, 603-9
antibiotic cover in, 605, 609
carditis in, 604
chorea in, 604, 607
drugs for, 606
erythema marginatum in, 604
nursing objectives, 605-9
subcutaneous nodules in, 604

rheumatic heart disease, infective
   endocarditis in, 391
rheumatoid foot, 595
rickets, 724-5
   vitamin D-resistant, 785
ringworm of scalp, 530-2
ritualism, 17, 18, 39
roentgenography, 781
rooting, 7
rooting reflex, 8, 11
roseola infantum, 28-9
rubella, 28-9
   vaccine, 44, 45-6
rubella syndrome, the, 29, 263
rubeola (measles), 28-31

safety, 48-56
salaam attacks, 655
salicylates, 606
scabies, 534-5
scarf sign, 245
scarletina rash, 34
school child *(5-12 years)*
   behaviour patterns, 21-5
   concept of death, 91-3
   hospitalized, 42, 63-5
   impact of hospitalization on the
      development of, 63-5
   intramuscular injections and, 112, 113
   nutrition, 41-2
   safety, 54-5
school-child, oral medications,
   administering to, 111
school health programme, 23
school nurse, 750
Schwachman syndrome, 439
scissoring, 619
separation from parents, problems of,
   infants, 58, 59, 60
   pre-school child, 61-3
   toddlers, 60, 61
separation of children and parents through
   hospitalization, 67-70, 83
septicaemia neonatorum, 286-93
   nursing objectives, 290-3
sequestrum, 607
shock, post-operative, 85
shock, from burn, 516, 518

short-bowel syndrome, 439
sickle cell disease (anaemia), 346, 351-8,
   784
   nursing objectives, 354-6
side-turning, in newborn, 8
skeletal traction, 223-8
skin infections, bacterial, 31
skin problems, 515-37
skull, percussion of in hydrocephalus, 628
   X-ray, 611, 744
small for gestational age, 262-8
   asphyxia neonatorum, 266-7
   congenital abnormalities in, 266
   hypoglycaemia in, 267
   nursing objectives, 266-8
   polycythaemia, 268
smallpox vaccination, 46
socialization and development, 9-14
sodium abnormalities, 154
sodium and fluid and electrolyte balance,
   152, 154, 155, 483
sodium bicarbonate, 199, 484
spasticity, 618-20
spica cast, 702, 717
spina bifida, 634-45, 635 (fig)
   see also meningomyelocele, 645-6
spina bifida occulta, 634, 635 (fig), 636
spinal cord tumour, 719
spinal fusion, 721-3
spinal tap, 148-9
Spitz-Holter valve, 629
sports, recreation and safety, 49-50
spread eagle position, 655
square window, in preterm infant, 244
Steinman pins, 227
Stensen's duct, 30
stepping reflex, 8, 11
steroids, for rheumatic fever, 606
   for Henoch-Schonlein purpura, 601
   for nephrotic syndrome, 487-8
   for rheumatoid arthritis, juvenile, 498
Still's disease, 594-5
stoma care, 450-4
stool, specimen collection, 146-8
story-telling and the hospitalized child,
   71-2
strabismus, 568-9
streptococcal pharyngitis, 34-5

strep throat, 34
strongyloidiasis, 439
structural scoliosis, 718-24
    nursing objectives, 721-4
Stryker frame, 722
subacute bacterial endocarditis, and dental
    caries, 407-410
subaortic stenosis, 367
subdural haemorrhage, 667-74
    nursing objectives in, 671-4
sucking reflex, 37, 261
suctioning, 179-83
    endotracheal, 82
    nasopharyngeal, 181-2, 502
    nasotracheal, 182-3, 502
    oral 180-1, 501
sudden infant death syndrome, 299-304
sulphaphurazole (Gantrisin), 496, 497,
    639
supravalvular aortic stenosis, 369
surface area, estimation of, 110, 151
surfactant, 328
surgery, care of child undergoing, 83-7
surma, 764
sympathetic ophthalmia, 571
syndactyly, 785

talipes equinovarus, see congenital clubfoot
Tay-Sachs disease, 784
Td (adult-type tetanus and diptheria
    toxins), 44
teeth, 46-7
teething, (gaining adult/permanent teeth),
    21, 47, 48
teething, (gaining milk/primary teeth),
    12, 13, 14, 17, 46
temper tantrums, 18
temperature, 99, 100, 101
temperature control, 74, 82
tetanus, 34-5
tetanus immune globulin, 35
tetanus, immunization against, 11, 12, 20,
    44
tetanus, vaccines, 11, 12, 20, 44
tetracycline, 35
thalassaemic syndromes, 344
Thomas splint, 704
threadworms, 474-5

thrush, 535-7
thyrotoxicosis see hyperthyroidism
L-thyroxine, 554
tinea capitis, 530-2
toddler (1-3 years)
    concept of death, 80
    development and growth of, 14-8
    hospitalized, 60-1
    impact of hospitalization on
        development of, 60-1
    intramuscular injections and, 112-3
    nutritional requirements, 39
    oral medication, administering to, 111
    reflexes of, 14, 16
    safety, 52-3
toilet-training, 16
tonic neck reflex, 7, 12
tonsillar diptheria, 30
tonsillectomy, 574-8
    nursing care, 575-7
tooth decay, 46, 47, 48
total parenteral nutrition see
    hyperalimentation
toxoplasmosis, 263
tracheo-oesophageal fistula and
    oesophageal atresia, 418-25
tracheostomy, 184-6
    nursing management, 184-6
traction, Bryant, 704
traction, 219, 228, 620
    cervical, 225-6
    Cotrel's, 266, 721
    gallows, 223-4, 704
    halofemural, 227-8, 620, 721, 722
    halopelvic, 721, 722
    Russel Hamilton, 224-5
    skeletal, 223
    skin, 223
    transcultural knowledge of, 87-88
transposition of great vessels (arteries),
    complete, 368, 369, 379-82, 399
Trendelenburg's sign, 710
tricuspid artesia, 369, 370, 371, 382-3
triplegia, 620
trisomy-21, 689
trisomy syndromes, 263, 783
truncus arteriosus, 367
tuberculin test, 45

tunnel vision, 562
tumours, 105, 343, 719, 727-54
tumours, renal, 750-4
Turner's syndrome, 784
turning bed frame, 520
tympanometry, 579
ultrasonography, 781
umbilical catheterization, 73
umbilical hernia, 461
undescended testis, 506-7
urachus, patent, 501
uraemia, 480
urinary tract, infection of, 494-9
    nursing objectives, 496-8
    obstruction of, 431-2, 502-3
urine, collection of, 141-146
    collecting bag, 141-142
    testing in diabetes mellitus, 544
urologic surgery, child requiring, 509-12

valium (Diazepam), 295, 659-60
vasopressin, 548, 549, 550, 551, 552
vasopressin sensitivity test, 549
venepuncture, 125-6, 139, 140, 152, 154, 159
ventilator, 191-6
ventilator care, 73, 82, 191-6
ventricular septal defect, 367, 368, 369, 370, 376, 377, 379, 398, 399, 403
ventriculogram, 611-2, 628
venturi masks, 188
verbalization, development of, 13-4
vincristine (Oncovin), 736, 739, 744, 753
vital signs, measurement of, 85, 99-105
vitamin B_{12}, malabsorption of, 440
vitamin B_{12}, anaemia, 343, 350
vitamin D supplements, 42
vitamin K_1 administration, 248
vitamin supplements
    for neonates, 36, 37
    for school children, 42
vocalization and development, 9-14
Volkmann's contracture, 232, 703

water, 153, 155
    deprivation test, 549
water and fluid and electrolyte balance, 149, 151, 152, 153, 155

Waterston shunt, 378, 383, 403
weaning, 38, 129
Wharton's duct, 30
whooping cough see pertussis
Wilm's tumour, 727, 750-4
    nursing objectives, 752-4
wisdom teeth, 47
withdrawal reflex, 8
Wood's light, 530, 531
Wright respirometer, 195

zaroutin (ethosuximide), 658